Vetiscan

About the Author

Dr. Sukdeb Nandi graduated in Veterinary Science and Animal Husbandry in 1986 from Bidhan Chandra Krishi Viswavidyalaya, Mohanpur, Nadia, W.B. and ranked first class third position. He did his Master Degree and Ph. D. in Veterinary Virology from Deemed University, Indian Veterinary Research Institute, Izatnagar, Bareilly, U.P. in 1988 and 1992 respectively. He had carried out research on important viral diseases of animals namely Rabies, FMD, Sheep Pox, Goat Pox, Bluetongue, Infectious Bovine Rhinotracheitis. Classical Swine Fever Virus, Canine Parvovirus, Canine Distemper Virus, Infectious Canine Hepatitis Virus and Avian Influenza or Birdflu. He had also developed and applied a galaxy ol" diagnostic techniques namely Polymerase Chain Reaction (PCR), Nested PCR, PCR and RE mapping, RT-PCR, SYBER GREEN based Real Time PCR, cloning and sequencing of PCR products for diagnosis and characterization of a number of important viral diseases of animals. He had also adopted Taqman based Real Time PCR for detection of bovine herpes virus -1 (BHV-1) in the semen and clinical samples. He had also developed live attenuated goat pox vaccine and inactivated bluetongue virus vaccines. He had also organized a DBT sponsored training programme entitled "Serological and PCR based Diagnosis of Economically Important Infectious Diseases of Domestic Animals" for the mid-career Scientists, Teachers, Assistant and Associate Professors in 2009. He was awarded with DBT sponsored National Biotechnology Associateship to carry out research on molecular biology at IICB, Kolkata. He was also deputed to United Kingdom (U.K.) to undergo 'Transfer of Molecular Biology Training' (TOMBIT) from 1998-1999. He had also attended a FAO sponsored international training on "Advanced Biorisk Training' at Australian Animal Health Laboratory (AAHL), Geelong, Australia in 2011. He had written a number of books, book chapters and many review and research articles in international and national journals of repute. He had also delivered many lead or concept papers in different national and international symposiums or seminars and received lot of applauses and appreciation. He had widely travelled different places in United Kingdom, Scotland, Netherland, France, Thailand and Australia. Presently, he is working as Principal Scientist at Centre for Animal Disease Research and Diagnosis, Indian Veterinary Research Institute, Izatnagar, U.P. He is actively involved in the diagnosis of viral diseases of animals and shouldering the responsibility of BSL-3 laboratory for routine surveillance of birdflu samples from different parts of the country. He is also the author of 'Manual of Viral Disease Investigation' - a book very much useful for the scientists, teachers, students, diagnosticians and others who are working in this area. Other books in his credit are Veterinary Virology : at a glance, Immunology - at a glance, Animal Cell Culture and Virology, Avian influenza or Birdflu, Rabies : a killer disease, Veterinary Vaccines -Concepts and application, Veterinary Public Health - at a glance. Poultry Diseases - at a glance, Infectious diseases of animals : Their identification and Treatment and Zoonotic diseases.

Vetiscan

Sukdeb Nandi

Principal Scientist
Centre for Animal Disease Research and Diagnosis
Indian Veterinary Research Institute
Izatnagar, U.P. (243122)

NEW INDIA PUBLISHING AGENCY

New Delhi – 110 034

NEW INDIA PUBLISHING AGENCY
101, Vikas Surya Plaza, CU Block, LSC Market
Pitam Pura, New Delhi 110 034, India
Phone: +91 (11)27 34 17 17 Fax: +91(11) 27 34 16 16
Email: info@nipabooks.com
Web: www.nipabooks.com

Feedback at feedbacks@nipabooks.com

ISBN 978-93-89130-01-0

Composed and Designed by NIPA

Dedicated to the
ALMIGHTY
for
Everything

Preface

Veterinary Science is an important branch devoted to caring for all species of animals. A galaxy of subjects just like human medicine is taught encompassing a large number of animals. Microbiology is an inherently valuable and useful discipline that offers an insight of an invisible world. There are a galaxy of infectious diseases of animal and human caused by a variety of microorganisms. Among them, viruses and bacteria are of paramount importance because of enormous economic losses due to high morbidity, high mortality, reduced productivity, impaired work ability, reproductive inefficiencies and disturbances of national and international trade. Micro-organisms are everywhere. They exist in a range of environments including in the air we breathe, in the food we eat and even within our own body. In fact we come in contact with countless numbers of micro-organisms every day. Although some microbes can cause disease, most are rather play a pivotal role in the processes that provide energy and make life possible. Some even prevent disease and others are used in an attempt to cure diseases. As microorganisms play diverse role in the world, microbiology continues to be an exciting and interesting discipline to study. The book 'VETISCAN' has been written to provide relevant and current informations on all the aspects of important viral and bacterial diseases of animals including immunology, famous scientist associated with discoveries, industrial microbiology, antibiotics, biochemistry, bacteriology, virology, genetic engineering, public health etc to the students, teachers, scientists, diagnosticians, researchers, policy makers etc. Further it will continue to be an important subject to study with lot of recent developments and areas to be explored.

In this book MCQ on all the aspects have been given keeping in view the latest examination system conducted by the different institutions, agencies, boards etc. With the implementation of new trimester/semester systems, the students have to face a number of quizzes, midterm and final examinations. This system evaluates the student's learning capability and teacher's teaching techniques on a regular basis. Again, in various competitive examinations namely IAS, IPS, IPS, CSIR, UGC, ICMR, ICAR, NET, JRF, SRF etc objective type as well as subjective type questions are set to evaluate the depth of knowledge of a particular subject of the students. This book has been written very nicely so that end users can grow a concept on the topic and easily overcome any challenge without any difficulty. Further, a number of organization/institutions hold regular examination for admission in various degree programmes, award of merit scholarships and appointment on various jobs based on objective type questions.

It is therefore hoped that the book will be extremely useful for teachers as well as students and personnel in the field of Virology, Immunology, Bacteriology, Biochemistry, Biotechnology, Public Health and other related disciplines of various institutions.

Lastly, the author will appreciate receiving comments on the quality of books and errors if any for further improvement of the book.

(S. **Nandi)**
E-mail: sukdebnandi@yahoo.in
Mob: 09412066583

Contents

1

Antibiotics

1. ———— is a synthetic antimicrobial drug against M. tuberculosis.

   A. Penicillin B. Tetracycline

   C. Erythromycin D. Isoniazid

Ans. D.

2. Which of the antibiotic is not used as a food preservative ?

   A. Pimaricin B. Nisin

   C. Tylosin D. β-lactam antibiotic

Ans. D.

3. Which of the following bacteria is susceptible to thiophen-2-carboxylic acid hydrazide?

   A. M. bovis B. M. tuberculosis

   C. M. chelonei D. M. fortuitum

Ans. A.

4. The most selective antibiotics are those that interfere with the synthesis of

   A. Bacterial DNA B. Bacterial RNA

   C. Bacterial cell wall D. Bacterial plasma membrane

Ans. C.

5. Cycloserine inhibits

   A. Alanine racemase B. D-alanyl - D-alanine synthetase

   C. Both A & B D. amidase

Ans. C.

6. Which antibiotic has a beta-lactam ring?

   A. Cephalosporin B. Penicillin

   C. Tetracycline D. Streptomycin

Ans. B.

7. Chemotherapeutic agents must

A. Prevent/destroy the activity of a parasite

B. Leave unaltered the host's natural defence mechanisms

C. Be able to come in contact with the parasite by penetrating the cells

D. All of the above

Ans. D.

8. Novobiocin can be used against

A. Gram +ve Staphylococci B. Gram -ve Meningococci & Gonococci

C. Haemophilus D. All of these

Ans. D.

9. Interference mechanism of ciprofloxacin and norfloxacin is due to their action on

A. Cell wall synthesis B. Cell membrane function

C. DNA function D. Protein synthesis

Ans. C.

10. By which of the following means antifungal chemotherapeutic agents may affect fungi?

A. Interfere with nuclear division by preventing the aggregation of microtubules needed for mitosis

B. Interfere with normal nucleic acid synthesis

C. Interfere with ergosterol biosynthesis and thus alter the structure of the cytoplasmic membrane as well as the function of several membrane-bound enzymes like those involved in nutrient transport and chitin synthesis

D. All of these

Ans. D.

11. Which of the following drugs involves modification of the drug by enzymatic modification or degradation of its active element to alter its/their resistance?

A. Pencillins B. Chloramphenicol

C. Aminoglycosides D. All of these

Ans. D.

12. When using alcohol as an antiseptic, which concentration is considered most effective?

A. 95% B. 50%

C. 70% D. 25%

Ans. C.

13. Fluoroquinolones are antibiotics which inhibit

A. DNA polymerase
B. RNA polymerase
C. DNA gyrase
D. Cross-linking of peptidoglycan

Ans. C.

14. Which of the following is used only in life-threatening situations when no other drug is adequate?

A. Penicillin
B. Tetracycline
C. Chloramphenicol
D. Streptomycin

Ans. C.

15. The susceptibility of a microorganism to antibiotics and other chemotherapeutic agents can be determined by using

A. Tube dilution technique
B. Paper disk plate
C. Both (a) and (b)
D. None of these

Ans. C.

16. Most antibiotics are isolated from

A. Viruses
B. Aquatic microorganisms
C. Soil microorganisms
D. Plants

Ans. C.

17. Which of the following group is not the carbohydrate containing antibiotic?

A. Streptomycin & Streptothricin
B. Vancomycin & Moenomycin
C. Everninomycin & Nogirimycin
D. Erythromycin & Candicidin

Ans. D.

18. The penicillin stable in gastric acid and suitable for oral administration is

A. Methicillin
B. Carbenicillin
C. Cloxacillin
D. Penicillin-G

Ans. C.

19. Which of the following is not an example of potent antitumor agents?

A. Anthramycin
B. Sibromycin
C. Neothramycin
D. Erythromycin

Ans. D.

20. A parenteral route of drug administration refers to

A. Oral
B. Nonoral
C. Intravenously
D. Intramuscularly

Ans. B.

21. Which of the following antibiotics can't be used for treatment of infections with b-lactamase-producing Staphylococcus aureus?

A. Vancomycin B. Ampicillin/Sulbactam
C. Cephalothin D. Piperacillin

Ans. D.

22. Which of the following is not an aminoglycoside antibiotic?

A. Streptomycin B. Neomycin
C. Kanamycin D. Cephalosporin

Ans. D.

23. The nitrofurans differ from the antibiotics in that they

A. Do not occur naturally B. Occur naturally
C. Are antimicrobial drugs D. All of these

Ans. A.

24. Quinolones are

A. Antimetabolites B. Penicillin derivatives
C. Bacteriostatic D. Broad-spectrum

Ans. D.

25. Which of the following is not a semi synthetic chemotherapeutic agent?

A. Ampicillin B. Carbenicillin
C. Penicillin D. Sulfonamide

Ans. C.

26. Which of the following tests is used to determine the minimal lethal concentration?

A. Broth dilution test B. Agar dilution test
C. Dilution susceptibility tests D. All of these

Ans. D.

27. The mode of action of Polymyxin is to

A. Inhibit protein synthesis B. Inhibit DNA synthesis
C. Injury to the plasma membrane D. Inhibit folic acid synthesis

Ans. C.

28. Polyene antibiotics are

A. Large ring structures B. B-lactam - thiazolidine ring
C. Small ring structures D. Any of these

Ans. A.

29. Which of the following may cause resistance to penicillin?
A. Impermeability of cell envelope
B. Production of b-lactamases by bacteria
C. Alteration or lack of penicillin-binding proteins
D. All of the above

Ans. D.

30. The third generation cephalosporin agents is
A. Cefotaxime
B. Cefoxitin
C. Cephalothin
D. Cephalexin

Ans. A.

31. The penicillin resistant to β-lactamases is
A. Carbenicillin
B. Closacillin
C. Penicillin-G
D. Ampicillin

Ans. B.

32. The antibiotics not clinically useful for Pseudomonas aeruginosa infection is
A. Aminoglycosides
B. Ceftazidime
C. Piperacillin
D. Trimethoprim-Sulphamethoxazole

Ans. D.

33. Which of the following drugs may show plasmid-mediated resistance?
A. Nalidixic acid
B. Ampicillin
C. Rifampicin
D. Methicillin

Ans. B.

34. The scientist who first discovered the substance penicillin was
A. Joseph Lister
B. Alexander Fleming
C. Paul Ehrlich
D. None of these

Ans. B.

35. The larger the __________, the better the chemotherapeutic agent.
A. Therapeutic index
B. Therapeutic dose
C. Selective toxicity
D. Spectrum

Ans. A.

36. Chelate forming peptide antibiotic are/is
A. Bleomycins
B. Sideromycins
C. Both (a) and (b)
D. Vancomycin

Ans. C.

37. With which of the following aminoglycosides interfere?

A. Protein synthesis B. DNA function

C. Cell wall synthesis D. Cell membrane function

Ans. A.

38. The antibiotics not having good activity against Enterobacteriaceae is

A. Clindamycin B. Cefoxitin

C. Trimethoprim-Sulphamethoxazole D. Ciprofloxacin

Ans. A.

39. Quinones and related antibiotics are

A. Tetracyclines B. Actinorhodin

C. Mitomycin D. All of these

Ans. D.

40. Both penicillin and fluoroquinolones

A. Bind to and inactivate a bacterial protein

B. Inhibit the cross-linking of peptidoglycan

C. Are inactivated by b-lactamase

D. Must be transported into the cytoplasm in order to act

Ans. A.

41. A broad-spectrum antibiotic such as Chloramphenicol is one that

A. Kills both gram positive and gram negative bacteria

B. Kills all bacteria

C. Kills numerous types of microbes

D. Kills all microorganisms

Ans. C.

42. Vancomycin inhibits peptidoglycan synthesis by binding

A. D-alanyl - D-alanine B. D- alanine racemase

C. D-alanyl - D-alanine synthetase D. Amidase

Ans. A.

43. Nystatin is a drug used for treatment of diseases caused by

A. Gram negative bacterium B. Gram positive bacterium

C. Yeast D. Protozoan

Ans. C.

44. Which is not an amino acid and peptide antibiotic?

A. Penicillin B. Actinomycin

C. Bacitracin D. Tetranactin

Ans. D.

45. Cephalosporins and Penicillins interfere with which of the following?.

A. Protein synthesis B. DNA function

C. Cell membrane function D. Cell wall synthesis

Ans. D.

46. Bacterial cells susceptible to Penicillium can be protected from destruction if the medium in which they are exposed is of

A. High osmotic pressure B. Low osmotic pressure

C. Moderate osmotic pressure D. High surface tension

Ans. A.

47. The compound(s) which act(s) as metabolic antagonist is/are

A. Trimethoprim B. Sulphonamides

C. both (a) and (b) D. none of these

Ans. C.

48. Amphotericin B and Polymyxin interfere with

A. Cell wall synthesis B. Protein synthesis

C. Cell membrane function D. DNA function

Ans. C.

49. Which of the following is not β-lactamase-resistant penicillin?

A. Oxacillin B. Nafcillin

C. Carbenicillin D. Methicillin

Ans. C.

50. The antibiotics which affords a broad spectrum of antimicrobial coverage against aerobic and anaerobic bacteria, rickettsiae, chlamydiae, and mycoplasmas is

A. Gentamicin B. Tetracycline

C. Metronidazole D. Vancomycin

Ans. B.

51. The PCR/sequencing approach to rRNA is most likely to give information about

A. The species to which the bacteria are most closely related

B. Morphology of the bacterium

C. The type of energy metabolism the bacterium has

D. Whether the bacterium is motile

Ans. A.

52. Which of the following chemotherapeutic agents may affect the growth of Campylobacter jejuni?

A. Vancomycin B. Polymyxin

C. Trimethoprim D. None of these

Ans. D.

53. Higher doses of Chloramphenicol affects the eukaryotic cells because

A. They have 30 S ribosomes B. They have mitochondria

C. They have 70 S ribosomes D. None of the above

Ans. B.

54. Penicillin is a

A. Primary metabolite B. Secondary metabolite

C. Tertiary metabolite D. None of the above

Ans. B.

55. Antibiotic produced from Streptomyces orientalis is

A. Streptomycin B. Penicillin

C. Vancomycin D. Both a and b

Ans. C.

56. The drug of choice for dermal, oral and vaginal candidiasis is

A. Griseofulvin B. Amphoterein B

C. Gentian violet D. Nystatin

Ans. D.

57. Chloramphenicol is obtained from

A. Streptomyces griseus B. Streptomyces venezuelae

C. Streptomyces pyrogenes D. None of these

Ans. B.

58. Streptomycin is obtained from

A. Streptococcus species B. Streptomyces griseus

C. Straphylococcus aureus D. None of these

Ans. B.

59. Ciprofloxacin acts by inhibiting

A. Cell wall synthesis B. RNA synthesis

C. Folate synthesis D. DNA gyrase

Ans. D.

60. The antibiotic acting on cell wall is

A. Bacitracin
B. Penicillin
C. Cyclosporine
D. All of these

Ans. D.

61. Erythromycin is obtained from

A. S.griseus
B. S. rimosus
C. S. scabies
D. S. erythraeus

Ans. D.

62. Antibiotics used for treatment of cholera are

A. Tetracyclines
B. Penicillins
C. Streptomycin
D. None of these

Ans. A.

63. Drugs used against tuberculosis (TB) are

A. Rifampicin, Isoniazid
B. Pyrazinamide, Streptomycin
C. Both A and B
D. None of these

Ans. C.

64. Penicillin is the drug of choice for

A. Scarlet fever
B. Whooping cough
C. Brucellosis
D. Cholera

Ans. A.

65. Penicillic acid is produced by

A. A. ochraceus
B. P. puberulum
C. Both a and b
D. None of the above

Ans. C.

66. Most important Penicillium toxins are

A. Citrinin
B. Patulin
C. Penicillic acid
D. All of the above

Ans. D.

67. Bacitracin sensitivity test is done for

A. Pneumococci
B. Group 'A' Streptococci
C. Gonococci
D. Staphylococci

Ans. B.

68. The antibiotic acting on cell wall is

A. Penicillin B. Bacitracin

C. Cyclosporin D. All of the above

Ans. D.

69. Erythromycin belongs to chemical class of antibiotics

A. Beta lactam B. Tetracyclines

C. Macrolides D. Aminoglycosides

Ans. C.

70. Resistant to drugs in tuberculosis develops by

A. Transduction B. Transformation

C. Conjugation D. Mutation

Ans. D.

71. Erythromycin inhibits protein synthesis by

A. Attaching to 30 S ribosome unit

B. Attaching to 50 S ribosome unit

C. By the attachment to t-RNA

D. By the attachment to m-RNA

Ans. B.

72. The function of (THFA) Tetrahydrofolic acid coenzyme include

A. Amino acid synthesis B. Thymidine synthesis

C. Protein synthesis D. Both a and b

Ans. D.

73. Which of the following is penicillinase resistant penicillin?

A. Amoxycillin B. Cloxacillin

C. Carbenicillin D. Methicillin

Ans. D.

74. Which of the following does not inhibit cell wall synthesis?

A. Penicillin B. Carbenicillin

C. Amikacin D. Vancomycin

Ans. C.

75. The anti tumour antibiotics act by inhibiting

A. Cell wall synthesis B. RNA synthesis

C. Cell membrane synthesis D. The DNA structure & function

Ans. D.

76. Drug resistance to sulphonamides is due to

A. Production of PABA

B. Folic acid synthetase

C. Drug alteration

D. Low affinity for drug synthesis by bacteria

Ans. B

77. Amoxycillin is combined with Clavulanic acid to inhibit

A. DNA gyrase

B. Cell wall synthesis

C. Protein synthesis

D. Beta lactamase enzymes

Ans. D

78. Drug of choice for Methicillin resistant Staph. aureus is

A. Ampicillin

B. Erythromycin

C. Neomycin

D. Vancomycin

Ans. D

79. Nalidixic acid activity is due to

A. The inhibition of DNA synthesis

B. Inhibition of protein synthesis

C. The inhibition of cell wall synthesis

D. Both b and c

Ans. A

80. The best test for the susceptibility of a microorganism to antibiotics and other chemotherapeutic agents:

A. Tube-dilution test

B. Paper-disc test

C. Both a and b

D. None of these

Ans. C

81. The smallest amount of chemotherapeutic agents required to inhibit the growth of the organism in vitro is known as

A. MIC (minimum inhibitory concentration)

B. Thermal death point (TDP)

C. Death rate

D. None of these

Ans. A

82. Clear-zones formation around antibiotic disc is due to

A. Growth of the bacterium surrounding of the disc

B. Lysis of the bacterial cells surrounding the disc

C. The destruction of paper disc (antibiotic)

D. None of these

Ans. B.

83. Bacitracin is obtained from

A. B. subtilis

B. B. anthracis

C. B. cereus

D. B. anthracoid

Ans. A.

84. Beta-lactum antibiotics are

A. Penicillin

B. Cephalosporin

C. Both a & b

D. None of these

Ans. C.

85. Following are the test organisms used for the I.P microbiological assay of antibiotics. Match them correctly:

1. Rifampicin — A. Escherichia Coli
2. Tetracyclin — B. Bacillus cereus
3. Streptomycin — C. Micrococcus luteus
4. Chloramphenicol — D. Bacillus subtilis

Ans. 1 D, 2 B, 3 A, 4 C.

86. The drugs mentioned below are produced by the species mentioned from A to D. Match them correctly :

1. Rifampicin — A. Streptomyces noursei
2. Nystatin — B. Streptomyes griseus
3. Amphotericin B — C. Streptomyces mediterranei
4. Candicidin — D. Streptomyces nodosus

Ans. 1 C, 2 A, 3 D, 4 B.

87. Match the following rickettsial disease with their respective organisms:

1. Epidemic typhus — A. Rickettsia typhus
2. Scrub typhus — B. Rickettsia prowazekii
3. Trench typhus — C. Rickettsia typhus
4. Murine typhus — D. Rickettsia Quintana

Ans. 1 B, 2 C, 3 D, 4 A.

88. Match the following antibiotics with their respective modes of administration :

1. Penicillin V	A. Intramuscular suspension
2. Benzathine Penicillin	B. Oral
3. Methicillin Sodium	C. Both as oral and injection
4. Ampicillin	D. Intramuscular injection

Ans. 1 B, 2 A, 3 D, 4 C.

89. Match the following antibiotics with respective strains used for their production :

1. Tetracyclin	A. Streptomyces erythreus
2. Chloramphenicol	B. Streptomyces garyphalous
3. Erythromycin	C. Streptomyces venezuelae
4. Cycloserine	D. Streptomyces viridifaciens

Ans. 1 D, 2 C, 3 A, 4 B.

90. Match the following strains with their respective produced antibiotics A to D:

1. Streptomyces griseus.	A. Oxytetracycline
2. Streptomyces aureofaciens	B. Streptomycin
3. Streptomyces rimosus	C. Viomycin
4. Streptomyces puniceus	D. Chlortetracycline

Ans. 1 B, 2 D, 3 A, 4 C.

91. Match the following antibiotics with their respective disease A to D to be cured :

1. Streptomycin	A. Staphylococcus infections
2. Cycloserine	B. Tuberculosis
3. Novobiocin	C. Fungal tuberculosis
4. Griseofulvin	D. Pulmonary tuberculosis

Ans. 1 B, 2 D, 3A, 4C.

92. Match the following antibiotics with their respective side effects A to D:

1. Novobiocin	A. Kidney problems
2. Neomycin	B. Damages CNS
3. Cycloserine	C. Damages haemopoietic system
4. Chloramphenicol	D. Skin rashes

Ans. 1D, 2 A, 3 B, 4 C.

93. Match the following antibiotics with their modes of action A to D:

1. Tetracyclines	A. Influences mitosis
2. Erythromycin	B. Chelation of light divalent salts
3. Novobiocin	C. Blocks protein synthesis
4. Griseofulvin	D. Interferes with the conjugation of bilirubin

Ans. 1 B, 2 C, 3 D, 4 A.

94. Match the following side effects with their respective antibiotics A to D:

1. Nephrotoxic	A. Triacetyloleandomycin
2. Rashes	B. Polymixin B sulphate
3. Hypersensitivity	C. Cephaloridine
4. Gastric irritation	D. Sodium fusidate

Ans. 1 B, 2 C, 3 A, 4 D.

95. The wonder drug of second world war is produced by

A. Algae B. Fungi
C. Bacteria D. Plants

Ans. B.

96. Name the source of the following antibiotics and their sources

S. No.	Name of antibiotic
1.	Erythromycin
2.	Aureomycin
3.	Teramycin
4.	Chloromycetin
5.	Streptomycin
6.	Penicillin
7.	Actinomycetin
8.	Tetramycin
9.	Neomycin, Novaboium

Ans.

S.No.	Name of antibiotic	Obtained from
1.	Erythromycin	Streptomyces erythaeraeus
2.	Aureomycin	Streptomyces aurofaciens
3.	Teramycin	Streptomyces ramosus
4.	Chloromycetin	Streptomyces venezuela
5.	Streptomycin	Streptomyces griseus
6.	Penicillin	Pencillium notatum
7.	Actinomycetin	Micromonospora spp
8.	Tetramycin	Streptomyces rimosus
9.	Neomycin	Streptomyces fradiae

97. Sulphonamide

A. Competitive inhibition of folic acid synthesis
B. Affects fungal nucleic acid synthesis
C. Inhibits functions of cell membrane
D. Inhibits RNA synthesis

Ans. A.

98. The mode of action of Cephalosporin :

A. Affects protozoal metabolism
B. Affects fungal nucleic acid synthesis
C. Inhibits RNA synthesis
D. Inhibits cell wall synthesis

Ans. D.

99. Erythromycin contains

A. Dimethyl amino sugar
B. Trimethyl amino sugar
C. Sterol and sugar
D. Glycerol and sugar

Ans. A.

100. Mode of action of quinolone antibiotics on growing bacteria was thought to be

A. Inhibition of β lactamase
B. Prevention of the cross linking of glycine
C. Inhibition of DNA gyrase
D. Inhibition of reverse transcriptase

Ans. C.

101. The discovery that leads to the development of first antibiotic was made by

A. Jenner
B. Pasteur
C. Fleming
D. Pauling

Ans. C.

102. The yield of the antibiotic depends upon

A. pH of the medium
B. Age of the inoculums
C. Composition of the medium
D. All of these

Ans. D.

103. Fermentation medium for oxytetracyclin (Terramycin) consist of

A. CSL, starch, $(NH_4)_2$ SO_4, sodium chloride and $CaCO_3$
B CSL, $(NH_4)_2$ SO_4, sodium chloride and $CaCO_3$
C CSL, starch,$(NH_4)_2$ SO_4, ammonium chloride and $CaCO_3$
D. CSL,$(NH_4)_2$ SO_4, ammonium chloride and $CaCO_3$

Ans. A.

104. pH of the fermentation medium for chlorotetracyclins is

A. 5-6
B. 6-7
C. 7-8
D. 8-9

Ans. A.

105. At normal pH, penicillin remains in

A. Aqueous phase
B. Solvent phase
C. Both A & B
D. Precipitates

Ans. A.

106. Chlorotetracycline is soluble in

A. Organic solvents
B. Water
C. Ether
D. All of these

Ans. B.

107. Penicillin is produced by

A. Aerobic fermentation
B. Anaerobic fermentation
C. Aerobic fermentation followed by anaerobic fermentation
D. Anaerobic fermentation followed by aerobic fermentation

Ans. A.

108. Penicillin is recovered after fermentation as

A. Potassium penicillin
B. Calcium penicillin
C. Sodium penicillin
D. Penicillin only

Ans. A.

109. Media composition for the production of streptomycin is

A. Soybean meal, glucose, peptone, malt extract, sodium chloride
B. Soybean meal, glucose, peptone, malt extract, ammonium chloride
C. Soybean meal, glucose, peptone, malt extract, calcium carbonate
D. Soybean meal, glucose, peptone, malt extract, ammonium sulphate

Ans. A.

110. Which of the following organism(s) produce(s) tetracycline?

A. Steptomyces aureofaciens
B. Steptomyces ramosus
C. Nocardia sulphurea
D. All of these

Ans. D.

111. Media used for the production of chlorotetracyclin consists of

A. Sugar, corn steep liquor, $CaCO_3$, $(NH_4)_2SO_4$ and NH_4Cl
B. Corn steep liquor, $CaCO_3$ and $(NH_4)_2SO_4$
C. Sugar, $CaCO_3$ and $(NH_4)_2SO_4$
D. Corn steep liquor, $CaCO_3$, $(NH_4)_2SO_4$ and NH_4Cl

Ans. A.

112. Which of the following precursor is added in the medium to get penicillin G?
A. Phenyl carbamic acid B. Phenyl acetic acid
C. Ammonium sulphate D. Ammonium chloride

Ans. B.

113. High yield of chlorotetracycline requires
A. No aeration
B. Continuous aeration
C. Aeration which does not affect the yield
D. Controlled aeration

Ans. B.

114. Streptomycin is produced by
A. S. griseus B. S. griseoflavus
C. S. aerofaciens D. S. ramosus

Ans. A.

115. Inoculum preparation for the fermentation medium of penicillin takes place on
A. Wheat seeds B. Barley seeds
C. Rice seeds D. All of these

Ans. B.

116. Antibiotics are typically produced in fed batch reactors because
A. Antibiotic yields are generally higher when cells enter the stationary phase
B. The precursors are often toxic to the cells
C. Antibiotic yields are generally higher when cell growth slows
D. All of these

Ans. D.

117. Which of the following event occurs during third phase of growth of P chrysogenum?
A. Concentration of antibiotic increases in the medium
B. Autolysis of the medium starts
C. Slight rise in pH due to liberation of ammonia
D. All of the above

Ans. D.

118. Vegetable oil, (corn oil or soybean oil) added in the fermentation medium for penicillin, act as
A. Source of nutrients B. Carbon source
C. Antifoam agent D. Both A & C

Ans. C.

119. Which of the following changes occur during first phase of growth of Penicillium chrysogenum?

A. Growth of mycelia occurs

B. Ammonia is liberated in the medium

C. Lactic acid present in the corn steep liquor is utilized at the maximum rate

D. All of the above

Ans. D.

120. The penicillin stable in gastric acid and suitable for oral administration is

A. Carbenicillin B. Methicillin

C. Penicillin-G D. Closacillin

Ans. D.

121. The antibiotics not clinically useful for Pseudomonas aeruginosa infection is

A. Ceftazidime

B. Aminoglycosides

C. Trimethoprim-sulphamethoxazole

D. Piperacillin

Ans. C.

122. Which of the antibiotic is not used as a food preservative ?

A. Nisin B. Primaricin

C. β lactam antibiotic D. Tylosin

Ans. C.

123. Quinones and related antibiotics are

A. Actinorhodin B. Tetracyclines

C. All of these D. Mitomycin

Ans. C.

124. The third generation cephalosporin agents is

A. Cefoxitin B. Cefotaxime

C. Cephalexin D. Cephalothin

Ans. B.

125. Polyene antibiotics are

A. b lactam-thiazolidine ring B. Large ring structures

C. Any of these D. Small ring structures

Ans. B.

126. Interference mechanism of ciprofloxacin and norfloxacin is due to their action on

A. Cell membrane function
B. Cell wall synthesis
C. Protein synthesis
D. DNA function

Ans. D.

127. Vancomycin inhibits peptidoglycan synthesis by binding

A. Alanine racemase
B. D-alanyl-D-alanine
C. Amidase
D. D-alanyl-D-alanine synthetase

Ans. D.

128. Which antibiotic has a beta-lactam ring?

A. Penicillin
B. Cephalosporin
C. Streptomycin
D. Tetracycline

Ans. A.

129. The antibiotics not having good activity against Enterobacteriaceae is

A. Cefoxitin
B. Clindamycin
C. Ciprofloxacin
D. Trimethoprim-sulphamethoxazole

Ans. B.

130. Which of the following antibiotics can't be used for treatment of infections with b-lactamase-producing Staphylococcus aureus?

A. Ampicillin/sulbactam
B. Vancomycin
C. Piperacillin
D. Cephalothin

Ans. C.

131. Bacterial resistance to antibiotics is transmitted by

A. Transduction
B. Transformation
C. Mutation
D. Plasmids

Ans. D.

2

Bacteriology

1. Eugonic growth on Lowenstein-Jensen medium is produced by

   A. M. bovis
   B. M. tuberculosis
   C. Both A & B
   D. None

Ans. B.

2. The causative agent of Buruli ulcer is

   A. M. chelonei
   B. M. marinum
   C. M. fortuitum
   D. M. ulcerans

Ans. D.

3. Which of the following bacteria is susceptible to thiophen-2-carboxylic acid hydrazide?

   A. M. bovis
   B. M. tuberculosis
   C. M. chelonei
   D. M. fortuitum

Ans. A.

4. Culture of tubercle bacilli may be positive if number of bacteria in the specimen is

   A. As few as 1-4 per ml
   B. As few as 5-9 per ml
   C. As few as 10-100 per ml
   D. As few as 125-200 per ml

Ans. C.

5. Example of a Saprophytic bacteria is

   A. M. xenopi
   B. M. smegmatis
   C. Mycobacterium chelonei
   D. M. marinum

Ans. B.

6. Culture of tubercle bacilli may be positive if number of bacteria in the specimen is

   A. As few as 1-4 per ml
   B. As few as 5-9 per ml
   C. As few as 10-100 per ml
   D. As few as 125-200 per ml

Ans. C.

7. Example of a Saprophytic bacteria is

A. M. xenopi B. M. smegmatis

C. M. chelonei D. M. marinum

Ans. B.

8. Which of the following can be identified by milk ring test?

A. Brucellosis B. Salmonellosis

C. Bovine tuberculosis D. All of these

Ans. A.

9. Human transmission of Brucellae occurs by

A. Ingestion of contaminated meat

B. Direct contact with animal tissues

C. Ingestion of infected milk

D. All of these

Ans. D.

10. The most pathogenic Brucella spp for man is

A. B. melitensis B. B. abortus

C. B. suis D. B. canis

Ans. A.

11. Brucella are

A. Cocci B. Rods

C. Coccobacilli D. Very short rods

Ans. D.

12. Which of the following bacteria can grow in acidic pH?

A. Vibrio cholerae B. Lactobacilli

C. Shigella D. Salmonella

Ans. B.

13. To select cholera-causing bacterium, Vibrio cholerae, the pH of the medium is maintained at a pH of

A. 8.5 B. 8.9

C. 6.79 D. 3.5

Ans. A.

14. For the selection of endospore-forming bacteria, a mixed culture can be heated at

A. 80°C for 10 minutes B. 70°C for 10 minutes

C. 60°C for 10 minutes D. 90°C for 10 minutes

Ans. A.

15. The concentration of agar to obtain semi solid media is

A. 1.5-20% B. 0.5% or less

C. >10% D. >10%but<20%

Ans. B.

16. Which of the following bacteria dies quickly after drying ?

A. Treponema pallidum B. Mycobacterium tuberculosis

C. Staphylococcus aureus D. Pseudomonas aeruginosa

Ans. A.

17. Mac-Conkey medium is an example of

A. Transport medium B. Enrichment medium

C. Differential medium D. All of these

Ans. C.

18. Pseudomonas aeruginosa forms a blue water soluble pigment called

A. Pyocyanin B. Chlororaphin

C. Pyoverdin D. β-carotene

Ans. A.

19. Agar is used for solidifying culture media because

A. It does not affect by the growth of bacteria

B. It does not add to the nutritive properties of the medium

C. The melting and solidifying points of agar solution are not the same

D. All of the above

Ans. D.

20. For the selection of lactobacilli present in cheddar cheese, the pH of the medium is maintained at

A. 6.35 B. 5.35

C. 4.35 D. 5.75

Ans. B.

21. A disease producing species occurring in a mixed culture can often be selected on the basis of its

A. Pathogenic properties B. Special carbon source

C. Special nitrogen source D. None of these

Ans. A.

22. A psychrophilic halophile would be a microbe that prefers

A. Cold temperatures and increased amounts of salt

B. Warm temperatures and increased amounts of pressure

C. Cold temperatures and the absence of oxygen

D. Warm temperatures and increased amounts of acid

Ans. A.

23. NaCl can act as
   A. Antagonist at optimal concentrations
   B. Synergistically if added in excess of optimum level
   C. Both (a) and (b)
   D. None of the above

Ans. C.

24. Most spoilage bacteria grow at
   A. Acidic pH
   B. Alkaline pH
   C. Neutral pH
   D. Any of the pH

Ans. C.

25. The microbiological examination of coliform bacteria in foods preferably use
   A. MacConkey broth
   B. Violet Red Bile agar
   C. Eosine Methylene Blue agar
   D. All of these

Ans. D.

26. Which of the following acid will have higher bacteriostatic effect at a given pH ?
   A. Acetic acid
   B. Tartaric acid
   C. Citric acid
   D. Maleic acid

Ans. A.

27. Which of the following is not true for the thermal resistance of the bacterial cells?
   A. Cocci are usually more resistant than rods
   B. Higher the optimal and maximal temperatures for growth, higher the resistance
   C. Bacteria that clump considerably or form capsules are difficult to kill
   D. Cells low in lipid content are harder to kill than other cells

Ans. D.

28. Water activity can act as
   A. An intrinsic factor determining the likelihood of microbial proliferation
   B. A processing factor
   C. An extrinsic factor
   D. All of the above

Ans. D.

29. Enumeration of microorganism refers to
   A. Either spiral plating, pour plate or spread plate of a food suspension on to a suitable selective agar, or non-selective plate, depending on the test
   B. Either spiral plating, pour plate or spread plate of a food suspension on to a suitable selective agar
   C. Non-selective plating, depending on the test
   D. None of the above

Ans. A.

30. The different ACC's between food categories reflect the
   A. Expected level of contamination of the raw material
   B. Potential for microbial growth during storage
   C. Potential shelf life
   D. All of the above

Ans. D.

31. Examination of the presence / absence of organisms refers to
   A. Incubation of a food suspension in an enrichment medium followed by inoculation on to a suitable selective medium
   B. Incubation of a food suspension in an enrichment medium followed by inoculation on to a non-selective medium
   C. Incubation of a food suspension in an enrichment medium
   D. None of the above

Ans. A.

32. Plate count of bacteria in foods generally use the plating medium consisting of
   A. Peptone, yeast extract, glucose, sodium chloride, agar and distilled water
   B. Yeast extract, glucose, sodium chloride, agar and distilled water
   C. Peptone, glucose, sodium chloride, agar and distilled water
   D. Peptone, yeast extract, glucose, sodium chloride and distilled water

Ans. A.

33. What are the intrinsic factors for the microbial growth?
   A. pH
   B. Moisture
   C. Oxidation-Reduction Potential
   D. All of these

Ans. D.

34. Food poisoning is caused by
   A. Clostridium tetani
   B. Clostridium welchii
   C. Diptheria
   D. Clostridium botulinum

Ans. D.

35. Listeriosis is a(an) ______ disease.
   A. Food borne
   B. Water borne
   C. Milk borne
   D. Air borne

Ans. A.

36. Lyme disease is caused by
   A. Bacteria
   B. Fungi
   C. Spirochaete
   D. Virus

Ans. C.

37. Toxic shock syndrome is caused by

A. Staph.albus B. Staph.aureus

C. Strep.viridana D. None of these

Ans. B.

38. Mantoux test detects

A. M.tuberculosis B. Cyanobacteria

C. Clostridia D. Both a and b

Ans. A.

39. The causative agent of scrub typhus:

A. R. quintana B. R. rickettsii

C. R. orientalis D. R. prowazekii

Ans. C.

40. Lymphogranuloma venereum (LGV) a sexually transmitted disease is caused by

A. C. ophthalmia B. C. trachomatis

C. C. pneumoniae D. C. psittasi

Ans. B.

41. Intradermal test employed for diagnosis of LGV is

A. Frei test B. Mantoux test

C. Schick test D. Dick test

Ans. A.

42. Which algae is pathogenic to human?

A. Cephaloeuros B. Ulothrix

C. Macrocystis D. Prototheca

Ans. D.

43. Salmonella typhi is causative organism of

A. Undulent fever B. Remittent fever

C. Dengue fever D. Enteric fever

Ans. D.

44. Which of the following Salmonella paratyphi is the commonest in India?

A. A B. B

C. C D. None of these

Ans. A.

45. In enteric fever, the organ lodging maximum number of the organism is

A. Liver B. Gall bladder

C. Small intestine D. Large intestine

Ans. B.

46. True about Enteric fever is

A. Bacteraemia in first week B. Carrier in 90%

C. All serotypes cause the disease D. Rosy spots on 18th day

Ans. A.

47. E. coli produces the following toxins:

A. Enterotoxins B. Endotoxins

C. Verocytotoxins D. Hemolysins

Ans. B.

48. Diphtheria is caused by

A. Corynebacterium diphtheriae B. C. Bovis

C. C. Jeikeium D. C. equi

Ans. A.

49. Corynebacterium is

A. Gram positive B. Resistant to Penicillin

C. Gram negative D. Resistant to Chloramphenicol

Ans. A.

50. Diphtheria virulence test is

A. Ascoli's thermoprecipitation test B. Eleck's gel precipitation test

C. C.R.P test D. M.R.T. test

Ans. B.

51. Diphtheria toxoid is prepared by using

A. Aldehyde B. Formalin

C. Phenols D. None of these

Ans. B.

52. Diphtheria is an example of

A. Bacteraemia B. Pyaemia

C. Septicaemia D. Toxaemia

Ans. D.

53. Bacilli Calmette Guerin (BCG) contains the avirulent strains of

A. Human tubercle bacilli
B. Avian tubercle bacilli
C. Bovine tubercle bacilli
D. A typical mycobacteria

Ans. C.

54. Histoid Hansen is a variety of

A. Tuberculoid Leprosy
B. Borderline tuberculoid
C. Borderline lepromatous
D. Lepromatous leprosy

Ans. D.

55. Causative agent of Scarlet fever:

A. Staphylococcus aureus
B. Streptococcus viridans
C. Streptococcus pyogenes
D. None of these

Ans. C.

56. Rheumatic fever is most commonly caused by

A. Streptococcus viridans
B. Streptococcus pyogenes
C. Staphylococcus aureus
D. None of these

Ans. B.

57. Mediterranean fever is caused by

A. M. tuberculosis
B. S. typhi
C. C. neoformans
D. Brucella

Ans. D.

58. Which of the following test is specific for Brucellosis?

A. Frei
B. Weil
C. Castaneda strip
D. Rose water

Ans. C.

59. Malignant pustule is caused by

A. Anthrax
B. Tetanus
C. Diphtheria
D. None of these

Ans. A.

60. The mode of spread of tetanus neurotoxin from blood to brain is

A. Via lymphatics
B. Arterial blood
C. Cranial nerves
D. None of these

Ans. C.

61. Tetanus is caused by spread of

A. Exotoxin in sympathetic system B. Exotoxin in parasympathetic system

C. Endotoxin in sympathetic system D. Endotoxin in parasympathetic system

Ans. A.

62. The first symptom of tetanus is

A. Lock jaw B. Trismus

C. Anorexia D. Dysphagia

Ans. B.

63. Of which clostridia, the neurotoxin is most powerful?

A. Cl. tetani B. Cl. welchii

C. Cl. botulism D. Cl. septicum

Ans. C.

64. Toxin produced by C.botulism is

A. Botulin B. Tetanospasmin

C. Tetanolysin D. Cholaragen

Ans. A.

65. "Toxic shock syndrome" is caused by the toxin of

A. Staphylococcus aureus B. Streptococcus pyogenes

C. Vibrio cholerae D. Candida

Ans. A.

66. Causative agent of syphilis

A. T. pallidum B. T. pertenue

C. T. carateum D. T. endemicum

Ans. A.

67. Specific test for syphilis is

A. VDRL test B. ELISA

C. FTA D. None of these

Ans. A.

68. VDRL test is a

A. Agglutination test B. Slide flocculation test

C. Precipitation test D. None of these

Ans. B.

69. Gonorrhoea is

A. Air borne disease

B. Water borne disease

C. Sexually transmitted venereal disease

D. Both a and c

Ans. C.

70. Bartholin cyst is caused by

A. Candida
B. Streptococcus
C. Staphylococcus
D. Gonococcus

Ans. D.

71. Neisseria gonorrhoeae causes

A. Urethritis
B. Conjunctivitis
C. Arthritis
D. All of the above

Ans. D.

72. Virulence in gonococcus is due to

A. Pili
B. Cell membrane
C. Its cellular location
D. Cyclic enzymes

Ans. A.

73. Splenomegaly is an important manifestation of

A. Kala-agar
B. Typhoid
C. Malaria
D. All of these

Ans. D.

74. Fungi producing mycelium are called

A. Moulds
B. Filamentous fungi
C. Both a and b
D. Yeasts

Ans. A.

75. Candidiasis is caused by

A. Candida albicans
B. Aspergillus spp.
C. E. floccosum
D. M. audouinii

Ans. A.

76. Aspergillus fumigatus can infect

A. A. niger
B. A. fumigatus
C. A. flavus
D. A. oryzae

Ans. D.

77. A. fumigatus can produce

A. Endotoxins
B. Exotoxins
C. Enterotoxins
D. None of these

Ans. A.

78. The following Penicillium species are pathogenic except

A. P. commune
B. P. bicolor
C. P. glaucum
D. P. notatum

Ans. D.

79. Tinea versicolor is caused by

A. Candida albicans
B. Malassezia furfur
C. Aspergillus niger
D. None of these

Ans. B.

80. Causative agent of Tinea nigra

A. Malassezia furfur
B. Exophiala werenekii
C. Candida albicans
D. Aspergillus flavus

Ans. B.

81. Causative agent of African histoplasmosis

A. Histoplasma capsulatum
B. Histoplasma duboissi
C. Aspergillus niger
D. Aspergillus flavus

Ans. B.

82. The effect of antibiotics on micro organisms is mainly due to

A. Inhibition of cell-wall synthesis
B. Damage to the cytoplasmic membrane
C. Inhibition of nucleic acid and protein synthesis
D. All of the above

Ans. D.

83. Match the following enzymes with their activities A to D:

1. Hyaluronidase	A. Inactivate leucocytes and aid bacterial invasion
2. Collagenase	B. Reversibly catalyzes the breakdown of a major component
3. Lecithinase	C. Disintegrates a constituent of muscle, cartilage and bone
4. Leucocidins	D. Haemolysis of erythrocytes and the necrosis of other cells

Ans. 1 B, 2 C, 3 D, 4 A.

84. Match the following aggresins with their respective modes of action from A to D:

1. Hyaluronidase	A. Destroys RBC's and other tissues
2. Haemolysis	B. Breaks down connective tissues, increases permeability of tissue space
3. Streptokinase	C. Causes lysis of RBC's and other tissues
4. Lecithinase	D. Digest the fibrin of blood

Ans. 1 B, 2A, 3 D, 4 C.

85. Match the following terms with their respective effects A to E:

1. Brucella melitensis	A. Causes trachoma, conjunctivitis and nongonococcal gamets
2. Flavobacterium	B. Causes influenza like fever species
3. Chlamydia	C. Causes Malta fever in goats
4. Leptospira	D. Weil's disease (jaundice)

Ans. 1C, 2B, 3A and 4 D.

86. The role that human play in the plague life cycle is

A. Secondary reservoir
B. Primary transmission vector
C. Primary host
D. Accidental intruder in rat flea cycle
E. None of these

Ans. D.

87. Which organism is responsible for causing fever to a man dealing with goats?

A. Treponema Pallidum
B. M. tuberculosis
C. Clostridium novyi
D. Brucella melitensis
E. None of these

Ans. D.

88. Diphtheria toxins are produced from the strains of C. diphtheriae, which are

A. Encapsulated
B. Sucrose fermentors
C. Glucose fermentors
D. Lysogenic for β prophase

Ans. D.

89. Which of the following is not related to congenital syphilis?

A. Aneurysm
B. Saddle nose
C. Still birth
D. Hutchiso's teeth

Ans. A.

90. Streptococcus pyogenes produce infection

A. Streptococcal sore throat
B. Acute glomerulonephritis
C. Rheumatic fever
D. None of these

Ans. A.

91. Salmonella which can cause prolong septicaemia.
   A. Salmonella anatum B. Salmonella cholerasuis
   C. Salmonella typhimurium D. Salmonella enteritidis

Ans. B.

92. E. coli produce which type of toxins?
   A. Exotoxins B. Endotoxins
   C. Leucocidin D. Both a and b

Ans. D.

93. Main causative organism of gas gangrene is
   A. B. anthracis B. Clostridium tetani
   C. Cl. deficile D. Cl. perfringens

Ans. D.

94. Causative organism of whooping cough is
   A. Bordetella pertussis B. Bordetella parapertussis
   C. Bordetella bronchiseptica D. None of these

Ans. A.

95. Pfeiffer phenomenon is related to
   A. Vibrio cholerae B. B. anthracis
   C. Rickettsial pox D. All of these

Ans. A.

96. Sporadic summer diarrhoea may be caused by
   A. E. coli B. Enterobacter
   C. Hafnia D. Serratia

Ans. A.

97. Biological false reaction in VDRL is related to
   A. Lepra bacilli B. Corynebacterium diphtheria
   C. Cl. welchii D. None of these

Ans. A.

98. A psychrophilic halophile would be a microbe that prefers
   A. Cold temperatures and increased amounts of salt
   B. Warm temperatures and increased amounts of pressure
   C. Cold temperatures and the absence of oxygen
   D. Warm temperatures and increased amounts of acid

Ans. A.

99. Most spoilage bacteria grow at

A. Acidic pH
B. Alkaline pH
C. Neutral pH
D. Any of the pH

Ans. C.

100. The microbiological examination of coliform bacteria in foods preferably use

A. MacConkey broth
B. Violet Red Bile agar
C. Eosine Methylene blue agar
D. all of these

Ans. D.

101. Which of the following acid will have higher bacteriostatic effect at a given pH?

A. Acetic acid
B. Tartaric acid
C. Citric acid
D. Maleic acid

Ans. A.

102. Which of the following is not true for the thermal resistance of the bacterial cells?

A. Cocci are usually more resistant than rods
B. Higher the optimal and maximal temperatures for growth, higher the resistance
C. Bacteria that clump considerably or form capsules are difficult to kill
D. Cells low in lipid content are harder to kill than other cells

Ans. D.

103. Water activity can act as

A. An intrinsic factor determining the likelihood of microbial proliferation
B. A processing factor
C. An extrinsic factor
D. All of the above

Ans. D.

104. Enumeration of microorganism refers to

A. Either spiral plating, pour plate or spread plate of a food suspension on to a suitable selective agar, or non-selective plate, depending on the test
B. Either spiral plating, pour plate or spread plate of a food suspension on to a suitable selective agar
C. Non-selective plating, depending on the test
D. None of the above

Ans. A.

105. Examination of the presence / absence of organisms refers to
A. Incubation of a food suspension in an enrichment medium followed by inoculation on to a suitable selective medium
B. Incubation of a food suspension in an enrichment medium followed by inoculation on to a non-selective medium
C. Incubation of a food suspension in an enrichment medium
D. None of the above

Ans. A.

106. Plate count of bacteria in foods generally use the plating medium consisting of
A. Peptone, yeast extract, glucose, sodium chloride, agar and distilled water
B. Yeast extract, glucose, sodium chloride, agar and distilled water
C. Peptone, glucose, sodium chloride, agar and distilled water
D. Peptone, yeast extract, glucose, sodium chloride and distilled water

Ans. A.

107. What are the intrinsic factors for the microbial growth?
A. pH
B. Moisture
C. Oxidation-Reduction Potential
D. All of these

Ans. D.

108. There are many different types of bacteria normally present in the oral cavity. Which of the following is the name of the one most likely to be associated with the onset of dental caries?
A. Actinomyces
B. Bacteroides
C. Lactobacillus
D. Staphylococcus
E. Streptococcus

Ans. E.

109. Elderly patients sometimes present with a fungal infection of the palate, beneath a denture, referred to as denture stomatitis. Which organism causes this condition?
A. Actinomyces
B. Borrellia vincenti
C. Candida albicans
D. Herpes simples
E. Staphylococcus aureus

Ans. C.

110. Many diseases are due to infection with one type of micro-organism or another. Which one of the following options is the most likely example of an infection that is not caused by a micro-organism?
A. Creutzfeldt–Jakob disease
B. Hepatitis C
C. Meningitis
D. Poliomyelitis
E. Swine influenza

Ans. A.

111. Which of the following options is the group of bacteria most likely to live in colonies arranged as chains of circular micro-organisms?

A. Bacilli
B. Lactobacilli
C. Spirochaetes
D. Staphylococci
E. Streptococci

Ans. E.

112. When the body tissues undergo a disease process, certain types of condition develop. Which term correctly describes that which appears as an abnormal fluid-filled sac within the tissues?

A. Benign tumour
B. Cyst
C. Infection
D. Malignant tumour
E. Ulcer

Ans. B.

113. When body tissues become infected, they exhibit five classic signs of inflammation. Which is the last of these five signs to occur?

A. Heat
B. Loss of function
C. Pain
D. Redness
E. Swelling

Ans. B.

114. Which of the following is most similar to Rickettsia and Chlamydia?

A. Bdellovibrio
B. Clostridium
C. Mycobacterium
D. Mycoldaima

Ans. C.

115. How would you distinguish pseudomonas species from E. coli?

A. Gram staining
B. Morphology
C. Glucose fermentation Vs Respiration
D. All of the above

Ans. C.

116. The colonies produced by Pseudomonas on Mac Conkey's medium are

A. Purple colored
B. Pink colored
C. Pale colored
D. Green colored

Ans. C.

117. Staining material of gram positive bacterium is

A. Fast green
B. Haematoxylin
C. Crystal violet
D. Safranin

Ans. C.

118. Endotoxin produced by gram negative bacteria is present in

A. Peptidoglycan
B. Lipopolysaccharide
C. Teichoic acid
D. Inner membrane

Ans. B.

119. Which one of the following was Gram negative, chemolithotrophic bacteria?

A. Siderococcus
B. E. coli
C. Spirillum
D. Mycoplasmas

Ans. B.

120. The mode of reproduction which occurs in mycoplasma is

A. Budding
B. Bursting
C. Binary fission
D. Binary fusion

Ans. C.

121. Which one of the following produce typical fried egg appearance colonies on solid media?

A. Mycobacteria
B. Mycoplasts
C. Mycoplasmas
D. Bacteroides

Ans. C.

122. An organism that is osmophilic and has a specific requirements for sodium chloride resembles

A. Halophile
B. Basophile
C. Barophile
D. Xerophile

Ans. A.

123. Heterolactic acid bacteria produce

A. Lactic acid only
B. Lactic acid + H_2O + CO_2
C. Lactic acid + CO_2
D. Lactic acid + alcohol + CO_2

Ans. D.

124. The pigment present in red algae is

A. Rhodochrome
B. Fucoxanthin
C. Chlorophyll only
D. Chlorophyll + phycobilin

Ans. D.

125. Citrus canker is caused by

A. Phytomonas B. Salmonella

C. Lactobacillus D. Hay bacillus

Ans. A.

126. Bacteria that are responsible for fermentation of dairy milk are

A. Azotobacter B. Rhizobium

C. Lactobacillus D. Hay bacillus

Ans. C.

127. The staining technique used to stain the metachromatic granules of Corynebacterium

A. Giemsa stain B. Alberts stain

C. Acid fast staining D. Both a and b

Ans. B.

128. The causative organism of cholera, i.e., Vibrio show the movement called

A. Gliding movement B. Darting movement

C. Pseudopoidal movement D. None of these

Ans. B.

129. Erythrocytes will get its ATP energy only by

A. Glycolysis B. Kreb's cycle

C. Electron Transport D. HMP shunt

Ans. A.

130. The bacterial pili mainly contain

A. Carbohydrates B. Lipids

C. Proteins D. Minerals

Ans. C.

131. Role of bacteria in carbon cycle is

A. Photosynthesis

B. Chemosynthesis

C. Breakdown of organic compounds

D. Assimilation of nitrogen compounds

Ans. C.

132. All prokaryotes are surrounded by a cell wall except

A. Mycoplasmas B. Spirochetes

C. Actinomycetes D. Methanogens

Ans. A.

133. Enzyme hydrolyzing bacterial cell wall

A. Lysozome
B. Reductase
C. Protease
D. Lysozyme

Ans. D.

134. Cows can digest straw because they contain

A. Cellulose hydrolyzing microorganisms
B. Protein hydrolyzing bacteria
C. Lipid hydrolyzing microorganisms
D. Amino acid degrading bacteria

Ans. A.

135. Which one of the following bacteria has found extensive use in genetic engineering work in plants?

A. Clostridium septicum
B. Xanthomonas oryzae
C. Bacillus coagulans
D. Agrobacterium tumefaciens

Ans. D.

136. Bioleaching is done by

A. Protozoa
B. Bacteria
C. Algae
D. All of the above

Ans. B.

137. Which of the following organisms capable of surviving high temperature?

A. Vibrio
B. Pseudomonas
C. Torula
D. Coxiella

Ans. C.

138. The test used to detect the deamination of the amino acids by bacteria

A. Nessler's reagent test
B. Proteolytic test
C. Lactose test
D. Rose indole reagent test

Ans. A.

139. Diphtheria is caused by

A. Corynebacterium
B. Staphylococcus
C. Streptococcus
D. None of these

Ans. A.

140. A bacterium containing prophage is called as

A. Lytic
B. Lysogen
C. Lytogen
D. None of these

Ans. B.

141. The most infectious food borne disease is

A. Tetanus
B. Dysentery
C. Gas gangrene
D. Botulism

Ans. D.

142. An example for common air borne epidemic disease

A. Influenza
B. Typhoid
C. Encephalitis
D. Malaria

Ans. A.

143. Rancidity of stored foods is due to the activity of

A. Toxigenic microbes
B. Proteolytic microbes
C. Saccharolytic microbes
D. Lipolytic microbes

Ans. D.

144. Virulence of the microorganisms can be reduced by

A. Attenuation
B. A virulence
C. Inactivation
D. Freezing

Ans. A.

145. The test used for detection of typhoid fever

A. WIDAL test
B. ELISA
C. Rosewaller test
D. Western blotting

Ans. A.

146. Diphtheria bacillus is otherwise known as

A. Fried-Landers bacillus
B. Klebs–Loeffler bacillus
C. Frchs bacillus
D. Koch's bacillus

Ans. B.

147. Acridine dyes are more effective against

A. Gram positive
B. Gram negative
C. Rickettsia
D. Mycoplasma

Ans. A.

148. In bacteria pigment bearing structures are

A. Chloroplast
B. Protoplast
C. Spheroplast
D. Chromatophores

Ans. D.

149. The procedure of differential staining of bacteria was developed by

A. A.H. Gram B. H. C. Gram

C. N. C. Gram D. H. A. Gram

Ans. B.

150. Intermediate group of pathogen between bacteria and viruses which are intracellular parasites are called

A. Mycoplasmas B. Rickettsias

C. Prions D. Virusoides

Ans. B.

151. Bacillus is an example of

A. Gram positive bacteria B. Gram negative bacteria

C. Virus D. Viroid

Ans. A.

152. Mordant used in grams staining is

A. Crystal violet B. Iodine

C. Saffranin D. All of these

Ans. B.

153. Following Cocci are non-motile except

A. Staphylococcus B. Meningococcus

C. Gonococcus D. Rhodococcus agilis

Ans. A.

154. Aspergillus fumigatus can infect

A. Birds B. Animals

C. Man D. All of them

Ans. D.

155. Enterotoxin responsible for food poisoning is secreted by

A. Enterococci B. Entamoeba histolytica

C. Enterobacteriaceae D. Staphylococci

Ans. D.

156. Autolysis is done by

A. Mitochondria B. Lysosomes

C. Golgi bodies D. Peroxisomes

Ans. B.

157. A facultative anaerobic is

A. Only grow anaerobically

B. Only grow in the presence of O2

C. Ordinarily an anaerobe but can grow with O2

D. Ordinarily an aerobe but can grow in absence of O2

Ans. D.

158. The percentage of O2 required by moderate anaerobe is

A. 0% B. < 0.5%

C. 2-8% D. 5-10%

Ans. C.

159. Cell wall of gram negative bacteria is

A. Thick B. Lipids are present

C. Teichoic acids are absent D. None of these

Ans. C.

160. Cytoplasmic streaming is present in

A. Prokaryotes B. Animals

C. Eukaryotes D. Both a and b

Ans. C.

161. The motile bacteria is

A. S. typhi B. K. pneumoniae

C. B. anthracis D. Shigella

Ans. A.

162. The stain used to demonstrate fungus

A. Albert B. Nigrosin

C. Lactophenol cotton blue D. None of these

Ans. C.

163. Exotoxins are

A. Heat labile B. Heat stable

C. Part of cell wall D. Polymerized complexes

Ans. A.

164. The bacterial cell multiplication is usually by

A. Mitosis B. Meiosis

C. Conjugation D. Binary-fission

Ans. D.

165. All the groups of bacteria have cell wall except

A. Mycobacteria B. Mycoplasmas

C. Clostridia D. Rickettsia

Ans. B.

166. Thickness of cell wall ranges from

A. 9-10 nm B. 12-13 nm

C. 10-25 nm D. 30-40 nm

Ans. C.

167. Teichoic acids and Teichuronic acids are found in

A. Gram positive bacteria B. Gram negative bacteria

C. Fungi D. None of these

Ans. A.

168. The characteristic shape of the bacteria is maintained because of

A. Capsule B. Cell wall

C. Cell membrane D. Slime layer

Ans. B.

169. Bacterial capsule is chemically composed of

A. Polypeptide B. Polynucleotides

C. Polysaccharides D. Polypeptides or polysaccharides

Ans. D.

170. The cell wall deficient form of bacteria is

A. Mycoplasma B. 'L' form

C. Protoplast D. Spheroplast

Ans. B.

171. The differences between Gram positive and Gram negative bacteria is shown to reside in the

A. Cell wall B. Nucleus

C. Cell membrane D. Mesosomes

Ans. A.

172. Capsule formation occurs in the presence of

A. Albumin B. Charcoal

C. Serum D. Starch

Ans. C.

173. The virulence determining antigens of microorganisms may be

A. Proteins and polysaccharides

B. Carbohydrate – protein complexes

C. Polysaccharide – Phospholipid – Protein complexes

D. All of these

Ans. D.

174. Organelles with hydrolytic enzymes are

A. Mitochondria B. Golgi complex

C. Lysosomes D. Ribosomes

Ans. C.

175. Bacterial locomotion is accomplished by

A. Fimbria B. Flagella

C. Cytoskeleton D. Both a and b

Ans. D.

176. Fimbriae are demonstrated by

A. Culture B. Gram stain

C. Biochemical reactions D. Haemagglutination test

Ans. D.

177. The motile bacteria is

A. Salmonella typhi B. Klebsiella pneumoniae

C. Bacillus anthracis D. Shigella flexneri

Ans. A.

178. Metachromatic granules are chemically composed of

A. Lipids B. Proteins

C. Polymetaphosphates D. Polysaccharide

Ans. C.

179. Metachromatic granules can be stained with

A. Safranin B. Methylene blue

C. Crystal violet D. Picric acid

Ans. B.

180. Bacterial spores are

A. Weakly acid fast B. Strongly acid fast

C. Alcohol fast D. Non acid fast

Ans. A.

181. Endospores can be stained with

A. Safranin
B. Crystal violet
C. Methylene blue
D. Malachite green

Ans. D.

182. The following bacteria produce pigment, except

A. Pseudomonas pyocyaneus
B. Serratia marcescens
C. K. pneumoniae
D. Staphylococcus aureus

Ans. C.

183. The order of stains in Gram-staining procedure is

A. Crystal violet, Iodine solution, Alcohol, Safranin
B. Iodine solution, Crystal Violet, Safranin, Alcohol
C. Alcohol, Crystal Violet, Iodine solution, Safranin
D. All of these

Ans. A.

184. The percentage of alcohol used in Gram staining is

A. 75%
B. 90%
C. 60%
D. 25%

Ans. B.

185. Gram positive bacteria appear as

A. Pink
B. Violet
C. Both a & b
D. None of these

Ans. B.

186. Gram negative bacteria appear as

A. Pink
B. Violet
C. Both a & b
D. None of these

Ans. A.

187. The action of alcohol during Gram staining is

A. Allows the color
B. It adds color
C. Decolorises the cells
D. None of these

Ans. C.

188. Lipid contents is more in

A. Gram negative bacteria
B. Gram positive bacteria
C. Same in both
D. None of these

Ans. A.

189. Cell-wall is

A. Thick in Gram positive than Gram negative

B. Thick in Gram negative than Gram positive

C. Equal in both

D. In Gram negative cell-wall is absent

Ans. A.

190. The Lipid content present in Gram positive bacterial cell-wall is

A. 1-10 % B. 1-5 %

C. 2-8 % D. None of these

Ans. B.

191. Rickettsiae stained by Gram staining appear as

A. Gram positive B. Gram negative

C. Between positive and negative D. None of these

Ans. B.

192. Chlamydiae occur in

A. Elementary bodies B. Reticulate bodies

C. Complex structures D. A and B

Ans. D.

193. Chlamydiae can be stained better with

A. Ziehl–Neelsen staining B. Castaneda & Machiavelli stain

C. Gimenez stain D. Both B and C

Ans. D.

194. The study of algae is known as

A. Algalogy B. Phycology

C. Mycology D. Bacteriology

Ans. B.

195. The free floating algae are known as

A. Phytoplankins B. Benthons

C. Sea weeds D. None of these

Ans. A.

196. In algae, advanced type of sexual reproduction is

A. Isogamy B. Anisogamy

C. Oogamy D. None of these

Ans. C.

197. Alginic acids and its salts are obtained from the wall of

A. Red algae
B. Brown algae
C. Green algae
D. Red and brown algae

Ans. B.

198. The molds obtained nutrition from dead and decaying matter which are called

A. Saphrophytes
B. Parasites
C. Commensals
D. None of these

Ans. A.

199. Most molds are capable of growing in the temperature range between

A. $0^{\circ} - 25^{\circ}C$
B. $0^{\circ} - 35^{\circ}C$
C. $10^{\circ} - 25^{\circ}C$
D. $10^{\circ} - 35^{\circ}C$

Ans. B.

200. Pellicle is found in only

A. Algae
B. Fungi
C. Bacteria
D. Protozoans

Ans. D.

201. If only one stain is used for staining a specimen

A. Simple staining
B. Negative staining
C. Differential staining
D. None of these

Ans. A.

202. Other than the sample (specimen) the remaining portion is stained then it is called

A. Simple staining
B. Negative staining
C. Differential staining
D. None of these

Ans. B.

203. If more than one stain is used, such staining is called

A. Simple staining
B. Negative staining
C. Differential staining
D. None of these

Ans. C.

204. 'Fluorescence' was first observed by

A. Kohler
B. Coons
C. Both a and b
D. None of these

Ans. A.

205. Fluorescent antibody technique was developed by

A. Kohler
B. Coons
C. Both a and b
D. None of these

Ans. B.

206. During staining for Electron Microscopy, the method which improves contrast of specimen is

A. Positive staining
B. Negative staining
C. Shadow staining
D. None of these

Ans. B.

207. The inorganic forms of nitrogen, which are accepted by bacteria are

A. Nitrates
B. Nitrites
C. Ammonium salts
D. All of these

Ans. D.

208. Archaeo bacteria are known as

A. Halophiles
B. Red extreme halophiles
C. Osmophiles
D. Extreme thermophiles

Ans. B.

209. Nitrite is converted into nitrate by the bacteria

A. Nitrosomonas
B. Nitrosocytes
C. Nitrobacter
D. Azatobacter

Ans. C.

210. Sulphur oxidizing bacteria is

A. Alcaligenes
B. Pseudomonas
C. Thiobacillus
D. None of these

Ans. C.

211. Bacillus Schlegelli is

A. Hydrogen – Oxidizing bacteria
B. Sulphur – Oxidizing bacteria
C. Iron-Oxidising bacteria
D. Nitrite oxidizing bacteria

Ans. A.

212. The group of bacteria which depends on organic sources in nature for their energy requirements. They are said to be

A. Chemotrophs
B. Phototrophs
C. Heterotrophes
D. Organotrophs

Ans. C.

213. Symbionts are
   A. Bacteria in symbiotic association
   B. The group of fungi in symbiotic association
   C. The groups participating in symbiotic association
   D. All of these

Ans. C.

214. The best example for symbiotic association is
   A. E.coli in intestine of man   B. Lichens
   C. Normal flora of skin   D. All of the above

Ans. B.

215. Urea is decomposed by the species
   A. Micrococcus sps.   B. Nitrosomonas sps.
   C. Proteus sps.   D. Both a and c

Ans. D.

216. Capsulated forms of bacteria are
   A. Virulent   B. A virulent
   C. Useful   D. Symbiotic

Ans. B.

217. The bacterial cells participating in conjugation are
   A. Conjugants   B. Fertile cells
   C. Exconjugants   D. None of these

Ans. A.

218. The natural reservoir of infection for cholera is
   A. Flies   B. Horse
   C. Man   D. None of these

Ans. C.

219. Main cause for Cholera is
   A. Poverty and insanitation   B. Mosquitoes
   C. Toxin produced by pesticides   D. None of these

Ans. A.

220. Vibrio cholera differs from Vibrio eltor by
   A. It shares some Inaba, Ogawa subtypes with eltor
   B. Resistant to polymyxin
   C. Eltor is non-motile
   D. Causes less subclinical infections as compared to eltor

Ans. D.

221. Cholera vaccine gives protection for

A. 1-3 months
B. 3-6 months
C. 6-9 months
D. 9-12 months

Ans. B.

222. Prophylaxis of cholera is

A. Protected water supply
B. Environmental sanitation
C. Immunisation with killed vaccines
D. All of these

Ans. D.

223. Sh. dysenteriae is also known as

A. Sh. shiga
B. Sh. schmitzi
C. Both a and b
D. Sh. paradysenteriae

Ans. C.

224. Acid fast bacteria are

A. Neisseria
B. Staphylococci
C. Mycobacteria
D. All of the above

Ans. C.

225. Mycobacteria are stained with

A. Gram's staining
B. Simple staining
C. Both a and b
D. Ziehl – Neelsen's staining

Ans. D.

226. Niacin test is positive in case of

A. Corynebacterium
B. M. tuberculosis
C. M. bovis
D. M. avium

Ans. B.

227. Lepromin test

A. Is negative in tubercular leprosy
B. Positive in lepromatous type
C. Indicated delayed hypersensitivity test
D. Indicates infection

Ans. C.

228. Streptococcus causes which type of infections?

A. Fever
B. Zoonotic
C. Pyogenic
D. None of these

Ans. D.

229. Streptococcus pyogenes classification is based on

A. Protein M
B. Protein T
C. Protein R
D. Polysaccharide C

Ans. A.

230. α-haemolytic streptococci are also known as

A. Str. pyogenes
B. Virulence group
C. Viridans group
D. None of these

Ans. C.

231. Streptolysin O is inactivated by

A. CO2
B. Nitrogen
C. Oxygen
D. Serum

Ans. C.

232. Streptolysin 'S' is

A. Oxygen unstable
B. Thermostable
C. Oxygen stable
D. None of these

Ans. C.

233. Glutamic acid is oxidized by the species except

A. B. abortus
B. B. melitensis
C. B. suis
D. B. canis

Ans. D.

234. Of the following, this is a capsulated organism

A. Bacillus anthracis
B. Escherichia-coli
C. Corynebacterium
D. Brucella

Ans. A.

235. Anthrax is a

A. Vector borne
B. Zoonotic infection
C. Wound bone
D. Soil borne

Ans. B.

236. Mc Fadyean's reaction is used to detect

A. Bacillus anthracis
B. Brucella
C. Corynaebacterium
D. None of these

Ans. A.

237. Gas gangrene bacillus is

A. Facultative anaerobe
B. Obligate anaerobe
C. Facultative aerobe
D. Obligate aerobe

Ans. B.

238. Those fungi which do not have a sexual stage are classified as

A. Phycomycetes
B. Ascomycetes
C. Basidiomycetes
D. Fungi imperfecti

Ans. D.

239. Tinea capitis is

A. Ring worm of the foot
B. Ring worm of scalp
C. Ring worm of non-hairy skin of body
D. Both a and c

Ans. C.

240. Diagnosis of bacterial disease can be made by

A. Finding bacteria in pathological fluids
B. Isolation of bacteria by culture from exudates or blood
C. Both a and b
D. None of these

Ans. C.

241. Staphylococcus aureus are characterized by

A. Formation of acid in sucrose, dextrose
B. Liquification of gelatin due to production of gelatinase
C. Strains are catalase positive
D. All of above
E. None of these

Ans. C.

242. Cholera occurs in _______ form

A. Endemic
B. Epidemic
C. Sporadic
D. all of these

Ans. D.

243. Endemic typhus is caused by

A. R. mooseri
B. R. quintana
C. R. prowazekii
D. any of them
E. None of these

Ans. A.

244. A man is usually infected with tick typhus due to

A. Drinking milk of sick animals
B. Tending cattle
C. Inhaling infected dust
D. All of these

Ans. C.

245. In Gram positive bacteria, ratio of RNA to DNA is

A. 8 : 1
B. 1 : 2
C. Almost equal
D. None of these

Ans. A.

246. Ziehl – Neelsen stain is a ______

A. Simple stain
B. Counter stain
C. Differential stain
D. None of them

Ans. C.

247. Wet mount slide preparations are used in microbiology as they allow to see

A. Size and shape of individual organisms
B. Characteristic arrangement or grouping of cells
C. Motility of the organism
D. All of these
E. None of these

Ans. D.

248. Organism resistant to degradative lysosomal enzymes includes

A. M. tuberculosis
B. Legionella pneumophila
C. M. leprae
D. Both a and b
E. Both b and c

Ans. E.

249. The properties common to Gram positive and negative cell walls are

A. Equal susceptibility to hydrolysis by lysozyme
B. Peptide crosslinks between polysaccharides
C. Rigid peptidoglycan activity
D. Greater resistance to drying than vegetative cell.
E. All of these

Ans. D.

250. The main difference in true bacteria and mycoplasma is that it does not possess

A. Flagella
B. Cell wall
C. ATP synthesis
D. A capsule

Ans. B.

251. The organism responsible for retarding penetration of host cell by an inhibitor of ATP synthesis.

A. M. pneumoniae
B. Rickettsia rickettsii
C. Chlamydia trachomatis
D. Chlamydia psitacci

Ans. B.

252. Mycoplasmas differ from Chalamydiae in that, it

A. Has ability to cause urinary tract infection
B. Lack of a true bacterial cell wall
C. Susceptible to penicillin
D. All of these
E. None of these

Ans. B.

253. Fungi differs with bacteria in that it

A. Contain no peptidoglycan
B. Are prokaryotic
C. Susceptible to griseofulvin
D. Have nuclear membranes
E. All of these

Ans. E.

254. A polysaccharide capsule is present on cryptococci which –

A. Inhibits phagocytosis
B. Is an aid to diagnose
C. Cross reacts with rheumatoid factor
D. All of these

Ans. A.

255. The bacteria, which is motile at 22°C but non-motile at 37°C is

A. Tranformation
B. Transduction
C. Conjugation
D. Cell fusion

Ans. D.

256. Teichoic acid is

A. Found in the walls of Gram positive bacteria
B. Provide receptors for phages
C. Make up outer wall of Gram negative bacteria
D. Influence the permeability of the membrane

Ans. A.

257. One flagellum at one end of the organ is called –

A. Monotrichate
B. Amphitrichate
C. Iophotrichate
D. Peritrichate

Ans. A.

258. What is the function of bacterial capsule?

A. Production of organism from phagocytosis
B. Helps in adherence of bacteria to surface in its environment
C. Both a and b
D. None of these

Ans. C.

259. Which of the following is the characteristic of bacterial spore?

A. Highly refractile
B. Usually dehydrated
C. Sensitive to formaldehyde
D. All of these

Ans. D.

260. Which of the following are acid fast structures?

A. Mycobacteria
B. Bacterial spores
C. Nocardia
D. All of these

Ans. D.

261. All of the following are acid fast structures except

A. Clostridium
B. Bacterium spores
C. Exoskeleton
D. None of these

Ans. A.

262. All of the following are energy source of bacteria except

A. Oxidation of inorganic compounds
B. Oxidation of organic compounds
C. Absorption of heat
D. Utilisation of visible light

Ans. C.

263. Identify the obligate anaerobes

A. Salmonella
B. Vibrio cholerae
C. Cl. tetani
D. Sarcinae

Ans. C.

264. Streptococci which are destroyed at 60°C for 30 minutes

A. Preptostreptococci
B. Streptococcus viridans
C. Streptococcus hemolyticus
D. All of these

Ans. D.

265. Toxins or enzymes which are not produced by Streptococcus pyogenes

A. Hyaluronides
B. Phosphate
C. Hemolysin
D. Streptokinase

Ans. B.

266. Cholera red reaction is identified by

A. Sulphuric acid
B. Nitric acid
C. Hydrochloric acid
D. Carbolic acid

Ans. A.

267. Diagnosis of carrier of Salmonella typhi may be shown by

A. Faecal culture
B. Bile culture
C. Urine culture
D. All of these

Ans. D.

268. Daisy head colony is associated with

A. M. tuberculosis
B. C. diphtheriae
C. Cl. tetani
D. None of these

Ans. B.

269. Neil Mooser reaction is related to

A. Rickettsiae
B. Chlamydiae
C. Spirochaetes
D. Clostridium perfringens

Ans. A.

270. Ricketssia are stained with

A. Giesna and Castaneda stains
B. Macchiavello and Gimnez stains
C. Both a and b
D. Malachite green

Ans. C.

271. Syphilis is caused by

A. Staphylococcus aureus
B. Yersinia pestis
C. Treponema pallidum
D. Streptococcus syphilitic

Ans. C.

272. Disease that affects many people at different countries is termed as

A. Sporadic
B. Pandemic
C. Epidemic
D. Endemic

Ans. B.

273. The minimum number of bacteria required to produce clinical evidence of death in a susceptible animal under standard condition is called

A. LD50
B. ID
C. MLD
D. All of these

Ans. C.

274. Botulinum toxin is a———.

A. Protein
B. Lipid
C. Sugar
D. Nucleic acid

Ans. A.

275. Tear drops are rich in ———

A. Amylase
B. Phosphatase
C. Lysozyme
D. Protease

Ans. C.

276. Microbes which are capable of growing over a wide range of temperature are called

A. Stenothermal
B. Thermotolerant
C. Thermophilic
D. Eurythermal

Ans. D.

277. Fragmentation of filamentous cyanobacteria generates small filaments called — that help in reproduction.

A. Trichomes
B. Hormogonia
C. Hetercysts
D. Akinetes

Ans. C.

278. Hopanoids in prokaryotes are the equivalents of ———— in eukaryotes

A. Steroids
B. Hormones
C. Antibiotics
D. Cholesterol

Ans. D.

279. Carbohydrates binding proteins are called ————.

A. Glycoproteins
B. Lectins
C. Alexins
D. Polysaccharide-proteins

Ans. B.

280. Mucopeptide is a component of cell wall in ———.

A. Brown algae B. Green Algae

C. Green Algae D. Blue Green Algae

Ans. D.

281. TB is the most common infectious cause of death worldwide surpassing both HIV and malaria (True/False).

Ans. True.

282. Which day is celebrated as 'World TB day' ?

Ans. 24th March.

283. ———(nos) of cases of MDR TB occur every year in the world.

Ans. 0.5 million.

284. 25% of the global multidrug resistant TB (MDR-TB) cases are reported in the European region particularly from the former Soviet Union countries (True/False).

Ans. True.

285. Prisons are hotspots for TB transmission (True/False).

Ans. True.

286. M. africanum is found primarily in West Africa and seems to progress less frequently to clinical disease and show lower transmissibility(True/False).

Ans. True.

287. Increased CMI to CMV and EBV antigens at the time of diagnosis of pulmonary TB were associated with increased survival after a standard 6 months anti-TB therapy(True/False).

Ans. True.

288. BCG is also used as immunotherapy in selected cases of bladder cancer(True/False).

Ans. True.

289. What is the full form of MDR-TB and XDR –TB ?

Ans. Multidrug resistant and Extensively drug resistant.

290. The co-infection with HIV greatly increases mortality and risk of treatment failure of TB(True/False).

Ans. True.

291. Diabetes mellitus (DM) increases the risk of developing TB by 2-3 fold and TB treatment failure, relapse and death(True/False).

Ans. True.

292. Yeast and mould count determination requires-

A. Nutrient agar
B. Acidified potato glucose agar
C. MacConkey agar
D. Violet Red Bile agar

Ans. B.

293. The time temperature combination for HTST Paterurization of 71.1°C for 15 sec is selected on the basis of

A. Coxiella Burnetii
B. E. coli
C. B. subtilis
D. Cl. botulinum

Ans. A.

294. Aerobic Colony Count (ACC), is also known as

A. Total viable count (TVC)
B. Aerobic plate count (APC)
C. Standard plate count (SPC)
D. All of these

Ans. D.

295. Which bacteria contain reverse transcriptase ?

Ans. E. coli and Myxobacteria.

296. Which of the following is used for the proper maintenance and preservation of pure cultures?

A. Periodic transfer to fresh media
B. Preservation by overlaying cultures with mineral oil
C. Preservation by lyophilization
D. All of the above

Ans. D.

297. The solidifying agent commonly used in preparation of media is/are

A. agar
B. silica gel
C. both (a) and (b)
D. none of these

Ans. C.

298. The identification of bacteria by serologic tests is based on the presence of specific antigens. Which of the following bacterial components is least likely to contain useful antigens?

A. Ribosomes
B. Cell wall
C. Capsule
D. Flagella

Ans. D.

299. Each of the following statements concerning the Gram stain is correct except
   A. Escherichia coli stains pink because it has a thin peptidoglycan layer
   B. Streptococcus pyogenes stains blue because it has a thick peptidoglycan layer
   C. Mycoplasma pneumoniae is not visible in the Gram's stain because it does not have a cell wall
   D. Mycobacterium tuberculosis stains blue because it has a thick lipid layer

Ans. D.

300. An outbreak of sepsis caused by Staphylococcus aureus has occurred in the newborn nursery. You are called upon to investigate. According to your knowledge of the normal flora, what is the most likely source of the organism?
   A. Nose
   B. Colon
   C. Vagina
   D. Throat

Ans. A.

301. Each of the following organisms is an important cause of urinary tract infections except:
   A. Klebsiella pneumoniae
   B. Escherichia coli
   C. Bacteriodes fragilis
   D. Proteus mirabilis

Ans. C.

302. A 30 year old woman has non bloody diarrhoea for the past 14 hours. Which one of the following organisms is least likely to cause this illness?
   A. Streptococcus pyogenes
   B. Clostridium difficile
   C. Shigella dysenteriae
   D. Salmonella enteritidis

Ans. A.

303. Each of the following agents is a recognized cause of diarrhoea except
   A. Clostridium perfringens
   B. Vibrio cholerae
   C. Enterococcus faecalis
   D. Escherichia coli

Ans. C.

304. Each of the following statements about the classification of streptococci is correct except
   A. Pneumococci (Streptococcus pneumoniae) are alpha-hemolytic and can be serotyped on the basis of their polysaccharide capsule
   B. Enterococci are group D streptococci and can be classified by their ability to grow 6.5% sodium chloride
   C. Viridans streptococci are identified by Lancefield grouping, which is based on the carbohydrate in the cell wall
   D. Although pneumococci and the viridans streptococci are alpha-hemolytic, they can be differentiated by the bile solubility test and their susceptibility to optochin

Ans. C.

305. Which of the following bacteria has the lowest 50% infective dose (ID50)?
A. Campylobacter jejuni
B. Salmonella typhi
C. Vibrio cholerae
D. Shigella sonnei

Ans. D.

306. Which of the following disease is best diagnosed by serologic means?
A. Pulmonary tuberculosis
B. Gonorrhoea
C. Actinomycosis
D. Q Fever

Ans. D.

307. The coagulase test is used to differentiate
A. Staphylococcus epidermidis from Neisseria meningitidis
B. Staphylococcus aureus from Staphylococcus epidermidis
C. Streptococcus pyogenes from Staphylococcus aureus
D. Streptococcus pyogenes from Enterococcus faecalis

Ans. B.

308. Which one is true for acid fast bacteria
A. Cell walls with mycolic acid
B. Exotoxin production
C. Skin infection that can lead to septicaemia
D. Diseases that comes in stages
E. Diarrhoea of varying degrees

Ans. A.

309. A rancher that has processed deer skin comes down with an eschar on his forearm. This could be
A. Tetanus
B. Listeriosis
C. Cutaneous anthrax
D. Tattoo

Ans. C.

310. Most fungi reproduce asexually to form haploid
A. Hypae
B. Spores
C. Asci
D. Basidia

Ans. B.

311. Typhoid fever affect the systems except
A. Respiratory
B. Urogenital
C. Gastrointestinal
D. Skin
E. Muscle

Ans. D.

312. The fungus candida causes
   A. vaginal yeast infections
   B. Thrash of the mouth
   C. Infection in Canadians
   D. A & B.

Ans. D.

313. What types of foods are associated with the diarrheal form of bacillus food poisoning?
   A. Starchy
   B. Meat
   C. Veggies
   D. Candy

Ans. B.

314. What age group is at most risk for legionellosis ?
   A. Young
   B. Teenagers
   C. Adults
   D. Old folks

Ans. D.

315. Pneumonia is simply
   A. A disease affecting the very young and the elderly
   B. Fluid in the lungs
   C. Caused by a wide variety of organisms
   D. All of the above
   E. B & C only

Ans. D.

316. Why are pseudomonas infection is difficult to treat and prevent ?
   A. The bacteria is highly resistant to detergents and antibiotics
   B. Metabolically versatile
   C. It is found everywhere
   D. Causes nosocomial infections

Ans. B.

317. A complication of Campylobacter jejuni infection is
   A. Ulcerative peritonitis
   B. Toxic megacolon
   C. Guillain-Barre syndrome
   D. All of the above

Ans. C.

318. The total magnification of a microscope is equal to
   A. The magnification of the objective lens x the number of eye piece
   B. The magnification of the objective x the magnification of the ocular
   C. The total of all the objectives
   D. The price of the microscope
   E. None of the above

Ans. B.

319. What percentage of population on the planet are infected with M. tuberculosis?

A. 10% B. 20%

C. 30% D. 50%

Ans. C.

320. Why is treatment of TB so difficult ?

A. Long time period of treatment

B. Drugs are expensive

C. MDR : TB is not treatable

D. Drugs have serious side effects that prevent many from completing treatment

Ans. A.

321. What is one of the biggest problems in preventing the spread gonorrhoeal and Chlamydia ?

A. People hate condoms

B. It is mainly spread by young irresponsible teenagers

C. Asymptomatic people do not realize they have it

D. Highly antibiotic resistant

Ans. C.

322. Gonorrhoea still a problem among teens in the form of

A. Outbreak B. Epidemic

C. Endemic D. Pandemic

Ans. C.

323. Which system is affected in Gonorrhoea ?

A. Respiratory B. Urogenital

C. Nervous, Fever, Eyes D. Gastrointestinal

E. Skin

Ans. C.

324. A man walks into a clinic and is complaining of an ulcerated lesion on his penis. It is painless and appears to be healing on its own. Which of the following would probably be the cause ?

A. Chancroid B. Syphilis

C. Gonorrhoea D. Chlamydia

Ans. B.

325. The diploid form of fungi is referred to as a zygospore.

A. True B. False

Ans. True.

326. In thioglycollate broth, a bacteria that are strictly anaerobic will grow

A. Throughout the medium B. Only at the top

C. Only at the bottom D. Only in the middle

Ans. C.

327. An experiment began with 4 cells and ended with 128 cells. How many generations did the cells go through

A. 64 B. 32

C. 6 D. 5

Ans. C.

328. What are some of the problems associated with BCG vaccine ?

A. Not very effective B. Results in positive skin test

C. Very expensive D. All of the above

E. A & B.

Ans. E.

329. Which of the following takes a bigger ID (infective dose) to cause illness ?

A. Salmonella enterica B. Salmonella typhi

Ans. A.

330. A patient comes to the doctor's office vomiting and very ill. She says that she had not eaten anything until about 2 hours ago she had leftover macaroni and cheese at her grandmother's house. What is she probably sick with ?

A. Gastrointestinal anthrax

B. Emetic form of bacillus food poisoning

C. S. aureus food poisoning

D. Something else

Ans. B.

331. One characteristic of fungal respiratory infections include all except which of the following ?

A. Moist, wet condition B. Presence of faecal material

C. Dry dusty soil D. Animals

Ans. B.

332. Which treatment is used for staphylococcal pneumonia ?
A. Supportive
B. Penicillin
C. Vancomycin
D. A &C

Ans. D.

333. One characteristic of typhoid fever is that after people become infected they
A. Recover completely
B. Feel fine but become carriers
C. Have S. typhi colonize their GI tract
D. All of the above

Ans. D.

334. E. coli 015:H7 is associated with
A. Respiratory
B. Urogenital
C. Nervous, fever, eyes
D. Gastrointestinal
E. Skin
F. Muscle

Ans. D.

335. Gas gangrene is a result of type 2 exotoxin. Which of the following describes this class of toxins ?
A. They are 2 part toxins
B. They are the outer LPS layer of Gm – bacteria
C. The cause of major overreactions of immune system
D. They damage cell membranes

Ans. D.

336. Most fungi grows best with oxygen at room temeprature and under — conditions.
A. Slightly acidic
B. Slightly basic
C. Neutral pH
D. Dark

Ans. A.

337. Which one of the following is a photosynthetic eukarya?
A. Fungus
B. Protozoa
C. Bacteria
D. Algae
E. Virus

Ans. D.

338. Anthrax is dose dependent. What does it mean ?
A. Different numbers of spores are needed for different portals of entry
B. To cure it requires different doses of ciprofloxacin
C. Differnt people require different doses to get infected
D. None of the above

Ans. A.

339. A major difference between EHEC and EPEC is

A. EHEC secretes a Shiga-like toxin and EPEC does not

B. EHEC possesses a type III secretion system and EPEC does not

C. EPEC rearranges host cell actin and EHEC does not

D. EPEC passes through the placenta to infect the fetus and EHEC does not

Ans. A.

340. Which of the following is true regarding anthrax?

A. Anthrax is caused by a virus

B. Anthrax is highly contagious

C. Inhalation anthrax and cutaneous anthrax are caused by separate strains of Bacillus anthracis

D. Inhalation Anthrax requires infection with a large number of spores

Ans. D.

341. The toxins produced by bacteria

A. Kill viruses

B. Encourage bacterial reproduction

C. Interfere with physiological processes in the body

D. All of the above

Ans. C.

342. Pseudomembraneous colitis is

A. Precipitated by the use of certain antibiotics

B. Caused by a gram-positive bacterium

C. Caused by a spore-forming bacterium

D. All of the above

Ans. D.

343. Both Mycobacterium tuberculosis and Streptococcus pneumonia

A. Are acquired by inhalation

B. Have cell walls that contain a high content of mycolic acids

C. Have polysaccharide capsules

D. Stay in the lung and rarely, if ever, enter the bloodstream

Ans. A.

344. Cholera toxin is an A-B type toxin in which the B portions bind to a receptor on a host cell and the A portion enters the cell to cause

A. ADP ribosylation of adenylate cyclase that stops production of cAMP

B. ADP ribosylation of a G protein that locks it into an active form that stimulates adenylate cyclase to make cAMP

C. cleavage of rRNA that results in disruption of ribosome function

D. ADP ribosylation of guanylate cyclase that stimulates production of cGMP

Ans. B.

345. Type III secretion systems are used to inject "effector" proteins directly into a host cell. Salmonella uses a type III secretion system to help the pathogen to

A. Survive the acid pH of the stomach

B. Secrete LT (heat labile toxin) and ST (heat stable toxin) into the lumen of the intestine

C. Secrete LT (heat labile toxin) and ST (heat stable toxin) into the lumen of the intestine

D. Activate T cells to proliferate and secrete cytokines

Ans. C.

346. The "A" subunit of diphtheria toxin

A. Binds host cell receptors found on heart cells

B. Cause ADP ribosylation of a factor involved in protein synthesis

C. Forms cAMP that leads to fluid accumulation

D. Lysis macrophages with the release of cytokines

Ans. B.

347. Prontosil is

A. An effective antibacterial when used in animals

B. An effective antibacterial when used in in-vitro cultures

C. An effective antibacterial both in animals as well as in in-vitro cultures

D. Not used as an antibacterial agent

Ans. C.

348. Immunization with which of the following toxoid induces high titer serum antibody, but does not protect from the corresponding disease?

A. Tetanus B. Botulism

C. Diphtheria D. Shigellosis

Ans. B.

349. Which of the following statements is not true regarding Mycobacterium tuberculosis and/or the disease it causes?

A. The pathogen contains mycolic acid in its cell wall

B. The pathogen can live inside macrophages

C. Antibodies to the pathogen are protective

D. None of these

Ans. C.

350. Which of the following can be identified by milk ring test?

A. Brucellosis B. Salmonellosis

C. Bovine tuberculosis D. All of these

Ans. A.

351. For brucellosis, 2 ME agglutination test is used to identify

A. IgG B. IgM

C. IgA D. IgE

Ans. A.

352. Human transmission of Brucellae occurs by

A. Ingestion of contaminated meat B. Direct contact with animal tissues

C. Ingestion of infected milk D. All of these

Ans. D.

353. Agglutination test for Brucella mainly identifies which class of antibodies?

A. IgG B. IgM

C. IgA D. IgE

Ans. B.

354. The most pathogenic Brucella spp for man is

A. B. melitensis B. B. abortus

C. B. suis D. B. canis

Ans. A.

355. Mycoplasmas are different from the other prokaryotes by

A. Presence of chitin in cell walls B. Presence of murrain in cell walls

C. Presence of proteins in cell walls D. Absence of cell wall itself

Ans. D.

356. Mycoplasmas, rickettsiae and chlamydiae are

A. Types of fungi B. Small bacteria

C. Species of protozoa D. Forms of viruses

Ans. B.

357. A characteristic of protein synthesis in both the archaea and eukarya is
   A. Transcription and translation are coupled
   B. Translation is inhibited by diphtheria toxin
   C. Proteins are synthesized from D-, rather than L-, isomers of amino acids
   D. The initiator tRNA is charged with N-formyl-methionine

Ans. C.

358. The membranes of which domains are chemically the most similar?
   A. Archaea and Bacteria
   B. Bacteria and Eukarya
   C. Eukarya and Archaea
   D. Membranes of all three domains are chemically identical

Ans. B.

359. Primary differences between cilia and flagella are
   A. Arrangement of microtubules
   B. Length and location of basal bodies
   C. How the microtubules are fused to each other
   D. Number, length and direction of force

Ans. D.

360. All membranes of free-living organisms have phospholipid bilayers, but exception is
   A. Bacteria B. Fungi
   C. Archaea D. Protozoa

Ans. C.

361. All of the following are features of prokaryotes except
   A. Nitrogen fixation B. Photosynthesis
   C. Sexual reproduction D. Locomotion

Ans. C.

362. Which of the following is/are included in Kingdom Prokaryotae?
   A. Bacteria B. Protozoa
   C. Fungi D. All of these

Ans. A.

363. What are Blue-Green bacteria called?
   A. Acquaobacteria B. Cyanobacteria
   C. Protozoa D. None of the above

Ans. B.

364. Which of the following is common in the disease caused by Corynebacterium diphtheriae and Bacillus anthracis?

A. Both organisms are gram-positive spore formers

B. Diphtheria toxin and edema toxin are ADP ribosylating toxins

C. The most serious disease symptoms are the direct result of toxin action

D. Both organisms cause skin and respiratory tract infections

Ans. C.

365. Which of the following disease is not caused by microbial protein toxin ?

A. Botulism B. Diphtheria

C. Shigella dysentery D. Tuberculosis

Ans. D.

366. In the human disease cholera, what is it that actually ends up killing the victim?

A. Faulty carrier proteins

B. Dehydration and loss of nutrients

C. Too little water in the food stream

D. the toxin produced by the bacterium

Ans. B.

367. Each of the 3 virulence factors of Bacillus anthracis i.e. the capsule, edema toxin and lethal toxin can affect the activity of

A. B cells B. Macrophages

C. Ciliated epithelial cells D. M cells

Ans. B.

368. Grinding and mixing of foods such as sausage and hamburger

A. Increase the food surface area

B. Alter cellular structure

C. Distribute contaminating microorganisms throughout the food

D. All of the above

E. None of the above

Ans. D.

369. Which is not true about aflatoxins?

A. Cause frameshift mutations B. Are carcinogenic

C. Are alkaloids D. Fluoresce

E. Have been found in beer

Ans. C.

370. There is an increased sensitivity to aflatoxins in individuals previously infected with

A. Hepatitis B
B. Measles
C. Mumps
D. Chickenpox
E. Rabies

Ans. A.

371. Complex algal toxins, most of which are temperature stable, are known to cause peripheral neurological system effects, often in less than ———- after ingestion

A. 1 hour
B. 2 hours
C. 3 hours
D. 4 hours
E. 5 hours

Ans. A.

372. Louis Pasteur established the modern era of food microbiology in 1857 when he showed that microorganisms cause——— spoilage.

A. Beer
B. Wine
C. Juice
D. Milk
E. Grain

Ans. D.

373. Several major brands of beer are ——- rather than pasteurized to better preserve the flavor and aroma of the original product

A. Centrifuged
B. Precipitated
C. Filtered
D. Heat Treated
E. All of the above

Ans. E.

374. Which of the following terms describes organisms that thrive in the cold?

A. Mesophiles
B. Thermophiles
C. Psychrophiles
D. Aerophiles
E. Basophiles

Ans. C.

375. Which is not true of the bacterium produced by Streptococcus lactis?

A. A small hydrophobic protein
B. Nontoxic to humans
C. Affects mainly Gram-negative bacteria
D. Improves inactivation of C. botulinum during the canning process
E. Inhibits germination of any surviving C. botulinum spores

Ans. C.

376. E. coli O157:H7 is thought to have acquired enterohemorrhagic genes from

A. Clostridium B. Bacillus

C. Campylobacter D. Shigella

E. Listeria

Ans. D.

377. The main reservoir of Staphylococcus aureus is

A. Human faeces B. Human nasal cavity

C. Human R.B.C. D. All of the above

E. None of the above

Ans. B.

378. Which type of fermentation is used to produce yogurt?

A. Mesophilic B. Thermophilic

C. Therapeutic D. Yeast-lactic fermentations

E. Mold-lactic fermentations

Ans. B.

379. Which of the following fungi is most likely to be found within reticuloendothelial cells.

A. Histoplasma capsulatum B. Sporothrix schenckii

C. Cryptococcus neoformans D. Candida albicans

Ans. A.

380. Aspergillosis is recognized in tissue by the presence of

A. Metachromatic granules B. Psuedohyphae

C. Septate hyphae D. Budding cells

Ans. C.

381. Fungi often colonize lesions due to other causes. Which of the following is least likely to be present as colonizer

A. Candida B. Sporothrix

C. Mucor D. Aspergillus

Ans. B.

382. A girl who pricked her finger while pruning some rose bushes develops a local pustule that progresses to an ulcer. Several nodules then develop along the local lymphatic drainage. The most likely agent is

A. Aspergillus fumigatus B. Sporothrix schenckii

C. Cryptococcus neoformans D. Candida albicans

Ans. B.

383. Immunocompromised persons are suffered from several fungal diseases. Which of the following is the least frequently associated

A. Cryptococcus neoformans B. Aspergillus fumigatus
C. Malassezia furfur D. Mucor species

Ans. C.

384. Each of the following statements concerning Cryptococcus neoformans are correct except

A. Its natural habitat is the soil, especially associated with pigeon faeces
B. Budding yeasts are found in the lesions
C. The initial site of infection is usually the lung
D. Pathogenesis is related primarily to the production of exotoxin A.

Ans. D.

385. Fungal cells that reproduce by budding are seen in the infected tissues of patients with

A. Candidiasis, cryptococcosis, and sporotrichosis
B. Mycetoma, candidiasis and mucormycosis
C. Tinea corporis, tinea unguium, and tinea versicolor
D. Sporotrichosis, mycetoma and aspergillosis

Ans. A.

386. Which of the following is not the characteristics of histoplasmosis

A. Person to person transmission B. Specific geographic distribution
C. Yeasts in tissue D. mycelial phase in the soil

Ans. A.

387. Infection with dermatophyte is most often associated with

A. Intravenous drug abuse
B. Inhalation of the organism from contaminated bird faeces
C. Adherence of the organism to perspiration moist skin
D. Faecal oral transmission

Ans. C.

388. Each of the following statements concerning Candida albicans is correct except

A. C. albicans is a budding yeast that forms psuedohyphae when it invades tissue
B. C. albicans causes thrush
C. C. albicans is transmitted primarily by respiratory aerosol
D. Impaired cell mediated immunity is an important predisposing factor to disease

Ans. C.

389. The most commonly encountered bacteria are roughly spherical. The microbiological term describing this shape is

A. Coccus
B. Bacillus
C. Pleomorphic

Ans. A.

390. Another common bacterial shape is that of a rod, often called

A. Coccus
B. Bacillus
C. Pleomorphic

Ans. B.

391. What is a plasmid ?

A. Self-replicating segment of double stranded DNA
B. Self-replicating segment of single stranded RNA
C. A bacterial chromosome

Ans. A.

392. Plasmids are important to the genetics of many bacteria. This is because

A. They are inherited from one generation to the next
B. They may carry genes that give their host a selective advantage
C. They can render bacteria drug-resistant
D. All of the above

Ans. D.

393. Bacteria do not always swim aimlessly but are attracted by such nutrients such as sugar and amino acids, and are repelled by harmful substances and bacterial waste products. Movement toward chemical attractants and away from repellents is called

A. Gliding motility
B. Tumbling
C. Chemotaxis

Ans. C.

394. Some bacteria are considered pleomorphic. This means

A. They are shaped like bent rods
B. They have a corkscrew shape
C. They do not have just shape
D. They are not either bacilli or cocci

Ans. C.

395. Poly-beta-hydroxybutyrate inclusion bodies

A. Protect bacteria from excessive drying
B. Store carbon from energy and biosynthesis
C. Turn reddish brown when stained with iodine
D. Are composed of polymers of glucose

Ans. B.

396. Gas vesicles in bacteria
   A. Help move cells to optimal nutrient levels
   B. Store oxygen for growth anaerobically
   C. Are bounded by a lipid bilayer membrane
   D. Are bounded by a membrane impervious to gas

Ans. A.

397. Magnetostomes in bacteria
   A. Help cells attach to metal objects
   B. Help cells to magnetically attach to each other
   C. Help cells to float on the surface of fresh water ponds.
   D. Help cells to orient in the earth's magnetic field

Ans. D.

398. The 70S prokaryotic ribosomes consist of
   A. Two 40S subunits
   B. A 50S and a 30S subunit
   C. A 40S and a 30S subunit
   D. A 50S and a 20S subunit

Ans. B.

399. Gram positive cells
   A. Have a second, outer membrane that helps retain the crystal violet stain
   B. Have multiple layers of peptidoglycan that help retain the crystal violet stain.
   C. Have a thick capsule that traps the crystal violet stain
   D. Have a periplasmic space that traps the crystal violet

Ans. B.

400. The presence of D-amino acids in the cross links of the peptidoglycan layer is most likely because
   A. Most peptidases can only cleave L-amino acids
   B. D- amino acids fit the structural constraints of the cell wall better than L amino acids.
   C. Most L-amino acids have already been used for protein synthesis
   D. D-amino acids are easier to crosslink in the absence of ribosomes

Ans. A.

401. The third amino acid in the peptidoglycan cross linking chain is either diaminopimilic acid or lysine because this amino acid must
   A. Be positively charged for a salt bridge to form
   B. Be hydrophilic
   C. Have a free amino group for peptide bond formation
   D. Have a large R-side chain to fill space in the cell wall

Ans. C.

402. Gram positive cells
   A. Have thick, homogeneous cell walls
   B. Have large amounts of teichoic acids
   C. Do not have an outer membrane
   D. All of the above

Ans. D.

403. The outer membrane of Gram negative cells is more permeable than the plasma membrane because
   A. LPS is larger than most membrane phospholipids
   B. Lipoproteins stretch the outer membrane
   C. Porin proteins establish holes in the outer membrane
   D. The core polysaccharide spans the lipid bilayer

Ans. C.

404. The most important role of the prokaryotic cell wall is to
   A. Maintain the shape of the cell
   B. Protect the cell from osmotic pressures
   C. Prevent ions from diffusing away from the cell
   D. Block the effects of antibiotics like penicillin

Ans. B.

405. Which of the following is not true about capsules and slime layers ?
   A. They consist of secreted material lying outside of the bacterial cell wall
   B. They can prevent desiccation of bacteria cells
   C. They are required for bacteria to grow normally in culture
   D. They help bacteria resist phagocytosis by macrophages

Ans. C.

406. Fimbriae
   A. Attach bacteria to various surfaces
   B. Cause bacteria more through fluids
   C. Sense changes in nutrient concentration
   D. Are pathways for the secretion of exoenzymes

Ans. A.

407. A bacillus bacterium with a single flagellum at each end is described as
   A. Monotrichous   B. Amphitrichous
   C. Lophotrichous   D. Peritrichous

Ans. B.

408. Which of the following is not true about bacterial flagella ?
   A. Most of their length consists of a hollow, rigid protein tube
   B. They are constructed largely of a single protein called flagellin
   C. They spin like wheels, either clockwise or counter clockwise
   D. They use cytoplasmic ATP as their primary energy source

Ans. D.

409. The flagellar filament grows by
   A. Enzymatic addition of subunits to the tip of the flagellum.
   B. Enzymatic addition of subunits to the base of the flagellum
   C. Self-assembly of subunits travelling through the hollow flagellum to the tip
   D. Self-insertion of subunits along the length of the filament

Ans. C.

410. How does a bacterium control the direction of swimming ?
   A. The length of the flagellum acts as a rudder to steer the bacterium
   B. The speed of rotation is faster when the bacterium is headed the correct way
   C. The bacterium can stop and spin until it is pointed the correct way
   D. The bacterium does not control the direction of its swimming

Ans. D.

411. The methyl-accepting chemotaxis proteins of bacteria
   A. Are directly connected to the flagellar motor to guide the bacterium
   B. Can only sense conditions that are favourable for bacterial growth
   C. Integrate multiple signals through a two components phosphor-relay system
   D. Tell the bacterium which way to go

Ans. C.

412. Bacteria accomplish chemotaxis by
   A. Steering toward better growth conditions
   B. Making long, uninterrupted runs when conditions are good
   C. Frequently stopping and tumbling to better sense good conditions
   D. Stopping movement when conditions are good

Ans. B.

413. What is the purpose of bacterial endospores?
   A. Allow the bacterium to make hundreds of "seeds" to spread on the wind
   B. Help the bacterium to differentiate into faster growing stages of bacteria
   C. Allow the bacterium to survive the absence of oxygen
   D. Allow the bacterium to survive extended periods of heat or dryness

Ans. D.

414. The Gram stain is used to classify cells based on differences in their ———.

A. Cell membrane B. Cytoplasm

C. Nucleus D. Cell wall

Ans. D.

415. A small ring of DNA independent from the bacterium's main genome that can be taken in and expressed by bacteria is –

A. Plasmid B. RNA

C. Mini-DNA D. Ribosome

Ans. A.

416. LPS is an endotoxin that is found on the outer membrane of Gram negative bacteria. LPS stands for ——.

A. Leading poison strand B. Lipopolysaccharide

C. Lactepeptosucrose D. Lagging poison strand

Ans. B.

417. One genus of bacteria that can be found in the bottom, black layer of a Winogradsky column is ———

A. Desulfovibrio B. Beggiatoa

C. Cyanobacteria D. Rhodobium

Ans. A.

418. Which of these is used as a mordant in the Gram stain ?

A. Safranin B. Alcohol

C. Iodine D. Crystal violet

Ans. C.

419. Which of these is not in the domain bacteria ?

A. Cyanobacteria B. Proteobacteria

C. Bacteroides D. Methanobacterium

Ans. D.

420. The genus Mycoplasma is resistant to the effects of ———.

A. Triclosan B. Sulfanomides

C. Streptomycin D. Penicillin

Ans. D.

421. Which type of plasmid, when taken up by bacteria, confers the ability to create a sex pilus ?

A. R-plasmid B. S-plasmid

C. Col-plasmid D. F-plasmid

Ans. D.

422. Which is least likely to kill bacteria ?

A. Extreme cold
B. Extreme acidity
C. Extreme heat
D. Extreme alkalinity

Ans. A.

423. Spirulina is a

A. Edible fungus
B. Bofertilizer
C. Biopesticide
D. Single cell protein

Ans. D.

424. Who showed that S. cerevisiae causes fermentation forming products such as beer and buttermilk ?

A. L. Pasteur
B. A. Fleming
C. Selman Waksman
D. Schatz

Ans. A.

425. Name the first organic acid produced by microbial fermentation

A. Citric acid
B. Lactic acid
C. Acetic acid
D. None of the above

Ans. B.

426. Vinegar is obtained from molasses with the help of———.

A. Rhizopus
B. Acetobacter
C. Yeast
D. Both B and C

Ans. D.

427. Agar Agar is obtained from ————.

A. Gelidium
B. Polysiphonia
C. Fucus
D. Laminaria

Ans. A.

428. Which are the most primitive group of algae ?

A. Blue green algae
B. Red algae
C. Brown algae
D. Green algae

Ans. C.

429. Which of the following is the most advanced group of algae ?

A. Cyanophyta
B. Rhodophyta
C. Phaeophyta
D. Chlorophyta

Ans. B.

430. Which algae is responsible for the red colour in the red sea ?

A. Chlamydomonas brauii B. Trichodesmium erythrium

C. Ulothrix zonata D. None of the above

Ans. B.

431. One of the following is present in blue green algae

A. Starch B. Cyanophacean granule

C. Any polysaccharide D. Floridian starch

Ans. B.

432. Ability to fix atmospheric nitrogen is found in ———.

A. Leaves of some crop plants B. Chlorella

C. Some marine red algae D. Some blue green algae

Ans. D.

433. Origin and evolution of sex in algae is best seen in ———.

A. Blue green algae B. Red algae

C. Brown algae D. Green algae

Ans. D.

434. In endospore staining which one is used ?

A. Basic Fuschin B. Indian ink

C. Methylene blue D. Malachite green

Ans. D.

435. Species of Mycoplasma is inhibited by

A. Penicillum B. Tetramycin

C. Both A and B D. None

Ans. B.

436. Actinomyces are

A. Gram negative aerobic B. Gram negative anaerobic

C. Gram positive anaerobic D. Gram positive aerobic

Ans. D.

437. Funaric acid is produced by

A. Aspergillus terrus B. Aspergillus niger

C. Aspergillus fumigatus D. Rhizopus nigricans

Ans. D.

438. Urea degrading bacteria

A. Bacillus pasturi

B. Aspergillus niger

C. Micrococcus sp.

D. Cl. Pasteurianum

Ans. A.

439. Fungi used for bioassay of pantothenic acid

A. Yeast

B. Neurospora

C. Aspergillus

D. Mucor

Ans. A.

440. Mesophillic bacteria involved in composting

i. Bacillus

ii. Cellulomonas

iii. Clostridium

iv. Myxococcus

A. 1, 3

B. 2, 4

C. 1, 4

D. All

Ans. B.

441. Murein is present in

A. Cyanobacteria

B. Methanobacterium

C. Halobacterium

D. None

Ans. A.

442. A diagnosis of diphtheria is confirmed by

A. Microscopic appearance of organisms stained by methylene blue

B. Isolation of a typical colony on tinsdale's agar

C. Isolation of typical organisms from materials such as blood showing invasiveness

D. Detection of beta phage plaques in cultures of suspicious isolates

E. Demonstration of toxin production by a suspicious isolate

Ans. E.

443. L. monocytogens shows which of the following characteristics ?

A. It can grow at refrigeration temperatures (4°C)

B. It is an extracellular pathogen

C. It is catalase negative

D. It is a gram negative coccus

E. It is strictly a human pathogen

Ans. A.

444. Which one of the following is characteristic of N. meningitidis but not N. gonorrhoeae

A. Ferments glucose

B. Contains a polysaccharide capsule

C. Is oxidase positive

D. Most isolates show resistance to penicillin

E. No effective vaccines are available

Ans. B. N. meningitides contains a polysaccharide capsule whereas N. gonorrhoeae does not. N. meningitides ferments both glucose and maltose but N. gonorrhoeae metabolizes only glucose. Most isolates of N. meningitides remain sensitive to penicillin, although resistance is increasing. Effective vaccines exist for N. meningitides serogroups A, C, W-135 and Y but not for N. gonrrhoeae.

445. Which of the following is true of H. Influenza ?

A. Invasive infections are most commonly associated with encapsulated strains

B. Mos invasive infections occur in infants during the neonatal period

C. Most human infections are acquired from domestic pets

D. The organisms can be readily cultured on sheep blood agar in an environment of elevated CO2

E. Older adults are rarely at risk for infection with this organism because they typically have a high level of immunity

Ans. A.

446. Which of the following organisms do not have any animal reservoir ?

A. Francisella tularensis

B. P. multocida

C. Bordetella pertussis

D. Brucella melitensis

E. Yersinia pestis

Ans. C.

447. A distinguishing feature of human mycoplasma species is that they

A. Stain well with giemsa but not by gram stain

B. Contain no bacterial peptidoglycan

C. Are not immunogenic because they mimic the host cell membrane components

D. Can not be cultivated in vitro

E. Are dependent on host source of ATP

Ans. B.

448. Which one of the following is most characteristic of Mycoplasma pneumoniae infection ?

A. Infection results in a fever of sudden onset accompanied by a productive cough

B. Infection most commonly occurs in the URT

C. Infection is definitely diagnosed by direct microscopic examination of sputum

D. Reinfection is rare and less severe than primary infection

E. Infection causes extensive scarring and calcification of affected lung tissue

Ans. B.

449. Which of the following describes both Chlamydia and Rickettsia ?

A. Motile
B. Gram positive
C. Obligate extracellular pathogens
D. Biphasic morphology

Ans. D.

450. Which of the following describes the membranes and cell wall of Chlamydia ?

A. Contain murein
B. Contain mycolic acid
C. Has LPS
D. No cytoplasmic membrane

Ans. C.

451. Which of the following bacteria are auxotropic and need ATP and amino acids from their host

A. Rickettsia
B. Chlamydia
C. Mycoplasma
D. A & B

Ans. D.

452. Lymphogranuloma venereum can be described as which of the following

A. A variant of the rickettsia bacteria

B. May be present with N. gonorrhoea infection

C. Occurs in children and may lead to blindness

D. Common cause of pneumonia

Ans. B.

453. Trachoma, an ocular disease affecting children and a possible cause of blindness is linked to which of the following bacteria?

A. Rickettsia
B. Neisseria
C. Chlamydia
D. Clostridium

Ans. C.

454. A patient presents with coronary artery disease. Which of the following findings may be expected?

A. Previous rickettsial infection B. C. trachomatis infection

C. M. tuberculosis infection D. Previous C. pneumoniae infection

Ans. D.

455. Which of the following similarities exist between Rickettsia and Chlamydia

A. Have a 2-form developmental cycle

B. Spread by arthropod vectors

C. Affect blood vessels

D. Murein in cell walls

Ans. C.

456. Which of the following describes an Elementary body?

A. Developmental form of Rickettsia

B. Noninfectious and found intracellularly in respiratory and GI mucosa

C. Metabolically active and does not attach to epithelium

D. Forms fused inclusions except forC. pneumonia

Ans. D.

457. Which of the following describes a reticulate body?

A. Developmental form of Rickettsia

B. Lives outside of inclusions by binding epithelial cells

C. Replicates by binary fission

D. Are infectious

Ans. C.

458. Chlamydia obtain nutrients through which of the following methods?

A. Straw like appendages similar to type III secretion system

B. Transform into elementary body and escape phagosome

C. Release siderophores and hydrilipases

D. None of the above

Ans. A.

459. Which of the following methods are used by the Chlamydia in persistence phase?

A. RBs are smaller and consume less nutrients

B. Produce protease to delay cell death

C. Intracellular invasion reduces inflammation

D. All of the above

Ans. B.

460. C. trachomatis damage is linked to which of the following?

A. Cell mediated host response to serovars

B. Bacterial release of protease that cause cell lysis

C. Reiter's syndrome in women

D. Serovars are immobile and no exudate is present

Ans. A.

461. Herpes like lesions are most likely due to which of the following

A. C. pneumoniae B. Rickettsia

C. LGV biovariant D. All of the above

Ans. C.

462. Which bacteria infects cells involved in atherogenesis?

A. C. trachomatis B. C. pneumoniae

C. Rickettsia D. Q fever

Ans. B.

463. Which of the following methods can sufficiently diagnose C. trachomatis ?

A. Direct fluorescent assay B. Culture from exudate

C. Nucleic amplification of urine D. A & C

E. All of the above

Ans. D.

464. C. Pneumoniae can be distinguished from M. pneumoniae because M. pneumoniae is positive for cold agglutinins

A. True B. False

Ans. A.

465. A patient with non-flulike symptoms reports to the hospital for C. pneumonia. After running routine tests you find out she is pregnant, What is the best drug therapy?

A. Azythromizin 7 days B. Doxycycline 7 days

C. Erythromycin D. 3 weeks of therapy

Ans. C.

466. After a host is inoculated by a tick bite, which of the following actions are taken by Rickettsia?

A. Disseminate via the lymphatic system

B. Avoid being engulfed by cells

C. Multiply in the lumen of the blood vessels

D. Attach to cell membrane of vascular endothelium

Ans. D.

467. Which of the following describes Rickettsia's ability to infect endothelial cells?

A. Release pore forming toxins
B. Type III secretion system
C. No cellular damage
D. Remain extracellularly

Ans. B.

468. Which of the following separates Rickettsia from Chlamydia ?

A. Affects the appearance of the skin
B. Multiply in phagosomes
C. Affects blood vessels
D. Can be cleared by strong host defence

Ans. D.

469. Patient presents with R. prowazekii infection. Which of the following disease may they develop?

A. Lyme disease
B. Typhus fever
C. Q fever
D. Rickettsia

Ans. B.

470. Which of the following does not need a living vector for transmission?

A. Typhus fever
B. Q fever
C. Ehrliciosis
D. Anaplasmosis

Ans. B.

471. Which of the following infects neutrophils ?

A. E. chaffeensis
B. E. ewingii
C. Anaplasma phagocytophilum
D. A & B
E. B & C

Ans. E.

472. Which of the following would rule out Q fever ?

A. Fever
B. Rash
C. Tick bite
D. High titers

Ans. B.

473. The drug of choice for Rickettsial infections is which of the following?

A. Tetracycline
B. Doxycycline
C. Fluoroquinolones
D. Trimethoprim

Ans. B.

474. Which of the following extracellular enzymes produced by Group A streptococci is called "spreading factor" an enzyme important in skin and soft tissue infection ?

A. Streptokinase
B. Hyaluronidase
C. M protein
D. DNase C
E. None of the above

Ans. D.

475. All of the statements are true about the M protein of Group A Streptococcus except

A. The amino terminal portion is variable accounting for more than 80 distinct serotypes
B. M protein allows streptococci to resists phagocytosis
C. antibodies to M protein confer type specific antibodies
D. M protein is the major virulence factor of Group A Streptococci
E. M protein is major constituents of capsule of Group A Streptococci

Ans. E.

476. Which of the following statements about Group B Streptococci (Strep. agalactiae) is not correct ?

A. They are important causes of toxic strep syndrome
B. They are frequent colonizers of female genital tract
C. Screening for this pathogen during pregnancy has reduced the incidence of neonatal sepsis
D. These organisms are beta haemolytic
E. These are important causes of urinary tract infections and bacteraemia in elderly and diabetic adults

Ans. A.

477. What is the O antigen of Enterobacteriaceae ?

A. Cell surface polysaccharide
B. A channel controlling substance taken into the organism
C. A flagellar protein
D. A peptidoglycan matrix important for cellular rigidity
E. Cell wall lipopolysaccharide

Ans. E.

478. All Enterobacteriaceae share all of the following characteristics except

A. Ferment glucose
B. reduces nitrates to nitrites
C. Oxidase positive
D. Gram negative
E. Rod shaped bacilli

Ans. C.

479. Which of the following virulence factors of E. coli is important for attachment to host epithelial cells in the pathogenesis of urinary tract infections ?

A. Aerobactin
B. Alpha hemolysis
C. Urease
D. K 1 antigen
E. Pili

Ans. E.

480. The urinary pathogen 'swarms' across agar surfaces and may cause bladder and renal calculi (stones).

A. Citrobacter freundii
B. Enterobacter aerogenes
C. Serratia marcescens
D. Klebsiella oxytoca
E. Proteus mirabilis

Ans. E.

481. Which of the following statements regarding Enterotoxigenic E. coli are correct ?

A. They are important causes of traveller's diarrhoea
B. Transmission occurs from ingestion of contaminated food and water
C. Disease is caused by production of one or both of two types of enterotoxins
D. None of the above are correct
E. All of the above are correct

Ans. E.

482. R factors

A. Are small plasmids which encode resistance to only one type of antibiotic
B. Contain plasmid elements (replication origins, incompatibility determinants etc) that were widespread in the preantibiotic era
C. Represent genetically engineered cloning vectors which have escaped into pathogenic bacteria
D. All of the above are correct

Ans. B.

483. Move of DNA from one bacteria to another through a tubular bridge or pilus

A. Conjugation
B. Transposition
C. Transfection
D. Transduction

Ans. A.

484. Which statement describing the potential advantages of DNA technologies over conventional culture based methods is not true ?

A. Greater stability of samples during transport

B. Potentially more sensitive detection

C. More complete and accurate determination of organism resistance to antibiotics

D. More rapid than culture

Ans. C.

485. The PCR

A. Has been adapted for accurate quantification of viruses

B. May yield false positive results when amplicons contaminate clinical samples

C. Offers detection sensitivity which often but not always exceed that of culture

D. All of the above

Ans. D.

486. Which of the following is not one of Koch's postulate ?

A. The organism is regularly found in lesions of the disease

B. The organism can be isolated from diseased tissues in pure culture on artificial media

C. Inoculation of this pure culture produces a similar disease in experimental animals

D. Treatment of the disease with a broad spectrum oral antimicrobial dependably eradicates the organism and cures the disease

Ans. D.

487. The diagnosis of septicaemia should be considered in patients who are at increased risk of blood strem infection (secondary to local disease such as urinary tract infection or pneumonia). All of the following are factors predisposing patients to septicaemia except

A. Underlying diseases that appear to compromise host defenses such as diabetes, lymphoma etc.

B. Patients with a polymorphonuclear leukocyte count less than 1000/mm3

C. Patients with a polymorphonuclear leukocyte count less than 10000-20000/mm3

D. Long term therapy with broad spectrum antimicrobials

Ans. C.

488. Physical findings and other factors that should suggest the presence of septicaemia in a particular patient are all of the following except

A. Shaking chills, spiking fevers

B. Conjunctivitis

C. Nausea, vomiting, diarrhoea

D. In elderly patients, decreased uring output or mental changes (confusion)

Ans. B.

489. A 45 year old woman who was complalining of shaking chills and fever went to the hospital. She has enlarged lymph nodes in the right axilla and there was an ulcer on the top of the patient's right hand. She told that she had been bitten by an insect resembling horse fly having yellow stripe on its abdomen. She denied any contact with rats or fleas. She was most likely suffering from :

A. Brucellosis

B. Ulceroglandular tularemia

C. Pneumonic plaque

D. Relapsing fever

Ans. B.

490. Which of the following diseases are not transmitted by ticks ?

A. Ulceroglandular tularemia

B. Bubonic plaque

C. Relapsing fever

D. Lyme disease

Ans. B.

491. A 20 year old patient comes to the homeless clinic with a skin abscess on the right arm. A swab from the intact skin overlying this abscess grows coagulase negative staphylococci. An aspirate obtained aseptically with a needle and syringe grows Staphylococcus aureus. About these 2 organisms in this patient you can say

A. Both are normal flora and contaminated the specimens sent to the lab.

B. The staphylococcus aureus is a pathogen and the coagulase negative staphylococcus is not

C. The coagulase negative staphylococcus is a pathogen

D. The coagulase negative Staphylococcus is an opportunistic pathogen

Ans. B.

492. A person with normal healthy immune system acquires a new strain of E. coli that now lives in his gastrointestinal tract. This individual is not ill. A second person with an acute leukaemia and no white blood cells acquires the same organism, develops diarrhoea followed by hypotension, bacteraemia, sepsis, and death. The organism is

A. Normal flora for both individuals

B. A pathogen for both individuals

C. An opportunistic pathogen for both individuals

D. One with a low degree of virulence

Ans. D.

493. The characteristics of a bacterial capsule include

A. All bacteria have one

B. It is composed of peptidoglycan

C. It is important mechanism for protecting a bacteria against ingestion by PMNs

D. It is what causes the Gram stain reaction

Ans. C.

494. A chemical that removes the cell wall of the bacteria but otherwise undamage D. The thing the bacteria will lose because of this include

A. The ability to stain gm positive : All will look gm negative

B. The ability to more

C. The ability to have a Gram stain result

D. The ability to attach to other cell

Ans. C.

495. A bacterium isolated from the mouth is having a polar flagellum stretching from one end looking like a tail under EM. A characteristic of the organism should be

A. An ability to stay at one place for long period of time

B. An ability to move one direction opposite to flagellum

C. An ability to avoid ingestion by pmns

D. An ability to induce large antibody response

Ans. B.

496. On clinical examination, it was found that both the human patients are infected with two strains of the same bacterial species. One is with pili on the surface the other does not. So, it indicates

A. The patient with the piliated strain is ill, the other is not

B. The patient with the piliated strain is not ill, the other is

C. Both the patients are ill since pili do not correlate with virulence

D. The patient with the piliated strain is a child the other patient is an adult

Ans. A.

497. A 19 year old mother delivers a healthy male child. Three days later the baby becomes lethargic has a high temperature and vomits. A lumber puncture shows that the infant has bacterial meningitis. A Gram stain of spinal fluid shows short Gram positive rods. The organism is

A. L. monocytogens
B. B. Group B Streptococcus
C. Most likely a contaminant
D. Anaerobic

Ans. A.

498. Infections caused by anaerobes are

A. Usually confined to the abdomen
B. Never seen in the lung because of its excellent blood supply
C. Mixed
D. Rapidly progressive

Ans. C.

499. Specific organisms that are considered strict anaerobes include

A. E. Coli and Streptococcus pneumoniae
B. Bacteroides and Klebsiella
C. Fusobacterium and Clostridium
D. Peptostreptococcus and Nocardia

Ans. C.

500. The single most important characteristic of diarrhoea caused by Vibrio cholerae is

A. Profuse watery diarrhoea
B. evere abdominal pain
C. Massive bloody diarrhoea
D. Renal insufficiency

Ans. A.

501. A 16 year old boy comes to the clinic with pain in his left ear. He swam daily 2 hours in the pool. Besides his ear is red and having watery greenish drainage from the ear. The organism responsible for this

A. Staphylococcus aureus
B. Viridans group of Streptococcus
C. Streptococcus pneumoniae
D. Pseudomonas aeruginosa

Ans. D.

502. Helicobacter pylori

A. Is the presumed cause of colon cancer
B. Causes most of the cases of acute food poisoning
C. Is the cause of peptic ulcer
D. Is urease negative

Ans. C.

503. Non fermentative Gram negative bacilli are

A. Strict aerobes

B. Catalase negative

C. Beta haemolytic on sheep blood agar

D. Spore forming

Ans. A.

504. The normal habitats of nonfermentative bacteria include the following except

A. Contact lens solutions
B. Hospital water sources
C. House plants
D. Reptiles

Ans. D.

505. Each of the following statements concerning Q fever is correct except

A. Rash is a prominent feature

B. It is transmitted by rrespiratory aerosol

C. Sheep and cattle are important reservoir

D. It is caused by C.burnetti

Ans. A.

506. Each of the following statement about epidemic typhus is correct except

A. The disease is characterized by a rash that begins on the trunk and moves distally

B. The recrudescent form of the disease is called Brill-Zinsser

C. It is caused by Rickettsia typhi

D. The causative organism is transmitted to humans through lice

Ans. C.

507. Which of the following statements is true concerning Q fever ?

A. The organism is transmitted by fleas

B. Headache, fever, and petechial rash are characteristic features of the disease

C. The chronic form of the disease is called brill-zinsser

D. It is caused by Coxiella burnetii

Ans. D.

508. Which of the following is true regarding Rickettsia rickettsii

A. Highest attack rates occur in colorado and utah in usa

B. It can be transmitted by flying squirrels

C. Sheep and cattle are important reservoirs

D. It is transmitted by ticks

Ans. D.

509. Which of the following is not transmitted by ticks ?

A. Rocky Mountain Spotted fever B. Ehrlichiosis

C. R. rickettsii D. Q fever

Ans. D.

510. Which of the following statements concerning Bartonella henselae is correct ?

A. Causes Trench fever

B. Causes Bacillary Angiomatosis in AIDS patients

C. Causes oroya fever

D. Causes Veruga Peruana

Ans. B.

511. The lesions of bacillary angiomatosis in AIDS patients are very similar to the hemangiomatous nodules caused by

A. R. prowazekii B. Ehrlichia chaffeensis

C. Bartonella baciliformis D. Coxiella burnetti

Ans. C.

512. Which of the following is transmitted by lice ?

A. R. prowazekii B. R. typhi

C. R. Rickettsii D. Rickettsia tsutsugamushi

Ans. A.

513. Which of the following is the metabolically active form of Chlamydia trachomatis?

A. Elementary body B. Jolley body

C. Extracellular body D. Reticulate body

Ans. D.

514. Which of the following pathogens is unlikely to be a cause of nongonococcal urethritis ?

A. Ureaplasma urealyticum B. Chlamydia trachomatis

C. Mycoplasma hominis D. Mycoplasma genitalium

E. Chlamydia pneumoniae

Ans. E.

515. A 25 year old pigeon rearer presents with fever to 40oC, severe, diffuse headache, malaise, dry hacking cough and muscle aches. Lung exam reveals bilateral crackles and there is hepatosplenomegaly. The most likely pathogen causing this person's infection is

A. Mycoplasma pneumoniae B. Chlamydia pneumoniae

C. Chlamydia psittaci D. Legionella penumophilia

Ans. C.

516. Which of the following statements concerning Chlamydia trachomatis infections is not correct ?

A. Serology is the diagnostic test of choice in the diagnosis of acute infection

B. 50% of infants born to infected mothers develop infections during labor

C. Tetracyclines are useful for treatment of C. trachomatis infections

D. the clinical spectrum of C. trachomatis sexually transmitted diseases is similar to N. Gonorrhoea

E. Endemic trachoma is a major cause of blindness worldwide

Ans. A.

517. Which of the following statements regarding mycoplasmas is not correct ?

A. Mycoplasmas are the smallest free living microorganisms

B. Mycoplasmas are resistant to cell wall active antibiotics

C. Mycoplasmas are the common commensals of the respiratory and urogenital tracts

D. Mycoplasmas stain well with the Gram's stain

E. Mycoplasmas grow slowly on enriched media

Ans. D.

518. Which of the following is the most common clinical syndrome associated with Mycoplasma pneumonia ?

A. Haemolytic anaemia
B. Lobar pneumonia
C. Tracheobronchitis
D. Bullous myringitis
E. Pericarditis

Ans. C.

519. Which of the following pathogens causes invasive joint disease in immunocompromised host ?

A. Mycoplasma pneumoniae
B. Mycoplasma hominis
C. Ureaplasma urealyticum
D. Chlamydia pneumoniae
E. None of the above

Ans. B.

520. Which of the following are characteristics that are shared by Mycoplasma hominis and Ureaplasma urealyticum ?

A. Both cause post partum fever

B. Ampicillin would be a reasonable choice for treatment

C. Both organisms are identified by production of urease

D. Both stimulate production of cold agglutinins

E. Both organism grow well on sheep blood agar

Ans. A.

521. A 5 year old child complains sore throat, swelling and difficulty breathing. On X ray there is swollen epiglottis. The organisms causing this condition is

A. Neisseria meningitides
B. Group A Streptococcous
C. Haemophilus influenzae
D. Candida albicans

Ans. C.

522. The major virulence factor of Haemophilus influenzae is

A. Its surface pili
B. Its surface polysaccharide
C. Its cell wall
D. Its cell membrane

Ans. B.

523. Important point to remember while detecting Haemophilus influenzae is

A. Beta haemolytic
B. Catalase positive
C. Anaerobic
D. Fastidious

Ans. D.

524. A common characteristic of Legionella species is that they

A. Are gram positive rods
B. Are acid fast
C. Require supplemental ingredients to grow them in laboratory media
D. Are excellular pathogens

Ans. C.

525. Most humans become infected with Legionella by

A. Water source
B. By tick exposure
C. By mosquito exposure
D. By direct contact with another infected person

Ans. A.

526. Legionella infection is more common in patients who

A. Are smokers with COPD
B. Are diabetics
C. Are premature infants
D. Are patients on broad spectrum antibiotics

Ans. A.

527. An important characteristic of mycobacteria is that they are

A. Gram negative
B. Rapid growing (doubling time 15 min)
C. Acid fast
D. Alpha haemolytic

Ans. C.

528. A 30 year old patient with advanced HIV infection (AIDS) is admitted to the hospital with a high fever. Blood cultures showed positive for Mycobacterium ...

A. M. leprae B. M. avium

C. M. kansasii D. M. marinum

Ans. B.

529. An important characteristic of all fungal infections is that

A. They are usually transmitted from person to person

B. They are usually simple and straightforward to treat

C. They cause serious disease in debilitated and/or immunocompromised patients

D. They are usually mixed infections with a combination of fungi and bacteria in the same tissue site

Ans. C.

530. Some fungi have two different morphological forms, yeast and molds. If they do it is likely that

A. The yeast form appears in the environment the mold form in tissue

B. The mold form appears in the environment the yeast form in tissue

C. Both forms appear in tissue

D. Neither forms appear in the tissues since both are non-pathogenic

Ans. B.

531. A 32 years old patient with advanced HIV infection comes into clinic complaining pain in the throat. On examination there were white coating which can be easily removed leaving a red base. He is likely to be infected with

A. Histoplamsa B. Candida albicans

C. Group A Strep D. Strongyloides

Ans. B.

532. The infection most often associated with Cryptococcus neoformans is

A. Septic arthritis B. Sinusitis

C. Pneumonia D. Meningitis

Ans. D.

533. People usually get the fungal infection through

A. Ingestion from meat

B. Ingestion from water

C. Contact with another infected person

D. Inhalation

Ans. D.

534. Which one of the following statement is false regarding Pneumocystis carinii ?

A. It lives as a commensal in most humans

B. It is a common cause of community acquired pneumonia

C. It is an aids defining illness in patients with hiv

D. It caused pneumonia in malnourished children

Ans. B.

535. Spirochetes can be differentiated from other bacteria because they :

A. Motile with axial filaments

B. Have a rigid cell wall

C. Unable to grow on artificial culture media

D. Have no cell wall

Ans. A.

536. All of the following characteristics are true for primary syphilis except:

A. There is a non-tender ulcer usually on genitalia

B. Treponema are demonstrated in the chancre by dark field examination

C. The spirochete is not limited to the primary site

D. The initial lesion appears one month after contact

Ans. C.

537. Secondary syphilis is characterized by all of the following except :

A. Skin and mucous membranes involvement

B. Onset 2 to 4 month after chancre

C. Inability to find spirochetes from lesions

D. There is blood stream dissemination

Ans. C.

538. The stage of syphilis characterized by granulomatous lesions in various organs of the body, including cardiovascular and neurological disorders, is :

A. Primary B. Secondary

C. Tertiary D. Congenital

Ans. C.

539. Primary syphilis is best diagnosed by :

A. Clinical signs and serum antibody testing

B. Clinical signs and dark field examination

C. Dark field examination and serum antibody testing

D. Growth on culture media and Gram stain

Ans. B.

540. A patient's serum yields a positive Rapid plasma reagin (RPR) and negative FTA test. These results most likely indicates :

A. Syphilis infection

B. False-negative FTA due to low sensitivity of the test

C. False-positive RPR due to cross-reacting antibodies

D. Patient in remission for syphilis

Ans. C.

541. Which statement does not accurately describe tertiary syphilis?

A. Occurs years after primary syphilis

B. Chronic granuloma in internal organs.

C. Presence of spirochetes in small numbers in the lesion

D. The patient is highly infectious in this stage

Ans. D.

542. A 22-year-old male presents to his physician, complaining of a sore on his penis. Physical examination shows a firm, raised, red, non-tender chancre of the genitalia. Which of the following is the most appropriate course of action for the physician?

A. Swab the chancre and culture on Thayer-Martin agar

B. Swab the chancre and perform a Gram stain

C. Perform a dark-field examination on a swab of the active lesion

D. Swab the chancre and culture on blood agar

Ans. C.

543. The probable cause for the relapsing nature of relapsing fever caused by Borrelia recurrentis is :

A. The appearance of new antibiotic resistant variants

B. Successive appearance of antigenic variants

C. Defect in cell-mediated immunity

D. Multiplication of the organisms in the blood

Ans. B.

544. The best diagnostic method for relapsing fever is :

A. Biochemical identification B. Giemsa stain of blood smears

C. Serological techniques D. Growth on culture media

Ans. B.

545. Which statement is incorrect for Leptospira icterohaemorrhagica?

A. Tightly coiled spiral with terminal hooks

B. Primarily pathogenic on vertebrates other than humans

C. Stain well with Gram stain

D. Infection may involve liver, kidney and CNS

Ans. C.

546. Leptospirosis is an occupational disease, which one of the following workers is the most likely to be exposed?

A. Butchers
B. Sewer workers
C. Woolsorters
D. Food handlers

Ans. B.

547. Non-gonococcal urethritis due to Ureaplasma urealyticum is treated with :

A. Tetracycline
B. Penicillin G
C. Chloramphenicol
D. Vancomycin

Ans. A.

548. Which is the most specific laboratory test used for diagnosis of Mycoplasma pneumoniae?

A. Detection of cold agglutinins

B. Gram stain

C. Detection of specific antibodies in serum by ELISA

D. Culture of sputum

Ans. C.

549. A distinguishing feature of human mycoplasma species is that :

A. Stain well with Giemsa and Gram stain

B. Contain no bacterial peptidoglycan

C. Cannot be cultivated in vitro

D. Rapid grower under microaerophilic condition

Ans. B.

550. Post-partum fever due to Mycoplasma hominis is treated with :

A. Tetracycline
B. Penicillin G
C. Gentamycin
D. Vancomycin

Ans. A.

551. Mycoplasma pneumoniae is sensitive to the antimicrobial action of :

A. Cycloserine B. Tetracycline

C. Penicillin D. Cephalosporin

Ans. B.

552. Each of the following correctly describes the mycoplasma except :

A. They contain both DNA and RNA

B. They do not have a cell wall

C. They cannot replicate outside host cells

D. They are the smallest free-living organisms known

Ans. C.

553. Mycoplasma pneumonia :

A. Is the etiologic agent of primary atypical pneumonia

B. It is mainly identified through culture and biochemical reactions

C. Responds well to penicillin therapy

D. All of the above

Ans. A.

554. Which of the following is true for cold agglutinins as indicative of current infection with Mycoplasma pneumoniae?

A. It is specific method for diagnosis of infection

B. It is IgG autoantibodies that agglutinate group A antibodies at 4°C

C. It is IgM autoantibodies that agglutinate group O antibodies at 4°C

D. It is IgM autoantibodies that agglutinate group O antibodies at 37°C

Ans. C.

555. Mycoplasma colonies are identified by the following :

A. Fried egg appearance B. Giemsa stain

C. IF technique D. All of the above

Ans. D.

556. Characteristics of Mycoplasma & Ureaplasma include :

A. The presence of a thin gram positive-like cell wall with no cell membrane

B. Rapid growth on Mac Conkey's agar, slow growth on basic nutrient agar

C. The presence of only a cell membrane with no cell wall

D. Rapid growth on Mac Conkey's medium & routine blood agar plates

Ans. C.

557. All of the following regarding Mycoplasma is true except :

A. Parasitic Mycoplasma requires 10% serum in its growth medium

B. Mycoplasma pneumoniae is responsible for 10% of all pneumonia

C. Ureaplasma urealyticum requires 10% of urea in its growth medium

D. Ureaplasma urealyticum is responsible for 10% of non-gonococcal urethitis cases

Ans. A.

558. Chlamydia resemble bacteria in all of the following except :

A. They possess both RNA and DNA

B. They multiply by binary fission

C. They can be inhibited by many antimicrobials effective against bacteria

D. They are closely related to Gram positive bacteria

Ans. D.

559. Which one of the following is characteristic of Chlamydia trachomatis?

A. Reticulate bodies are infectious, extracellular form of the organism

B. Produce granular conjunctivitis

C. Inclusion bodies are formed from division of elementary bodies

D. Sensitive to B-lactam antibiotics

Ans. B.

560. All the followings are true statements about Chlamydia trachomatis except :

A. Can grow on artificial culture media

B. It has a number of serotypes (about fifteen) that correlate with the syndrome produced on infection

C. It causes sexually-transmitted disease

D. It can be detected by direct IF examination of pathological specimen

Ans. A.

561. A feature of Chlamydia that is unique to this genus is

A. It is obligate intracellular parasite

B. Its replicative cycle is distinguished by two morphologic forms in infected cells

C. They lack muramic acid in its cell envelope

D. Cannot grow on artificial culture media

Ans. B.

562. Which of the following statements does not describe trachoma?

A. It causes mucopurulent conjunctivitis

B. It can lead to blindness

C. It is caused by C.trachomatis serotype D-K

D. It is diagnosed by isolation of the organism on yolk sac

Ans. C.

563. Trachoma is diagnosed by detection of inclusion bodies in conjunctival scraping smear stained by

A. Gram stain B. Methylene blue stain

C. Giemsa stain D. Modified ZN stain

Ans. C.

564. Which statement correctly describes the genus Chlamydia?

A. Classified as viruses B. Do not contain both DNA and RNA

C. Obligate intracellular bacteria D. Smallest free-living organisms

Ans. C.

565. Each of the following conditions has been associated with C. trachomatis except

A. Lymphogranuloma venereum B. Non-gonococcal urethritis

C. Atypical pneumonia D. Granular conjunctivitis

Ans. C.

566. Which of the following serotypes are associated with Chlamydia diseases acquired through the venereal route?

A. A, B, Ba and C B. D-K

C. L4, L5 and L6 D. All of the above

Ans. B.

567. Which of the following is true about Chlamydia and separates them from Rickettsiae?

A. Is an obligate intracellular parasite

B. It has a complicated growth cycle

C. Contains both types of nucleic acid DNA & RNA

D. It is sensitive to antibiotics like tetracycline

Ans. B.

568. Chlamydia can be recognized by all the following laboratory procedures except:

A. Microscopic examination of Giemsa-stained scrapings from infected tissues

B. Culture on agar medium

C. Culture in tissue culture cells

D. Polymerase chain reaction

Ans. B.

569. A 45-year-old woman is admitted to the hospital following a sudden onset of fever, malaise, severe headache and prostration. She has a dry cough. WBC is normal. Her husband states that her parrot died 3 days before the onset of the patient's illness. The diagnosis that is most strongly suggested is :

A. Tuberculosis

B. Psittacosis

C. Rickettsial pox

D. Q fever

E. Epidemic typhus

Ans. B.

570. If the patient has psittacosis

A. The respiratory tract is the main portal of entry

B. She must have been bitten by a mite

C. A rising of specific antibody titre is not essential for diagnosis

D. Tetracycline would be ineffective

Ans. A.

571. Which of the following statements is true assuming that the correct diagnosis is psittacosis?

A. Chlamydia psittaci can cause severe pneumonia

B. Chlamydia psittaci cannot be isolated from clinical specimens like sputum

C. Chlamydia psittaci can be isolated from the blood

D. It can be cultured on ordinary media

Ans. A.

572. If the condition is Psittacosis :

A. Infection from man to man is common

B. The organism can grow well in tissue culture

C. The drug of choice for treatment is sulphonamides

D. Gram stained film is done to detect elementary bodies

Ans. B.

573. All of the following statements are true concerning rickettsial pox except :

A. Mite serves as the vector

B. It is caused by R. rickettsii

C. It is characterized by inward spreading rash

D. It is diagnosed by detection of Rickettsia antigen in skin biopsy by IF

Ans. B.

574. All of the following statements describe the Rickettsiae except :

A. They are small Gram negative bacilli

B. They are obligate intracellular parasites

C. They cannot be isolated on ordinary culture media

D. They all produce fever and rash in humans

Ans. D.

575. Which of the following is true concerning Rocky Mountain spotted fever?

A. It produces widespread vascular endothelial damage

B. It can be transmitted only from mite bite

C. Humans are the only known host

D. It is characterized by outward spreading rash

Ans. A.

576. Which of the following is not true concerning epidemic typhus?

A. It produces vascular endothelial damage

B. It is transmitted only by louse

C. Rodents are the only known reservoir

Ans. C.

577. Rickettsiae :

A. Grow only extracellularly

B. Are eukaryotic cells

C. Are sensitive to penicillin

D. Generally invade the endothelial lining of capillaries causing haemorrhages

Ans. D.

578. The vector of epidemic typhus is :

A. Dog tick B. Rat flea

C. Human body louse D. Mite

Ans. C.

579. Choose incorrect statement regarding Coxiella burnetii

A. It can survive outside the host

B. It can affect humans as well as animals

C. It is sensitive to tetracycline

D. Manifested by trunk rash that spreads to the extremities

Ans. D.

580. Choose incorrect statement regarding epidemic typhus :

A. Disease characterized by centrifugal rash

B. Disease is caused by Rickettsia prowazekii

C. Patients who recover from this disease may develop later Brill's disease

D. The causative organisms is transmitted from rodents to human by tick

Ans. D.

581. A 10-year-old boy is admitted to a teaching hospital because of severe chills, fever, headache, malaise, joint pains and myalgia. A rash appeared on the extremities, then on the trunk and becomes generalized. On clinical examination, liver and spleen show enlargement. The most likely diagnosis is :

A. Influenza B. Typhus fever

C. Rocky Mountain spotted fever D. Q fever

Ans. C.

582. Assume that this patient has Rocky Mountain spotted fever, it has been transmitted by

A. Mite bite B. Flea faeces

C. Louse faeces D. Tick bite

Ans. D.

583. There is four fold rise in titre in the immunofluorescent antibody test. The rise in titre indicates :

A. There is no infection

B. A recent rickettsial infection

C. The patient is completely recovered

D. The patient has developed immunity

Ans. B.

584. The treatment of choice for Rocky Mountain spotted fever is :

A. Penicillin B. Tetracycline

C. Sulfonamides D. Antitoxic serum

Ans. B.

585. Neisseria species are positive for the enzyme :

A. Coagulase
B. DNase
C. Oxidase
D. Catalase

Ans. C.

586. Which statement correctly describes the toxins associated with Neisseria?

A. The toxins are released by the living bacterial cell
B. The toxins are composed of lipopolysaccharide - components of the cell wall
C. The toxins are categorized as exotoxins
D. The toxins are similar to the enzymes of Staph. aureus

Ans. B.

587. Virulence of Neisseria gonorrheae is due to :

A. Pili
B. Outer membrane protein
C. Lipopolysaccharides
D. Protease enzyme
E. All of the above

Ans. E.

588. The most appropriate specimen for diagnosis of acute gonorrhoea

A. Mid-stream urine
B. High vaginal swab in females
C. Prostatic secretion in males
D. Urethral discharge

Ans. D.

589. One of the following is not considered a virulent factor of N. gonorrhoea :

A. Pili
B. Capsule
C. IgA protease
D. Outer membrane protein

Ans. B.

590. Regarding N. gonorrhoea, choose the correct statement :

A. Carriers in the general population are 5%
B. Repeated gonococcal infections are uncommon
C. Serotyping is based on capsular polysaccharide
D. Differentiated from N. meningitidis by its inability to ferment maltose

Ans. D.

591. The causative agent in strangles is

A. Rhodococcus
B. Corynebacterium
C. Streptococcus
D. Actinobacillus

Ans. C.

592. Distemper in horses refers to which disease:

A. Herpes
B. Strep. equi (strangles)
C. Rhodococcus equi
D. Influenza
E. Equine Viral arteritis

Ans. B.

593. Clostridium botulinum does not cause harm in the normal animal because:

A. It is in spore form
B. It only grows in necrotic tissue
C. It only grows in dead waterfowl
D. It can only grow once it encounter air
E. The normal animal can readily neutralize any toxins produced

Ans. B.

594. There is an available vaccine for botulism. (True or false)

Ans. True.

595. There is an available antitoxin for treating botulism (true or false)

Ans. True.

596. Botulism causes:

A. CNS signs
B. rigid paralysis
C. flaccid paralysis
D. both a and b
E. both a and c

Ans. C.

597. Of the following species least likely to be affected by, or to be a carrier/shedder of Leptospirosis is:

A. cats
B. dogs
C. ruminants (cattle, moose, elk, goats, sheep)
D. hogs
E. Rodents

Ans. A.

598. Tuberculosis (TB) is an example of

A. Pandemic
B. Prodemic
C. Endemic
D. Epidemic

Ans. C.

599. People who are infected with, likely to live their whole life

A. Acquired Immune Deficiency Syndrome (AIDS)

B. HIV

C. Lungs cancer

D. All of above

Ans. D.

600. Vancomycin is

A. An infectious disease B. Is a virus

C. Is an antibiotic D. Is an antiviral

Ans. C.

601. Annual worldwide incidence of cholera is

A. 1-2 million B. 1-3 million

C. 1-5 million D. 3 -5 million

Ans. D.

602. Polio is known as humans haunt after eradication of

A. Tuberculosis B. Measles

C. Chickenpox D. Smallpox

Ans. D.

603. Oral rehydration therapy largely consists of water and

A. Sodium ions B. Glucose

C. Potassium magnate solution D. All of above

Ans. B.

604. Which statement is incorrect? Effective antibiotics

A. Show selective toxicity B. Kill host cell

C. Kill pathogens D. Are useless against virus

Ans. B.

605. Childhood blindness can be caused due to

A. Acquired Immune Deficiency Syndrome (HIV/AIDS)

B. Malaria

C. Measles

D. Tuberculosis

Ans. C.

606. Rice water is clinical name of

A. Diarrhoea B. Measles

C. Chronic Bronchitis D. Emphysema

Ans. A.

607. Drug is Isoniazid for treatment of

A. Cholera B. Tuberculosis (TB)

C. Measles D. Malaria

Ans. B.

608. Which strain of cholera is more virulent?

A. Classical strain B. El Tor

C. V Cholerae 0139 D. All of above

Ans. C.

609. Total pandemics have been caused by Cholera virus

A. 5 B. 6

C. 7 D. 8

Ans. D.

610. Infectious diseases include

A. Malnutrition B. Cystic fibrosis

C. Retinoblastoma D. Tuberculosis

Ans. D.

611. Causes of cholera do not include

A. Poor sanitation B. Unclean water

C. Genetic disorder D. Infectious pathogens

Ans. C.

612. A sudden increase in number of people having disease is called as

A. Pandemic B. Prodemic

C. Endemic D. Epidemic

Ans. D.

613. Toxin choleragen causes

A. Increase in pulmonary constrictions

B. Salt and water leave blood

C. Stomach lining gets disrupted

D. An increase in salt and water

Ans. B.

614. Bacteria are known to cause

A. Cholera

B. Acquired Immune Deficiency Syndrome (HIV/AIDS)

C. Malaria

D. Measles

Ans. A.

615. Incubation period of Vibrio cholerae has duration of
A. Few hours to four days
B. Two hours to five days
C. Two hours to fifteen days
D. None of above

Ans. B.

616. Action site of cholera virus is
A. Small intestine
B. Large intestine
C. Faeces of infected person
D. Stomach

Ans. A.

617. Cholera can be fatal if it is not treated within
A. 12 hours
B. 24 hours
C. 36 hours
D. 48 hours

Ans. B.

618. Transmission cycle of cholera can be broken by
A. Treating with medications
B. By destroying small intestine lining were cholera virus grows
C. By boiling all vegetables and fruits before consuming
D. Chlorination of water

Ans. D.

619. Number of people who have disease at any one time is refer to as
A. Incidence
B. Coincidence
C. Transmission cycle
D. Prevalence

Ans. D.

620. Vibrio cholerae bacterium can not survive if the
A. pH is below 4.5
B. pH is between 4.5 and 7
C. pH is between 7 and 11
D. pH is above 11

Ans. A.

621. Bacterial and fungal infections
A. Are non-infectious diseases
B. Can be cured by antibiotics
C. Need to be helped through transmission cycle
D. None of above

Ans. B.

622. Function of Penicillinases is to
A. Act as narrow spectrum antibiotic.
B. Act as broad spectrum antibiotic.
C. Resist and destroy penicillin.
D. Destroy cross-links of peptidoglycan polymers in bacterial cell wall.

Ans. C.

623. Almost unknown disease in developed countries is

A. Malaria B. Measles

C. Smallpox D. Chickenpox

Ans. B.

624. A rapid increase in cases around world is called

A. Pandemic B. Prodemic

C. Endemic D. Epidemic

Ans. A.

625. In India, El Tor strain of cholera replaced classical strain in a time period of

A. 2 to 14 days B. 6 months

C. 12 months D. 24 months

Ans. D.

626. In Cholera, body can be rehydrated

A. Intravenously B. Orally

C. Both A and B D. None of above

Ans. C.

627. El Tor strain cholera has been replaced by

A. V Cholerae 0142 B. V Cholerae 0149

C. V Cholerae 0139 D. V Cholerae 0134

Ans. C.

628. Bacteria are known to cause

A. Acquired Immune Deficiency Syndrome (HIV/AIDS)

B. Malaria

C. Measles

D. Tuberculosis

Ans. D.

629. Name some Acid Fast organisms (Other than Mycobacteria)

Ans. 1. **Nocardia spp: Partial Acid Fast**

2. Rhodococcus spp: Partial Acid Fast
3. Legionella micdadei: Partially acid fast in tissue
4. Cyst of Cryptosporidium: Acid Fast
5. Cyst of Isospora: Acid Fast

630. All of the following statements regarding M. tuberculosis are correct except
   A. Mycobacteria are obligate aerobes
   B. Can grow in cell free media
   C. Doubling time of tubercle bacilli is about 18 hours
   D. Increased CO2 tension enhances growth

Ans. D.

631. Swimming pool granuloma is caused by
   A. M. tuberculosis
   B. M. marinum
   C. M. ulcerans
   D. M. chelonei

Ans. B.

632. Which of the following statements is incorrect
   A. Risk of developing TB disease is highest in first 2 years after infection
   B. People with TB infection may or may not develop TB disease
   C. Every individual exposed to TB develops disease
   D. People who are exposed to TB may or may not develop TB infection

Ans. C.

633. Cord growth seen on mycobacterial culture is characteristic of
   A. Saprophytic strains
   B. Avirulent strains
   C. Atypical mycobacteria
   D. Virulent strains

Ans. D.

634. MDR TB is defined as resistance to
   A. Isoniazid and Rifampicin irrespective of resistance to any other drug
   B. more than three anti tubercular drugs
   C. Isoniazid, Pyrazinamide and Rifampicin
   D. fluoroquinolones and at least one of the three injectable second-line drugs used to treat TB

Ans. A.

635. XDR is defined as
   A. MDR TB that is resistant to either one of the injectable second line drugs or second-line therapeutic fluoroquinolones
   B. resistant to two most effective first-line therapeutic drugs, Isoniazid and rifampicin irrespective of resistance to any other drug
   C. Strain resistant to more than one drug (excluding co resistance to INH and rif)
   D. MDR TB that also is resistant to fluoroquinolones and at least one of the three injectable second-line drugs used to treat TB (Amikacin, Kanamycin, or Capreomycin)

Ans. D.

636. The scientist who discovered M. tuberculosis was

A. Robert Koch
B. Calmette and Guerin
C. Louis Pasteur
D. Jean-Antoine Villemin

Ans. A.

637. Mutations in katG gene of M. tuberculosis are responsible for resistance to

A. Pyrazinamide
B. isoniazid (INH)
C. Streptomycin
D. Rifampicin

Ans. B.

638. Tubercular granulomas are made up of

A. Organized aggregates of immune cells that surround foci of infected tissues
B. Damaged tissue cells and bacilli only
C. Fibrous and damaged tissue and bacilli only
D. Necrotic tissue and damaged tissue and bacilli only

Ans. A.

639. After TB has been transmitted, how long does it take for the body's immune system to be able to react to tuberculin ?

A. 48 to 72 hours
B. 7 to 10 days
C. 2 to 8 weeks
D. 6 months or more

Ans. C.

640. Buruli ulcer is caused by

A. M. marinum
B. M. chelonei
C. M. tuberculosis
D. M. ulcerans

Ans. D.

641. Which of the following environmental factors do not increase the probability that M. tuberculosis will be transmitted ?

A. Exposure in small enclosed spaces
B. Inadequate local or general ventilation that results in insufficient dilution or removal of infectious droplet nuclei.
C. Recirculation of air containing infectious droplet nuclei
D. Improper specimen handling procedures that generate infectious droplet nuclei.
E. Negative pressure in an infectious TB patient's room

Ans. E.

642. Which of the following is a non cultivable mycobacteria ?

A. M. tuberculosis B. M. leprae

C. M. avium intracellulare D. M. bovis

Ans. B.

643. A case of leprosy with good cell mediated immunity usually presents as following form of disease

A. Borderline B. Indeterminate

C. Lepromatous D. Tuberculoid

Ans. D.

644. During which phase of growth of Penicillium chrysogenum maximum antibiotic production takes place

A. During the first phase B. During the second phase

C. During the third phase D. Same in all the phases

Ans. B.

645. Which of the following is the causative agent of fowl cholera ?

A. Vibrio cholera B. E. coli

C. Salmonella pullorum D. Pasteurella multocida

Ans. D.

646. In order to combat bacteria, types of viruses used are called as

A. Tobacco mosaic virus B. Hybrid virus

C. Bacteriophages D. Influenza virus

Ans. C.

647. In adverse conditions, bacteria

A. Start dividing B. Start copying DNA

C. Form a thick walled spore D. All of these

Ans. C.

648. Temperature of fermenter to produce Fusarium is maintained at

A. 20 °C B. 30 °C

C. 40 °C D. 50 °C

Ans. B.

649. In fungi, starch $(C_6H_{10}O_5)_n$ is converted to maltose $(C_{12}H_{22}O_{11})$ through

A. Protease B. Deamination process

C. Maltase D. Amylase

Ans. C.

650. Walls of spores may be broken only through

A. Very drastic conditions B. If it settles on a growth suitable medium

C. Both of these D. None of these

Ans. C.

651. Fungi stores carbohydrates ($C_nH_{2m}O_m$) in form of

A. Spores B. Glucose

C. Galactose D. Glycogen

Ans. D.

652. In fungi, enzymes are secreted through

A. Slime capsule B. Hypha

C. Cytoplasm D. Multiple nucleoli

Ans. B.

653. In fermented dough, cavities appear due to

A. Carbon monoxide B. Carboxy acids

C. Carbon dioxide D. Oxygen

Ans. C.

654. Flagellum is not found in

A. Non-motile bacterium B. Motile bacterium

C. Non-motile virus D. Motile virus

Ans. A.

655. Cytoplasm of bacteria contains smaller rings of DNA (Deoxyribonucleic Acid) called as

A. Chromatains B. Chromatids

C. Plasmids D. Pyramids

Ans. C.

656. Rhizopus is a form of

A. Unicellular fungi B. Multicellular fungi

C. Bicellular fungi D. Tricellular fungi

Ans. B.

657. Glucose ($C_6H_{12}O_6$) and amino acids are diffused in hypha through

A. Osmosis B. Diffusion

C. Concentration gradient D. Selective reabsorption

Ans. B.

658. Comma shaped bacteria are called as

A. Cocci B. Bacilli

C. Spirilla D. Vibrio

Ans. D.

659. Each hypha is divided into

A. Many cells B. Few cells

C. No cell D. A tissue

Ans. C.

660. Slime capsule often covers the

A. Bacterium B. Virus

C. Fungi D. All of these

Ans. A.

661. Motile-bacterium moves with help of

A. A whip B. A tail

C. A flagellum D. All of these

Ans. C.

662. Under suitable conditions, mycelia threads grow

A. In host cells B. Undergo binary fissions

C. Grow over substratum D. Form spores for later reproduction

Ans. C.

663. Spherical-shaped bacteria are referred as

A. Cocci B. Bacilli

C. Spirilla D. Vibrio

Ans. A.

664. Athletes foot is caused due to

A. Fungi B. Bacteria

C. Virus D. Excess of adrenaline

Ans. A.

665. Hyphhas has

A. No nucleus B. One nucleus

C. No true nucleus D. Many nucleoli

Ans. D.

666. Saprophytes do not include

A. Fungi B. Virus
C. Bacteria D. All of these

Ans. B.

667. Fungi play a role as decomposers through enzyme

A. Protease B. Lactase
C. ADH D. Insulin

Ans. A.

668. Bacteria capable to produce their own food are called as

A. Saprophytes B. Parasites
C. Autotrophs D. Penicillin

Ans. C.

669. In fungi, enzyme protease digests proteins into

A. Peptones B. Amino acids
C. Substrate D. Sugars

Ans. B.

670. Bacterium does not have a

A. Cytoplasm B. True nucleus
C. Protoplasm D. DNA (Deoxyribonucleic Acid)

Ans. B.

671. Bacteria

A. Can be seen with naked eye
B. Are in form of pupa
C. Are larger than virus
D. Can only be controlled through bacteriophages

Ans. C.

672. Bacteria may be

A. Aerobic B. Anaerobic
C. Viral or fungal D. Both A and B

Ans. D.

673. When growth of fungal cells slows down in culture medium

A. Carbon dioxide is given off B. Carbon monoxide is given off
C. Fungal cells excrete penicillin D. Process is stopped

Ans. C.

674. To form cheese, a mixture of bacteria and fungi act upon

A. Fermented milk sugar B. Lactic acid

C. Fats D. All three

Ans. D.

675. Yeasts are

A. Unicellular fungi B. Multicellular fungi

C. Bicellular fungi D. Tricellular fungi

Ans. A.

676. Lactobacillus is used to convert milk sugar (lactose: $C_{12}H_{22}O_{11}$) into

A. Glucose B. Glycogen

C. Lactic acid D. Citric acid

Ans. C.

677. Parasitic fungi

A. Act as decomposer

B. Actively forms spores

C. Lives in living tissues of plants and animals

D. Secretes hormones like maltase

Ans. C.

678. For optimal growth of fungus, process shall be

A. Anaerobic

B. Aerobic

C. Oxygen supply should be cut off after some time

D. Oxygen should not be supplied since beginning

Ans. B.

679. Saprophytic bacteria feed

A. In intestines of animals B. By producing their own food

C. Feed on decaying organic matter D. All of these

Ans. C.

680. Fungal diseases in man commonly appear as

A. Hook worms B. White spores

C. Tapeworms D. Ringworms

Ans. D.

681. Vibrio bacteria are a variation of

A. Cocci
B. Bacilli
C. Spirilla
D. Vibrious

Ans. B.

682. Enzymes found in fungi are

A. Protease
B. Amylase
C. Maltase
D. All of these

Ans. D.

683. During milk fermentation, lactose is converted to lactic acid through

A. Lactobacillus
B. Streptococcus
C. Lactococcus
D. Streptobacillus

Ans. A.

684. Restriction enzymes

A. Protect bacteria from viral infection
B. Cut DNA in a staggered fashion
C. Cut DNAs producing a blunt end
D. All of the above

Ans. D.

685. Eukaryotic cells are more efficient than prokaryotes because their internal compartmentalization

A. Makes each compartment nutritionally independent of all others
B. Allows for specialization through the subdivision of particular tasks
C. Allows for specialization through merging of different tasks
D. Reduces overall cell size

Ans. B.

686. The simplest way to differentiate a prokaryotic cell from a eukaryotic one is to

A. Look for a plasma membrane
B. See if a nucleus is present
C. Check for the presence of DNA
D. Determine if the cell is an entire organism or not

Ans. B.

687. Which of the following is the best criterion for deciding whether a cell is prokaryotic or eukaryotic?

A. The cell came from a single-celled or multicelled organism
B. The cell has a nucleus or not
C. The cell has cytosol or not
D. DNA is present in the cell or not

Ans. B.

688. Lysosomes are specialized vesicles in ———— that contain digestive enzymes for the breakdown of food. A related organelle known as a vacuole, which is found in ————, also contains enzymes but in addition may act as a storage organelle for nutrients or water.

A. Animals; plants and fungi
B. Plants; animals and fungi
C. Plants and fungi; animals
D. Animals and plants; fungi

Ans. A.

689. Which of the following statements about prokaryotes is false?

A. Prokaryotic cells concentrate important materials for the cells survival
B. The substance known as cytosol is found within the bacterial nucleus
C. Prokaryotic cells are much smaller than most eukaryotic cells
D. Ancient prokaryotes may have given rise to some eukaryotic organelles

Ans. B.

690. What do dystrophin, utrophin, actin, and tubulin have to do with eukaryotic cell structure and function?

A. They are components in the reactions of photosynthesis
B. They all participate in the degradation of large amounts of ATP
C. They all participate in the production of large amounts of ATP
D. They are all embedded proteins in plasma membranes

Ans. C.

691. Which of the following is present in both prokaryotes and eukaryotes?

A. Lysosome
B. Chloroplast
C. Plasma membrane
D. Vacuole

Ans. C.

692. Human transmission of Brucellae occurs by

A. Direct contact with animal tissues
B. Ingestion of contaminated meat
C. Ingestion of infected milk
D. All of these

Ans. D.

693. Brucella are

A. Rods
B. Cocci
C. very short rods
D. Coccobacilli

Ans. A.

694. Which of the following can be identified by milk ring test?

A. Salmonellosis
B. Brucellosis
C. All of these
D. Bovine tuberculosis

Ans. B.

695. The most pathogenic Brucella spp for man is

A. B. abortus
B. B. melitensis
C. B. canis
D. B. suis

Ans. B.

696. In chilled shrimp __________ is chiefly responsible for spoilage.

A. Pseudomonas
B. Achromobacter
C. Molds or yeasts
D. Micrococcus or Bacillus species

Ans. B.

697. The predominant kind of bacteria causing spoilage in fish at chilling temperature is

A. Micrococcus
B. Pseudomonas sp.
C. None of these
D. Bacillus

Ans. B.

698. At higher temperatures, the souring of Oysters may be the result of the fermentation of sugars by

A. Streptococci
B. Coliform bacteria
C. All of these
D. Lactobacilli and yeast

Ans. A.

699. The chief spoilage organisms on smoked fish are

A. Bacteria
B. Molds
C. fungi
D. Both A and B

Ans. D.

700. Normally, due to the holding of the chilled fish

A. Achromobacters decrease
B. Pseudomonas increase in numbers
C. All of the above
D. Flavobacteria increase temporarily and then decrease

Ans. B.

701. A bacterial food intoxication refers to

A. Food borne illness caused by the presence of a bacterial toxin formed in food
B. Illness caused by presence of pathogens
C. None of the above
D. Both A and B

Ans. A.

702. The Bacillus cereus causes gastroenteritis by the production of an exoenterotoxin which is released in food as a result of

A. Cell autolysis B. Cell growth

C. Cell damage D. Cell permeation

Ans. A.

703. The botulism intoxication occurs due to

A. Neurotoxin B. An enterotoxin

C. All of these D. Mycotoxin

Ans. A.

704. The staphylococcal intoxication refers to presence of

A. Neurotoxin B. An enterotoxin

C. All of these D. Mycotoxin

Ans. B.

705. The milk streptococci produce acetoin that gets spontaneously oxidized yielding a flavourings agent (responsible for aroma of butter) that is

A. Acetyl CoA B. Acetone

C. Dicacetyl D. Butyric acid

Ans. C.

706. The application of Gamma rays destroys botulism toxin. The dose of gamma rays required for this purpose is

A. 73 Rad B. 73 Gy

C. 173 Rad D. 7.3 Mrad

Ans. D.

707. Stormy clot reaction is useful in identification of

A. C. botulinum B. C. tetani

C. C. difficile D. C. perfringens

Ans. D.

708. Food poisoning strains of Clostridium perfringens belong to

A. Type B B. Type A

C. Type D D. Type C

Ans. B.

709. Types of Clostridium exotoxin, most commonly associated with botulism in man, is/are?

A. Type B B. Type A

C. All of these D. Type E

Ans. C.

710. The micro-organism which is present in both fresh and frozen juices is

A. Enterobacter aerogens B. E. coli

C. None of these D. P. chrysogenum

Ans. A.

711. Under what conditions food poisoning bacteria may grow and produce toxins in vegetables?

A. When thawed vegetables are held at room temperature for any considerable period

B. When thawed vegetables are held at refrigerated temperature for any considerable period

C. None of the above

D. When thawed vegetables are held below refrigerated temperature for any considerable period

Ans. A.

712. Species of __________ are predominant on thawing vegetables like sweet corn and peas when the temperature of thawing is fairly low.

A. Micrococcus B. Streptococcus

C. None of the above D. Both A and B

Ans. A.

713. Watery soft rot is found mostly in

A. Vegetable B. Fruits

C. All of these D. Cereals

Ans. A.

714. Bacterial soft rot is caused due to

A. Fermentation of sugars B. Fermentation of pectin

C. Formation of amino acids D. Formation of ketones

Ans. B.

715. Saprophytic bacteria cause

A. Brown rot in vegetables

B. Sliminess or souring in piled, wet and heating vegetables

C. Bacterial soft rot

D. Black rot in fruits

Ans. B.

716. Concentrate of fruits and vegetable juices

A. Favour the growth of yeast and of acid and sugar tolerant Leuconostoc and Lactobacillus species

B. Favor the growth of niger and flavus species

C. None of the above

D. Favour the growth of saprophytic bacteria

Ans. A.

717. Black mold rot is caused by

A. A. Niger B. A. Flavus

C. Trichothecium roseum D. Tricoderma

Ans. A.

718. Hyphomycete fungi

A. Grow in leaves and the infected leaves are the preferred food source for some aquatic insects

B. Produce nonmotile tetaradiate conidia

C. None of the above

D. Both A and B

Ans. D.

719. All of the following species are considered coliforms except

A. Klebsiella pneumoniae B. Enterobacter aerogenes

C. E. coli D. S. typhi

Ans. D.

720. Which of the following species in water reveal the presence of fecal pollution of human or animal origin?

A. Faecal Streptococci B. E. coli

C. All of these D. Cl. perfringens

Ans. A.

721. Example of a Saprophytic bacteria is

A. M. smegmatis B. M. xenopi

C. M. marinum D. M. chelonei

Ans. A.

722. Eugonic growth on Lowenstein-Jensen medium is produced by

A. M. tuberculosis B. M. bovis

C. None of the above D. Both A and B

Ans. A.

723. False negative Mantoux test is observed in

A. Advanced tuberculosis
B. Early tuberculosis
C. All of these
D. Severe malnutrition

Ans. C.

724. Which of the following bacteria is sensitive to pyrazinamide?

A. M. bovis
B. M. tuberculosis
C. None of these
D. M. fortuitum

Ans. B.

725. Which of the following bacteria is susceptible to thiophen-2-carboxylic acid hydrazide?

A. M. tuberculosis
B. M. bovis
C. M. fortuitum
D. M. chelonei

Ans. B.

726. Rough and buff colonies on LJ medium are characteristic of

A. M. bovis
B. M. chelonei
C. M. fortuitum
D. M. tuberculosis

Ans. D.

727. Humans become infected with Mycobacterium tuberculosis most frequently by

A. Ingestion
B. Inhalation
C. Inoculation
D. Contact

Ans. B.

728. The substance(s) which can be produced by strains of Pseudomonas aeruginosa is/are

A. Elastase
B. Exotoxin A and S
C. All of these
D. Haemolysis

Ans. C.

729. Pseudomonas aeruginosa can be diagnosed from the pigment, known as

A. Pyoverdin
B. Pyocyanin
C. Pyorubrin
D. Pyomelanin

Ans. C.

730. Coagulase-reacting factor is necessary for

A. Tube coagulase test
B. Slide coagulase test
C. None of these
D. Precipitation test

Ans. A.

731. Staphylococcal food poisoning usually manifests itself following ingestion of contaminated food after

A. 8-12 hours
B. 2-6 hours
C. 18-36 hours
D. 12-18 hours

Ans. B.

732. Which of the following Staphylococcal haemolysins does not cause lysis of human RBCs?

A. γ haemolysin
B. β haemolysin
C. δ haemolysin
D. α haemolysin

Ans. D.

733. Bacteria which produces coagulase is

A. S. saprophyticus
B. S. epidermidis
C. S. hominis
D. S. aureus

Ans. D.

734. Which of the following condition is non-suppurative sequelae of Streptococcus pyogenes infections?

A. Acute glomerulonephritis
B. Acute rheumatic fever
C. All of these
D. Erythema nodosum

Ans. C.

735. Which of the following cross-reacts with cell wall carbohydrate of Streptococcus pyogenes?

A. Synovial fluid
B. Cardiac valves
C. Vascular intima
D. Myocardium

Ans. B.

736. Which of the following test indicates the susceptibility to streptococcal pyrogenic exotoxin?

A. Disk test
B. Schick test
C. Precipitation test
D. ASO test

Ans. A.

737. Crystal violet blood agar is a selective medium for

A. Staphylococcus aureus
B. β haemolytic streptococci
C. M. tuberculosis
D. C. diphtheriae

Ans. B.

738. Cell wall protein of Streptococcus pyogenes cross reacts with human

A. Cardiac valves
B. Synovial fluid
C. Vascular intima
D. Myocardium

Ans. D.

739. Individuals suffering from primary atypical pneumonia have agglutinins to

A. S. avium
B. Streptococcus MG
C. Enterococcus faecalis
D. S. mutans

Ans. B.

740. Streptococcus pyogenes can be differentiated from other haemolytic Streptococci on the basis of

A. Erythromycin sensitivity
B. Bacitracin sensitivity
C. Penicillin sensitivity
D. Aminoglycosides sensitivity

Ans. B.

741. In Yersinia pestis, capsule is best demonstrated in cultures grown at

A. 29°C
B. 25°C
C. 45°C
D. 37°C

Ans. D.

742. Which of the following is the commonest species of Salmonella for causing zoonotic disease?

A. S. Newport
B. S. Indiana
C. S. enteritidis
D. S. typhimurium

Ans. D.

743. The bacteria which produce(s) β-galactosidase is/are

A. Enterobacter
B. Citrobacter
C. All of the above
D. Serratia

Ans. C.

744. The most common cause of urinary tract infection in the community is

A. Proteus vulgaris
B. Klebsiellla pneumoniae
C. Citrobacter freundii
D. E. coli

Ans. D.

745. Dysentery may be caused by

A. Enteroinvasive E. coli
B. Enteropathogenic E. coli
C. Verotoxigenic E. coli
D. Enterotoxigenic E. coli

Ans. D.

746. Xylose lysine deoxycholate (XLD) agar is better selective medium than the deoxycholate citrate agar (DCA) because

A. It imparts better growth

B. It is selective

C. It is less inhibitory to S. Dysenteriae and S. Flexneri

D. It contains high salt concentration

Ans. C.

747. In Widal test the significant titres for H agglutinins is

A. 1:100 or more B. 1:50 or more

C. 1:400 or more D. 1:200 or more

Ans. D.

748. Pseudomembraneous colitis is

A. Caused by a gram positive bacterium

B. Precipitated by the use of certain antibiotics

C. All of the above

D. Caused by a spore forming bacterium

Ans. C.

749. The toxins produced by bacteria

A. Encourage bacterial reproduction

B. Kill viruses

C. All of the above

D. Interfere with physiological processes in the body

Ans. D.

750. Fatalities following influenza infection are usually due to the

A. Bacterial superinfection

B. Dehydration

C. Formation of granulomas in the lung

D. Damage to the heart muscle

Ans. B.

751. Which is not a major defence mechanism in the stomach?

A. Low pH B. Proteolytic enzymes

C. All of these D. Dense normal flora

Ans. D.

752. The nature of the poliovirus gives for oral vaccination (Sabin vaccine) as part of the eradication programme is

A. Live attenuated strains of all three immunological types

B. Heat killed virus

C. Formalin inactivated virus

D. Small dosage of wild type live viruses

Ans. A.

753. Both mycobacterium tuberculosis and streptococcus pneumoniae

A. Have cell walls that contain a high content of mycolic acid

B. Are acquired by inhalation

C. Stay in the lung and rarely, if ever, enter the bloodstream

D. Have polysaccharide capsules

Ans. B.

754. Novobiocin can be used against

A. Gram –ve Meningococci and Gonococci

B. Gram +ve Staphylococci

C. All of these

D. Haemophilus

Ans. C.

755. Which of the following methods would be most appropriate for sterilizing an antibiotic solution?

A. Microfiltration B. Dry heat sterilization

C. Desiccation D. Autoclaving

Ans. A.

756. Which of the following medium are used to differentiate the colonies of Vibrio cholerae and V. parahaemolyticus?

A. Thiosulphate citrate bile sucrose B. Alkaline bile salt

C. All of the above D. MacConkey

Ans. A.

757. The test(s) used for the assay of cholera toxin is/are

A. ELISA

B. RIA

C. All the above

D. Morphological changes in CHO (Chinese hamster ovary) cells

Ans. C.

758. Which of the following toxin resembles cholera toxin?

A. Diphtheria toxin
B. Stable toxin of E. coli
C. Tetanus toxin
D. Labile toxin of E. coli

Ans. D.

759. The DNA coding for the production of cholera toxin in Vibrio cholerae is on the

A. Plasmid
B. Phage
C. Transposon
D. Chromosome

Ans. D.

760. The transport medium for Vibrio cholerae can be

A. Selenite F broth
B. Venkatraman-Ramakrishnan medium
C. Nutrient broth
D. Tetrathionate broth

Ans. B.

761. Coliform bacteria on fermentation of carbohydrates yields

A. Acetic acid
B. Lactic acid
C. All of these
D. Formic acid

Ans. C.

762. The gram-positive bacteria lack ———— structure/component?

A. Murein
B. Outer membrane
C. Plasma membrane
D. Teichoic acid

Ans. B.

763. Which of the following is/are not a gram-positive bacteria?

A. Pseudomonas
B. Streptococci
C. None of the above
D. Mycobacteria

Ans. A.

764. Bacterial spoilage is identified by which of the following morphological characteristics?

A. Endospores
B. Encapsulation
C. All of these
D. Cell aggregation

Ans. C.

765. Which of the following bacteria can be typed by phage typing method?

A. Staphylococcus aureus
B. Salmonella typhi
C. Vibrio cholera
D. All of these

Ans. D.

3

Biochemistry

1. The macromolecules that require a template for their synthesis are

   A. Carbohydrate
   B. Lipids and carbohydrates
   C. Proteins
   D. Proteins and nucleic acids

Ans. D.

2. The macromolecules whose monomers are bound only by noncovalent forces are

   A. carbohydrates
   B. Lipids
   C. Carbohydrates and lipids
   D. Lipids and nucleic acid

Ans. B.

3. A nucleotide base not present in DNA is

   A. Adenine
   B. Guanine
   C. Uracil
   D. Thymine

Ans. C.

4. The polarity of DNA chains is represented by

   A. 3'-5'
   B. 2'-5'
   C. 1'-6'
   D. 2'-3'

Ans. A.

5. An amino acid that has a secondary amine and disrupts α helix formation is

   A. Glycine
   B. Phenylalanine
   C. Serine
   D. Proline

Ans. D.

6. Adenosine is

   A. A nitrogenous base
   B. A ribonucleotide
   C. A deoxyribonucleotide
   D. None of these

Ans. A.

7. The kind of nucleic acid that is represented by a clover leaf model

A. Mitochondrial DNA B. mRNA

C. tRNA D. rRNA

Ans. C.

8. Which of the following is not a characteristic of most DNA under physiological conditions?

A. A pairs with T by hydrogen atoms

B. 20 A° diameter

C. 3.4 A° pitch

D. 10 base pairs per turn of the helix

Ans. C.

9. RNA molecules differ from DNA molecules in all but which one of the following respects

A. Kinds of purine B. Kind of pyramidines

C. Number of strands per molecule D. Type of sugar

Ans. A.

10. What type of function do protein porins perform

A. Cytoskeletons B. Transport

C. Structural D. None of the above

Ans. B.

11. The degree of inhibition for non competitive inhibition of an enzyme catalysed reaction ?

A. Increase with increase in substrate concentration

B. Reaches with increase in substrate concentration

C. Reaches a maxima with increase in substrate concentration and then decreases

D. Decrease with increase in substrate concentration

Ans. C.

12. Enzyme papain is used with success to

A. To increase meat production B. Ripen papaya fruit

C. Leaven bread D. Tenderize meat

Ans. D.

13. Which one of the following reactions used for the purpose of recycling enzymes in bioprocesses

A. Isomerisation B. Phosphorylation

C. Immobolization D. Polymerization

Ans. C.

14. Which one of the following techniques is not ideal immobilized cell free enzymes?

    A. Physical entrapment by encapsulation

    B. Physical bonding by flocculation

    C. Covalent chemical bonding by cross linking the precipitate

    D. Covalent surface bonding to surface carriers

Ans. B.

15. Most industrial enzymes are obtained from

    A. Plants B. Microbes

    C. Insects D. Animal tissues

Ans. B.

16. Ki indicates

    A. Reaction velocity B. Competition inhibition

    C. Denaturation of enzyme D. All the above

Ans. B.

17. The phenomenon by which the synthesis of a set of enzyme leading to a product is

    A. Repression B. Suppression

    C. Depression D. None of the above

Ans. A.

18. de novo synthesis of an enzyme promoted by the substrate on which it acts is characterized by the term

    A. Induction B. Activation

    C. Gratuity D. Derepression

Ans. A.

19. Out of total enzymes present in the cell mitochondria alone has

    A. 4% B. 70%

    C. 95% D. Non enzyme

Ans. B.

20. Enzymes, vitamins and hormones can be classified into a single category of biological chemicals because all of them

    A. Aid in regulating metabolism B. Are synthesised in organism

    C. Are proteins D. Enhance the oxidation metabolism

Ans. C.

21. A nucleoside is

A. A nucleotide without sugar

B. A nucleotide without phosphate

C. A nucleotide without nitrogenous base

D. None of the above

Ans. B.

22. The adjacent nucleotides are joined by

A. Ionic bond

B. Hydrogen bond

C. Phosphodiester bond

D. All of these

Ans. C.

23. According to Chargaff's rule, in a DNA molecule

A. The amount of Adenine and Thymine = the amount of Guanine and Cytosine

B. Amount of Guanine and Cytosine = the amount of Adenine and Cytosine

C. The amount of Adenine and Guanine = the amount of Thymine and Cytosine

D. All of the above

Ans. C.

24. Watson and Cricks double helical DNA is a

A. A-DNA

B. B-DNA

C. Z-DNA

D. D-DNA

Ans. B.

25. The two strands in a DNA double helix are joined by

A. Hydrogen bonds between sugars

B. Phosphodiester bonds between sugars

C. Hydrogen bonds between bases

D. None of the above

Ans. C.

26. Who all got the Nobel prize for discovering the structure of DNA double helix

A. Watson and Crick

B. Watson, Crick and Wilkins

C. Watson, Crick and Franklin

D. Watson, Crick and Pauling

Ans. B.

27. The diameter of DNA helix is

A. 10 A°

B. 21 A°

C. 1 nm

D. 2 nm

Ans. D.

28. The distance between two adjacent nucleotide is
A. 6.8 A° B. 3.4 A°
C. 1.7 A° D. 10 A°

Ans. B.

29. DNA is
A. Positively charged B. Negatively charged
C. Neutral D. None of these

Ans. B.

30. Which of the following statement is true
A. The two DNA strands are parallel and complementary
B. The two DNA strand are antiparallel and non complementary
C. The two DNA strand are antiparallel and complementary
D. None of these

Ans. C.

31. Enzymes are
A. Carbohydrate B. RNA
C. Protein D. Fats

Ans. C.

32. The term enzymes are coined by
A. Pasteur B. Buchner
C. Urey Miller D. Kuhne

Ans. D.

33. The fastest enzymes is
A. Pepsin B. Carbonic anhydrase
C. DNA gyrase D. DNA polymerase

Ans. B.

34. Fat is hydrolysed by the enzyme known as
A. Trypsin B. Lipase
C. Pepsin D. Amylase

Ans. B.

35. The term apoenzyme is applicable to
A. Simple enzyme
B. Protein part of conjugate enzyme
C. Organic cofactor of a conjugate enzyme
D. Inorganic cofactor of a conjugate enzyme

Ans. B.

36. Enzymes
   A. Do not require activation energy
   B. Do not change requirement of activation energy
   C. Need increase requirement of activation energy
   D. Need lowest requirement of activation energy

Ans. D.

37. Zymogen is
   A. Enzyme poison
   B. Enzyme modulator
   C. Enzyme precursor
   D. Enzyme inhibitor

Ans. C.

38. Allosteric enzyme possesses
   A. Active site and an allosteric site
   B. Active site and two types allosteric sites
   C. Active site and three types allosteric sites
   D. Three types allosteric sites

Ans. B.

39. Enzymes generally have
   A. Same pH and temeprature optima
   B. Same pH but different temeprature optima
   C. Different pH but same temeprature optima
   D. Different pH and different temeprature optima

Ans. A.

40. The enzyme which forms the peptide bond is known as
   A. Carbonic unhydrase
   B. Peptidase
   C. Carbohydrase
   D. Peptidyl transferase

Ans. D.

41. The enzyme tyrosinase is activated by
   A. Iron
   B. Copper
   C. Zinc
   D. Potassium

Ans. B.

42. Lock and key theory of enzyme action was proposed by
   A. Fischer
   B. Koshland
   C. Kuhne
   D. Arrhenius

Ans. A.

43. Trypsin are active in

A. Acidic
B. Alkaline
C. Neutral
D. None of these

Ans. B.

44. Koshland's theory of enzyme action is known as

A. Reduced fit theory
B. Lock and key theory
C. Induced fit theory
D. Enzyme coenzyme theory

Ans. C.

45. The enzymes involved in feedback inhibition are called

A. Allosteric enzymes
B. Holoenzymes
C. Apoenzymes
D. Coenzymes

Ans. A.

46. Which one of the following is a group of proteolytic enzymes ?

A. Bromelin and Papain
B. Cellulase and myrosinase
C. Maltase and Diastase
D. Phosphatase and Chlorophyliase

Ans. A.

47. Enzymes having slightly different molecular structures but performing identical activity are

A. Holoenzymes
B. Apoenzymes
C. Isoenzymes
D. Coenzymes

Ans. C.

48. Which factor is responsible for inhibition enzymatic process during feed back ?

A. Enzymes
B. End products
C. Temperatures
D. Substrate

Ans. B.

49. Which one of the following statements regarding enzyme inhibition is correct ?

A. Competition inhibition is seen when a substrate competes with an enzyme for binding to a inhibitor protein

B. Noncompetitive inhibition of an enzyme can be overcome by adding large amount of substrate

C. Noncompetitive efficiency inhibitors often bind to the enzyme irreversibly

D. Competitive inhibition is seen when the substrate and the inhibitor compete for the active site on the enzyme

Ans. D.

50. The catalytic efficiency of two different enzymes can be compared by the

A. Formation of the product B. Km value

C. Molecular size of the enzymes D. pH of optimum value

Ans. B.

51. The nuclease enzyme which begins its attack from free of a polynuclotide is

A. Polymerase B. Kinase

C. Exonuclease D. Endonuclease

Ans. C.

52. The enzyme enterokinase helps in the conversion of

A. Caseinogens into casein B. Trypsinogen into trypsin

C. Pepsinogen into pepsin D. Protein into polypeptides

Ans. B.

53. Which of the following is a typical example 'feed back inhibition' ?

A. Cyaninde and cytochrome reaction

B. Sulpha drugs and folic acid synthesizer bacteria

C. Allosteric inhibition of hexokinase by glucose-6-phosphate

D. Reaction between succinic dehydrogenase and succinic acid

Ans. C.

54. Some of the enzymes which are associated in converting fats into carbohydrates are present in

A. Liposomes B. Golgi bodies

C. Glyoxysomes D. Microsomes

Ans. C.

55. In which one of the following enzymes, is copper necessarily associated as an activator ?

A. Tyrosinase B. Lactic dehydrogenase

C. Carbonic unhydrase D. Trypsinase

Ans. D.

56. A peptide bond

A. Has a partial double bond character

B. Is ionized at physiological pH

C. Is stable to heating in strong acids

D. Occurs most commonly in the cis configuration

Ans. A.

57. At neutral pH, a mixture of amino acids in solution would be predominantly

A. Hydrophobic
B. Negative and monovalent
C. Hydrophobic
D. Dipolar ions

Ans. D.

58. Which one of the following states of haemoglobin (Hb) binds oxygen with the greatest affinity

A. Hb
B. Hb(O)2
C. Hb(O2)2
D. Hb(O2)4

Ans. D.

59. Which of the following amino acids is most compatible with an α helical structure?

A. Proline
B. Tryptophan
C. Alanine
D. Cysteine

Ans. C.

60. Which of the following techniques is used to separate proteins based upon their mass ?

A. Isoelectric focussing
B. Western blotting
C. Ion exchange chromatography
D. SDS gel electrophoresis

Ans. D.

61. The greatest buffering capacity at physiologic pH would be provided by a protein rich in which of the following amino acids ?

A. Lysine
B. Aspartic acid
C. Valine
D. Histidine

Ans. D.

62. The site of enzyme modification by phosphorylation is the amino acid

A. Arginine
B. Cysteine
C. Phenylalanine
D. Serine

Ans. D.

63. Which of the following reagents would be most useful in determining the N terminal amino acid of polypeptide ?

A. Trypsin
B. Cyanogen bromide
C. 1 mol/L HCl
D. Phenylisothiocyanate

Ans. D.

64. Which of the following statements is correct ?

A. The helix can be composed of more than one polypeptide chain

B. β sheets exists only in the antiparallel form

C. Motifs are a type of secondary structure

D. β bends often contain proline

An D.

65. The highest concentration of cystine can be found in

A. Melanin B. Keratin

C. Myosin D. Collagen

Ans. B.

66. If the percentage of adenine in a DNA sample is 20% what would be the

A. T-30%, G-20%, C-30% B. T-40%, G-20%, C-20%

C. T-20%, G-30%, C-30% D. T-20%, G-20%, C-40%

Ans. C.

67. Which of the following statement is incorrect ?

A. DNA is the only biomolecules with self repair mechanism

B. DNA is autocatalytic

C. DNA is heterocatalytic

D. Increasing temperature to 90-100°C breaks phosphodiester bonds in DNA

Ans. D.

68. In a DNA sample, the percentage of bases is G-30% and C-40%. The most probable explanation is

A. Mutation might have occurred

B. The DNA sample may be a bacterial genome

C. The DNA sample may be a viral genome

D. None of the above

Ans. C.

69. Which of the following statement is true ?

A. DNA bases varies from one species to another

B. DNA bases of a species does not change with age, nutritional state and environment

C. DNA base remains same in different tissues of the same individual

D. All of these

Ans. D.

70. The negative charge of DNA is due to
   A. Sugar, phosphate and amino acids
   B. Deoxyribose sugar
   C. Nitrogenous bases specifically adenine
   D. Phosphate group

Ans. D.

71. The amount of DNA in a cell can be altered by
   A. Ecological factors
   B. Environmental factors
   C. Physiological factors
   D. can not be altered

Ans. D.

72. The amount of DNA of a cell at the beginning of mitosis is
   A. Half of the amount found in cells at G1 stage
   B. Same as the amount found in cells at G1 stage
   C. Twice the amount found in cells at G1 stage
   D. Four times the amount found in cells at G1 stage

Ans. C.

73. The DNA found in all living organism is
   A. Left handed DNA
   B. Right handed DNA
   C. Both A and B
   D. Z- DNA

Ans. B.

74. The DNA strand is directly involved in the formation of all except
   A. Protein
   B. Another DNA strand
   C. mRNA molecules
   D. tRNA molecules

Ans. A.

75. Which of the following statement is wrong ?
   A. A DNA is the dehydrated form of DNA
   B. The naturally occurring DNA is B-DNA and is also called as wet DNA
   C. Z DNA is also called zig-zag DNA and is a right handed helix
   D. Z DNA occurs in dehydrated high salt concentration

Ans. C.

76. RNA is the genetic material in
   A. Viruses only
   B. In some viruses and some prokaryotes
   C. In some viruses and some prokaryotes and rarely in eukaryotes
   D. Only in some viruses

Ans. D.

77. RNA is

A. Single stranded
B. Double stranded
C. Triple stranded
D. Both A and B

Ans. A.

78. The sugar in RNA is

A. Deoxyribose
B. Ribose
C. Hexose
D. Fructose

Ans. B.

79. Nucleotides in RNA are joined by

A. 3'-5' phosphodiester bond
B. 3'-4' phosphodiester bond
C. 3'-2' phosphodiester bond
D. 3'-6' phosphodiester bond

Ans. A.

80. Thymine in DNA is replaced by

A. Guanine in RNA
B. Adenine in RNA
C. Cytosine in RNA
D. Uracil in RNA

Ans. D.

81. The most abundant type of RNA in the cell is

A. rRNA
B. mRNA
C. tRNA
D. hnRNA

Ans. A.

82. Which of the following RNA serves as adaptor molecule during protein synthesis?

A. rRNA
B. mRNA
C. tRNA
D. hnRNA

Ans. C.

83. rRNA is synthesized in

A. Nucleus
B. Cytoplasm
C. RER
D. Nucleolus

Ans. D.

84. cDNA is

A. Complementary to mRNA
B. Complementary to rRNA
C. Complementary to tRNA
D. Complementary to hnRNA

Ans. A.

85. Amino acids are attached to the

A. Acceptor arm of tRNA
B. Anti-codon arm of tRNA
C. Codon arm of tRNA
D. None of these

Ans. A.

86. Ribozymes are

A. Enzymes with catalytic activity
B. RNAs with catalytic activity
C. Problems with catalytic activity
D. Nucleic acid with catalytic activity

Ans. B.

87. RNA is primarily seen in

A. Nucleus
B. Cytoplasm
C. RER
D. SER

Ans. B.

88. Ribose sugar in RNA is

A. D-ribose
B. L-ribose
C. Both L and D form
D. None of these

Ans. A.

89. Which of the virus has double stranded RNA as genetic material ?

A. Coronavinus
B. Reovinus
C. Adenovius
D. Picornavinus

Ans. B.

90. Fats are abundantly found in

A. Reproductive tissue
B. Vegetative tissue
C. Both A and B
D. None of these

Ans. A.

91. Natural lipids are readily soluble in

A. Oil
B. Mercury
C. Water
D. None of these

Ans. D.

92. Which of the following is/are unsaturated fatty acids ?

A. Linoleic acid
B. Oleic acid
C. Palmitoleic
D. All of these

Ans. D.

93. Fats can be stored in the cell without disturbing their

A. Hydroxyl bond
B. Aleurone layer
C. Osmotic relations
D. None of these

Ans. C.

94. Liquid form of triglycerides at ordinary room temperature are called

A. Oils
B. Solid
C. Fats
D. None of these

Ans. A.

95. The synthesis of glucose from fat is called

A. Glycolysis
B. Kreb's cycle
C. Saponification
D. Gluconeogenesis

Ans. D.

96. Hydrolysis of fats by alkalies into fatty acids and glycerol is called

A. Coagulation
B. Saponification
C. Suspension
D. Colloidal

Ans. B.

97. The fats and oils are respectively rich in

A. Unsaturated fatty acids
B. Saturated fatty acids
C. Saturated and unsaturated fatty acids
D. None of these

Ans. C.

98. β oxidation takes place in

A. Mitochondria
B. cytoplasm
C. chloroplasts
D. nucleus

Ans. A.

99. Which is a phospholipid ?

A. Lecithin
B. Cholesterol
C. Sterol
D. Steroid

Ans. A.

100. The number of double bonds in Arachidonic acid

A. 1
B. 2
C. 3
D. 4

Ans. D.

101. Essential fatty acids are

A. Linoleic acid
B. Arachidonic acid
C. Linolenic acid
D. All of these

Ans. D.

102. Which of the following is not a phospholipid ?

A. Sphingomyelin
B. Lecithin
C. Cephalin
D. Cerebroside

Ans. D.

103. Which one of the following is a monosaturated fatty acid ?

A. Oleic acid
B. Arachidonic acid
C. Palmitic acid
D. Linolenic acid

Ans. A.

104. High content of Triglycerides are seen in

A. LDL
B. HDL
C. VLDL
D. Chylomicrons

Ans. D.

105. The repeating units of proteins are

A. Glucose units
B. Amino acids
C. Fatty acids
D. Peptides

Ans. B.

106. Amino acids are joined by

A. Peptide bond
B. Hydrogen bond
C. Ionic bond
D. Glycosidic bond

Ans. A.

107. The primary structure of protein represents

A. Linear sequence of amino acids joined by peptide bond
B. 3 –dimensional structure of protein
C. Helical structure of protein
D. Subunit structure of protein

Ans. A.

108. Peptide bond is

A. Rigid with partial double bond character

B. Planer, covalent

C. Covalent

D. All of the above

Ans. D.

109. Enzymes are

A. Protein
B. Carbohydrate
C. Nucleic acids
D. DNA molecules

Ans. A.

110. The first protein sequenced by F. Sanger is

A. Haemoglobin
B. Myoglobin
C. Insulin
D. Myosin

Ans. C.

111. A dipeptide has

A. 2 amino acids and 1 peptide bond

B. 2 amino acids and 2 peptide bond

C. 2 amino acids and 3 peptide bond

D. 2 amino acids and 4 peptide bond

Ans. A.

112. The most common secondary structure is

A. α helix
B. β pleated sheet
C. β pleated sheet parallel
D. β pleated sheet anti-parallel

Ans. A.

113. Myoglobin is a

A. Protein with primary structure
B. Protein with secondary structure
C. Protein with tertiary structure
D. Protein with quaternary structure

Ans. C.

114. Fibrous protein such as silk fibroin consists of polypeptide chains arranged in

A. α helix
B. β pleated sheet
C. β helix
D. None of the above

Ans. B.

115. Tertiary structure is maintained by

A. Peptide bond
B. Hydrogen bond
C. Di-sulphide bond
D. All of the above

Ans. D.

116. Haemoglobin has

A. Primary structure
B. Secondary structure
C. Tertiary structure
D. All of the above

Ans. D.

117. Disulphide bonds are formed between

A. Cysteine residues that are close together
B. Cystine residues that are close together
C. Proline residues that are close together
D. Histidine residues that are close together

Ans. A.

118. The 3-D structure of protein can be determined by

A. Nuclear magnetic resonance
B. X ray crystallography
C. Both A and B
D. Spectroscopy

Ans. C.

119. 4-hydroxy proline is present in

A. Collagen
B. Plant cell wall
C. Keratin
D. Both Plant cell wall and Collagen

Ans. D.

120. Peptide bonds between amino acids are highly stable and have a half life of seven years in intracellular condition. This is due to

A. High activation energy required for hydrolysis
B. Low activation energy required for hydrolysis
C. Peptide bond is a covalent bond
D. Peptide bond is rigid and planar

Ans. A.

121. Tri-peptide consists

A. 3 amino acids and 3 peptide bonds
B. 2 amino acids and 3 peptide bonds
C. 3 amino acids and 2 peptide bonds
D. 3 amino acids and 4 peptide bonds

Ans. C.

122. All the following statements are true except

A. Ornithine and citruline are uncommon amino acids

B. Ornithine is an intermediate in Urea cycle

C. Ornithine and citruline are uncommon amino acids present in many proteins

D. Both Ornithine and citruline are intermediates in Urea cycle

Ans. C.

123. The characteristic strong absorbance of 280 nm of proteins is due to

A. All amino acids can absorb at 280 nm

B. Only tryptophan and tyrosine can absorb at 280nm

C. Tryptophan is responsible for the absorbance

D. Tryptophan, tyrosine and phenylalanine can absorb at 280nm

Ans. D.

124. The formation of cystine occurs at

A. ER B. Golgi

C. Cytosol D. Mitochondria

Ans. A.

125. Which of the following interaction contributes most in protein folding

A. Covalent bond B. Ionic bond

C. Hydrophobic interaction D. Van der walls interaction

Ans. C.

126. Which of the following amino acid has pKa near neutrality ?

A. Tryptophan B. Arginine

C. Histidine D. Asparagine

Ans. C.

127. Desmosine is an unusual amino acid found in

A. Myosin B. Elastin

C. Troponin D. Actin

Ans. B.

128. How many small peptides are formed upon cleavage by trypsin if a protein has 5 lysine residues

A. 4 B. 5

C. 6 D. 7

Ans. C.

129. EF-1 α and EF-Tu are

A. Analogs
B. Homologs
C. Paralogs
D. Syllogs

Ans. B.

130. All statements regarding peptide bond are true except

A. Peptide bond is a covalent bond
B. Peptide bond is rigid and planar
C. Peptide bond has partial double bond character
D. Peptide bond is formed by noncondensation reaction

Ans. D.

131. Alpha helix has

A. 3.6 residues per turn and is a right handed helix
B. 3.8 residues per turn and is a right handed helix
C. 3.6 residues per turn and is a left handed helix
D. 3.8 residues per turn and is a left handed helix

Ans. A.

132. Which of the following amino acids are rarely present in alpha helix

A. Glycine and proline
B. Proline and tryptophan
C. Tryptophan and glycine
D. Proline only

Ans. A.

133. PDI is an enzyme involve in

A. Protein synthesis
B. Protein degradation
C. Protein folding
D. Protein quaternary structure formation

Ans. C.

134. A prosthetic part of a protein in a non protein structure that is

A. A ligand of the protein
B. A part of the secondary structure of the protein
C. A substrate of the protein
D. Permanently associated with the protein

Ans. D.

135. In the bonding of oxygen to myoglobin, the relationship between the concentration of oxygen and the fraction of binding sites occupied can best be described as

A. Hyperbolic
B. Linear with a negative slope
C. Linear with a positive slope
D. Sigmoidal

Ans. A.

136. Myoglobin and subunits of hemoglobin have

A. No obvious structural relationship

B. Very different primary and tertiary structures

C. Very similar primary and tertiary structures

D. Very similar tertiary structures but different primary structures

Ans. D.

137. In hemoglobin the transition from T state to R state (low to high affinity) is triggered by

A. Fe2+ binding

B. Heme binding

C. Oxygen binding

D. Subunit association

Ans. C.

138. Which of the following is not correct concerning cooperative binding of a ligand to a protein ?

A. It is usually a form of allosteric interaction

B. It is usually associated with proteins with multiple subunits

C. It rarely occurs in enzymes

D. It results in a nonlinear Hill Plot

Ans. C.

139. The fundamental cause of sickle cell disease is a change in the structure of

A. Blood

B. Capillaries

C. Hemoglobin

D. Red cells

Ans. C.

140. The protein of the MHC bind and display

A. Antigen segments

B. B cells fragments

C. Immunoglobulin fragments

D. Macrophage fragments

Ans. A.

141. A monoclonal antibody differs from a polyclonal antibody in that monoclonal antibodies

A. Are labeled with chemicals that can be visualized

B. Are produced by cells from the same organism that produced the antigen

C. Are synthesized by a population of identical or cloned cells

D. Are synthesized only in living organisms

Ans. C.

142. The predominant structural feature in myosin molecules is

A. A β structure
B. An α helix
C. The Fab domain
D. The light chain

Ans. B.

143. During muscle contraction, hydrolysis of ATP results in a change in the

A. Conformation of actin
B. Conformation of myosin
C. Structure of myofibrils
D. Structure of sarcoplasmic reticulum

Ans. B.

144. The process of sorting and transporting newly synthesized proteins to correct destination in a cell is called

A. Protein sorting
B. Protein targeting
C. Protein trafficking
D. All of these

Ans. D.

145. Proteins required in the cytosol like the enzymes of glycolysis are synthesized on

A. Ribosomes on endoplasmic reticulum
B. SER
C. Free ribosomes in the cytosol
D. Ribosomes on nuclear membrane

Ans. C.

146. Secretory protein are synthesized by

A. Free ribosome
B. Ribosomes on endoplasmic reticulum
C. Ribosomes on nuclear membrane
D. all of the above

Ans. B.

147. Choose the correct order of transport of protein in a secretory pathways ?

A. Protein synthesized in the cytoplasm→SER lumen→RER lumen→cis golgi→median golgi→trans golgi→vesicles→fusion of vesicles with plasma membrane→exocytosis

B. Protein synthesized in the cytoplasm→RER lumen→cis golgi→median golgi→trans golgi→vesicles→fusion of vesicles with plasma membrane→ exocytosis

C. Protein synthesized in the cytoplasm→vesicles→SER→RER lumen→cis golgi→median golgi→trans golgi→vesicles→fusion of vesicles with plasma membrane→exocytosis

D. Protein synthesized in the cytoplasm→RER lumen→trans golgi→median golgi→cis golgi→vesicles→fusion of vesicles with plasma membrane→ exocytosis

Ans. B.

148. According to signal hypothesis, the signal peptide for a secretory protein is

A. Rich in hydrophobic amino acids at the centre of the signal peptide and is attached to the N terminal of the protein

B. Rich in hydrophilic amino acids at the centre of the signal peptide and is attached to the N terminal of the protein

C. Rich in hydrophobic amino acids at the centre of the signal peptide and is attached to the C terminal of the protein

D. Rich in sulphur containing amino acids at the centre of the signal peptide and is attached to the N terminal of the protein

Ans. A.

149. Signal sequences are

A. Short peptide sequences that serves as an address for transporting newly synthesized protein to the correct location

B. Glycoproteins that serves as an address for transporting newly synthesized protein to the correct location

C. Short peptide sequences to transport a protein to the nucleus

D. Short peptide sequences attached to a protein that initiates its degradation by digestive enzymes

Ans. A.

150. The retention signal of proteins of endoplasmic reticulum consists of amino acids

A. Gly-Asp-Glu-Leu at the N terminus

B. Lys-Asp-Glu-Leu at the N terminus

C. Gly-Asp-Glu-Leu at the C terminus

D. Lys-Asp-Glu-Leu at the C terminus

Ans. D.

151. Protein tagged with mannose 6-phosphate are transported to

A. Nucleus
B. Lysosome
C. Mitochondrion
D. Golgi apparatus

Ans. B.

152. Nuclear localization signal that ensures transport of a protein to nucleus is rich in

A. Lysine and arginine
B. Glutamine and asparagines
C. Serine and threonine
D. Tryptophan and histidine

Ans. A.

153. Proteins targeted to mitochondrial matrix are tagged with matrix targeting sequence rich in

A. Serine and threonine

B. Serine, threonine, lysine and arginine

C. Serine, threonine , glutamine and asparagine

D. Serine, threonine, tryptophan and histidine

Ans. B.

154. Protein purification refers to the

A. Purification of proteins

B. Separation of protein from other biomolecules

C. Separation of a particular protein from other contaminating proteins

D. All of these

Ans. C.

155. Protein separation techniques are often based on the following properties except

A. Solubility of the protein

B. Viscosity of protein

C. Charge of protein

D. Specific binding affinity of the protein

Ans. B.

156. Primary steps in protein purification includes

A. Homogenization

B. Differential centrifugation

C. Solubilization

D. All of these

Ans. D.

157. Which of the following detergent is commonly used to release integral proteins from its membranes ?

A. Urea

B. Dimethyl sulphoxide

C. TritonX100

D. Cyanogens bromide

Ans. C.

158. Salting out process involves

A. Precipitation of proteins using ammonium sulphate

B. Precipitation of proteins using copper sulphate

C. Precipitation of proteins using sodium chloride

D. None of these

Ans. A.

159. Which of the following separation method is suited for a protein sample with large differences in molecular mass

A. Dialysis
B. Salting out process
C. Density gradient centrifugation
D. Rate zonal centrifugation

Ans. D.

160. In which of the following separation method, proteins are separated on the basis of their charges ?

A. Affinity chromatography
B. Ion exchange Chromatography
C. Dialysis
D. Gel filtration chromatography

Ans. B.

161. In gel filtration chromatography, separation of proteins are based on their

A. Size and net charge
B. Size and shape
C. Size and specific affinity
D. Shape and net charge

Ans. B.

162. The use of insulin hormone to purify its receptor is an example of

A. Ion exchange Chromatography
B. Affinity chromatography
C. Gel filtration chromatography
D. Ligand mediated chromatography

Ans. B.

163. In anion exchange chromatography

A. The column contains negatively charged beads where positively charged proteins bind
B. The column contains positively charged beads where negatively charged proteins bind
C. The column contains both positively and negatively charged beads where proteins bind depending on their net charge
D. All of these

Ans. B.

164. For the study of a protein in detail, first an effort is usually made to

A. Conjugate the protein to a known molecule
B. Determine its amino acid composition
C. Determine its amino acid sequence
D. Determine its molecular weight
E. Purify of protein

Ans. E.

165. In a mixture of the five proteins listed below, which should elute second in size exclusion (gel filtration) chromatography ?

A. Cytochrome C Mr =13000 B. IgG Mr = 145000

C. Ribonuclease A Mr = 13700 D. RNA polymerase Mr =450000

E. Serum albumin Mr =68500

Ans. B.

166. By adding SDS during the electrophoresis of protein, it is possible to

A. Determine a protein's isoelectric point

B. Determine an enzyme's specific activity

C. Determine the determine composition of the protein

D. Preserve a protein's native structure and biological activity

E. Separate protein's exclusively on the basis of molecular weight

Ans. E.

167. To determine the isoelectric point of a protein first establish that a gel

A. Contains a denaturing detergent that can distribute uniform negative charges over the protein's surface

B. Exhibits a stable pH gradient when ampholytes become distributed in an electric field

C. Is washed with an antibody specific to the protein of interest

D. Neutralizes all ionic groups on a protein by titrating them with strong bases

E. Relates the unknown protein to a series of protein markers with known molecular weights Mr

Ans. B.

168. The first step in two dimensional gel electrophoresis generates a series of protein bands by isoelectric focusing. In a second step, a strip of this is turned 90o placed on another gel containing SDS and electric current is again applied. In this second step

A. Protein with similar isoelectric points become further separated according to their molecular weights

B. The individual bands become stained so that the isoelectric focus pattern can be visualized

C. The individual bands undergo a second more intense isoelectric focusing

D. The proteins in the bands separate more completely because the second electric current in the opposite polarity to the first current

Ans. A.

169. The term specific activity differs from the term activity in that specific activity

A. Is measured only under optimal conditions

B. Is the activity (enzyme units) in a milligram of protein

C. Refers only to a purified protein

D. Refers to proteins other than enzyme

Ans. B.

170. In isoelectric focusing separation of proteins are based on

A. Relative content of positively charged groups

B. Relative content of negatively charged groups

C. Both A and B

D. d. pH

E. None of the above

Ans. C.

171. Which of the following statement is incorrect ?

A. In affinity chromatography, lectins are used to purify a glycoprotein

B. The separation in gel filtration chromatography is based on size, shape and net charge of the protein

C. In ion exchange chromatography, the bound protein are eluted using NaCl solution

D. In affinity chromatography, the binding of a protein to a ligand is by specific non-covalent interactions

E. All of these

Ans. B.

172. Carbohydrates are organic compounds made up of

A. Carbon and hydrogen

B. Carbon, hydrogen and oxygen

C. Carbon, hydrogen, oxygen and nitrogen

D. Carbon and oxygen

Ans. C.

173. The most common monomer of carbohydrate is

A. Nucleotides

B. Glucose

C. Amino acids

D. Maltose

Ans. B.

174. Monosaccharides are

A. Aldoses B. Ketoses

C. Both A and B D. none of these

Ans. C.

175. The minimum number of carbon in a monosaccharide is

A. 1 B. 2

C. 3 D. 4

Ans. C.

176. All the following are monosaccharides except

A. Glucose B. Fructose

C. Maltose D. Galactose

Ans. C.

177. Two monosaccharides are joined by

A. Peptide bond B. Phosphodiester bond

C. Glycosidic bond D. Hydrogen bond

Ans. C.

178. All the following are reducing sugars except

A. Glucose B. Maltose

C. Sucrose D. Lactose

Ans. C.

179. Sucrose is disaccharide made up of

A. Glucose and fructose B. Glucose and lactose

C. Glucose and glucose D. Glucose and galactose

Ans. A.

180. All the following are storage polysaccharides except

A. Starch B. Cellulose

C. Glycogen D. Dextran

Ans. D.

181. Carbohydrates occur naturally in

A. D-form B. L-form

C. Both A and B D. None of these

Ans. B.

182. Amino acids are

A. Building blocks of carbohydrates B. Building blocks of nucleic acids

C. Building blocks of lipids D. Building blocks of proteins

Ans. D.

183. Amino acids has

A. Both amino group and carboxyl group

B. both amino group and keto group

C. amino group only

D. carboxyl group only

Ans. A.

184. The simplest amino acid is

A. Proline B. Methionine

C. Glycine D. Serine

Ans. C.

185. Which of the following amino acid is α helix terminator ?

A. Tryptophan B. Phenylalanine

C. Tyrosine D. Proline

Ans. D.

186. The first amino acid in a polypeptide chain is

A. Serine B. Valine

C. Alanine D. Methionine

Ans. D.

187. Which of the following amino acid has buffering capacity ?

A. Tryptophan B. Cysteine

C. Histidine D. Arginine

Ans. C.

188. Which of the following is an α imino acid ?

A. Serine B. Threonine

C. Valine D. Proline

Ans. D.

189. The naturally occurring form of amino acid in proteins

A. L-amino acids only B. D- amino acids only

C. Both L and D amino acids D. None of these

Ans. A.

190. Sulphur containing amino acids are

A. Cysteine and methionine
B. Methionine and threonine
C. Cysteine and threonine
D. Cysteine and serine

Ans. A.

191. Aromatic amino acids include

A. Phenylalanine, tyrosine and tryptophan
B. Phenylalanine, serine and tryptophan
C. Threonine, tyrosine and tryptophan
D. Asparagine, tyrosine and tryptophan

Ans. A.

192. Positively charged basic amino acids are

A. Lysine and arginine
B. Lysine and asparagine
C. Glutamine and arginine
D. Lysine and Glutamine

Ans. A.

193. Acidic amino acids include

A. Asparagine and glutamate
B. Aspartate and asparagine
C. Aspartate and lysine
D. Aspartate and glutamate

Ans. D.

194. Amino acids with hydroxyl groups are

A. Serine and alanine
B. Alanine and valine
C. Serine and threonine
D. Valine and isoleucine

Ans. C.

195. The 21st amino acid is

A. Hydroxylysine
B. Hydroxylproline
C. Selenocysteine
D. Citruline

Ans. C.

196. Absorbance at 260 nm exhibited by protein is due to

A. Aliphatic amino acid
B. All amino acids
C. Non polar amino acids
D. Aromatic amino acids

Ans. D.

197. Which of the following statement is true when a cell is kept in hypotonic solution?

A. Water moves out of the cell

B. Size of the cell remains same

C. No movement of water takes place

D. Size of the cell increases

Ans. D.

198. Which one of the following amino acids has a higher propensity for cis peptide bond formation ?

A. Histidine
B. Cysteine
C. Glycine
D. Proline

Ans. D.

199. The length of an alpha helix composed of 36 amino acid residues is

A. 10A°
B. 54A°
C. 27A°
D. 360A°

Ans. D.

200. Which one of the following amino acid residues is specifically recognized by chymotrypsin during peptide bond cleavage ?

A. Phe
B. Leu
C. Val
D. Asp

Ans. A.

201. During the biosynthesis of urea in the urea cycle, the two nitrogen atoms are derived from

A. Two free ammonium groups

B. Free ammonium group and aspartate

C. Both nitrogen atoms are derived from arginine

D. One nitrogen atom is derived from citrulline and one from glutamate

Ans. B.

202. An enzyme has two binding sites for an inhibitor molecule. When the inhibitor binds to the first site, the dissociation constant of the inhibitor for the second site increases, leading to negative co-operativity. The Hill coefficient for such an inhibitor is

A. Equal to one
B. Greater than 1
C. Less than one
D. Less than zero

Ans. C.

203. In different types of tissue transplantations, the rate of graft rejection in decreasing order is

A. Isograft> Xenograft> Allograft B. Allograft> Isograft> Xenograft

C. Xenograft> Autograft> Allograft D. Xenograft> Allograft> Isograft

Ans. D.

204. Arrange the following in the decreasing order of their permeability coefficients across a lipid bilayer membrane

(i) Urea (ii) Glucose

(iii) H2O (iv) Na+

(v) Tryptophan

A. (i), (iii), (v), (ii), (iv) B. (iii), (v), (ii), (iv), (i)

C. (iii), (i), (v), (ii), (iv) D. (i), (iii), (iv), (v), (ii)

Ans. C.

205. Match the following enzymes with their regulatory mechanism

(a) Phosphofructokinase 1. Product inhibition

(b) Glycogen synthetase 2. Control of enzyme synthesis

(c) Beta galatosidase 3. Allosteric interaction

(d) Lactate dehydrogenase 4. Covalent modification

A. (a)3, (b) 2, (c) 1 (d) 4 B. (a)3, (b) 4, (c) 2 (d) 1

C. (a)4, (b) 3, (c) 1 (d) 2 D. (a) 4, (b) 1, (c) 2 (d) 3

Ans. B.

206. A researcher wants to clone 3 DNA fragments of sizes 1.1 Mb, 0.097 Mb and 0.045 Mb. The choice of the vectors for cloning

A. Cosmid, bacteriophage lambda, bacteriophage P1

B. Yeast artificial chromosome, bacteriophage lambda, cosmid

C. Bacterial artificial chromosome, bacteriophage lambda, Yeast artificial chromosome

D. Only plasmids

Ans. B.

207. Which of the four restriction enzymes given below cut the following DNA sequence? 5' CCGATATCTCGAGGGC 3'

1. BamHI (3'CCTAG^G-5') 2. Xho I (3' GAGCT^C5')

3. Eco RI (3' CTTAA^G5') 4. EcoRV (3' CTA^TAG5')

A. 1 and 2 B. 1, 3 and 4

C. 2 and 4 D. 1, 2 and 3

Ans. C.

208. An enzyme of 40 kDa is added to a substrate solution in a molar ratio of 1:3. The concentration of the enzyme in the mixture is 12 mg/ml. What would be the corresponding substrate concentration ?

A. 0.4 mM
B. 0.12 mM
C. 0.9 mM
D. 0.3 mM

Ans. C.

209. Which of the following mineral element facilitates insulin binding to cell receptor site ?

A. Zinc
B. Selenium
C. Copper
D. Chromium

Ans. D.

210. Which of the following is a folate analog?

A. Carnosine
B. Aniserine
C. Azaserine
D. Methotrexate

Ans. D.

211. ATP concentration is maintained relatively constant during muscle contraction by

A. Increasing the metabolic activity
B. The action of creatine phosphokinase
C. The action of adenylate phosphokinase
D. All of the above

Ans. D.

212. The cone of retina

A. Are responsible for colour vision
B. Are much more numerous than rods
C. Have red, blue and green light sensitive pigment that differ because of small difference in the retinal prosthetic group
D. Do not use transduction in signal transduction

Ans. A.

213. The major protein responsible for the storage of iron

A. Ferredoxin
B. Ferritin
C. Hemosiderine
D. Transferrin

Ans. B.

214. Which of the following is an excitatory neurotransmitter ?

A. Glutamate
B. GABA
C. Glycine
D. Taurine

Ans. A.

215. The preferred substrate for hexokinase is

A. Glucose
B. Fructose
C. Glucose and fructose are equally preferred
D. None of these

Ans. A.

216. The general chemical formula of carbohydrate is

A. $(CH_2O)n$
B. $(CH_2O)2n$
C. (CHO)n
D. Cn H_2n O

Ans. A.

217. Which of the following is an aldotriose ?

A. Dihydroxyacetone
B. Glyceraldehyde
C. Ribulose
D. Erythrose

Ans. B.

218. What is the molecular formula of sucrose ?

A. $C_{12}H_{22}O_{11}$
B. $C_{10}H_{20}O_{10}$
C. $C_6H_{12}O_6$
D. $C_{12}H_{20}O_{11}$

Ans. A.

219. The glycosidic linkage between glucose molecule is

A. β1-4
B. α 1-2
C. α 1-4
D. β1-2

Ans. C.

220. A keto pentose will have ——— sterioisomers.

A. 4
B. 6
C. 8
D. 10

Ans. A.

221. The reserve food material of green algae is

A. Laminarin
B. Chrysolaminarin
C. Floridian starch
D. Starch

Ans. D. Laminarin – reserve food material of brown algae. Chrysolaminarin-reserve food material of diatoms. Floridian starch -reserve food material of red algae.

222. The only carbohydrate which is not having any chiral carbon atom is

A. Glutaraldehyde B. Erythrose
C. Dihydroxyacetone D. Erythrulose

Ans. C. All carbohydrates except dihydroxyacetone (a ketotriose) will have atleast one chiral centre.

223. Select the odd one from the following

A. Arabinose B. Xylose
C. Lyxose D. Erythrose

Ans. D. Erythrose is an aldo tetrose. Rest are aldo pentoses.

224. A pentose sugar reported to be present in heart cell

A. Xylose B. Arabinose
C. Lyxose D. Xylulose

Ans. C.

225. Which of the following is an epimeric pair ?

A. D-glucose and D-mannose B. D-glucose and D-galactose
C. D-glucose and D-glucose D. Both A and B

Ans. D.

226. Select the odd one from the following

A. Xylulose B. Dihydroxyacetone
C. Glyceraldehyde D. Ribulose

Ans. C.

227. Which of the following sugar give a positive result with Seliwanoff test ?

A. Sucrose B. Glucose
C. Galactose D. Mannose

Ans. A.

228. Which of the following is a keto tetrose ?

A. Erythrulose B. Xylulose
C. Sorbose D. Psicose

Ans. A.

229. The glycosidic linkage between two glucose molecules in isomaltose is

A. α1-4 B. β1-4
C. α1-6 D. β1-6

Ans. C.

230. Which of the following is an alpha lactone ?

A. Vit C B. Vit D

C. Vit A D. Vit K

Ans. A.

231. A sweetener used in sugar less gums and candies

A. Ribitol B. Xylitol

C. Inositol D. Mannitol

Ans. B. Ribitol, Xylitol, Inositol and Mannitol are sugar alcohols.

232. The glycosidic linkage in cellobiose is

A. α 1-4 B. β1-4

C. α 1-6 D. β1-6

Ans. B.

233. Pick out the odd one from the following

A. Deoxyribose B. Rhamnose

C. Fucose D. Altrose

Ans. D. Altrose is aldo hexose sugar. Rest are deoxysugars.

234. Lectins are ———.

A. Sugars specific to proteins

B. Proteins specific to sugars

C. Enzymes specific to carbohydrates

D. Carbohydrates specific to enzymes

Ans. B.

235. Which of the following is a keto triose ?

A. Dihydroxyacetone B. Glyceraldehyde

C. Ribulose D. Erythrose

Ans. A.

236. Maltose is a disaccharide of ———

A. Glucose and galactose B. Glucose and glucose

C. Glucose and lactose D. Fructose and lactose

Ans. B.

237. Glycosidic bond in sucrose is ———.

A. α 1-4 B. β 1-4

C. α 1-2 D. β 1-2

Ans. C.

238. Minimum number of carbon required for a ketose sugar to have cyclic structure is

A. 3 B. 4

C. 5 D. 6

Ans. C.

239. An aldo hexose will have ——— stereoisomers

A. 8 B. 10

C. 14 D. 16

Ans. D.

240. Minimum number of carbon required for a monosaccharide

A. 1 B. 2

C. 3 D. 4

Ans. C.

241. The vitreous humor of eye is composed of———.

A. Heparin B. Hyaluronic acid

C. Keratan sulphate D. Chondroitin sulphate

Ans. B.

242. N acetyl glucosamine (NAG) and N acetyl muramic acid (NAM) in peptidoglycan is connected by——— glycosidic linkage.

A. α 1-4 B. β 1-4

C. α 1-2 D. β 1-2

Ans. B.

243. Sulbactam is a ————.

A. β lactam antibiotic B. β lactamase

C. β lactamase inhibitor D. A class of penicillin

Ans. C.

244. Which of the following is not a sugar molecule of the O antigen of gram negative bacteria ?

A. Tyvelose B. Abequose

C. 2Keto-3-deoxyoctanoate D. Teichoic acid

Ans. D.

245. Glycosidic bond between galactose and glucose in lactose is ———.

A. α 1-4 B. β 1-4

C. α 1-2 D. β 1-2

Ans. B.

246. Which one of the following is a sugar alcohol ?

A. Arabitol
B. Manitol
C. Sorbitol
D. All of these

Ans. D.

247. Minimum number of carbons required for an aldose sugar to have a cyclic structure is ——.

A. 3
B. 4
C. 5
D. 6

Ans. B.

248. The reserve food materials of red algae is ————.

A. Laminarin
B. Chrysolaminarin
C. Floridian starch
D. Starch

Ans. C.

249. Reserve food material of fungi is ———.

A. Glucose
B. Starch
C. Laminarin
D. Glycogen

Ans. D.

250. Glycosidic bond in trehalose is ———.

A. α 1-4
B. α 1-2
C. α 1-1
D. β 1-2

Ans. C.

251. Which of the following is a non-reducing sugar ?

A. Maltose
B. Lactose
C. Trehalose
D. Cellobiose

Ans. C.

252. A disaccharide of galactose and fructose joined by β 1-4 glycosidic linkage :

A. Trehalose
B. Lactulose
C. Gentiobiose
D. Melibiose

Ans. B.

253. Which of the following sugar do not form cyclic structure ?

A. Erythrulose
B. Dihydroxyacetone
C. Both A and B
D. Erythrose

Ans. C.

254. A disaccharide of two glucose molecules joined by β 1-6 glycosidic linkage :

A. Trehalose
B. Gentiobiose
C. Lactulose
D. Melibiose

Ans. B.

255. Glycerol moieties in Teichoic acid of bacterial cell wall are linked each other by ——

A. Ether bonds
B. Ester bonds
C. Phosphodiester bonds
D. Glycosidic bonds

Ans. C.

256. A disaccharide of galactose and glucose in a α1-6 glycosidic linkage :

A. Lactose
B. Melibiose
C. Gentiobiose
D. Vasbascose

Ans. B.

257. Which of the following sequence correctly represent the sweetness of glucose, sucrose and fructose ?

A. Glucose $<$ Sucrose $<$ Fructose
B. Sucrose $<$ Glucose $<$ Fructose
C. Glucose $\leq$ Sucrose $<$ Fructose
D. Glucose $>$ Fructose $>$ Sucrose

Ans. A.

258. After osazone test, the sample sugar gave needle shaped crystals, the sample sugar will be——.

A. Glucose
B. Fructose
C. Maltose
D. Cellulose

Ans. A.

259. Partial fermentation of cane sugar by Leuconostoc mesenteroides produce :

A. Glucose and fructose
B. Glucose and gluconic acid
C. Fructose and gluconic acid
D. Dextran

Ans. D.

260. Which of the following commonly acts as the precursor for the synthesis of Vitamin C in plants ?

A. Fructose
B. Ribose
C. Glucose
D. Ribulose

Ans. C.

261. Which of the following is an example for a trisaccharide ?

A. Verbascose
B. Stachyose
C. Raffinose
D. Sucralose

Ans. C.

262. Chrysolaminarin is ——————.

A. A storage polysaccharide of green algae
B. A storage polysaccharide of brown algae
C. A storage polysaccharide of red algae
D. A storage polysaccharide of diatoms

Ans. D.

263. Which of the following is an example for an artificial sweetener of saccharide origin ?

A. Sucralose
B. Saccharin
C. Stachyose
D. All of these

Ans. D.

264. In a chemical reaction 'X' is able to convert Cu2+ ions to Cu+ ions. If X is a carbohydrate, which of the following best explains to be the 'X' ?

A. X is a reducing sugar
B. X is a non reducing sugar
C. X is a monosaccharide
D. Both A and B
E. Both A and C

Ans. E.

265. Which of the following is a reducing sugar ?

A. Glucose in closed ring form
B. Glucose in open chain form
C. Sucrose

Ans. B.

266. Most prominent carbohydrate component of hemicelluloses is

A. Pectin
B. Arabinose
C. Arabinoxylan
D. Suberin

Ans. C.

267. Which of the following is an example for heteropolysaccharide ?

A. Hyaluronic acid
B. Gelatin
C. Glycogen
D. Both A and B

Ans. A.

268. Glucose on oxidation with bromine water form

A. Glucuronic acid B. Glucosaccharic acid

C. Gluconic acid D. Mannose

Ans. C.

269. Dextrin is a branched bacterial homopolysaccharide of — linked D-glucose with —— branches.

A. α 1-6 and α 1-3 B. β1-6 and β1-3

C. β1-6 and α 1-3 D. α 1-6 and β 1-3

Ans. A.

270. Laminarin is ——

A. A storage polysaccharide of red algae

B. A storage polysaccharide of brown algae

C. A structural polysaccharide of red algae

D. A structural polysaccharide of brown algae

Ans. B.

271. Which of the following statements are true about agarose ?

A. It is a branched polysaccharide

B. It is a linear polysaccharide

C. It is made up of arabionose

D. Agarose is one of the principal components of agar

Ans. B.

272. Caramelization of sucrose yields

A. Glucose B. Fructose

C. Glucose and Fructose D. Charcoal

Ans. C.

273. Which of the following reaction is called 'Maillard reaction' ?

A. Reaction between amino group and hydroxyl group

B. Reaction between amino group and keto group

C. Reaction between amino group and aldehyde group

D. Reaction between amino group and carboxylic group

Ans. D.

274. Bial's test is used to detect the presence of ———

A. Triose B. Tetrose

C. Pentose D. Hexose

Ans. C.

275. Which of the following animal possess cellulose ?

A. Coelenterates B. Sponges

C. Tunicates D. Protozoans

Ans. C.

276. Glucose residues in amylase are linked by

A. α 1-4 B. β 1-4

C. α 1-6 D. β 1-6

Ans. A.

277. Chitin is a ———

A. Homopolysaccharide of N acetyl glucosamine

B. Heteropolysaccharide of N acetyl glucosamine and N acetyl muramic acid

C. A complex polymer of many sugars

D. A branched homopolysaccharide of N acetyl glucosamine

Ans. A.

278. The branched points of amylopectin are connected by

A. α 1-4 B. β 1-4

C. α 1-6 D. β 1-6

Ans. C.

279. Which of the following is an example for homopolysaccharide ?

A. Cellulose B. Starch

C. Glycogen D. All of these

Ans. D.

280. Which amino acid, among the 20 standard protein coding amino acids, is most abundantly occurs in proteins ?

A. Glycine B. Methionine

C. Serine D. Leucine

Ans. D.

281. Which of the following amino acid is having more polarity ?

A. Lysine B. Arginine

C. Histidine D. Aspartate

Ans. B.

282. Majority of enzyme's active site usually contain one or more —— residues.

A. Glycine B. Tryptophan

C. Histidine D. Arginine

Ans. C.

283. The following is the amino acid sequence of an alien polypeptide : AGQHIKXSKPWYVGLBUFF. The X represents

A. Asparagine B. Isoleucine

C. An ambiguous amino acid D. An unknown amino acid

Ans. D.

284. Amino acid acting as a defensive molecule in plants

A. Canavanine B. Con-canavalin

C. Proline D. All of these

Ans. A.

285. Which amino acid act as the precursor for the synthesis of the neurotrnamitter serotonin ?

A. Tyrosine B. Tryptophan

C. Glycine D. Arginine

Ans. B.

286. —— is an exclusively ketogenic amino acid in human.

A. Valine B. Methionine

C. Leucine D. Proline

Ans. C. Leucine and lysine are two amino acids in human which are exclusively ketogenic.

287. pI of —— is near to physiological pH.

A. Lysine B. Histidine

C. Arginine D. Glutamic acid

Ans. B.

288. Which amino acid act as the precursor of dopamine ?

A. Glycine B. Aspartatae

C. Valine D. Tyrosine

Ans. D.

289. What is the molecular weight of tryptophan ?

A. 202 $g.mol^{-1}$ B. 204 $g.mol^{-1}$

C. 206 $g.mol^{-1}$ D. 208 $g.mol^{-1}$

Ans. B.

290. Amino acid which act as the precursor of IAA (indole 3 acetic acid) biosynthesis in plants is —.

A. Tyrosine B. Phenylalanine

C. Tryptophan D. Methionine

Ans. C.

291. Amino acid involved in urea cycle ——.

A. Ornithine B. Citrulline

C. Arginine D. Both A and B

E. All of these

Ans. E.

292. Which of the following amino acid have the buffering capacity at physiological pH ?

A. Lysine B. Arginine

C. Histidine D. Aspartic acid

Ans. C.

293. Which amino acid acts as the precursor of epinephrine synthesis ?

A. Glycine B. Aspartate

C. Tyrosine D. Valine

Ans. C.

294. Which amino acid acts as the precursor of nitric oxide biosynthesis in animals ?

A. Phenyl alanine B. Arginine

C. Aspartate D. Ornithine

Ans. B.

295. Which of the following is an essential amino acid ?

A. Aspartic acid B. Alanine

C. Leucine D. Asparagine

E. All of these

Ans. C.

296. Which of the following is a nonessential amino acid ?

A. Alanine B. Histidine

C. Lysine D. Methionine

E. All of these

Ans. A.

297. Which of the following amino acid is coded by a single codon ?

A. Lysine B. Arginine

C. Tryptophan D. Phenylalanine

Ans. C.

298. First discovered amino acid is ———.

A. Asparagine B. Aspartate

C. Glutamate D. Glutamine

Ans. B.

299. Among the 20 standard protein coding amino acids, which one was last discovered?

A. Leucine B. Isoleucine

C. Threonine D. Serine

Ans. C.

300. pH below pI amino acids will be ——.

A. Anionic B. Cationic

C. Net charge zero D. No change

Ans. B.

301. Naturally occurring proteins are usually polymers of———.

A. D- amino acids

B. L- amino acids

C. A mixture of D and L amino acids

D. Either D or L amino acids

Ans. B.

302. At zwitterionic form, an amino acid will act as ——.

A. Proton donor B. Proton acceptor

C. Proton donor and acceptor D. None of these

Ans. C.

303. Which of the following amino acid is more likely to occupy the interior of a globular protein ?

A. Methionine
B. Aspartate
C. Lysine
D. Arginine
E. All of these

Ans. A.

304. Proteins absorb UV light at 280 nm and show a characteristic peak at this wavelength. Which amino acid residue in the protein is responsible for this absorption ?

A. Methionine
B. Valine
C. Glutamic acid
D. Tryptophan

Ans. D.

305. Glycine is ———.

A. A stimulatory neurotransmitter
B. An inhibitory neurotransmitter
C. Both A and B
D. Not a neurotransmitter

Ans. B.

306. Selenocysteine is a rare amino acid which contain ———.

A. Selenium
B. Selenium and sulphur
C. Sulphur
D. Selenium and Nickel

Ans. A.

307. Which of the following amino acid contains a thioether group in the side chain ?

A. Cysteine
B. Cystine
C. Glycine
D. Methionine

Ans. D.

308. An amino acid with a sulfydryl group in the side chain.

A. Methionine
B. Cystine
C. Cysteine
D. All of these

Ans. C.

309. Which among the following is the largest amino acid ?

A. Phenylalanine
B. Tyrosine
C. Tryptophan
D. Histidine

Ans. C.

310. Which of the following amino acid is completely non-polar ?

A. Phenylalanine
B. Tyrosine
C. Tryptophan
D. All of these
E. None of these

Ans. A.

311. Which amino acid is known as "the 22nd amino acid" ?

A. Selenocysteine B. Pyrrolysine

C. N-formylmethionine D. Selenomethionine

Ans. B.

312. Cystine is ——

A. Highly polar B. Highly nonpolar

C. Partially polar D. Partially nonpolar

Ans. B.

313. The side chain of Histidine contain——.

A. Indole ring B. Phenol group

C. Imidazole ring D. Guanidino ring

Ans. C.

314. Taurine, the major constituent of bile is derived from ——.

A. Cysteine B. Methionine

C. Tryptophan D. Lysine

Ans. A.

315. Selenocysteine is derived from ———

A. Cysteine B. Serine

C. Methionine D. Cystine

Ans. B.

316. Example for selenocysteine containing protein

A. Glutathione peroxidase B. Thioredoxin reductase

C. Glycine reductase D. All of these

E. None of these

Ans. D.

317. A fully protonated glycine can release ——— protons.

A. 1 B. 2

C. 3 D. 4

Ans. B.

318. —— is the only amino acid which is optically inactive

A. Valine B. Glycine

C. Selenocysteine D. Proline

Ans. B.

319. Selenocysteine is coded by——— codon.

A. UAA B. UAG

C. UGA D. AUG

Ans. C.

320. Which group of a fully protonated glycine first release a 'proton' when it is titrated against –OH ions ?

A. Carboxyl group B. Amino group

C. Both at the same time D. It can not be predicted

Ans. A.

321. pKa is the measure of a group to ——— proton.

A. Take up B. Release

C. Combine D. Consume

Ans. B.

322. Which of the following amino acid bears a guanidine group in the side chain ?

A. Lysine B. Arginine

C. Histidine D. Proline

Ans. B.

323. The precursor of glycine synthesis in microbes and plants is ——.

A. Serine B. Leucine

C. Valine D. None of these

Ans. A.

324. Single letter code of selenocysteine is ——.

A. B B. J

C. U D. O

Ans. C.

325. Which of the following amino acid has an imino group in the side chain ?

A. Proline B. Asparagine

C. Glutamate D. Histidine

Ans. A.

326. 4 hydroxy proline (a derivative of proline) is abundantly present in ———.

A. Keratin B. Myoglobin

C. Haemoglobin D. Collagen

Ans. D.

327. Desmosine is a complex derivative of five ——— residues.

A. Lysine | B. Arginine
C. Histidine | D. Methionine

Ans. A.

328. Isoelectric pH is designated as——.

A. pKa | B. pI
C. Pi | D. None of these

Ans. B.

329. Which of the following amino acid is biosynthesized from Ribose 5-phosphate ?

A. Histidine | B. Serine
C. Glycine | D. All of these

Ans. A.

330. Amino acid biosynthesized from pyruvate of glycolysis is —.

A. Alanine | B. Valine
C. Leucine | D. All of these

Ans. D.

331. Aromatic amino acids (phenylalanine, tyrosine and tryptophan) are derived from phosphoenol pyruvate and ————.

A. Ribose 5 phosphate | B. Erythrose 4 phosphate
C. Oxaloacetate | D. α ketoglutarate

Ans. B.

332. Isoleucine is derived from——.

A. Methionine | B. Threonine
C. Lysine | D. Leucine

Ans. B.

333. Blood clotting protein thrombin usually contain which of the following modified amino acid ?

A. 4-hydroxy proline | B. 5 hydroxy lysine
C. 6Nmethyl lysine | D. γ carboxy glutamate

Ans. D.

334. Cysteine is not an essential amino acid in human since we have the machinery to synthesize cysteine from other two amino acids namely ——— and serine.

A. Methionine | B. Selenocysteine
C. Citrulline | D. Hydroxyproline

Ans. A.

335. Which of the following contain a disulfide bridge ?

A. Cysteine B. Cystine

C. Methionine D. None of these

E. All of these

Ans. B.

336. Which of the following protein contain a modified amino acid –desmosine ?

A. Keratin B. Gelatin

C. Elastin D. Collagen

Ans. C.

337. During biosynthesis, Methionine and threonine are derived from a common intermediate

A. Chorismate B. Citrulline

C. Homoserine D. Cystathione

Ans. C.

338. N methyl lysine is a derivative of lysine, present in ——.

A. Keratin B. Collagen

C. Myosin D. Myoglobin

Ans. C.

339. A common intermediate branch point in the synthesis of all aromatic amino acids such as tryptophan, phenylalanine and tyrosine is ——.

A. Homoserine B. Chorismate

C. Cystathione D. None of these

Ans. B.

340. Sarcosine, a ubiquitous non protenacius amino acid in animals and plants is—

A. N-methylglycine B. N-methylvaline

C. N-methylserine D. N-methylmethionine

Ans. A.

341. Which of the following molecule can act as molecular chaperons for assisting the folding of protein ?

A. Carbohydrates B. Vitamins

C. Lipids D. Amides

Ans. C.

342. Which of the following macromolecule can be most structurally diverse among living world ?

A. Carbohydrates B. Proteins

C. Nucleic acid D. Lipids

Ans. D.

343. Fat storing cells of vertebrates are called

A. Hepatocytes B. Asterocytes

C. Adipocytes D. Melanocytes

Ans. C.

344. The enzyme abundantly distributed in adipocytes and germinating seeds are

A. Proteases B. Lipase

C. Cellulose D. Nuclease

Ans. B.

345. Rancidity of lipids in lipid rich food stuffs is due to

A. Hydrogenation of unsaturated fatty acids

B. Reduction of fatty acids

C. Oxidation of fatty acids

D. Dehydrogenation of saturated fatty acids

Ans. C.

346. Main function of preen glands in birds is

A. Hormone secretion B. Fatty acid degradation

C. Wax secretion D. Pigment synthesis

Ans. C.

347. Which of the following statement is true ?

A. Oxidative rancidity is observed more frequently in animal fats than vegetable fats

B. Oxidative rancidity is observed more frequently in vegetable fats than animal fats

C. Plant fats do not undergo oxidative rancidity

D. Oxidative rancidity can be effectively checked by dehydrogenation of fatty acids

Ans. A.

348. Number of milligrams of KOH required to neutralize fatty acid present in 1 g of fat is called

A. Potassium number B. Acid number

C. Saponification number D. Iodine number

Ans. B.

349. Saponification number is the number of milligrams of KOH required to saponify 1g fat. Which of the following statement is true about saponification number ?

A. The shorter is the chain length of fatty acids the higher is the saponification number

B. The shorter is the chain length of fatty acids the lower will be the saponification number

C. The higher the chain saturation of fatty acid, the lower will be saponification number

D. The lower is the chain saturation of fatty acid, the higher will be saponification number

Ans. A.

350. The degree of unsaturation of lipid can be measured as ——.

A. Saponification B. Iodine number

C. Polenske number D. Reichert Meissil number

Ans. B.

351. The number of OH group in fats can be expressed as———.

A. Polenske number B. Reichert Meissil number

C. Acetyl number D. Iodine number

Ans. C.

352. Polenske value of fatty acid indicates ———.

A. How much unsaturation is there in the fatty acid

B. Level of saturation in the fatty acid

C. Indication of branching of fatty acid in the fat

D. How much volatile fatty acid can be extracted through saponification

Ans. D.

353. Which of the following is an example for derived lipids ?

A. Steroids B. Terpenes

C. Carotinoids D. All of these

Ans. D.

354. Naturally occurring fats are

A. L type

B. D type

C. An equimolar mixture of L and D type

D. Symmetric

Ans. A.

355. Generally fats with unsaturated fatty acids are —— at room temperature (25oC).

A. Solid
B. Liquid
C. Liquid in presence of O2
D. Liquid in absence of O2

Ans. B.

356. Carnauba wax is an example for ———.

A. Liquid wax
B. Soft wax
C. Hard Wax
D. Archaebacterial wax

Ans. C.

357. Specific gravity of lipid is ———

A. 0.2
B. 0.8
C. 1.0
D. 1.5

Ans. B.

358. Greater the number of carbon atom in chain of fatty acid

A. The boiling point will be higher
B. The boiling point will be lower
C. The melting point will be higher
D. The melting point will be lower

Ans. C.

359. Dietary fats are transported as

A. Chylomicrons
B. Liposomes
C. Lipid globules
D. Oil droplets

Ans. A.

360. Beta oxidation of fatty acids takes place at

A. Peroxisome
B. Mitochondria
C. Mitochondria and Peroxisome
D. Mitochondria, Peroxisome and ER

Ans. B.

361. Most commonly occurring fatty acids in nature are

A. Even number of carbon atoms in an unbranched chain of 12-24 carbons
B. Odd number of carbon atoms in an unbranched chain of 12-24 carbons
C. Even number of carbon atoms in a branched chain of 12-24 carbons
D. Odd number of carbon atoms in a branched chain of 12-24 carbons

Ans. A.

362. In most of the naturally occurring monounsaturated fatty acids, the double bonds will be placed between ———.

A. C6-C7
B. C7-C8
C. C8-C9
D. C9-C10

Ans. D.

363. Which of the following molecule acts as a sugar carrier in animals ?

A. Warfarin B. Ubiquinone

C. Plastoquinone D. Dolichol

Ans. D.

364. The best source of trans fatty acid in diet is———.

A. Vegetables B. Ground nut

C. Dairy products D. Fruits

Ans. C.

365. LDL and HDL are commonly known as ——— and —— respectively.

A. Good cholesterol and bad cholesterol

B. Bad cholesterol and good cholesterol

C. Assimilatory cholesterol and oxidative cholesterol

D. Oxidative cholesterol and assimilatory cholesterol

Ans. B.

366. The solubility of fatty acids in water ———

A. Increase with increase in chain length and fewer the double bonds

B. Increase with increase in chain length and increase in double bonds

C. Decrease with chain length and decrease in number of double bonds

D. Decrease with chain length and increase in number of double bonds

Ans. C.

367. At room temperature (25oC) a fat with saturated fatty acid of 12-20 carbon have

A. Liquid consistency B. Solid consistency

C. Can not be predicted

Ans. B.

368. Carbon atoms in fatty acid are —— than those of sugars.

A. Less reduced B. More reduced

C. Less oxidized D. More oxidized

Ans. B.

369. In naturally occurring unsaturated fatty acids, the double bonds are in — conformation.

A. Cis conformation

B. Trans conformation

C. A mixture of cis and trans conformation

D. Cis and trans conformation alternatively

Ans. A.

370. Increased dietary uptake of fatty acid causes —— in blood.
A. Increase of HDL
B. Increase of LDL
C. Increase of LDL and decrease of HDL
D. Increase of HDL and decrease of LDL

Ans. C.

371. Which of the following is a cyclic fatty acid ?
A. Cerebronic acid
B. Ricinoleic acid
C. Chaulmoorgic acid
D. Oleic acid

Ans. C.

372. Which one of the following is not an essential amino acid ?
A. Linoleic acid
B. Linolenic acid
C. Arachidonic acid
D. Picrie acid

Ans. D.

373. Which of the following statement is true ?
A. Cholesterols are present in both plants and animals
B. Sterol is the only type of cholesterol in plants
C. Cholesterol is not found in plants
D. Cholesterol is totally absent in the liver cells of cold blooded animals.

Ans. C.

374. Heart problem in women is less than men because
A. Blood HDL level in women is more than men
B. Blood HDL level in women is less than men
C. Blood of women do not contain HDL
D. Blood of women do not contain LDL

Ans. A.

375. At room temperature(25°C) , an unsaturated fatty acid will have ——.
A. Liquid consistency
B. Soild consistency
C. Waxy consistency
D. Can not be predicted

Ans. A.

376. Which of the following statement is true ?
A. Sodium salt of higher fatty acid is called soft soaps
B. Potassium salt of higher fatty acid is called soft soaps
C. Sodium salt of higher fatty acid is called hard soaps
D. Potassium salt of higher fatty acid is called hard soaps
A. a
B. a, b, c
C. b, c
D. b, d

Ans. C.

377. The number of OH groups in fatty acids can be expressed as

A. Polenske number B. Reichert-Meissl number

C. Acetyl number D. Iodine number

Ans. C.

378. The triterpenoid which acts as the precursor of all animals sterols

A. Lanosterol B. Cholesterol

C. Cycloartenol D. Isoprenoids

Ans. A.

379. The precursor of all fungal sterols is——.

A. Lanosterol B. Cholesterol

C. Cycloartenol D. Isoprenoids

Ans. A.

380. The triterpenoid which acts as the precursor of almost all plants sterols

A. Lanosterol B. Cholesterol

C. Cycloartenol D. Isoprenoids

Ans. C.

381. A sterol present in the plasma membrane of fungi and protozoans instead of cholesterol is —.

A. Lanosterol B. Cholesterol

C. Ergosterol D. Cycloartenol

Ans. C.

382. A sterol which acts as the precursor of Vit D2 (provitamin D2) is

A. Colcalciferol B. Lanosterol

C. Cholesterol D. Ergosterol

Ans. D.

383. Which of the following is an example for phytosterol ?

A. β sitosterol B. Campesterol

C. Brassicasterol D. All of these

E. None of these

Ans. D.

384. A naturally occurring fatty acid with C-C triple bond in the hydrocarbon chain

A. Digitoxin B. Oubain

C. Nemotinic acid D. None of these

Ans. C. Santalbic acid found in sandal wood oil also contain one C-C triple bond.

385. Which of the following is not an omega 6 fatty acid ?

A. Alphalinolenic acid
B. Linoleic acid
C. Eicosadienoic acid
D. Arachidonic acid

Ans. A.

386. A genetic disorder caused by mutation in the hexosaminidase enzyme A which hydrolyse the GM2 to GM3 during membrane lipid turnover :

A. Tay-sachs syndrome
B. Fabryi disease
C. Gauche's disease
D. Niemann Pick disease

Ans. A.

387. The simplest hydrophilic moiety present in the membrane lipid is

A. Phosphate group
B. Hydroxyl group
C. Amino group
D. Glucose

Ans. B.

388. Which of the following cellular event can be best regulated by prostaglandins ?

A. Synthesis of inter cellular cyclic AMP
B. Synthesis of intra cellular cyclic AMP
C. Synthesis of inter cellular cyclic GMP
D. Synthesis of intra cellular cyclic GMP

Ans. B.

389. Which of the following statement is true regarding the solubility of steroids in biological fluids ?

A. Steroids and cholesterol are equally soluble
B. Steroids are more soluble than cholesterol
C. Cholesterol are more soluble than steroids
D. Cholesterol and steroids are completely insoluble

Ans. B.

390. The potent molecular signal molecule Platelet Activating Factor is an example for

A. Glycolipid
B. Phospholipid
C. Ether lipid
D. Ceramide

Ans. C.

391. Thylakoid membrane of chloroplast are rich in

A. Galactolipids
B. Phospholipids
C. Cardiolipin
D. Sphingolipids

Ans. A.

392. How many double bonds occur in Arachidonic acid ?

A. 1 B. 2

C. 3 D. 4

Ans. D.

393. —— is considered as the structural parent of all sphingolipids.

A. Sphingosine B. Ceramide

C. Lecithin D. Sphyngomylein

Ans. B.

394. Which among the following is the most complex sphingolipid ?

A. Cerebroside B. Ganglioside

C. Globoside D. Ceramide

Ans. B.

395. A genetic disorder caused by the accumulation of sphingomyelin in brain is called

A. Tay-sachs syndrome B. Gout

C. Niemann Pick disease D. Gauche's disease

Ans. C.

396. Lipid molecule involved in the biosignalling pathway that include membrane turnover and exocytosis is

A. Phosphatidylinositol B. Phosphatidylglycerol

C. Myoinositol D. Phosphatidylglycerol and Myoinositol

Ans. A.

397. The precursor of eicosanoids, a paracrine hormone in human is——.

A. Squaline B. Cholesterol

C. Arachidonic acid D. Ceramide

Ans. C.

398. Which of the following is not an eicosanoic acid in human ?

A. Prostaglandin E1 B. Thromboxane A2

C. Leukotriene A4 D. Arachidonic acid

Ans. D.

399. Which of the following is not an NSAID (nonsteroidal anti-inflammatory drug) ?

A. Aspirin B. Ibuprofen

C. Meclofenamate D. Omeprazole

Ans. D.

400. NSAIDs inhibit cellular inflammation by inhibiting — enzyme ?
A. Prostaglandilin H2 synthase B. Cyclooxygenase
C. COX D. All of these

Ans. D.

401. NSAIDs inhibit inflammation by preventing the conversion of
A. Membrane phospholipid to arachidonic acid
B. Arachidonic aicd to prostaglandin E2
C. Prostaglandin E2 to thromboxane A2
D. All of these

Ans. B.

402. Most abundant membrane lipid in the biosphere is
A. Phospholipid B. Galactolipid
C. Sphingolipid D. Ether lipid

Ans. B.

403. Enzymes for beta oxidation of fatty acids are located in
A. Mitochondria B. Mitochondria and Cytoplasm
C. Mitochondria and Golgi D. Mitochondria and Peroxisome

Ans. A.

404. For the detection of which biological compound, the Salkowski test is done ?
A. Fatty acids B. Glycerol
C. Ceramide D. Cholesterol

Ans. D.

405. Receptors for steroid hormones usually reside at ———.
A. Plasma membrane B. Cytoplasm
C. Nuclear membrane D. Nucleoplasm
E. Plasma membrane and nuclear membrane

Ans. D.

406. Prednisolone and Prednisone are anti-inflammatory drugs, they are chemically —
A. Glycerol derivatives B. Steroids
C. Amino alcohols D. NSAIDS

Ans. B.

407. Cerebroside is a
A. Phospholipid B. Sphingolipid
C. Aminolipid D. Glycolipid

Ans. D.

408. Glycosphingolipids are a combination of

A. Glycerol with two galactose residues

B. Ceramide with one or more sugar residues

C. Sphingosine with galactose and ceramide

D. Sphingosine with glucose

Ans. B.

409. What is the molecular formula of cholesterol ?

A. $C_{27}H_{45}OH$ B. $C_{28}H_{47}OH$

C. $C_{29}H_{47}OH$ D. $C_{23}H_{41}OH$

Ans. A.

410. Water is liquid at room temperature, the most important reason for this is the

A. High boiling point of water

B. High melting point of water

C. High heat of vaporization of water

D. Cohesive forces due to hydrogen bonds in water

Ans. D.

411. Water is a ———.

A. Polar solvent B. Non polar solvent

C. An amphipathic solvent D. Non polar uncharged solvent

Ans. A.

412. Polar molecules can readily dissolve in water. This is because

A. Polar molecules can form hydrogen bonds with water

B. Polar molecules can replace water -water interaction with more energetically favourable water solute interactions

C. Polar charged water can interact with the charge polar molecules

D. All polar molecules are amphipathic in nature

Ans. B.

413. Most important reason for the unusual properties of water is

A. The covalent bonding pattern in water molecule

B. The bond angle between the two hydrogen atoms in water

C. Hydrogen bonding between water molecules

D. Water can be immediately ionized at room temperature

Ans. C.

414. The H-O-H bond angle in water molecule is

A. 104°
B. 104.5°
C. 105°
D. 105.5°

Ans. **B.**

415. Which of the following statement is true regarding the electronegativity of atoms in water molecule ?

A. Hydrogen is more electronegative than oxygen
B. Hydrogen is less electronegative than oxygen
C. Electronegativity of oxygen and hydrogen is same
D. Oxygen and hydrogen do not have significant electronegativity in water

Ans. **B.**

416. Which of the following represent the current melting point, boiling point and heat of vaporization of water ?

A. O°C, 100°C, 2260J/g
B. 10O°C, 0°C, 2260J/g
C. O°C, 100°C, 1260J/g
D. 10O°C, 0°C, 1260J/g

Ans. **A.**

417. Hydrogen bond is best represented as the electrostatic attraction between

A. A hydrogen covalently bounded to an electronegative atom and another hydrogen atom
B. A hydrogen covalently bounded to an electronegative atom and another electronegative atom
C. Two electronegative atom and a hydrogen atom
D. two hydrogen atoms

Ans. **B.**

418. The bond dissociation energy of hydrogen bonds in water molecule is

A. 10 KJ/mol
B. 23 KJ/mol
C. 470 KJ/mol
D. 348 KJ/mol

Ans. **B.**

419. Which of the following statement is correct regarding the hydrogen bonds in water ?

A. Hydrogen bond is 10% covalent and 90% electrostatic
B. Hydrogen bond is 25% covalent and 75% electrostatic
C. Hydrogen bond is 50% covalent and 50% electrostatic
D. Hydrogen bond is 100% electrostatic

Ans. **A.**

420. A single water molecule can form how many hydrogen bonds at a time ? (theoretically possible value)

A. 1 B. 2

C. 3 D. 4

Ans. 4.

421. The life span of a hydrogen bond between two water molecule in liquid water is

A. 1-20 seconds B. 1-20 microseconds

C. 1-20 nanoseconds D. 1-20 picoseconds

Ans. D.

422. The bond dissociation energy of O-H bond in water

A. 470 kj/mol B. 348 kj/mol

C. 23 kj/mol D. 10 kj/mol

Ans. A.

423. What is the bond length of hydrogen bond between two water molecules in liquid water ?

A. 0.0177 nm B. 0.177 nm

C. 1.177 nm D. 17.70 nm

Ans. B.

424. Bond length between H and O atoms in water is

A. 0.00965 nm B. 0.0965 nm

C. 0.965 nm D. 9.650 nm

Ans. B.

425. The van der Waals radius of oxygen atom in water molecule is

A. 1.2 A° B. 1.4A°

C. 1.6A° D. 1.8A°

Ans. B.

426. At room temperature and atmospheric pressure, a single water molecule can be hydrogen bonded with ——— water molecules.

A. 3.4 B. 3.0

C. 2.4 D. 1.4

Ans. A.

427. Non polar molecules are insoluble in water. This is because

A. Non polar molecules are uncharged

B. Non polar molecues can not be ionized

C. Non polar molecules are unable to form water solute interaction

D. Hydrogen bond formation is not possible with nonpolar molecules

Ans. C.

428. Which of the following is the correct for the formation of a hydrogen bond ? (Hydrogen bond is represented as ...)

A. –O-H-O-H-X B. –O-H...O-X

C.- O-H...H-O-X D. –O-H...C-O-X

Ans. B.

429. Which of the following statement is true ? The number of inter-molecular hydrogen bonds between water molecules will be

A. Maximum in ice and minimum in water vapour

B. Maximum in liquid water and minimum in water vapour

C. Minimum in liquid water and maximum in water vapour

D. Same in ice, liquid water and water vapour

Ans. A.

430. What is the concentration of H+ ion in a solution of 0.1 M NaOH ?

A. 10^{-13}M B. 9^{-13}M

C. $10^{-13}M^2$ D. $9^{-13}M^2$

Ans. A.

431. As the Ka of an acid decreases, the acid will be

A. More weaker B. More stronger

C. Converted to neutral solution D. Converted to basic solution

Ans. A.

432. Which of the following molecule do not form hydrogen bond with water ?

A. –O-H B. –N-H

C. –C-H D. –S-H

Ans. C.

433. Hydrogen bond will be strongest when the bonded molecules oriented to maximize the electrostatic interaction, which can occur when

A. The hydrogen atom and the two atoms that share it are in the same molecule

B. The hydrogen atom and the two atoms that share it are in separate molecule

C. The hydrogen atom and the two atoms that share it are in very close contact

D. The hydrogen atom and the two atoms that share it are in a straight line

Ans. D.

434. Which of the following statement is true ?

A. CO2, O2 and N2 are non polar and completely insoluble in water

B. CO2, O2 and N2 are polar and soluble in water

C. CO2, O2 and N2 are partially soluble in water

D. CO2, O2 are polar and soluble in water but N2 is non polar and insoluble in water

Ans. A.

435. CO_2 in our body is transported through the blood primarily as

A. CO_2 bubbles

B. CO_2 hemoglobin complex

C. CO_2 myoglobin complex

D. As bicarbonate

Ans. D.

436. Which of the following statement is true regarding the solubility of NH3, NO and H2S in water ?

A. All are completely nonpolar and insoluble in water

B. All are polar and completely soluble in water

C. NH2 and H2S are polar but NO is non polar

D. NH2 and H2S are nonpolar but NO is polar

Ans. B.

437. When amphipathic compounds are mixed with water

A. It can be readily dissolved in water

B. It can form two separate layers in water

C. It can form micelles in water

D. It can increase the solubility of water

Ans. C.

438. Movement of H+ ions in water to negatively charge electrode (cathode) is extremely faster than Na+ or K+ ions this is because

A. H+ ions are smaller than Na+ or K+ ions

B. H+ ions are more positive than Na+ or K+ ions

C. H+ ions can move in water very fast by proton hopping

D. H+ ions can move in water very fast by proton tunneling

Ans. C.

439. What is the molecular weight of water ?

A. 10g/mol

B. 15g/mol

C. 18g/mol

D. 20g/mol

Ans. C.

440. What is the H^+ ion concentration in pure water ?

A. $1X10^{-7}$ m
B. $1X10^{7}$ m
C. $1X10^{-14}$ m
D. $1X10^{14}$ m

Ans. A.

441. The equilibrium constant of ionization reaction of pure water is

A. $1.8X10^{-14}$ M
B. $1.8X10^{-16}$ M
C. $1.8X10^{-7}$ M
D. $1.8X10^{-7}$ M

Ans. B.

442. The pH of pure water is neutral, the best explanation for this is

A. The pH of pure water is 7
B. In pure water the concentration of H+ and OH- are same
C. Water do not contain free H+ and OH-
D. Water will never ionize

Ans. B.

443. What is the concentration of OH^- ions in a solution with an H+ ion concentration of $1.3X10^{-4}$M

A. $7.7X10^{-11}$ M
B. $7.7X10^{-10}$ M
C. $1.4X10^{-11}$ M
D. $1.4X10^{-10}$ M

Ans. A.

444. As the pKa of an acid increases, the acid will be

A. More weaker
B. More stronger
C. Converted to neutral solution
D. Converted to basic solution

Ans. A.

445. Buffers are mixtures of

A. Strong acid and strong base
B. Strong acid and weak base
C. Weak acid and their conjugate base
D. Weak base and their conjugate acid

Ans. C.

446. If a solution has to be a buffer, its pH should be

A. At its pKa value
B. At its Ka value
C. At 7
D. At 14

Ans. A.

447. The most important peculiarity of water when compared to other solvents is that water

A. High boiling point, high melting point and high heat of vaporization

B. High boiling point, low melting point and low heat of vaporization

C. Low boiling point, high melting point and low heat of vaporization

D. Low boiling point, low melting point and low heat of vaporization

Ans. A.

448. According to Henderson-Hasselbatch equation, when the pH of a solution becomes equal to its pKa, the solution becomes a buffer. This condition is achieved when ——.

A. The concentration of proton donor equals the concentration of proton acceptor

B. The concentration of proton donor becomes zero

C. The concentration of proton acceptor become zero

D. The concentration of proton donor become log $1/10^{th}$ of concentration of proton acceptor

Ans. A.

449. Normal pH of human blood is

A. 7.0 B. 7.2

C. 7.3 D. 7.4

Ans. D.

450. The heat of vaporization of water molecule at atmospheric temperature is

A. 2260J/g B. 1260J/g

C. 2260 kcal D. 1260kcal

Ans. A.

451. The water level in the human body is regulated by the hormone ——.

A. ACTH B. Oxytocine

C. FSH D. Epinephrine

Ans. D.

452. The polarity of water molecule is due to

A. Difference in electronegativity of oxygen and hydrogen atoms in water

B. The readily ionizing behaviour of water

C. The positive charge of water molecule

D. The negative charge of water molecule

Ans. A.

453. The van der Walls radius of hydrogen atom in water molecule is

A. 1.2 A° B. 1.4 A°

C. 1.6 A° D. 1.8A°

Ans. A.

454. Fructose is metabolized by

A. Fructose 1-phosphate pathway

B. Fructose 6 phosphate pathway

C. Glyceraldehyde 3 phosphate pathway

D. Both A and B

Ans. D.

455. A common way that cells capture the energy released during the breakdown of large molecules is to add electrons to smaller, specialized molecules that can accept them. This process of electron acceptance is otherwise known as

A. biosynthesis B. metabolism

C. reduction D. catalysis

Ans. C.

456. Humans are unable to digest

A. Starch B. Complex carbohydrate

C. denatured proteins D. Cellulose

Ans. D.

457. How many ATP equivalents per mole of glucose input are required for gluconeogenesis?

A. 2 B. 6

C. 8 D. 4

Ans. B.

458. Which of the following compounds is responsible for coordinated regulation of glucose and glycogen metabolism?

A. NAD+ B. Fructose 2,6 bisphosphate

C. Acetyl-CoA D. Fructose 1,6 bisphosphate

Ans. B.

459. Gluconeogenesis requires a higher amount of ATP equivalents as compared to that produced by glycolysis because

A. Gluconeogenesis releases energy as heat

B. Glycolysis releases energy as heat

C. Glycolysis occurs in the mitochondria while gluconeogenesis occurs in the cytosol

D. All of the above

Ans. B.

460. Which of the following is carried out when cAMP functions as a second messenger?

A. Acts second in importance to AMP

B. Activates all cytosolic protein kinases

C. Activates the cAMP-dependent protein kinase

D. Acts outside the cell to influence cellular processes

Ans. C.

461. The production or break down of———— is often coupled with the metabolic reactions of biosynthesis and catabolism.

A. Aspirin B. DNA

C. ATP D. CO_2

Ans. C.

462. The cells dependent solely on glucose as an energy source are

A. Muscle cells B. Brain cells

C. Kidney cells D. Liver cells

Ans. B.

463. The main site for gluconeogenesis is

A. Kidney B. Liver

C. Brain D. Muscle

Ans. B.

464. Which of the following statements about the energy needs of cells is false?

A. Without a continuous input of energy, cell disorder will increase

B. The laws of thermodynamics force cells to acquire energy

C. Many cellular reactions have an associated activation energy

D. The most usable energy for cells comes from the rapid combustion of glucose

Ans. D.

465. In lysozyme catalysis, which of the following does not contribute?

A. The abnormally high pK_a of Glu35

B. The strained conformation of the D sugar

C. Formation of a covalent intermediate at Asp52

D. Formation of a covalent intermediate at Ser195

Ans. D.

466. Cellulose fibers resemble with the protein structure in the form of

A. β-sheets B. α-helices

C. β-turns D. None of these

Ans. A.

467. During vigorous exercise, pyruvate produced by glycolysis is converted to

A. Acetate B. Lactate

C. Monosodium phosphate D. Pyruvic acid

Ans. B.

468. Glucagon and epinephrine

A. Inhibits gluconeogenesis and stimulates glycolysis

B. Stimulates gluconeogenesis and glycolysis

C. Stimulates gluconeogenesis and inhibits glycolysis

D. Inhibits gluconeogenesis and glycolysis

Ans. C.

469. Gluconeogenesis uses

A. 3 ATPs and 2 GTPs per glucose B. 2 ATPs and 1 GTPs per glucose

C. 3 ATPs and 3 GTPs per glucose D. 4 ATPs and 2 GTPs per glucose

Ans. D.

470. Saliva contains all of the following except

A. Hormones B. Amylase

C. Bacteria killing enzymes D. Antibodies

Ans. A.

471. The conversion of pyruvate to oxaloacetate

A. Requires biotin B. Involves the fixation of carbon dioxide

C. Occurs in the mitochondria D. All of the above

Ans. A.

472. Gluconeogenesis is the

A. Formation of glycogen

B. Breakdown of glucose to pyruvate

C. Breakdown of glycogen to glucose

D. Synthesis of glucose from non-carbohydrate precursors

Ans. D.

473. Hydrolysis of lactose yields

A. Galactose and fructose B. Galactose and glucose

C. Glucose and fructose D. Fructose and fructose

Ans. B.

474. Two major products of pentose phosphate pathway are

A. Nicotinamide adenine dinucleotide and ribose 5-phosphate

B. Flavine adenine dinuclueotide and glucose 5-phosphate

C. FAD and CoA

D. NADPH and NAD

Ans. A.

475. A catabolic intermediate which stimulates phosphofructokinase would stimulate

A. Gluconeogenesis

B. Glycolysis

C. Glycogen synthesis

D. None of these

Ans. B.

476. Pyruvate is initially converted to which of the following in the gluconeogenesis?

A. Glycerol

B. Phosphoenol pyruvate

C. Oxaloacetate

D. Acetyl CoA

Ans. C.

477. Boat and chair conformations are found

A. In pyranose sugars

B. In any sugar without axial -OH groups

C. In any sugar without equatorial -OH groups

D. Only in D-glucopyranose

Ans. A.

478. The conversion of pyruvate to lactate is catalysed by

A. Pyruvate carboxylase

B. Lactate dehydrogenase

C. Pyruvate dismutase

D. Pyruvate decarboxylase

Ans. B.

479. Which of the following can act as precursors for gluconeogenesis?

A. Lactate

B. Glycerol

C. Alanine

D. All of these

Ans. D.

480. α amylase is similar to

A. β sheets

B. β turned coils

C. α helices

D. The hydrophobic core

Ans. C.

481. Storage polysaccharide made by animals is

A. Amylopectin
B. Glycogen
C. Cellulose
D. Collagen

Ans. B.

482. The glycosidic bond

A. In maltose is not hydrolyzed in lactose intolerant humans
B. In sucrose is hydrolyzed by bees
C. Joins glucose and fructose to form sucrose
D. Both B and C

Ans. D.

483. Under aerobic condition pyruvate is converted by pyruvate dehydrogenase to

A. Phosphoenol pyruvate
B. Acetyl CoA
C. Lactate
D. Glyceraldehyde 3 phosphate

Ans. B.

484. Which of the following is not a disaccharide?

A. Amylose
B. Cellobiose
C. Lactose
D. None of the above

Ans. A.

485. Hexokinase activity in glycolysis is inhibited by

A. Glucose 6- phosphate
B. Fructose 6-phosphate
C. Fructose 1,6 biphosphate
D. Phosphofructokinase

Ans. A.

486. The ultimate source of energy that sustains living systems is

A. Glucose
B. Oxygen
C. Sunlight
D. Carbon dioxide

Ans. C.

487. Citric acid accumulation would

A. Stimulate phosphofructokinase activity
B. Stimulate fructose 1,6 diphosphatase activity
C. Inhibit phosphofructokinase activity
D. Both B and C

Ans. D.

488. Which of the following is not involved in the biosynthesis of DNA?

A. Energy from ATP
B. Mononucleotides
C. Carbonic anhydrase
D. Enzyme

Ans. C.

489. Which of the following would be considered a part of metabolism?

A. Biosynthetic pathways that build DNA
B. Catabolic pathways that break down complex carbohydrates
C. The capture of light energy for use in making glucose
D. All of the above

Ans. D.

490. Insulin

A. Stimulates gluconeogenesis and glycolysis
B. Stimulates gluconeogenesis and inhibits glycolysis
C. Inhibits gluconeogenesis and glycolysis
D. Inhibits gluconeogenesis and stimulates glycolysis

Ans. D.

491. What is present in the stomach to prevent self-digestion?

A. Mucus
B. Acid
C. Enzymes
D. Hormones

Ans. A.

492. The key enzyme in the regulation of fatty acid synthesis is

A. Acetyl CoA carboxylase
B. AMP activated proteinkinase
C. Protein phosphatise
D. None of these

Ans. A.

493. Arachidonate has 20 carbon atoms with

A. 3 double bonds
B. 2 double bonds
C. 4 double bonds
D. 8 double bonds

Ans. C.

494. In the intestine, the dietary fats are hydrolysed by

A. Triacylglycerol lipase
B. Adenylate cyclise
C. Pancreatic lipase
D. Protein kinase

Ans. C.

495. HDLs are synthesized in

A. Blood
B. Liver
C. Intestine
D. Pancreas

Ans. B.

496. Triacylglycerols are

A. Soluble in water
B. Insoluble in water
C. Soluble in water at elevated temperature
D. Soluble in water

Ans. B.

497. Animals cannot convert fatty acids into glucose because

A. Acetyl CoA can not be converted to pyruvate
B. Absence of malate synthase
C. Absence of dehydrogenase
D. Absence of α-ketoglutarate dehydrogenase

Ans. A.

498. In eukaryotes fatty acid breakdown occurs in

A. Mitochondrial matrix
B. Cytosol
C. Cell membrane
D. Endoplasmic reticulum

Ans. A.

499. What is the major protein constituent of high-density lipoprotein (HDL)?

A. Apolipoprotein A-l
B. Apolipoprotein C-l
C. Apolipoprotein E
D. None of these

Ans. A.

500. Phospholipid contains

A. Hydrophilic heads and hydrophobic tails
B. Long water-soluble carbon chains
C. Positively charged functional groups
D. Both B and C

Ans. A.

501. Micelles of fatty acids in water are organized such that the __________ faces the solvent and the __________ are directed toward the interior

A. Carboxylic acid groups, hydrocarbon chains heads
B. Hydrophilic heads, hydrophobic tails
C. Hydrocarbon chains, carboxylic acid groups
D. Both A and B

Ans. D.

502. Cholesterolemia means
A. Lack of functional LDL receptors
B. Lack of functional HDL receptor
C. High sensitivity to fatty food intake
D. None of these

Ans. A.

503. VLDLs are synthesized in
A. Blood B. Liver
C. Intestine D. Pancreas

Ans. B.

504. Chylomicrons are synthesized in
A. Blood B. Liver
C. Intestine D. Pancreas

Ans. C.

505. How many types of lipoproteins are there?
A. 2 B. 6
C. 8 D. 5

Ans. D.

506. Fatty acid synthesis takes place in
A. Mitochondria B. Cell membrane
C. Cytosol D. Endoplasmic reticulum

Ans. C.

507. Cholesterol is the precursor of
A. Steroid hormones B. Vitamin A
C. Bile salts D. Both A and C

Ans. D.

508. Atherosclerosis can cause blood
A. Thining B. Clotting
C. Thickening D. None of these

Ans. B.

509. Palmitate has 16 carbon atoms with

A. 2 double bonds
B. 3 double bonds
C. 1 double bond
D. None of these

Ans. D.

510. How many ATPs are formed during complete oxidation of palmitate?

A. 35
B. 96
C. 129
D. 131

Ans. C.

511. The lowest energy value lipid for human nutrition is

A. Olive oil
B. Olestra
C. Margarine
D. Cardilipin

Ans. B.

512. How many classes of steroid hormones are there ?

A. 3
B. 2
C. 4
D. 5

Ans. D.

513. The number of water molecules consumed by the formation of phosphatidyl serine are

A. 0
B. 1
C. 2
D. 4

Ans. A.

514. Synthesis of fatty acid takes place when

A.. Fatty acid are plentiful
B. Carbohydrate is plentiful
C. Carbohydrate and energy are plentiful
D. None of these

Ans. C.

515. Which of the following is called milk ejection hormone?

A. Prolactin
B. Vasopressiin
C. Oxytocin
D. All of these

Ans. C.

516. Which of the following two organelles look most alike structurally?

A. Nucleus and vesicle
B. Golgi apparatus and smooth endoplasmic reticulum (ER)
C. Vacuole and cytoskeleton
D. Lysosome and chloroplast

Ans. B.

517. In terms of basic cell structure, what do an elephant and an oak tree have in common?

A. They both are eukaryotes
B. They both have a cell nucleus
C. They both have mitochondria
D. All of the above

Ans. D.

518. Where in a eukaryotic cell, DNA can be found?

A. Nucleus
B. Mitochondrion
C. Vacuole
D. Both A and B

Ans. D.

519. Which of the following structures is expected in a bacterium?

A. Nucleus
B. Plasma membrane
C. Golgi apparatus
D. Endoplasmic reticulum

Ans. B.

520. Which of the following organelles is directly connected to the outer membrane of the nucleus in a eukaryotic cell?

A. Mitochondrion
B. Lysosome
C. Golgi apparatus
D. Endoplasmic reticulum

Ans. D.

521. Microtubules, motor proteins, and actin filaments are all parts of

A. The mechanism of photosynthesis that occurs in chloroplasts
B. The rough ER in prokaryotic cells
C. The cytoskeleton of eukaryotic cells
D. The process that moves small molecules across cell membranes

Ans. C.

522. A certain cell organelle which is made of a double phospholipid bilayer that has many large pores in it, is most likely

A. The nuclear envelope
B. The plasma membrane
C. The mitochondrion
D. The cytoskeleton

Ans. A.

523. Which of the following cell organelles are expected to be associated with motor proteins?

A. Smooth ER
B. Vesicles
C. Plasma membrane
D. Chloroplasts

Ans. B.

524. Eukaryotic cells are more efficient than prokaryotes because their internal compartmentalization

A. Makes each compartment nutritionally independent of all others

B. Allows for specialization through the subdivision of particular tasks

C. Allows for specialization through merging of different tasks

D. Reduces overall cell size

Ans. B.

525. An organism's first line of defence against attack by an invader such as a virus or bacterium is usually

A. To flee of hide

B. Its body wall

C. A specific immune response

D. A non specific immune response

Ans. B.

526. According to the fluid mosaic model of cell membranes,

A. The most common type of molecules in the membrane are proteins

B. Basic membrane structure results from how the proteins interact with water

C. The membrane is a highly mobile mixture of phospholipids and proteins

D. The unique properties of cell types are determined by their phospholipids

Ans. C.

527. The simplest way to differentiate a prokaryotic cell from a eukaryotic one is to

A. Look for a plasma membrane

B. See if a nucleus is present

C. Check for the presence of DNA

D. Determine if the cell is an entire organism or not

Ans. B.

528. Lysosomes are specialized vesicles in ———— that contain digestive enzymes for the breakdown of food. A related organalle known as a vacuole, which is found in ————, also contains enzymes but in addition may act as a storage organelle for nutrients or water.

A. Animals; plants and fungi

B. Plants; animals and fungi

C. Plants and fungi; animals

D. Animals and plants; fungi

Ans. A.

529. Which of the following statements about prokaryotes is false?

A. Prokaryotic cells concentrate important materials for the cells survival

B. The substance known as cytosol is found within the bacterial nucleus

C. Prokaryotic cells are much smaller than most eukaryotic cells

D. Ancient prokaryotes may have given rise to some eukaryotic organelles

Ans. B.

530. In which of the following cell organelles, it is expected to find the biochemical reactions that harness energy from the breakdown of sugar molecules to synthesize large amounts of ATP?

A. Lysosome B. Vesicles
C. Mitochondria D. Plasma membrane

Ans. C.

531. Which of the following macromolecules are found in the plasma membrane?

A. Lipids and proteins only B. Lipids, proteins, and carbohydrates
C. Proteins and carbohydrates only D. Proteins only

Ans. B.

532. Clearly defined nucleus, mitochondria in a large central vacuole and chloroplasts, indicate the group of organisms from

A. Bacteria B. Fungi
C. Plants D. Animals

Ans. C.

533. Which of the following is present in both prokaryotes and eukaryotes?

A. Lysosome B. Chloroplast
C. Plasma membrane D. Vacuole

Ans. C.

534. Thin layer chromatography is

A. Partition chromatography B. Electrical mobility of ionic species
C. Adsorption chromatography D. None of the above

Ans. C.

535. In gas chromatography, the basis for separation of the components of the volatile material is the difference in

A. Partition coefficients B. Conductivity
C. Molecular weight D. Molarity

Ans. A.

536. In reverse phase chromatography, the stationary phase is made

A. Non polar B. Polar
C. Either nonpolar or polar D. None of these

Ans. A.

537. Ion exchange chromatography is based on the

A. Electrostatic attraction B. Electrical mobility of ionic species
C. Adsorption chromatography D. Partition chromatography

Ans. A.

538. A combination of paper chromatography and electrophoresis involves

A. Partition chromatography
B. Electrical mobility of ionic species
C. Both A and B
D. None of the above

Ans. C.

539. For gene transfer to be effective, transforming DNA must be

A. Incorporated into the bacterial chromosome
B. Incorporated into a viral genome
C. Free in the bacterial cytoplasm
D. None of the above

Ans. A.

540. Double stranded DNA denaturation with specified limit of temperature is

A. Reversible reaction
B. Irreversible reaction
C. Either A or B
D. None of these

Ans. A.

541. From a single molecule of DNA, PCR can make

A. 1 additional copy
B. Hundreds of copies
C. Thousands of copies
D. Millions of copies

Ans. D.

542. Genomic libraries are made from

A. Genomic DNA of an organism
B. Genomic RNA of an organism
C. Genomic cDNA of an organism
D. Genomic mRNA of an organism

Ans. A.

543. Bacteriophages are

A. Cells in the blood that eat bacteria
B. A class of bacteria
C. Bacterial viruses
D. None of these

Ans. C.

544. Specialized transduction occurs when

A. The bacteriophage incorporates randomly in the bacterial chromosome
B. The bacteriophage never incorporates into the bacterial chromosome
C. The bacteriophage always incorporates at the same position in the bacterial chromosome
D. None of the above

Ans. C.

545. PCR is used

A. To diagnose genetic diseases B. To solve crimes

C. To study gene function D. All of these

Ans. D.

546. To clone into a plasmid vector, both the plasmid and the foreign DNA are cut

A. With the same restriction enzyme and mixed together

B. With different restriction enzyme and mixed together

C. With the combination of enzymes and then separated

D. With the combination of enzymes and mixed together

Ans. A.

547. PCR can be used to amplify a specific fragment of DNA from which of the following?

A. A drop of blood B. A hair follicle

C. A fragment of skin D. All of these

Ans. D.

548. Transformation means

A. Formation of a pilus

B. Acquiring DNA from the environment by bacterial cell

C. Plasmid containing a F factor

D. F+ and F- strains of bacteria

Ans. B.

549. Restriction maps

A. Allows comparison between DNA molecules without the need to determine nucleotide sequence

B. Allows comparison between DNA molecules but requires to determine nucleotide sequence

C. Does not allow comparison between DNA molecules

D. None of the above

Ans. A.

550. Which of the following is correct?

A. HIV is a retrovirus that kills human helper T cells

B. Causes acquired immune deficiency syndrome (AIDS)

C. Cripples the immunity systems

D. All the above

Ans. D.

551. A PCR cycle consists of

A. Three steps, denaturation, primer annealing and elongation

B. Three steps, denaturation, initiation and elongation

C. Three steps, primer annealing, elongation and termination

D. Three steps, initiation, elongation and termination

Ans. A.

552. How many ds DNA molecule can be produced, which comprise precisely the target region in double strand form during 4th cycle of PCR?

A. Two ds DNA molecule

B. Three ds DNA molecule

C. Eight ds DNA molecule

D. Four ds DNA molecule

Ans. D.

553. PCR can be used in

A. Cloning

B. Sequencing

C. Medical diagnosis and forensic medicine

D. All of the above

Ans. D.

554. PCR (Polymerase Chain Reaction) can make multiple copies of

A. DNA

B. RNA

C. Protein

D. Carbohydrate

Ans. A.

555. PCR is an abbreviation for

A. Protein Change Reaction

B. Polymerase Chain Reaction

C. Positive Charge Reaction

D. Preliminary Change Rate

Ans. B.

556. PCR amplifies millions of copies of

A. A short fragment of DNA

B. The entire genome (all the DNA in a sample)

C. Both A and B

D. Short chain RNA

Ans. A.

557. Southern blotting involves

A. Electrophoresis of DNA molecules and then blotting the separated DNA bands followed by incubation

B. Electrophoresis of DNA molecules and then blotting the separated RNA bands followed by incubation

C. Electrophoresis of DNA molecules followed by incubation

D. Electrophoresis of RNA molecules and then blotting the separated RNA bands followed by incubation

Ans. A.

558. Bactriophages absorb to a bacterial surface and inject the phage DNA through the

A. Cell wall into cytosol

B. Cell wall into plasma membrane

C. Both A and B

D. Cell wall into endoplasmic reticulum

Ans. A.

559. In a PCR reaction after four cycles, each molecule of a duplex DNA will give rise to

A. 16 single strands of DNA
B. 16 double stranded DNA

C. 18 single strands of DNA
D. 18 double stranded DNA

Ans. A.

560. Additional mono saccharides are added in Golgi to produce

A. Either high mannose type oligosaccharide or a complex type

B. Either fructose type monosaccharide or a complex type

C. Either high sucrose type polysaccharide or a complex type

D. None of the above

Ans. A.

561. The PCR, polymerase chain reaction is becoming the method of choice for

A. Alteration of gene
B. Screening gene

C. Sterilization of gene
D. All of these

Ans. B.

562. Northern blotting is

A. Widely different than southern blotting

B. Another name for southern blotting

C. Analogous to southern blotting

D. None of the above

Ans. C.

563. What technique can be used to determine the murderer who left blood with the victim?

A. DNA sequencing B. PCR amplification
C. Western blot D. RFLP mapping

Ans. B.

564. DNA fragments in a restriction digest can be separated by electrophoresis in

A. Polyacrylamide B. Agarose gel
C. Both A and B D. None of these

Ans. C.

565. Beta pleated sheets are examples of protein's

A. Primary structure B. Secondary structure
C. Tertiary structure D. Quaternary structure

Ans. B.

566. BRACl, an inherited form of breast cancer, regulates cell division by

A. Binding to a DNA sequence
B. Complexing with cyclins
C. Binding to the cell outer membrane
D. Binding to the protein RAD 51 which repairs DNA damage

Ans. D.

567. Metastasis involves

A. Ability of cells to dissolve cellular matrix
B. Metalloprotein levels
C. Decreased levels of proteins that regulate metalloproteins
D. All of the above

Ans. D.

568. Signal sequences are part of a protein that

A. Signal folding of the protein
B. Signal the protein synthesis on the ribosomes is ended
C. Transport proteins to other sites within the cell
D. Refold proteins in prion-associated diseases

Ans. C.

569. Individuals with PKU disease are mentally retarded unless

A. Phenylalanine in the diet is restricted
B. Tyrosine in the diet is restricted
C. Homogentisic acid in the diet is restricted
D. None of the above

Ans. A.

570. Marfan's syndrome is thought to be a mutation affecting

A. Haemoglobin synthesis

B. Collagen synthesis

C. Metabolism homogentisic acid

D. Insufficient thyroid production

Ans. B.

571. Cyclins are proteins that

A. Regulate ability of cells to invade tissue

B. Regulate passage from one stage of cell division to another

C. Regulate apoptosis of damaged cells

D. None of the above

Ans. B.

572. Over 50% of common cancers are associated with damage to a protein, p53. This protein

A. Is a cyclin

B. Is a tumor supressor

C. Is an oncogene

D. Regulates apoptosis

Ans. B.

573. Protein folding is

A. Automatic, mediated by the protein itself

B. Mediated by other proteins called chaperones

C. Mediated by the ribosomes

D. None of these

Ans. B.

574. Sickle cell disease is due to

A. A mutation in the beta chain of Hb

B. A mutation in the alpha chain of Hb

C. Infection with a parasite

D. None of these

Ans. A.

575. The four subunits of the hemoglobin (Hb) gene represent protein's

A. Primary structure

B. Secondary structure

C. Tertiary structure

D. Quaternary structure

Ans. D.

576. Which of the following techniques was carried out by Nirenberg and Matthaei in 1961 to determine the first codon?

A. In vitro synthesis of a polypeptide using UUUUU
B. Labeled peptide binding to a ribosome
C. Mixed co-polymer mRNA synthesis
D. None of these

Ans. **A.**

577. Bacterial protein called catabolic activator protein (CAP) is an example of

A. Negative control of gene expression
B. Positive control of gene expression
C. Second type of positive control of gene expression
D. None of the above

Ans. **C.**

578. How many different codons are possible?

A. 3
B. 20
C. 64
D. An infinite number

Ans. **C.**

579. The genetic code is

A. Universal
B. Universal except for rare exceptions in mitochondria and some protozoa
C. Species specific
D. Kingdom specific

Ans. **B.**

580. Which of the following has been used as an evidence that primitive life forms lacked both DNA and enzymes?

A. RNA can both code genetic information and act as a catalyst
B. DNA and enzymes are only present in the most advanced cells
C. Advanced cells lack RNA
D. All of the above

Ans. **A.**

581. Crick demonstrated that the genetic code involved three bases and suggested that the code was degenerated. What experimental technique Crick conducted to suggest genetic code degeneration?

A. Gel electrophoresis
B. Density gradient centrifugation
C. Frameshift mutagenesis
D. Restriction digests of the rII gene

Ans. **C.**

582. Codon that specify the amino acids often differs in the

A. First base
B. Second base
C. Third base
D. None of these

Ans. C.

583. In some organelles in eukaryotes, the genetic code for some codons

A. Differ from that used in prokaryotes
B. Are same
C. Are partially same
D. None of the above

Ans. A.

584. The codons which do not specify an amino acid are called

A. Initiation code
B. Termination code
C. Propagation code
D. None of these

Ans. B.

585. The genetic code is degenerated. Which of the following codons represents the principle of degeneracy?

A. UAA and UAC
B. AUG and AUA
C. CAU and CAC
D. UUA and UUC

Ans. C.

586. The sequence of one strand of DNA is: 5' ATTGCCA 3', what is the sequence of the other strand?

A. 5' TAACGGT 3'
B. 5' TGGCAAT 3'
C. 5' ATTGCCA 3'
D. 5' UAAGCCU3'

Ans. B.

587. In prokaryotes, AUG encodes

A. Methionine
B. N-formyl methionine
C. a stop codon
D. Alanine

Ans. B.

588. How many amino acids will be encoded by 5' GAU GGU UGA UGU 3' sequence?

A. One
B. Two
C. Three
D. Four

Ans. B.

589. In protein synthesis of prokaryotes

A. The initiating amino acid is N- formyl methionine

B. The initiating amino acid is methionine

C. The initiating amino acid is phenyl alanine

D. None of these

Ans. A.

590. AUG codes for methionine act as a

A. Initiation code B. Elongation code

C. Termination code D. Propagation code

Ans. A.

591. Translation begins

A. At the replication fork B. On the lagging strand

C. At the start codon D. In nucleus

Ans. C.

592. Sex lethal (sxl) in Drosophila is transcribed when

A. The X autosome balance is less than 0.5

B. The X autosome balance is 1 or greater

C. The X autosome balance equals 0.5

D. None of the above

Ans. B.

593. A mutation in the tip binding site of the repressor would result in

A. Constitutive trp operon expression B. Inducible trp operon expression

C. No operon expression D. None of the above

Ans. A.

594. The first protein complex to bind to the TATA box is

A. Transcription factor IIA B. Transcription factor IIB

C. Transcription factor IID D. All of these

Ans. C.

595. Which of the following is not part of the lac operon?

A. I B. O

C. P D. None of these

Ans. A.

596. The lac operon is transcribed in which segments ?

A. 1 B. 2

C. 3 D. 4

Ans. A.

597. A frameshift mutation occurs in the sigma subunit gene transcribed as part of SPOl early genes. What will be the immediate result?

A. Early genes will not be translated

B. Middle genes will not be transcribed

C. The bacterial host will lyse immediately

D. Infection will proceed as usual

Ans. C.

598. In the presence of high levels of tryptophan

A. Attenuator allows transcription of TRP structural genes

B. Attenuator propogates transcription

C. Attenuator terminates transcription

D. None of these

Ans. C.

599. Tubulin is regulated by

A. Binding of tubulin to tubulin mRNA

B. Splicing of the tubulin transcript

C. Binding of tubulin to the tubulin translational product

D. Binding of tubulin to DNA

Ans. C.

600. Transcription factors are

A. Regions of DNA in the promoter area

B. Regions of DNA in the enhancer area

C. Any protein which binds to DNA

D. Proteins which bind DNA and initiate transcription

Ans. D.

601. Genes which need to be coordinately regulated but are not in operons may be regulated by

A. Common transcription factor binding domains

B. TATA boxes

C. CAAT regions

D. GC regions

Ans. A.

602. What are genes?

A. The functional unit of inheritance B. A fragment of DNA

C. A portion of a chromosome D. All of the above

Ans. D.

603. Which of the following is not a transcription factor?

A. Helix-turn-helix proteins B. Zinc finger proteins

C. Leucine zipper proteins D. Steroid hormones

Ans. D.

604. Sex determination in Drosophila involves

A. Alternate splicing B. Methylation

C. Gene amplification D. None of these

Ans. A.

605. Enhancers differ from promoters in that

A. They initiate transcription

B. They are adjacent to the start codon

C. Their orientation can be inverted without effect

D. They are restricted to a specific gene

Ans. C

606. Methylated genes are

A. Active B. Silent

C. Dynamic D. Either A or B

Ans. B.

607. Which of the following occur in the presence of glucose?

A. lac Z gene expression is increased

B. cAMP increases

C. Binding of CAP-cAMP complex to the promoter area decreases

D. None of the above

Ans. C.

608. Sex hormones activate transcription of specific genes by

A. Binding to a transcription factor B. Binding to RNA polymerase

C. Binding to DNA enhancer region D. Binding to DNA promoter region

Ans. A.

609. The Lac operon is translated into ——— proteins.

A. 1
B. 2
C. 3
D. 4

Ans. C.

610. In the presence of tryptophan in the cell, the repressor is —————.

A. Bound to tryptophan
B. Bound to DNA
C. Bound to both DNA and tryptophan
D. Bound to neither tryptophan nor DNA

Ans. C.

611. Catabolite activating protein exerts —— control on transcription of the lac operon genes.

A. Positive
B. Negative
C. May be positive or negative
D. None of these

Ans. A.

612. DNA is methylated at

A. AC sequences
B. TATA sequences
C. CAAT sequences
D. CG sequences

Ans. D.

613. Why are several structural genes regulated as a unit in bacteria?

A. An accident of evolution
B. It allows coordinating regulation of genes with a common function
C. The bacteria chromosome is so small; many different genes must be controlled by the same promoter
D. None of the above

Ans. B.

614. Alternate splicing of RNA transcripts is a mechanism to regulate

A. Tubulin
B. Tachykinins
C. DNA methylation
D. Leucine zippers

Ans. B.

615. Agarose gel electrophoresis and pulsed field gel electrophoresis may be used to resolve respectively

A. 2000 kb and 20kb DNA
B. 1000 kb and l0kb DNA
C. 20 kb and 2000 kb DNA
D. 10 kb and 1000 kb DNA

Ans. C.

616. The IPTG is a gratuitous inducers of β-galactosidase, and x-gal is a chromogenic substrate. When α-complementation occurs which colour is produced?

A. Blue
B. White
C. Brown
D. No color is produced

Ans. A.

617. The competitive immunoassay can be used

A. To detect very small amounts of antigen
B. To detect antibody associated with allergies (IgE)
C. Both A and B
D. Commonly to detect trace amounts of drugs.

Ans. C.

618. Which of the following is an immunodiffusion test?

A. Double diffusion
B. Gel diffusion
C. Ouchlerloney technique
D. All of these

Ans. D.

619. In Counter immunoelectrophoresis

A. Electrophoresis will drive the antibody and antigen parallel to each other
B. Electrophoresis will drive the antibody and antigen toward each other
C. The antibody will migrate towards anode
D. The antibody will migrate towards cathode

Ans. B.

620. What is the ELISA test intended to measure?

A. Antibody to HIV only
B. Antigen to HIV only
C. Presence of free, circulating virus in the patient
D. Antibodies directed against HLA molecules

Ans. A.

621. Immunoaffinity chromatography can be used in biochemical applications to

A. Break down antibody structure
B. Purify protein antigen
C. Break down antigen and analyze quantitatively
D. None of the above

Ans. B.

622. Different form of a plasmid, on an agarose gel, after electrophoresis may be resolved in which of the following sequence in decreasing molecular weight?

A. Open circular, super coiled, linear plasmid DNA

B. Linear plasmid, open circular, super coiled plasmid

C. Open circular, super coiled, linear plasmid DNA

D. Open circular, linear plasmid, super coiled plasmid

Ans. B.

623. In Rocket Immunodiffusion the length of the rocket is

A. Proportional to the amount of antibody placed in each well

B. Inversely proportional to the amount of antibody placed in each well

C. Inversely proportional to the amount of antigen placed in each well

D. Proportional to the amount of antigen placed in each well

Ans. D.

624. Radial immunodiffusion is similar to

A. Double diffusion
B. Gel diffusion

C. Ouchterloney technique
D. All of these

Ans. A.

625. Agarose a porous matrix used in various molecular biology technique is made by repetitive units of

A. Maltose
B. Agarobiose

C. Agar
D. None of these

Ans. B.

626. What radioactive molecule is used to end-label an oligonucleotide?

A. (alpha)-^{32}P-ATP
B. (alpha)-^{32}P-dUTP

C. (gamma)-^{32}P-ATP
D. Any of these

Ans. C.

627. Which of the following radioactive element is generally involved in RIA?

A. Tritium
B. Carbon-14

C. Iodine-125
D. All of these

Ans. D.

628. What is approximate half life of 32-Phosphorus?

A. 14 days
B. 28 days

C. 42 days
D. 30 days

Ans. A.

629. Rocket Immunodiffusion is also known as

A. Gel diffusion
B. Electroimmunodiffusion
C. Double diffusion
D. None of these

Ans. B.

630. DNA- footprinting is a suitable technique for identifying which of the following?

A. Particular mRNA in mixture
B. Particular t-RNA in mixture
C. Introns within DNA
D. Protein binding site within DNA

Ans. D.

631. What would happen if serum is omitted from the ELISA, but all other steps remain same?

A. Anti-human Ig-conjugate would not bind and be washed away
B. The OD values would be nearly the same as the assay control
C. Both A and B
D. Anti-human Ig-conjugate would bind non-specifically to the ELISA plate

Ans. C.

632. RAST test (radio allergosorbent test) is often used to detect

A. Antibodies associated with allergies (IgE)
B. Antigen associated with allergies (IgE)
C. Bacteriophages
D. None of the above

Ans. A.

633. What would happen if the anti-human Ig-conjugate is not washed free of the well before the substrate is added?

A. The ELISA would not develop when the substrate was added
B. The ELISA would develop normally
C. All wells would show uniform color-development due to unbound and excess anti-human Ig enzyme conjugate
D. None of the above

Ans. C.

634. An antigen preparation and an antibody preparation are tested by immunodiffusion. Three bands are found, indicating that

A. There was more than one antigen
B. The antibody was impure
C. The temperature was too high
D. There was one antibody and one antigen

Ans. A.

635. Immunoelectrophoresis techniques are designed to separate the mixture components from each other by using electrophoresis

A. Prior to reaction with antibody B. Prior to reaction with antigen

C. After reaction with antibody D. After reaction with antigen

Ans. A.

636. Which of the following is a positively charged matrix for ion exchange chromatography?

A. CM cellulose B. DEAE cellulose

C. Phosphocellulose D. None of these

Ans. B.

637. Which of the following is an immunoelectrophoresis technique?

A. Two-dimensional immunoelectrophoresis

B. Counterimmunoelectrophoresis

C. Coimmunoelectrophoresis

D. Both A and B

Ans. D.

638. The complex of RNA polymerase, DNA template and new RNA transcript is called

A. Transcription bubble B. Replication bubble

C. A translation bubble D. None of these

Ans. A.

639. RNA polymerase in prokaryotes has a removable

A. Alpha subunit B. Beta subunit

C. Both A and B D. Sigma subunit

Ans. D.

640. Promoters for tRNAs are located

A. Upstream from the start codon B. Downstream from the start codon

C. Both A and B D. None of these

Ans. B.

641. The binding of lac repressor to DNA could be considered to be analogous to

A. Competitive inhibition of an enzyme

B. Mixed-type inhibition of an enzyme

C. Uncompetitive inhibition of an enzyme

D. Allosteric effects in enzyme regulation

Ans. A.

642. Rho-dependent termination of transcription in *E.coli*

A. Requires ATP

B. Requires about 50 nucleotides of uncomplexed mRNA

C. Both A and B

D. Removes mRNA and holoenzyme from the DNA

Ans. C.

643. Enhancers are regions that

A. Bind RNA polymerase B. Are adjacent to the TATA box

C. Are CAT box binding proteins D. Modulate transcription

Ans. D.

644. Transcription by *E. coli* polymerase occurs in

A. Four phases known as initiation, propagation, elongation and termination

B. Three phases known as initiation, elongation and termination

C. Two phases known as initiation and termination

D. None of the above

Ans. B.

645. Which of the following is necessary for transcription to occur ?

A. DNA molecule B. RNA molecule

C. DNA polymerase D. Both DNA and RNA polymerase

Ans. D.

646. Multiple copies of 5S genes, located at a chromosomal site distinct from the other rRNA genes

A. Are transcribed by rRNA polymerase III and the 5S rRNA

B. Are transcribed by rRNA polymerase II

C. Are transcribed by rRNA polymerase I and the 5S rRNA

D. Are transcribed by DNA polymerase I

Ans. A.

647. Each tRNA molecule has a cloverleaf secondary structure consisting of

A. Three stem loops B. Two stem loops

C. Four stem loops D. Either A or B

Ans. A.

648. What is a promoter?

A. A specific sequence of DNA to which a catabolic repressor binds

B. A specific sequence of DNA to which RNA polymerase binds

C. A specific DNA sequence to which a restriction endonuclease binds

D. None of the above

Ans. B.

649. The function of the sigma factor of RNA polymerase is to

A. Assure that transcription begins at the proper point

B. Assure that transcription ends at the proper point

C. Assure that translation begins at the proper point

D. Assure that translation ends at the proper point

Ans. A.

650. In both eukaryotes and prokaryotes, a promoter region that is rich in AT bases is called as

A. CATT

B. Shine Dalgarno region

C. TATA box

D. SV40 region

Ans. C.

651. The RNA polymerases that transcribe bacterial DNA are

A. Multisubunit enzymes

B. Only active inside the cell

C. Interchangable with DNA polymerases

D. Highly glycosylated in their active forms

Ans. A.

652. Immediately after transcription

A. A methylated guanine cap is added to the 5' end of the transcript

B. A methylated guanine cap is added to the 3' end of the transcript

C. Both A and B

D. A poly adenylation signal is added

Ans. A.

653. Transcription factors are

A. Promoters

B. Proteins which bind to DNA and regulate transcription

C. TATA boxes

D. CATT boxes

Ans. B.

654. The major function of RNA polymerase's sigma factor is
   A. Recognition of the translational stop sequence
   B. Recognition of the transcriptional start sequence
   C. Recognition of the transcriptional stop sequence
   D. Recognition of the translational start sequence

Ans. B.

655. Most transcripts of protein coding genes are cleaved
   A. At the 3' end just after a poly adenylation signal
   B. At the 3' end just before a poly adenylation signal
   C. At the 5' end immediately after a poly adenylation signal
   D. At the 5' end immediately before a poly adenylation signal

Ans. A.

656. RNA is synthesized on a DNA template in a process called———, which utilizes the enzyme ——-.
   A. Translation, RNA polymerase   B. Transcription, DNA polymerase
   C. Transcription, RNA polymerase   D. Replication, DNA polymerase

Ans. C.

657. The closed complex at bacterial promoters is
   A. In equilibrium with free RNA polymerase and the promoter
   B. Not affected by promoter mutations
   C. Bound more tightly when repressors are present
   D. Not affected by activator proteins

Ans. A.

658. Transcription begins
   A. At the start codon   B. Upstream from the start codon
   C. Downstream from the start codon   D. None of these

Ans. B.

659. Transcription results in
   A. An amino acid chain   B. Messenger RNA
   C. Complementary DNA   D. Okazaki fragments

Ans. B.

660. RNA polymerase holoenzyme initiates transcription which involves
   A. Recognition of the -10 sequence and -35 sequence
   B. Recognition of the -10 sequence only
   C. Recognition of the -35 sequence only
   D. None of the above

Ans. A.

661. The transcriptional regulatory proteins in eukaryotes which induce transcription usually have

A. At least two distinct domains of protein structure, a DNA binding domain and an activation domain

B. At least two distinct domains of protein structure and a DNA binding domain

C. At least one distinct domains of protein structure, a DNA binding domain and an activation domain

D. None of these

Ans. A.

662. In prokaryotes, transcription is

A. Terminated by the stop codon
B. Terminated by a protein called rho
C. Terminated by a poly A sequence
D. Terminated by a start codon

Ans. B.

663. In eukaryotes, there are three different RNA polymerases. The RNA polymerase responsible for transcription of mRNA is

A. RNA polymerase I
B. RNA polymerase II
C. RNA polymerase III
D. None of the above

Ans. B.

664. The nucleus of eukaryotic cell has

A. RNA polymerase I
B. RNA polymerase II
C. RNA polymerase III
D. All of these

Ans. D.

665. Upstream regions which are essential for correct transcription are called

A. Enhancers
B. Start codons
C. Promoters
D. Transcription factors

Ans. C.

666. Transcription of each set of rRNA genes by RNA polymerase l produces

A. A single 45S rRNA precursor molecule

B. A single 5S rRNA precursor molecule

C. A single 18S rRNA precursor molecule

D. A single 28S rRNA precursor molecule

Ans. A.

667. The regions of a gene located at -10 and -35, with respect to the start of transcription, are termed

A. Start codons
B. oriC regions
C. Shine Dalgarno sequences
D. Promoters

Ans. D.

668. Which of the following conditions would cause the release of the lac repressor protein from the lac operator site on DNA?

A. Presence of glucose in the growth media

B. Presence of lactose in the growth media

C. Presence of IPTG (isopropyl thiogalactoside) in the growth media

D. Both B and C

Ans. D.

669. On the ribosome, mRNA binds

A. Between the subunits B. To the large subunit

C. To the small subunit D. None of these

Ans. C.

670. Type I proteins (plasma membrane) have a

A. Cleavage N- terminal signal sequence and a hydrophobic stop transfer sequence

B. Cleavaged N- terminal signal sequence that doubles as the membrane anchoring sequence

C. Multiple signal sequence and a hydrophobic stop transfer sequence

D. Multiple signal sequence that doubles as the membrane anchoring sequence

Ans. A.

671. Which of the following is not a necessary component of translation?

A. Anticodon B. mRNA

C. Ligase D. Amino aicd

Ans. C.

672. A polysome could be best described as

A. An active site of DNA synthesis B. An active site of protein synthesis

C. An active site of lipid synthesis D. All of the above

Ans. B.

673. Eukaryotic mRNA binding to the ribosomes is facilitated by ——————.

A. The Shine Dalgarno sequence B. The 7-methyl guanosine cap

C. tRNA D. poly A tail

Ans. B.

674. Amino acids are joined together into a protein chain by which of the following?

A. tRNA B. DNA polymerase

C. Hydrogen bonds D. mRNA

Ans. A.

675. Phosphorus is taken up by the cell during the process of

A. Carbohydrate synthesis
B. Protein synthesis
C. Lipid synthesis
D. ATP synthesis

Ans. D.

676. Protein synthesis rates in prokaryotes are limited by the rate of mRNA synthesis. If RNA synthesis occurs at the rate of 50 nucleotides/sec, then rate of protein synthesis occurs at

A. 10 amino acids/sec
B. 17 amino acids/sec
C. 25 amino acids/sec
D. 50 amino acids/sec

Ans. B.

677. The site of protein synthesis is

A. Ribosome
B. Nucleus
C. Endoplasmic reticulum
D. Chromosome

Ans. A.

678. The structure in a bacterium that indicates an active site for protein synthesis is

A. A chromosome
B. A cell membrane
C. A flagellum
D. A polysome

Ans. D.

679. The lac operon contains the z, y and a structural genes

A. Encoding p-galactosidase, galactose permeases and thio-galactosidase transacetylase respectively
B. Encoding p-galactosidase and galactose permeases
C. Encoding P-galactosidase only
D. None of the above

Ans. A.

680. Proteins contain ——— different amino acids, whereas DNA and RNA are composed of——— different nucleotides.

A. 20, 64
B. 3, 20
C. 4, 20
D. 20, 4

Ans. D.

681. Which of the following is not necessary for protein synthesis to occur, once transcription is completed?

A. tRNA
B. Ribosomes
C. mRNA
D. DNA

Ans. D.

682. Ribosomes select the correct tRNAs
   A. Then bind to the appropriate mRNA
   B. Solely on the basis of their anticodons
   C. Depending on their abundance in the cytosol
   D. With the least abundant anticodons

Ans. B.

683. Signal peptide protein removal that is translocated across a membrane is accomplished by
   A. Met aminopeptidase
   B. Trypsin
   C. Signal peptidase
   D. Chymotrypsin

Ans. C.

684. The direction of amino acid transfer to the growing polypeptide chain is
   A. From the A (aminoacyl tRNA site) site to the P (peptidyl tRNA site) site on the ribosome
   B. From the P site to the A site on the ribosome
   C. From the A site to the E (exit tRNA site) site on the ribosome
   D. From the P site to the E site on the ribosome

Ans. B.

685. The pathway of a tRNA during polypeptide elongation on the ribosome is
   A. A site→P site→E site
   B. P site→entry site→exit site
   C. A site→P site→entry site
   D. P site→A site→E site

Ans. A.

686. Which of the following has unusual bases?
   A. mRNA
   B. tRNA
   C. rRNA
   D. hnRNA

Ans. B.

687. The site on a bacterial chromosome that marks the termination point for chromosome replication is called
   A. *ter*
   B. A stop codon
   C. A stem loop
   D. *pau*

Ans. A.

688. Degenerated codon differs mostly in
   A. The identities of their second base
   B. The identities of their third base
   C. The wobble position
   D. Both B and C

Ans. D.

689. Translation in prokaryotes begins by the formation of a 30S initiation complex between the

A. 30S ribosomal subunit, mRNA, initiation factors and N-fMet tRNA

B. 30S ribosomal subunit, tRNA and initiation factors

C. 30S ribosomal subunit and mRNA only

D. 30S ribosomal subunit, mRNA and initiation factors

Ans. A.

690. The anticodon of tRNA

A. Binds to rRNA

B. Binds to an amino acid

C. Binds to the Shine Dalgarno sequence

D. Binds to an mRNA codon

Ans. D.

691. The peptidyl transferase reaction occurs

A. On the large subunit B. On the small subunit

C. Between the subunit D. None of these

Ans. A.

692. Processive synthesis is a characteristic feature of

A. All DNA polymerases

B. DNA Pol III at a replication fork

C. Removal of RNA primers on Okazaki fragments

D. DNA mismatch pair

Ans. B.

693. Which site of the tRNA molecule binds to the mRNA molecule?

A. Anticodon B. Codon

C. Amino aicd D. 5 prime end

Ans. A.

694. The first step in translation is

A. Binding of the two ribosomal subunits to each other

B. Binding of mRNA to the two ribosomal subunits

C. Binding of tRNA to the small ribosomal subunit

D. Binding of mRNA to the small ribosomal subunit

Ans. D.

695. Which of the following amino acid starts all proteins synthesis?

A. Glycine B. Proline

C. Thymine D. Methionine

Ans. D.

696. The growing polypeptide chain is released from the ribosomes when

A. A chain terminating codon is reached

B. Achain terminating tRNA binds to the ribosome

C. The 7-methyl guanosine cap is reached

D. The poly A tail is reached

Ans. A.

697. Which of the following RNAs bind to an amino acid?

A. mRNA B. tRNA

C. rRNA D. hnRNA

Ans. B.

698. How many bases of nucleic acid determine a single amino acid?

A. Four B. One

C. Two D. Three

Ans. D.

699. The ribosomes are composed of

A. Proteins B. RNA

C. Both A and B D. Lipids

Ans. C

700. Which is required for protein synthesis?

A. tRNA B. mRNA

C. rRNA D. All of these

Ans. D.

701. Glycolytic pathway regulation involves

A. Allosteric stimulation by ADP

B. Allosteric inhibition by ATP

C. Feedback, or product, inhibition by ATP

D. All of the above

Ans. D.

702. During catabolism, only about 40% of the energy available from oxidizing glucose is used to synthesize ATP. Remaining 60%

A. Is lost as heat

B. Is used to reduce NADP

C. Remains in the products of metabolism

D. Is stored as fat

Ans. A.

703. Why does the glycolytic pathway continue in the direction of glucose catabolism?

A. There are essentially three irreversible reactions that act as the driving force for the pathway

B. High levels of ATP keep the pathway going in a forward direction

C. The enzymes of glycolysis only function in one direction

D. Glycolysis occurs in either direction

Ans. A.

704. The released energy obtained by oxidation of glucose is stored as

A. a concentration gradient across a membrane

B. ADP

C. ATP

D. NAD+

Ans. C.

705. A kinase is an enzyme that

A. Removes phosphate groups of substrates

B. Uses ATP to add a phosphate group to the substrate

C. Uses NADH to change the oxidation state of the substrate

D. Removes water from a double bond

Ans. B.

706. For every one molecule of sugar glucose which is oxidized ———— molecule of pyruvic acid are produced.

A. 1 B. 2

C. 3 D. 4

Ans. B.

707. In the glycogen synthase reaction, the precursor to glycogen is

A. Glucose-6-P B. UTP – glucose

C. UDP-glucose D. Glucose-1-P

Ans. C.

708. The active form of glycogen phosphorylase is phosphorylated, while the dephosphorylation of which active form occurs?

A. Glycogen synthase B. Glycogen semisynthase

C. Glycogen hydrolase D. Glycogen dehydrogenase

Ans. A.

709. The amount of energy received from one ATP is

A. 76 kcal B. 7.3 kcal

C. 760 kcal D. 1000 kcal

Ans. B.

710. The enzymes of glycolysis in a eukaryotic cell are located in the

A. Intermembrane space B. Plasma membrane

C. Cytosol D. Mitochondrial matrix

Ans. C.

711. When concentration of the reactants is higher than the equilibrium concentration then

A. The gibbs free energy will be positive

B. The gibbs free energy will be negative

C. More products will be formed

D. Both B and C

Ans. D.

712. Which of the following is not true of glycolysis?

A. ADP is phosphorylated to ATP via substrate level phosphorylation

B. The pathway does not require oxygen

C. The pathway oxidizes two moles of NADH to NAD^+ for each mole of glucose that enters

D. The pathway requires two moles of ATP to get started catabo-lizing each mole of glucose

Ans. C.

713. In glycolysis, ATP is formed by the transfer of a high-energy phosphate from 1,3-bisphosphoglycerate to ADR. No such high-energy phosphate donor has ever been isolated in mitochondria because

A. The techniques for isolating the phosphate donor are not refined enough

B. No such phosphate donor exists

C. The high-energy phosphate donor is very short-lived and difficult to isolate

D. None of these

Ans. B.

714. ATP is from which general category of molecules?

A. Polysaccharides B. Proteins

C. Nucleotides D. Amino acids

Ans. C.

715. The glycolytic pathway (glucose→2 pyruvate) is found

A. In all living organisms

B. Primarily in animals excluding particles

C. Only in eukaryotes

D. Only in yeast

Ans. A.

716. Phosphofructokinase, the major flux-controlling enzyme of glycolysis is allosterically inhibited and activated respectively by

A. ATP and PEP B. AMP and Pi

C. ATP and ADP D. Citrate and ATP

Ans. C.

717. Which of the following regulates glycolysis steps?

A. Phosphofructokinase B. Hexose kinase

C. Pyruvate kinase D. All of these

Ans. D.

718. During glycolysis, the major energy generating step involves

A. Pyruvate kinase B. Phosphoglycerate kinase

C. Glyceraldehyde-3 –dehydrogenase D. Phosphofructokinase

Ans. C.

719. Fructose-2,6-bisphosphate

A. Activates fructose-1,6-bisphosphatase

B. Activates phosphofructokinase

C. Inhibits fructose-1,6-bisphosphatase

D. Both B and C

Ans. D.

720. Glucose from the breakdown of glycogen is obtained in

A. The liver by phosphorolysis B. The muscles by phosphorolysis

C. The muscles by hydrolysis D. Both A and B

Ans. D.

721. Glycogen has

A. α-1,4 linkage
B. α-1,6 linkages
C. α-1,4 and α-1,6 linkages
D. α-1,4 and β-1,6 linkage

Ans. C.

722. The symptoms of retinol excess are

A. Bone fragility
B. Nausea
C. Weakness
D. All of these

Ans. D.

723. Main function of insulin hormone is to

A. Increase glycogen in liver
B. Decrease glycogen in liver
C. Increase blood sugar
D. Decrease blood sugar

Ans. D.

724. Ascorbic acid acts as an

A. Reducing agent
B. Oxidizing agent
C. Both oxidizing and reducing agent
D. None of the above

Ans. A.

725. A deficiency of thiamin produces the disease known as

A. Beri-beri
B. Scurvy
C. Cataract
D. Anemia

Ans. A.

726. Acyl carrier protein (ACP) plays an important role in the biosynthesis of

A. Fatty acids
B. Amino acids
C. Sugars
D. Carbohydrates

Ans. A.

727. Vitamin B_{12} (Cobalamin) is only synthesized by

A. Fishes
B. Micro-organisms
C. Plants
D. Animals

Ans. B.

728. Which of the following are reduced coenzymes?

A. NADH and FADH2
B. NAD^+ and FAD
C. ATP and GTP
D. Coenzyme A and ubiquinone

Ans. A.

729. The absence of ascorbic acid in the human diet gives rise to

A. Rickets
B. Pernicious anemia
C. Cataract
D. Beri-beri

Ans. B.

730. Vitamins are essential because the organism

A. Can't synthesize these compounds at all
B. Can synthesize these compounds partially
C. Can't synthesize these compounds in the adequate amounts
D. None of the above

Ans. A.

731. The prosthetic group biotin is a carrier of which type of molecule?

A. Activated carbon dioxide (CO_2)
B. Ammonia
C. Methyl group
D. Sulfhydryl group

Ans. A.

732. Lipoic acid exists in

A. Oxidized form
B. Reduced form
C. Oxidized and reduced form both
D. None of these

Ans. C.

733. Vitamin B_{12} is useful in the prevention and treatment of

A. Pernicious anemia
B. Scurvy
C. Cataract
D. Beri-beri

Ans. A.

734. An example of a digestive hormone is

A. Lipase
B. Pepsin
C. Amylase
D. Gastrin

Ans. D.

735. In the co-enzyme B_{12} the position occupied by a cyanide ion in vitamin B_{12} is bonded directly to the ———— of the ribose of adenosine.

A. Adenine
B. 5-6 Dimethylbenzimidazole
C. Hydroxycobalamin
D. Cyanocobalamin

Ans. A.

736. The reductant, NADH, transfers the electrons via a flavo-proteins to the specific disulfide (S-S) protein to form a dithiol (SH,SH) protein which converts vitamin

A. $B_{12}(Co^{2+})$to $B_{12}(Co)$
B. $B_{12}(Co)$ to $B_{12}(Co^{2+})$
C. $B_{12}(Co^{2+})$to $B_{12}(Co^{+})$
D. $B_{12}(Co^{+})$to $B_{12}(Co^{2+})$

Ans. C.

737. An early sign of retinol deficiencies in man is

A. Night blindness
B. Keratinization
C. Xeropthalmia
D. None of these

Ans. A.

738. An enzyme, L-folate reductase reduces folic acid to

A. Hydrofolic acid
B. Dihydrofolic acid
C. Trihydrofolic acid
D. Tetrahydrofolic acid

Ans. B.

739. What compound of raw egg white causes a syndrome similar to vitamin B deficiency?

A. Avidin
B. Betabindin
C. Ovalbumin
D. Albumin

Ans. A.

740. The disease Beriberi is due to a dietary deficiency in

A. Vitamin B_1 (thiamine)
B. Vitamin B_2 (riboflavin)
C. Vitamin B_6 (pyridoxine)
D. Vitamin B_{12}

Ans. A.

741. Which of these is a symptom of vitamin A deficiency?

A. Osteoporosis
B. Impaired taste perception
C. Blindness
D. Impaired blood clotting

Ans. C.

742. Vitamin-C is considered as a

A. Water soluble
B. Fat soluble
C. Fat and water soluble
D. None of these

Ans. A.

743. The vitamin niacin is part of the __________ molecule.

A. Ferredoxin
B. Pyridoxal phosphate
C. Pyrophosphate
D. NAD^+

Ans. D.

744. Which of these hormones is a catecholamine?

A. Follitropin
B. Norepinephrine
C. Tetraiodothyronine
D. Tetrahydrofolate

Ans. B.

745. Dihydroorotate dehydrogenase contains

A. 4 flavins and 4 atoms of iron per molecule

B. 2 flavins and 4 atoms of iron per molecule

C. 2 flavins and 2 atoms of iron per molecule

D. 4 flavins and 2 atoms of iron per molecule

Ans. A.

746. *E.coli* ACP has its molecular weight as around

A. 9000 B. 19000

C. 39000 D. 90,000

Ans. A.

747. The vitamin riboflavin is part of the __________ molecule.

A. Ferredoxin B. FAD

C. Pyridoxal phosphat D. Pyrophosphate

Ans. B.

748. The most prominent role that tocopherol has in *in-vitro* systems is as a strong

A. Antioxidants B. Reducing agent

C. Oxidizing agent D. All of these

Ans. A.

749. Biotin occurs mainly in combined forms bound to protein through

A. ε-N-lysine moiety B. ε-S-lysine moiety

C. ε-N-biotinyl-L-lysine D. ε-N-lipoyl - L-lysine

Ans. A.

750. Lipoic acid is a co-factor of the

A. Pyruvic dehydrogenase B. α-ketoglutaric dehydrogenase

C. Both (a) and (b) D. Di-hydroorotate dehydrogenase

Ans. C.

751. β-carotene together with α-carotene, γ-carotene and cryptoxanthine are synthesized by

A. Plants B. Animal

C. Plants and animals both D. None of these

Ans. A.

752. Vitamin-D deficiency can cause

A. Rickets B. Pernicious anemia

C. Cataract D. Beri-beri

Ans. A.

753. A deficiency of Vitamin K results in a decreased level of

A. Prothrombin B. Thrombin

C. Fibrin D. Fibrinogen

Ans. A.

754. The vitamin riboflavin, which occurs as a yellow pigment in egg yolk and milk become

A. Colorless on reduction with Zn in acid and regained its color on re-oxidation

B. Colorless on oxidation and regained its color on reduction with Zn in acid

C. More deep in color on reduction with Zn in acid and regained its color on re-oxidation

D. More deep in color on oxidation and regained its color on reduction with Zn in acid

Ans. A.

755. Which of the following compounds/(s) belong/(s) to the vitamin B_6 group?

A. Pyridoxal B. Pyridoxine

C. Pyridoxamine D. All of these

Ans. D.

756. What metal ion is specifically bound by vitamin B_{12}?

A. Cobalt B. Copper

C. Zinc D. Iron

Ans. A.

757. A fat-soluble vitamin that regulates blood clotting is

A. Vitamin A B. Vitamin K

C. Vitamin C D. Niacin

Ans. B.

758. Which of these is a vitamin A precursor?

A. Cobalamin B. Pyridoxine

C. Beta-Carotene D. Thiamine

Ans. C.

759. In one iron-metalloflavoprotein, the iron is present as a

A. Heme-protein B. Nonheme type

C. Both (a) and (b) D. Flavin moiety

Ans. A.

760. Vitamin K_1 was first isolated from alfalalfa and has the phytyl side chain consisting of

A. Four isoprene units
B. Six isoprene units
C. Nine isoprene units
D. Four isoprene units

Ans. A.

761. Which of these molecules is vitamin H?

A. Biotin
B. Carnitine
C. Folic acid
D. None of these

Ans. A.

762. The occurrence of metals such as iron or molybdenum in some flavoproteins can

A. Stabilize the semiquinone
B. De-stabilize the semiquinone
C. Form chelation
D. All of these

Ans. A.

763. Models of end-linked Osaka VI Fibrinogen dimers, a bilayer dimer is linked at

A. Both ends by one disulfide bond
B. Either end via two disulfide bonds
C. Either end via a single disulfide bond
D. Both ends by two disulfide bonds

Ans. D.

764. A deficiency of niacin causes

A. Pellagra
B. Scurvy
C. Cataract
D. Anemia

Ans. A.

765. Selenium is an essential component of the enzyme glutathione peroxidase which

A. Scavenges toxic hydoperoxy compounds in tissues
B. Reduces toxic hydoperoxy compounds in tissues
C. Oxidizes toxic hydoperoxy compounds in tissues
D. None of the above

Ans. A.

766. Who discovered vitamin C (ascorbic acid)?

A. Paul Berg
B. Linus Pauling
C. Albert Szent-Gyorgyi
D. Kerry Mull is

Ans. C.

767. Which of the following mineral is involved in protein metabolism and oxidation reactions?

A. Molybdenum B. Manganese
C. Magnesium D. Calcium

Ans. A.

768. Which of the following mineral deficiency may result into impaired growth and development, skin lesions and loss of appetite?

A. Zinc B. Cobalt
C. Iron D. Magnesium

Ans. A.

769. Which of the following is not a function of iron?

A. Oxygen transport B. Immune function
C. Brain function D. Gene regulation

Ans. D.

770. Consumption of which nutrient leads to the multiplication of oral bacteria?

A. Fat B. Carbohydrate
C. Protein D. Fluoride

Ans. B.

771. Examples of goitrogenic foods are ———— and ————.

A. Turnips and corn B. Rutabagas and okra
C. Raw cabbage and turnips D. Cassava and lettuce

Ans. C.

772. Which of the following carbohydrate is effective in promoting the calcium absorption?

A. Lactose B. Maltose
C. Sucrose D. Xylose

Ans. A.

773. What condition is caused by iodine deficiency during pregnancy and is characterized by stunted growth, deafness, and mental retardation?

A. Cretinism B. Keshan disease
C. Multiple sclerosis D. Crohn's disease

Ans. A.

774. Iodine is a part of thyroid hormone and is essential for the prevention of

A. Goiter B. Osteoporosis
C. Muscle weakness D. Diarrhea

Ans. A.

775. What transports copper from the intestinal cells to the liver?

A. Ceruloplasmin B. Secretin

C. Acrolein D. Albumin

Ans. A.

776. Which group is most often affected with copper deficiency?

A. Elderly woman B. Alcoholics

C. Active toddlers with limited D. Preterm infants food variety

Ans. A.

777. What is the main source of natural fluoride?

A. Mushrooms B. Potatoes

C. Meat D. Water

Ans. D.

778. Which of the following mineral is involved in the enzyme -controlled energy yielding reactions of metabolism?

A. Calcium B. Phosphorus

C. Iron D. Copper

Ans. B.

779. The mineral which aids in the utilization of iron and in hemoglobin synthesis is

A. Calcium B. Phosphorus

C. Cobalt D. Copper

Ans. D.

780. The mineral which is considered important in maintaining electrical potential in nerves and membranes is

A. Magnesium B. Manganese

C. Calcium D. Iron

Ans. A.

781. Wilson's disease is an example of——— and Menkes' syndrome is an example of————.

A. Zinc deficiency; zinc toxicity

B. Zinc toxicity; zinc deficiency

C. Copper deficiency; copper toxicity

D. Copper toxicity; copper deficiency

Ans. D.

782. Which of the following is correct?

A. Cobalt is part of vitamin B_{12}.

B. Cobalt will not replace the need for vitamin B_{12} in humans

C. Both A and B

D. Cobalt will replace the need for vitamin B_{12} in humans

Ans. C.

783. Which of the following is required as a component of blood hemoglobin?

A. Iron B. Magnesium

C. Calcium D. Copper

Ans. A.

784. Adding ———— to a breakfast of cereal will help your body absorb iron.

A. Milk B. Orange juice

C. Coffee D. Water

Ans. B.

785. Which of the following ion is required for the development of sound teeth with resistance to tooth decay?

A. Fluoride ion B. Sodium ion

C. Chloride ion D. Magnesium ion

Ans. A.

786. Which of the following two beverages contribute 20 to 30 percent of our daily manganese intake?

A. Milk or tea B. Cola or coffee

C. Tea or orange juice D. Milk or orange juice

Ans. A.

787. An endemic disease of cardiomyopathy in children is attributed to

A. Low Se in the environment B. Low intake of iron

C. High Se in the environment D. High intake of iron

Ans. A.

788. Which of the following statement is correct?

A. Sodium and chloride are the chief extracellular ions of the body

B. Sodium and chloride are primarily involved in maintaining osmotic equilibrium and body fluid volume.

C. Chloride ion is necessary for the production of hydrochloric acid of gastric juice.

D. All of these

Ans. D.

789. Which of the following is necessary for the clotting of blood, functions of certain enzymes and control of fluids through cell membranes?

A. Calcium
B. Magnesium
C. Copper
D. Cobalt

Ans. A.

790. Selenium deficiency leads to

A. Liver necrosis
B. Diarrhea
C. Multiple sclerosis
D. Crohn's disease

Ans. A.

791. Manganese is a key component of all of the following enzymes except

A. Arginase
B. Pyruvate carboxylase
C. Ceruloplasmin
D. Mn-superoxide dismutase

Ans. C.

792. Which of the following vitamin is essential for the absorption of calcium from the intestinal tract?

A. Vitamin D
B. Vitamin E
C. Vitamin B_{12}
D. Vitamin B_6

Ans. A.

793. Which trace mineral is a component of the enzyme that activates vitamin A in the eye?

A. Zinc
B. Iron
C. Iodine
D. Chromium

Ans. A.

794. Chronic consumption of excess selenium can lead to

A. Brittle hair and nails.
B. Muscle weakness,
C. TPN
D. Diarrhea.

Ans. B.

795. Normal glucose metabolism requires

A. Chromium
B. Manganese
C. Magnesium
D. Calcium

Ans. A.

796. Manganese is needed for

A. Normal bone structure
B. Reproduction and functioning of central nervous system
C. Both (a) and (b)
D. Muscle strengthening

Ans. C.

797. Which of these restriction enzymes produce blunt ends?

A. SalI B. EcoRV
C. XhoI D. HindIII

Ans. B.

798. The RP13 gene of chromosome 17 codes for a protein ————- .

A. Involved in glucose transport
B. That is a component of hair and nails
C. Involved in eye development
D. Involved in the determination of personality

Ans. C.

799. Isoschizomers recognize

A. Same recognition sequence but different recognition site
B. Same recognition site and recognition sequence
C. Same recognition site and different recognition sequence
D. Different recognition site and different recognition sequence

Ans. B.

800. Restriction enzymes are named for

A. The person who discovered B. The bacterium they are derived from
C. The viral DNA that they attack D. None of the above

Ans. B.

801. Which of these genes codes for a protein that plays a role in white blood cell function?

A. DCP1 B. MPO
C. GLUT4 D. RP13

Ans. B.

802. When populations are small, gene frequencies can change from generation to generation and some alleles may become fixed in a population. This is called—.

A. Assortative mating B. Inbreeding
C. Heterosis D. Genetic drift

Ans. D.

803. Which of the following is correct in terms of determination of location of genetic traits?

A. Known protein coding sequences are too far apart to allow linkage determination for most new genes
B. Restriction sites allow DNAs to be digested
C. Protein-coding genes are always associated with a restriction pattern
D. None of the above

Ans. A.

804. In gel electrophoresis, DNA molecules migrate from ——— to ——— ends of the gel.

A. Negative ... positive
B. Basic ... acidic
C. Long ... short
D. Positive to negative

Ans. A.

805. The transfer of antibiotic-resistant genes from genetically engineered bacteria to disease-causing bacteria ———.

A. Would be of no concern if it occurred.
B. Has occurred
C. Can never occur
D. Seems unlikely

Ans. D.

806. Both DNA gel electrophoresis and SDS-PAGE of proteins are similar because

A. In both cases molecules migrate to the anode
B. Both techniques rely on a constant charge to mass ratio
C. Both techniques utilize the sieving properties of gels
D. All of the above

Ans. D.

807. The TP53 gene of chromosome 17 codes for a protein ———.

A. That plays a role in the digestive process
B. Involved in glucose transport
C. Involved in the regulation of the cell cycle
D. That is like a white blood cell protein

Ans. C.

808. Reverse transcriptase from HIV does not

A. Uses RNA as a template
B. Have a 5' to 3' polymerase activity
C. Have a 3'- 5' exonuclease activity
D. Requires a primer

Ans. C.

809. Which of the following amino acids can interact with the DNA or RNA nucleotide bases via hydrogen bonding?

A. Asn and Gln
B. Cys and Met
C. Lys and Leu
D. Ile and Val

Ans. A.

810. Different DNA polymerases play distinct roles in DNA replication and repair in both prokaryotic and eukaryotic cells. All known DNA polymerases synthesize DNA only in the ——— by the addition of dNTPs to a performed primer strand of DNA.

A. Positive direction
B. 3' to 5' direction
C. 5' to 3' direction
D. Negative direction

Ans. C.

811. Which of the following amino acids interact with the DNA or RNA backbone (i.E. phosphate)?

A. Ile and Val
B. Lys and Arg
C. Leu and Ala
D. Cys and Met

Ans. B.

812. Unpaired H-bond donors and acceptors are found in the hydrophobic core of a protein

A. Only at the ends of α-helices
B. Only at the turns connecting p-strands
C. Only on Pro residues
D. Rarely

Ans. D.

813. Attractive Vander Waals forces occur between

A. Apolar molecules in the liquid state
B. Any pair of nearby atoms
C. Polar molecules in the solid state
D. Only if other forces are less favorable

Ans. B.

814. Which of the following forces is the most favorable for protein folding?

A. Conformational entropy
B. Hydrophobic Interactions
C. Vander Waals interactions
D. Hydrogen bonds

Ans. B.

815. Which of the following is the most correct?

A. Charged amino acids are never buried in the interior of a protein
B. Charged amino acids are seldom buried in the interior of a protein
C. All hydrophobic amino acids are buried when a protein folds
D. Tyrosine is only found in the interior of proteins

Ans. B.

816. Which of the following forces is the most unfavorable for protein folding?

A. Conformational entropy
B. Hydrophobic interactions
C. Vander Waals interactions
D. Electrostatic interactions

Ans. A.

817. The correlation between free energy ΔG transfer between the aqueous/organic phases and the surface area of amino acid residues

A. Reflects the reduction in solvent-accessible area during protein folding
B. Is only meaningful for the polar amino acids
C. Ignores the important contribution of the peptide bond
D. Is similar to effects seen with SDS denaturation

Ans. A.

818. If the egg white protein, ovalbumin, is denatured in a hard-boiled egg, then which of the following is least affected?

A. The primary structure of ovalbumin
B. The secondary structure of ovalbumin
C. The tertiary structure of ovalbumin
D. The quaternary structure of ovalbumin

Ans. A.

819. Buried hydrophobic side chains in a globular protein fit into a hole formed by the side chains of

A. 1-3 other amino acids
B. 5-7 other amino acids
C. 9-12 other amino acids
D. 13-15 other amino acids

Ans. B.

820. Enzyme-driven metabolic pathways can be made more efficient by

A. Concentrating enzymes within specific cellular compartments
B. Grouping enzymes into free-floating, multienzyme complexes
C. Fixing enzymes into membranes so that they are adjacent to each other
D. All of the above

Ans. D.

821. Which of the following (s) is/are serine proteases?

A. Chymotrypsin
B. Trypsin
C. Elastase
D. All of these

Ans. D.

822. Which of the following statements about enzymes or their function is true?
A. Enzymes do not alter the overall change in free energy for a reaction
B. Enzymes are proteins whose three-dimensional form is key to their function
C. Enzymes speed up reactions by lowering activation energy
D. All of the above

Ans. D.

823. Tryprotophan synthetase of *E.coli*, a typical bifunctional oligomeric enzyme consist of
A. A protein designated A
B. Two proteins designated A and B
C. A protein A and one-subunit a
D. A protein designated B

Ans. B.

824. What is the specificity of the Clostripain protease?
A. It cleave after Arg residues
B. It cleave after His residues
C. It cleave after Lys residues
D. None of the above

Ans. A.

825. The proteolysis rate enhancement by chymotrypsin (~10^{10} folds) corresponds to a reduction in activation energy of about
A. 40 kJ/mol
B. 49 kJ/mol
C. 58 kJ/mol
D. 88 kJ/mol

Ans. C.

826. Which of the following is false statement with regard to comparison between Serine and HIV proteases?
A. Both use nucleophilic attack to hydrolyze the peptide bond
B. Both require water to complete the catalytic cycle
C. Both forms an acyl-enzyme intermediate
D. Both show specificity for certain amino acid sequences

Ans. C.

827. The nucleophile in serine proteases is
A. Serine
B. Water
C. Both (a) and (b)
D. Asparagine

Ans. C.

828. The role of Asp 102 and His 57 during trypsin catalysis is to
A. Neutralize the charge on the other's side chain
B. Keep the specificity pocket open
C. Function as a proton shuttle
D. Clamp the substrate into the active site

Ans. C.

829. The cleavage specificity of trypsin and chymotrypsin depend in part on the

A. Proximity of Ser 195 to the active site or specificity pocket

B. Size, shape, and charge of the active site or specificity pocket

C. Presence of a low-barrier hydrogen bond in the active site or specificity pocket

D. Absence of water in the active site

Ans. B.

830. The *E.coli* pyruvic acid dehydrogenase complex is reported to

A. Decatalyze the oxidation of pyruvic acid to acetyl Co A and CO_2

B. Catalyze the oxidation of pyruvic acid to acetyl Co A and CO_2

C. Retard the reduction of pyruvic acid to acetyl Co A and CO_2

D. Catalyze the reduction of pyruvic acid to acetyl Co A and CO_2

Ans. B.

831. Which of the common features are shared between serine and aspartate proteases?

A. Both require water to complete the catalytic cycle

B. Both use a base to activate the nucleophile

C. Both show specificity for certain amino acid sequences

D. All of the above

Ans. D.

832. Before they can react, many molecules need to be destabilized. This state is typically achieved through

A. Changing the three-dimensional shape of the molecule

B. Oxidizing the molecules by removing electrons

C. Changing the reaction from a biosynthetic to a catabolic pathway

D. The input of a small amount of activation energy

Ans. D.

833. Common feature in all serine proteases is a

A. Hydrophobic specificity pocket B. Hydrophilic specificity pocket

C. Cluster of reactive serine residues D. Single reactive serine residue

Ans. D.

834. How is the enzyme COX-1 important in human health?

A. It helps to transport carbon dioxide in the blood

B. It is critical for the biosynthesis of DNA

C. It is a chemical derivative of aspirin

D. It catalyzes the production of hormones that maintain the stomach lining

Ans. D.

835. A nicked RNA molecule can be ligated by

A. T4 RNA ligase
B. DNA polymerase
C. T4 DNA ligase
D. all of these

Ans. C.

836. The tertiary structure of yeast tRNA

A. Involves extensive base stacking interactions
B. Resembles the 3-dimensional structure of other tRNAs
C. Is maintained mostly by non-Watson-Crick base pairing
D. All of the above

Ans. D.

837. Which of following RNA characteristically contains unusual purines and pyrimidmes?

A. rRNA
B. nRNA
C. mRNA
D. tRNA

Ans. D.

838. The anticodon is a structure on

A. mRNA.
B. tRNA.
C. aribosome.
D. rRNA.

Ans. B.

839. During RNA synthesis, the DNA template sequence 5'Tp Ap Gp Cp 3' would be transcribed to produce which of the following RNA sequence?

A. 5'-Ap Tp Cp Gp-3'
B. 5'-Gp Cp Up Ap-3'
C. 5'-Gp Cp Tp Ap-3'
D. 5'-Ap Up Cp Gp-3'

Ans. B.

840. RNA instability in alkaline solutions is due to

A. adenine
B. Ribose
C. Uracil
D. Single strand nature

Ans. B.

841. In RNA, uracil pairs with

A. Adenine
B. Cytosine
C. Thymine
D. Guanine

Ans. A.

842. Two features of the tRNA molecule associated, in converting the triplet codon to an amino acid, are

A. In the T Loop and D stem and loop

B. In the anticodon loop and D stem loop

C. In the anticodon loop and the 3' CCA end

D. None of the above

Ans. C.

843. Which of the following is the smallest of the RNAs?

A. Messenger RNA B. Transfer RNAs

C. Ribosomal RNAs D. All of these

Ans. B.

844. The mRNA from which of the following would contain a poly-A tail?

A. A restriction endonuclease from *E. coli*

B. Bacterial alpha-amylase

C. Human insulin

D. Bacteriophage DNA ligase

Ans. C.

845. What is the average size (in bp) of a mature t-RNA?

A. 80 bp B. 100 bp

C. 120 bp D. 140 bp

Ans. A.

846. What modified base is at the 5' extremity of a capped eukaryotic m-RNA?

A. 1-methyl-adenosine B. 2'-O-methyl-guanosine

C. 7-methyl-guanosine D. 1-methyl-guanosine

Ans. C.

847. What is the function of messenger RNA?

A. It carries amino acids

B. It is a component of the ribosomes

C. It is a direct copy of a gene

D. It is the genetic material of some organisms

Ans. C.

848. Hydrogen bonds in a-helices are

A. More numerous than Vander Waals interactions

B. Not present at Phe residues

C. Analogous to the steps in a spiral staircase

D. Roughly parallel to the helix axis

Ans. D.

849. The peptide bond in proteins is

A. Only found between proline residues

B. Usually cis unless proline is the next amino acid

C. Usually trans unless proline is the next amino acid

D. Is planar because of steric hinderance

Ans. C.

850. The molecular formula for glycine is $C_2H_5O_2N$. What would be the molecular formula for a linear oligomer made by linking ten glycine molecules together by condensation synthesis?

A. $C_{20}H_{50}O_{20}N_{10}$

B. $C_{20}H_{32}O_{11}N_{10}$

C. $C_{20}H_{40}O_{10}N_{10}$

D. $C_{20}H_{68}O_{29}N_{10}$

Ans. B.

851. Which of the following is an example of tertiary structure in a protein?

A. A multimeric protein

B. An α-helix

C. A β-pleated sheet

D. A globular domain

Ans. D.

852. The peptide, Val-Lys-Glu-Met-Ser-Trp-Arg-Ala, was digested with cyanogen bromide (CNBr) to produce:

A. Val-Lys + Glu-Met-Ser + Trp-Arg-Ala

B. Val-Lys-Glu-Met-Ser-Trp + Arg-Ala

C. Val-Lys-Glu-Met + Ser-Trp-Arg-Ala

D. Val-Lys-Glu + Met-Ser-Trp-Arg-Ala

Ans. C.

853. In deoxy hemoglobin (Hb), the Fe (II) is coordinated to

A. Four nitrogens of heme, the proximal His, and a water molecule

B. Four nitrogens of heme and to a water molecule

C. Two nitrogens of heme and to three His residues in Hb

D. Two nitrogens of heme and to three water molecules

Ans. A.

854. In the β-pleated sheet

A. Hydrogen bonds are formed between the peptide bonds

B. Adjacent polypeptide chains can either be parallel or antiparallel

C. The polypeptide chain is fully extended

D. All of the above

Ans. D.

855. The Ramachandran Plot illustrates the fact that

A. The peptide bond is planar

B. The F & Y angles can assume any value in a peptide

C. The F & Y angles can assume only a single value in a protein

D. The F & Y angles can assume approximately three different values

Ans. D.

856. The resonance structures that can be drawn for the peptide bond indicate that the peptide bond

A. Is stronger than an ordinary single bond

B. Has partial double bond character

C. Both (a) and (b)

D. Is still not completely understood

Ans. C.

857. The major element of secondary structure in myoglobin and hemoglobin is

A. The P-strand B. The α-helix

C. The reverse turn D. All of these

Ans. B.

858. An oil drop with a polar coat is a metaphor referring to the three dimensional structure of

A. Fibrous proteins B. Collagen

C. Globular proteins D. Silk protein

Ans. C.

859. What was the first protein whose complete tertiary structure was determined ?

A. Lysozyme B. Myoglobin

C. Pancreatic ribonuclease D. Pancreatic DNase

Ans. B.

860. The peptide bond in proteins is

A. Planar, but rotates to three preferred dihedral angles

B. Nonpolar, but rotates to three preferred dihedral angles

C. Nonpolar, and fixed in a trans conformation

D. Planar, and usually found in a trans conformation

Ans. D.

861. In β-pleated sheet structures neighbouring

A. Chains lie in a flat plane

B. Neighboring residues are hydrogen bonded

C. Neighboring chains are connected by a-helices

D. Neighboring chains are hydrogen bonded

Ans. D.

862. The same peptide, Val-Lys-Glu-Met-Ser-Trp-Arg-Ala was digested with chymotrypsin to produce

A. Val-Lys + Glu-Met-Ser + Trp-Arg-Ala.

B. Val-Lys-Glu-Met-Ser-Trp + Arg-Ala.

C. Val-Lys-Glu-Met-Ser + Trp-Arg-Ala.

D. Val-Lys-Glu-Met + Ser-Trp-Arg-Ala.

Ans. B.

863. Disulfide bonds most often stabilize the native structure of

A. Extracellular proteins

B. Dimeric proteins

C. Hydrophobic proteins

D. Intracellular proteins

Ans. A.

864. Secondary structure in protein refers to

A. Linear sequence of amino acids joined together by peptide bond

B. Three dimensional arrangement of all amino acids in polypeptide chain

C. Regular folding of regions of the polypeptide chain

D. Protein made up of more than one polypeptide chain

Ans. C.

865. Heme is the binding pocket of myoglobin and hemoglobin and is composed of

A. Negatively charged residues

B. Polar residues

C. Hydrophobic residues

D. Positively charged residues

Ans. C.

866. What is the effect of a decrease in pH on hemoglobin oxygen affinity?

A. Decrease in oxygen affinity

B. Increase in oxygen affinity

C. No effect on oxygen affinity

D. Increase affinity in muscle cell otherwise decrease

Ans. A.

867. What is the proportion of glycine residues in collagenous regions?

A. One-fourth

B. One-third

C. Half

D. One-tenth

Ans. B.

868. Which of the following statements is incorrect?

A. Protein G contains both α-helix and β-sheet

B. Protein G contains only α-helix

C. Fatty acid binding protein contains largely β-sheet

D. Hemoglobin contains four sub-units

Ans. B.

869. The oxygen binding curves of hemoglobin and myoglobin

A. Allow maximum transfer of oxygen to the tissues

B. Are a consequence of the quaternary structure of hemoglobin

C. Both (a) and (b)

D. Are identical

Ans. C.

870. The nature of peptide bond can be best explained as

A. Partial double bond

B. Truly double bond

C. Hydrogen bond

D. Van der waals force

Ans. A.

871. Which of the following statement is incorrect?

A. Hemoglobin and myoglobin are the two oxygen binding proteins

B. Hemoglobin transports O_2 in the blood

C. Myoglobin stores O_2 in muscles

D. None of the above

Ans. D.

872. Which hemoglobin chain replaces the beta chain in embryonic hemoglobulin?

A. Delta
B. Epsilon
C. Gamma
D. Alfa

Ans. B.

873. Hemoglobin has quaternary structure and is made up of

A. Six polypeptide chains, two α-chains and four β-chains
B. Two polypeptide chains, one α-chains and one β-chains
C. Four polypeptide chains, two α-chains and two β-chains
D. Five polypeptide chains, two α-chains and three β-chains

Ans. C.

874. The oxygen in hemoglobin and myoglobin is bound to

A. The iron atom in the heme group
B. The nitrogen atoms on the heme
C. Histidine residues in the protein
D. Lysine residues in the protein

Ans. A.

875. Which of the three subunits of the G proteins binds GDP and GTP?

A. Alpha
B. Beta
C. Gamma
D. Delta

Ans. A.

876. If the F and Y angles of each peptide unit in a protein are known, which of the following may also be determined?

A. Complete secondary structure
B. Complete tertiary structure
C. Complete quaternary structure
D. Thermodynamic stability

Ans. A.

877. The different orders of protein structure are determined by all of the following bond types except

A. Peptide bonds
B. Phospho-diester bonds
C. Disulfide bridges
D. Hydrogen bonds

Ans. B.

878. The heme is held in place by a bond between

A. The Fe^{2+} and cysteine
B. The Fe^{3+} and histidine
C. The Fe^{3+} and cysteine
D. The Fe^{2+} and histidine

Ans. D.

879. When the amino acid alanine (R-group is CH_3) is added to a solution with a pH of 7.3, alanine becomes

A. A cation
B. Nonpolar
C. A zwitterions
D. An isotope

Ans. C.

880. What is the end product of leucine metabolism?

A. Acetyl-CoA
B. Pyruvic acid
C. Oxaloacetic acid
D. Acetyl carnitine

Ans. A.

881. What is the heaviest of the twenty amino acids?

A. Phenylalanine
B. Tryptophan
C. Tyrosine
D. Histidine

Ans. B.

882. Which of the following amino acids can form hydrogen bonds with their side (R) groups?

A. Asparagine
B. Aspartic acid
C. Glutamine
D. All of these

Ans. D.

883. The isoelectric point of an amino acid is defined as the pH

A. Where the molecule carries no electric charge
B. Where the carboxyl group is uncharged
C. Where the amino group is uncharged
D. Of maximum electrolytic mobility

Ans. A.

884. Molecules that bear charged groups of opposite polarity are known as

A. Zwitterions
B. Ambions
C. Ion conversion
D. Amphions

Ans. A.

885. What is the product of the catabolic breakdown of Arginine?

A. Alpha-ketoglutarate
B. Fumarate
C. Oxaloacetate
D. Succinate

Ans. A.

886. Which amino acids would most likely reside in the membrane-anchoring domain of a membrane embedded protein?

A. Isoleucine, valine and phenylalanine

B. Phenylalanine, valine, and aspartate

C. Leucine, threonine, and lysine

D. Lysine, arginine and histidine

Ans. A.

887. An essential amino acid is one that

A. Is essentially easy to synthesize

B. Is essential to flagella motion

C. The body cannot synthesize

D. The body can synthesize under essential conditions

Ans. C.

888. D-Alanine and L-Alanine are technically known as

A. Anomers
B. Enantiomers
C. Epimers
D. Polymer

Ans. B.

889. Which of the following pairs of amino acids would carry a negative charge on their side chain at pH 8.0?

A. Asparagine & Glutamine
B. Leucine & Glycine
C. Histidine & Lysine
D. Aspartate & Glutamate

Ans. D.

890. In a polypeptide average mass of an amino acid residue is

A. 110 daltons
B. 118 daltons
C. 80 daltons
D. 150 daltons

Ans. A.

891. Which pair of amino acids absorbs the most UV light at 280 nm?

A. Threonine & Histidine
B. Trp & Tyrosine
C. Cystein & Asparagine
D. Phenylalnine & Proline

Ans. B.

892. Which of the following is a nonstandard amino acid?

A. Cysteine
B. Isoleucine
C. Hydroxyproline
D. Histidine

Ans. C.

893. Which of the following is an essential amino acid?

A. Tryptophan B. Methionine

C. Lysine D. All of these

Ans. D.

894. Protein fluorescence arises primarily from which residue?

A. Arginine B. Tryptophan

C. Tyrosine D. Phenylalanine

Ans. B.

895. Which of the following amino acid is known as half-cystine residue?

A. Cysteine B. Isoleucine

C. Valine D. Histidine

Ans. A.

896. Which of the following is not an essential amino acid?

A. Aspartic acid B. Glutamic acid

C. Glycine D. All of these

Ans. D.

897. Which of the following is not a sensible grouping of amino acids based on their polarity properties?

A. Ala, Leu, and Val B. Arg, His, and Lys

C. Phe, Trp, and Tyr D. Asp, Ile, and Pro

Ans. D.

898. Proteins and macromolecular structures take on their higher order structures

A. By self-assembly

B. With the help of molecular chaperons

C. With the help of precursor sequences that are removed from the final structures

D. All of the above

Ans. D.

899. What is the product of the catabolic breakdown of Alanine?

A. Fumarate B. Oxaloacetate

C. Pyruvate D. Malate

Ans. C.

900. How many different amino acids are there?

A. 3 B. 20

C. 100 D. An infinite number

Ans. B.

901. Amino acids required in the human diet and not synthesized by the body are called

A. Specialized B. Trace

C. Essential D. Accessory

Ans. C.

902. Which of the following amino acid contain an imidazolium moiety?

A. Alanine B. Valine

C. Cysteine D. Histidine

Ans. D.

903. The sequence of letters 'WYQN' will represent

A. Tryptophan, tyrosine, glutamic acid, asparagine

B. Tryptophan, tyrosine, glutamine, asparagine

C. Tryptophan, glutamine, tryptophan, asparagine

D. Glutamine, tyrosine, tryptophan, aspartic acid

Ans. B.

904. The sulphur containing side chain of cysteine is

A. Ampiphillic, highly reactive and capable of reacting with another cysteine

B. Hydrophillc, highly reactive and capable of reacting with another cysteine

C. Hydrophobic, highly reactive and capable of reacting with another cysteine

D. None of the above

Ans. C.

905. Which of the following is a nonprotein amino acid?

A. Dopamine B. Hydroxylysine

C. Cystine D. None of these

Ans. A.

906. Serine and threonine are polar amino acids due to

A. Reactive hydroxyl group in the side chain

B. Reactive alcoholic group in the side chain

C. Reactive keto group in the side chain

D. Reactive aldehyde group in the side chain

Ans. A.

907. Which of the following is not the hydrophobic and aromatic amino acid?

A. Phenylalanine B. Tyrosine

C. Tryptophan D. None of these

Ans. D.

908. Stereo chemical configuration of all α-amino acids derived from proteins is

A. L
B. D
C. L and D
D. None of these

Ans. A.

909. The α-amino acids have a carboxyl group with a pK around ——————, and an amino group with a pK near ——————.

A. 1.1, and 12.1
B. 6.5, and 8.0
C. 3.3, and 10.5
D. 2.2, and 9.4

Ans. D.

910. Coomassie Blue stains the proteins by reacting with

A. Arginine residues
B. Free c-termini
C. Peptide bonds
D. Aromatic ring

Ans. A.

911. Which amino acid when exposed to ninhydrin produces a brown color?

A. Asparagine
B. Proline
C. Alanine
D. Valine

Ans. A.

912. Specific translocations are associated with

A. Colon cancer
B. Breast cancer
C. Pancreatic cancer
D. Some leukemias

Ans. D.

913. How many molecules of ATPs are synthesized per NADH oxidation?

A. 2
B. 1
C. 3
D. 4

Ans. C.

914. Why is the TCA cycle the central pathway of metabolism of the cell?

A. It occurs in the center of the cell
B. Its intermediates are commonly used by other metabolic reactions
C. All other metabolic pathways depend upon it
D. None of the above

Ans. B.

915. In what form does the product of glycolysis enter the TCA cycle?

A. AcetylCoA
B. Pyruvate
C. NADH
D. Glucose

Ans. A.

916. Malate-asparatate shuttle operates in

A. Lungs and liver B. Heart and liver

C. Pancreas and liver D. None of these

Ans. B.

917. Oxidation of a molecule involves

A. Gain of electron B. Loss of electron

C. Gain of proton D. Loss of proton

Ans. B.

918. During cellular respiration, most of the ATP made, is generated by

A. Oxidative phosphorylation B. Photophosphorylation

C. Glycolysis D. Substrate-level phosphorylation

Ans. A.

919. Important function of cholesterol is to

A. Modulate fluidity B. Enhance blood circulation

C. Prevent bile salts formation D. None of these

Ans. A.

920. To stop ATP synthesis which chemical is generally used?

A. DNSA B. 2,4 dinitrophenol

C. DDT

D. None of the chemical can stop ATP synthesis

Ans. B.

921. The enzymes of the TCA cycle in a eukaryotic cell are located in the

A. Nucleus B. Mitochondria

C. Plasma membrane D. Lysosomal bodies

Ans. B.

922. Citric acid cycle occurs in

A. Cytoplasm B. Mitochondria

C. Endoplasmic reticulum D. Golgi bodies

Ans. B.

923. Most multi-cellular organisms obtain energy for the synthesis of ATP during oxidative phosphorylation from

A. High energy phosphate compounds

B. A proton gradient across the inner mitochondrial membrane

C. A proton gradient across the cell membrane

D. A proton gradient across the outer mitochondrial membrane

Ans. B.

924. Standard redox potential for a substance is measured under standard condition and is expressed as

A. Mili-Ampere
B. Volt
C. Without unit
D. Ohm

Ans. B.

925. Most of the enzymes of the citric acid cycle in a eukaryotic cell are located in the

A. Inner mitochondrial membrane
B. Cytosol
C. Mitochondrial matrix
D. Intermembrane space

Ans. C.

926. A positive redox potential means substance has

A. Lower affinity for electron
B. Higher affinity for electron
C. Lower affinity for proton
D. Higher affinity for proton

Ans. B.

927. The end product of glycolysis is pyruvate, which enters the citric acid cycle after being converted to

A. Acetic acid
B. Acetyl-CoA
C. Acetaldehyde
D. None of these

Ans. B.

928. Energy that is released from glucose during respiration but not transferred to ATP bonds can be detected as

A. CO_2
B. AMP
C. ADP
D. heat

Ans. D.

929. Which of the following is involved in energy production?

A. Generation of proton gradients across membranes
B. Transport of electrons on organic molecules
C. Conversion of compounds with high energy to those of low energy
D. All of the above

Ans. D.

930. Which of the following enzyme does not take part in the TCA cycle?

A. Citrate synthase
B. Iso-citrate dehydrogenase
C. Pyruvate dehydrogenase
D. Malate dehydrogenase

Ans. C.

931. The first intermediate in TCA cycle is

A. Succinate
B. Fumerate
C. Citrate
D. Malate

Ans. C.

932. Cholesterol can be synthesized *de novo* in

A. Pancreas
B. Intestine
C. Liver
D. Cell membrane

Ans. C.

933. Which one of the following is not the intermediate of Kreb's cycle?

A. Isocitrate
B. Succinate
C. Fumarate
D. Stearate

Ans. D.

934. Which one is not the main protein in electron transport chain?

A. NADH dehydrogenase
B. Cytochrome bc1 complex
C. Cytochrome oxidase
D. Citrate synthease

Ans. D.

935. How many ATPs are produced during citric acid cycle?

A. 10
B. 13
C. 12
D. 8

Ans. C.

936. The $FADH_2$ and NADH produced by the oxidation of one acetyl-CoA results in the synthesis of about-

A. 3 ATPs
B. 6 ATPs
C. 11 ATPs
D. 15 ATPs

Ans. C.

937. In eukaryotes, electron transport occurs in

A. Membranes and mitochondria
B. Endoplasmic reticulum
C. Cytoplasm
D. All of the above

Ans. A.

938. The catabolism of sugars and fatty acids is similar because

A. Both of these compounds are funnelled through the TC A/citric acid cycle
B. Both of these compounds generate redox energy during catabolism
C. Both of these compounds generate chemical energy during catabolism
D. All of the above

Ans. A.

939. Okazaki fragments are associated with which essential process ?

A. DNA replication B. Protein synthesis

C. Cellular respiration D. Amino acid synthesis

Ans. A.

940. Wood sugar is

A. Glucose B. Mannose

C. Arabinose D. Xylose

Ans. D.

941. Which of the following amino acid has indole ring in its side chain

A. Phenyl alanine B. Tyrosine

C. Histidine D. Tryptophan

Ans. D.

942. Amino aicds with hydroxyl OH group include

A. Serine B. Threonine

C. Tyrosine D. All of these

Ans. D.

943. Which of the following amino acid has amide group in its side chain ?

A. Cysteine B. Lysine

C. Glutamine D. Isoleucine

Ans. C.

944. Aspartamine, an artificial sweetner is made of

A. Aspartate and glutamate B. Asparagine and Glutamate

C. Aspartate and phenylalanine D. Aspartate and glycine

Ans. C.

945. Which of the following amino acids are considered as semi-essential amino acids

A. Asparagine and Histidine B. Tryptophan and arginine

C. Histidine and arginine D. Histidine, arginine and tryptophan

Ans. C.

946. D- amino acids occur naturally in small amounts in

A. Bacterial peptidoglycan cell wall B. Fungal chitinous cell wall

C. Cellulose plant cell wall D. All of these

Ans. A.

947. Which of the following is an imino acid ?

A. Glycine
B. Proline
C. Lysine
D. Histidine

Ans. B.

948. Tryptophan is a precursor of plant hormone

A. Auxin
B. Cytokinin
C. Kinetin
D. Gibberellins

Ans. A.

949. Ornithine and citrulline for urea synthesis are derivatives of

A. Cysteine
B. Arginine
C. Histidine
D. Methionine

Ans. B.

950. Which of the following is considered as the 21st amino acid ?

A. Hydroxylysine
B. Ornithine
C. Citruline
D. Selenocysteine

Ans. D.

951. Chitin is a form of

A. Complex peptone
B. Complex DNA
C. Complex plasmids
D. Complex carbohydrates

Ans. D.

952. In anaerobic (without O_2) environment, sugar ($C_nH_{2m}O_m$) in dough is converted into

A. Glucose
B. Water
C. Alcohol
D. Carbon Monoxide

Ans. C.

953. Fusarium is made through a culture medium of

A. Lactose
B. Glucose
C. Galactose
D. Maltose

Ans. B.

954. Inorganic salts released during decomposition include

A. Nitrate
B. Sulphate
C. Phosphate
D. All of these

Ans. D.

955. Inorganic gases released during decomposition include

A. Carbon dioxide B. Hydrogen sulphide

C. Water vapours D. All of these

Ans. D.

956. A drug which prevents uric acid synthesis by inhibiting the enzyme xanthine oxidase is

A. Aspirin B. Allopurinol

C. Colchicine D. Probenecid

Ans. B.

957. Which of the following is required for crystallization and storage of the hormone insulin?

A. Mn++ B. Mg++

C. Ca++ D. Zn++

Ans. D.

958. Synthesis of prostaglandins is inhibited by

A. Aspirin B. Arsenic

C. Fluoride D. Cyanide

Ans. A.

959. HDL is synthesized and secreted from

A. Pancreas B. Liver

C. Kidney D. Muscle

Ans. B.

960. Which of the following phospholipids is localized to a greater extent in the outer leaflet of the membrane lipid bilayer?

A. Choline phosphoglycerides B. Ethanolamine phosphoglycerides

C. Inositol phosphoglycerides D. Serine phosphoglycerides

Ans. A.

961. Which one is the heaviest particulate component of the cell?

A. Nucleus B. Mitochondria

C. Cytoplasm D. Golgi apparatus

Ans. A.

962. Which one is the largest particulate of the cytoplasm?

A. Lysosomes B. Mitochondria

C. Golgi apparatus D. Entoplasmic reticulum

Ans. B.

963. The degradative processes are categorized under the heading of

A. Anabolism
B. Catabolism
C. Metabolism
D. None of the above

Ans. B.

964. The average pH of human urine is

A. 7.0
B. 6.0
C. 8.0
D. 0.0

Ans. B.

965. The pH of blood is 7.4 when the ratio between H2CO3 and NaHCO3 is

A. 1 : 10
B. 1 : 20
C. 1 : 25
D. 1 : 30

Ans. B.

966. The surface tension in intestinal lumen between fat droplets and aqueous medium is decreased by

A. Bile Salts
B. Bile acids
C. Conc. H2SO4
D. Acetic acid

Ans. A.

967. Which of the following is located in the mitochondria?

A. Cytochrome oxidase
B. Succinate dehydrogenase
C. Dihydrolipoyl dehydrogenase
D. All of these

Ans. D.

968. The most active site of protein synthesis is the

A. Nucleus
B. Ribosome
C. Mitochondrion
D. Cell sap

Ans. B.

969. Mitochondrial DNA is

A. Circular double stranded
B. Circular single stranded
C. Linear double helix
D. None of these

Ans. A.

970. The cellular organelles called "suicide bags" are

A. Lysosomes
B. Ribosomes
C. Nucleolus
D. Golgi's bodies

Ans. A.

971. The ability of the cell membrane to act as a selective barrier depends upon

A. The lipid composition of the membrane

B. The pores which allows small molecules

C. The special mediated transport systems

D. All of these

Ans. D.

972. A lipid bilayer is permeable to

A. Urea B. Fructose

C. Glucose D. Potassium

Ans. A.

973. The Golgi complex

A. Synthesizes proteins

B. Produces ATP

C. Provides a pathway for transporting chemicals

D. Forms glycoproteins

Ans. D.

974. Enzymes catalyzing electron transport are present mainly in the

A. Ribosomes B. Endoplasmic reticulum

C. Lysosomes D. Inner mitochondrial membrane

Ans. D.

975. Mature erythrocytes do not contain

A. Glycolytic enzymes B. HMP shunt enzymes

C. Pyridine nucleotide D. ATP

Ans. C.

976. In mammalian cells rRNA is produced mainly in the

A. Endoplasmic reticulum B. Ribosome

C. Nucleolus D. Nucleus

Ans. C.

977. The power house of the cell is

A. Nucleus B. Cell membrane

C. Mitochondria D. Lysosomes

Ans. C.

978. The digestive enzymes of cellular compounds are confined to

A. Lysosomes B. Ribosomes

C. Peroxisomes D. Polysomes

Ans. A.

979. The general formula of monosaccharides is

A. CnH2nOn B. C2nH2On

C. CnH2O2n D. CnH2nO2n

Ans. A.

980. The general formula of polysaccharides is

A. (C6H10O5)n B. (C6H12O5)n

C. (C6H10O6)n D. (C6H10O6)n

Ans. A.

981. The aldose sugar is

A. Glycerose B. Ribulose

C. Erythrulose D. Dihydoxyacetone

Ans. A.

982. A triose sugar is

A. Glycerose B. Ribose

C. Erythrose D. Fructose

Ans. A.

983. A pentose sugar is

A. Dihydroxyacetone B. Ribulose

C. Erythrose D. Glucose

Ans. B.

984. The pentose sugar present mainly in the heart muscle is

A. Lyxose B. Ribose

C. Arabinose D. Xylose

Ans. A.

985. Polysaccharides are

A. Polymers B. Acids

C. Proteins D. Oils

Ans. A.

986. The number of isomers of glucose is

A. 2 B. 4

C. 8 D. 16

Ans. D.

987. Two sugars which differ from one another only in configuration around a single carbon atom are termed

A. Epimers B. Anomers

C. Optical isomers D. Stereoisomers

Ans. A.

988. Isomers differing as a result of variations in configuration of the —OH and —H on carbon atoms 2, 3 and 4 of glucose are known as

A. Epimers B. Anomers

C. Optical isomers D. Steroisomers

Ans. A.

989. The most important epimer of glucose is

A. Galactose B. Fructose

C. Arabinose D. Xylose

Ans. A.

990. α-D-glucose and β -D-glucose are

A. Stereoisomers B. Epimers

C. Anomers D. Keto-aldo pairs

Ans. C.

991. Compounds having the same structural formula but differing in spatial configuration are known as

A. Stereoisomers B. Anomers

C. Optical isomers D. Epimers

Ans. A.

992. In glucose the orientation of the —H and —OH groups around the carbon atom 5 adjacent to the terminal primary alcohol carbon determines

A. D or L series B. Dextro or levorotatory

C. α and β anomers D. Epimers

Ans. A.

993. The carbohydrate of the blood group substances is

A. Sucrose B. Fucose

C. Arabinose D. Maltose

Ans. B.

994. A sugar alcohol is

A. Mannitol
B. Trehalose
C. Xylulose
D. Arabinose

Ans. A.

995. The major sugar of insect hemolymph is

A. Glycogen
B. Pectin
C. Trehalose
D. Sucrose

Ans. C.

996. The sugar found in DNA is

A. Xylose
B. Ribose
C. Deoxyribose
D. Ribulose

Ans. C.

997. The sugar found in RNA is

A. Ribose
B. Deoxyribose
C. Ribulose
D. Erythrose

Ans. A.

998. The sugar found in milk is

A. Galactose
B. Glucose
C. Fructose
D. Lactose

Ans. D.

999. Invert sugar is

A. Lactose
B. Sucrose
C. Hydrolytic products of sucrose
D. Fructose

Ans. C.

1000. Sucrose consists of

A. Glucose + glucose
B. Glucose + fructose
C. Glucose + galactose
D. Glucose + mannose

Ans. B.

1001. The monosaccharide units are linked by 1 ’! 4 glycosidic linkage in

A. Maltose
B. Sucrose
C. Cellulose
D. Cellobiose

Ans. A.

1002. Which of the following is a non-reducing sugar?

A. Isomaltose B. Maltose

C. Lactose D. Trehalose

Ans. D.

1003. Which of the following is a reducing sugar?

A. Sucrose B. Trehalose

C. Isomaltose D. Agar

Ans. C.

1004. A dissaccharide formed by 1,1-glycosidic linkage between their monosaccharide units is

A. Lactose B. Maltose

C. Trehalose D. Sucrose

Ans. C.

1005. Mutarotation refers to change in

A. pH B. Optical rotation

C. Conductance D. Chemical properties

Ans. B.

1006. A polysacchharide which is often called animal starch is

A. Glycogen B. Starch

C. Inulin D. Dextrin

Ans. D.

1007. The constituent unit of inulin is

A. Glucose B. Fructose

C. Mannose D. Galactose

Ans. B.

1008. The polysaccharide found in the exoskeleton of invertebrates is

A. Pectin B. Chitin

C. Cellulose D. Chondroitin sulphate

Ans. B.

1009. Which of the following is a heteroglycan?

A. Dextrins B. Agar

C. Inulin D. Chitin

Ans. B.

1010. The glycosaminoglycan which does not contain uronic acid is

A. Dermatan sulphate
B. Chondroitin sulphate
C. Keratan sulphate
D. Heparan sulphate

Ans. C.

1011. Keratan sulphate is found in abundance in

A. Heart muscle
B. Liver
C. Adrenal cortex
D. Cornea

Ans. D.

1012. Repeating units of hyaluronic acid are

A. N-acetyl glucosamine and D-glucuronic acid
B. N-acetyl galactosamine and D-glucuronic acid
C. N-acetyl glucosamine and galactose
D. N-acetyl galactosamine and L- iduronic acid

Ans. A.

1013. The approximate number of branches in amylopectin is

A. 10
B. 20
C. 40
D. 80

Ans. D.

1014. In amylopectin the intervals of glucose units of each branch is

A. 10–20
B. 24–30
C. 30–40
D. 40–50

Ans. B.

1015. The homopolysaccharide used for intravenous infusion as plasma substitute is

A. Agar
B. Inulin
C. Pectin
D. Starch

Ans. A.

1016. The polysaccharide used in assessing the glomerular fittration rate (GFR) is

A. Glycogen
B. Agar
C. Inulin
D. Hyaluronic acid

Ans. C.

1017. A polymer of glucose synthesized by the action of leuconostoc mesenteroids in a sucrose medium is

A. Dextrans
B. Dextrin
C. Limit dextrin
D. Inulin

Ans. A.

1018. Glucose on reduction with sodium amalgam forms

A. Dulcitol B. Sorbitol

C. Mannitol D. Mannitol and sorbitol

Ans. B.

1019. Glucose on oxidation does not give

A. Glycoside B. Glucosaccharic acid

C. Gluconic acid D. Glucuronic acid

Ans. A.

1020. Oxidation of galactose with concentrated HNO_3 yields

A. Mucic acid B. Glucuronic acid

C. Saccharic acid D. Gluconic acid

Ans. A.

1021. A positive Benedict's test is not given by

A. Sucrose B. Lactose

C. Maltose D. Glucose

Ans. A.

1022. Starch is a

A. Polysaccharide B. Monosaccharide

C. Disaccharide D. None of these

Ans. A.

1023. A positive Seliwanoff's test is obtained with

A. Glucose B. Fructose

C. Lactose D. Maltose

Ans. B.

1024. Osazones are not formed with the

A. Glucose B. Fructose

C. Sucrose D. Lactose

Ans. C.

1025. The most abundant carbohydrate found in nature is

A. Starch B. Glycogen

C. Cellulose D. Chitin

Ans. C.

1026. Impaired renal function is indicated when the amount of PSP excreted in the first 15 minutes is

A. 20%
B. 35%
C. 40%
D. 45%

Ans. A.

1027. An early feature of renal disease is

A. Impairment of the capacity of the tubule to perform osmotic work
B. Decrease in maximal tubular excretory capacity
C. Decrease in filtration factor
D. Decrease in renal plasma flow

Ans. A.

1028. ADH test is based on the measurement of

A. Specific gravity of urine
B. Concentration of urea in urine
C. Concentration of urea in blood
D. Volume of urine in ml/minute

Ans. A.

1029. Addis test is the measure of

A. Impairment of the capacity of the tubule to perform osmotic work
B. Secretory function of liver
C. Excretory function of liver
D. Activity of parenchymal cells of liver

Ans. A.

1030. Maltose can be formed by hydrolysis of

A. Starch
B. Dextrin
C. Glycogen
D. All of these

Ans. D.

1031. α–D–Glucuronic acid is present in

A. Hyaluronic acid
B. Chondroitin sulphate
C. Heparin
D. All of these

Ans. C.

1032. Fructose is present in hydrolysate of

A. Sucrose
B. Inulin
C. Both of the above
D. None of these

Ans. C.

1033. Ribulose is a

A. Ketotetrose B. Aldotetrose

C. Ketopentose D. Aldopentose

Ans. C.

1034. A carbohydrate, commonly known as dextrose is

A. Dextrin B. D-Fructose

C. D-Glucose D. Glycogen

Ans. C.

1035. A carbohydrate, known commonly as invert sugar, is

A. Fructose B. Sucrose

C. Glucose D. Lactose

Ans. B.

1036. A heteropolysacchraide among the following is

A. Inulin B. Cellulose

C. Heparin D. Dextrin

Ans. C.

1037. The predominant form of glucose in solution is

A. Acyclic form B. Hydrated acyclic form

C. Glucofuranose D. Glucopyranose

Ans. D.

1038. An L-isomer of monosaccharide formed in human body is

A. L-fructose B. L-Erythrose

C. L-Xylose D. L-Xylulose

Ans. D.

1039. Hyaluronic acid is found in

A. Joints B. Brain

C. Abdomen D. Mouth

Ans. A.

1040. The carbon atom which becomes asymmetric when the straight chain form of monosaccharide changes into ring form is known as

A. Anomeric carbon atom B. Epimeric carbon atom

C. Isomeric carbon atom D. None of these

Ans. A.

1041. The smallest monosaccharide having furanose ring structure is

A. Erythrose B. Ribose

C. Glucose D. Fructose

Ans. B.

1042. Which of the following is an epimeric pair?

A. Glucose and fructose B. Glucose and galactose

C. Galactose and mannose D. Lactose and maltose

Ans. B.

1043. α-Glycosidic bond is present in

A. Lactose B. Maltose

C. Sucrose D. All of these

Ans. B.

1044. Branching occurs in glycogen approximately after every

A. Five glucose units B. Ten glucose units

C. Fifteen glucose units D. Twenty glucose units

Ans. B.

1045. N–Acetylglucosamnine is present in

A. Hyaluronic acid B. Chondroitin sulphate

C. Heparin D. All of these

Ans. A.

1046. Lactate formed in muscles can be utilized through

A. Rapoport-Luebeling cycle B. Glucose-alanine cycle

C. Cori's cycle D. Citric acid cycle

Ans. C.

1047. Glucose-6-phosphatase is not present in

A. Liver and kidneys B. Kidneys and muscles

C. Kidneys and adipose tissue D. Muscles and adipose tissue

Ans. D.

1048. The highest concentrations of fructose are found in

A. Aqueous humor B. Vitreous humor

C. Synovial fluid D. Seminal fluid

Ans. D.

1049. Glucose uptake by liver cells is

A. Energy-consuming
B. A saturable process
C. Insulin-dependent
D. Insulin-independent

Ans. D.

1050. Renal threshold for glucose is decreased in

A. Diabetes mellitus
B. Insulinoma
C. Renal glycosuria
D. Alimentary glycosuria

Ans. C.

1051. Active uptake of glucose is inhibited by

A. Ouabain
B. Phlorrizin
C. Digoxin
D. Alloxan

Ans. B.

1052. Glucose-6-phosphatase is absent or deficient in

A. Von Gierke's disease
B. Pompe's disease
C. Cori's disease
D. McArdle's disease

Ans. A.

1053. Iodine gives a red colour with

A. Starch
B. Dextrin
C. Glycogen
D. Inulin

Ans. C.

1054. Amylose is a constituent of

A. Starch
B. Cellulose
C. Glycogen
D. None of these

Ans. A.

1055. Gluconeogenesis is decreased by

A. Glucagon
B. Epinephrine
C. Glucocorticoids
D. Insulin

Ans. D.

1056. Debranching enzyme is absent in

A. Cori's disease
B. Andersen's disease
C. Von Gierke's disease
D. Her's disease

Ans. A.

1057. McArdle's disease is due to the deficiency of

A. Glucose-6-phosphatase
B. Phosphofructokinase
C. Liver phosphorylase
D. muscle phosphorylase

Ans. D.

1058. Tautomerisation is

A. Shift of hydrogen
B. Shift of carbon
C. Shift of both
D. None of these

Ans. A.

1059. In essential pentosuria, urine contains

A. D-Ribose
B. D-Xylulose
C. L-Xylulose
D. D-Xylose

Ans. C.

1060. Action of salivary amylase on starch leads to the formation of

A. Maltose
B. Maltotriose
C. Both of the above
D. Neither of these

Ans. C.

1061. Congenital galactosaemia can lead to

A. Mental retardation
B. Premature cataract
C. Death
D. All of the above

Ans. D.

1062. Uridine diphosphate glucose (UDPG) is

A. Required for metabolism of galactose
B. Required for synthesis of glucuronic acid
C. A substrate for glycogen synthetase
D. All of the above

Ans. D.

1063. Catalytic activity of salivary amylase requires the presence of

A. Chloride ions
B. Bromide ions
C. Iodide ions
D. All of these

Ans. A.

1064. The following is actively absorbed in the intestine:

A. Fructose
B. Mannose
C. Galactose
D. None of these

Ans. C.

1065. An amphibolic pathway among the following is

A. HMP shunt
B. Glycolysis
C. Citirc acid cycle
D. Gluconeogenesis

Ans. C.

1066. Cori's cycle transfers

A. Glucose from muscles to liver
B. Lactate from muscles to liver
C. Lactate from liver to muscles
D. Pyruvate from liver to muscles

Ans. B.

1067. Excessive intake of ethanol increases the ratio:

A. NADH : NAD+
B. NAD+ : NADH
C. FADH2 : FAD
D. FAD : FADH2

Ans. A.

1068. Ethanol decreases gluconeogenesis by

A. Inhibiting glucose-6-phosphatase
B. Inhibiting PEP carboxykinase
C. Converting NAD+ into NADH and decreasing the availability of pyruvate
D. Converting NAD+ into NADH and decreasing the availability of lactate

Ans. C.

1069. Glycogenin is

A. Uncoupler of oxidative phosphorylation
B. Polymer of glycogen molecules
C. Protein primer for glycogen synthesis
D. Intermediate in glycogen breakdown

Ans. C.

1070. During starvation, ketone bodies are used as a fuel by

A. Erythrocytes
B. Brain
C. Liver
D. All of these

Ans. B.

1071. Animal fat is in general

A. Poor in saturated and rich in polyunsaturated fatty acids
B. Rich in saturated and poor in polyunsaturated fatty acids
C. Rich in saturated and polyunsaturated fatty acids
D. Poor in saturated and polyunsaturated fatty acids

Ans. B.

1072. In the diet of a diabetic patient, the recommended carbohydrate intake should preferably be in the form of

A. Monosaccharides B. Dissaccharides

C. Polysaccharides D. All of these

Ans. C.

1073. Obesity increases the risk of

A. Hypertension B. Diabetes mellitus

C. Cardiovascular disease D. All of these

Ans. D.

1074. The most common vitamin deficiency around the world is

A. Ascorbic acid B. Folic acid

C. Vitamin A D. Vitamin D

Ans. B.

1075. Consumption of iodised salt is recommended for prevention of

A. Hypertension B. Hyperthyroidism

C. Endemic goitre D. None of these

Ans. C.

1076. Restriction of salt intake is generally recommended in

A. Diabetes mellitus B. Hypertension

C. Cirrhosis of liver D. Peptic ulcer

Ans. B.

1077. Specific gravity of urine is raised in all of the following except

A. Diabetes mellitus B. Diabetes insipidus

C. Dehydration D. Acute glomerulonephritis

Ans. D.

1078. Specific gravity of urine is decreased in

A. Diabetes mellitus B. Acute glomerulonephritis

C. Diarrhoea D. Chronic glomerulonephritis

Ans. B.

1079. Heavy proteinuria occurs in

A. Acute glomerulonephritis B. Acute pyelonephritis

C. Nephrosclerosis D. Nephrotic syndrome

Ans. B.

1080. Bence-Jones protein precipitates at

A. 20°–40° C
B. 40–-60° C
C. 60°–80° C
D. 80°–100° C

Ans. B.

1081. Serum cholesterol is decreased in

A. Endemic goitre
B. Thyrotoxicosis
C. Myxoedema
D. Cretinism

Ans. B.

1082. The general formula for polysaccharide is

A. (C6H12O6)n
B. (C6H10O5)n
C. (C6H12O5)n
D. (C6H19O6)n

Ans. B.

1083. Honey contains the hydrolytic product of

A. Lactose
B. Maltose
C. Inulin
D. Starch

Ans. C.

1084. On boiling Benedict's solution is not reduced by

A. Sucrose
B. Lactose
C. Maltose
D. Fructose

Ans. A.

1085. Galactose on oxidation with conc. HNO_3 produces

A. Gluconic acid
B. Saccharic acid
C. Saccharo Lactone
D. Mucic acid

Ans. D.

1086. The distinguishing test between monosaccharides and dissaccharides is

A. Bial's test
B. Selwanoff's test
C. Barfoed's test
D. Hydrolysis test

Ans. C.

1087. Cellulose is made up of the molecules of

A. α-glucose
B. β-glucose
C. Both of the above
D. None of these

Ans. A.

1088. Iodine solution produces no color with

A. Cellulose B. Starch

C. Dextrin D. Glycogen

Ans. A.

1089. Glycogen structure includes a branch in between–glucose units:

A. 6–12 B. 8–14

C. 6–10 D. 12–18

Ans. D.

1090. Amylose contains glucose units

A. 100–200 B. 200–300

C. 300–400 D. 500–600

Ans. C.

1091. Each branch of amylopectin is at an interval of glucose units:

A. 14–20 B. 24–30

C. 34–40 D. 44–50

Ans. B.

1092. N-acetylneuraminic acid is an example of

A. Sialic acid B. Mucic acid

C. Glucuronic acid D. Hippuric acid

Ans. C.

1093. In place of glucuronic acid chondroitin sulphate B contains

A. Gluconic acid B. Gulonic acid

C. Induronic acid D. Sulphonic acid

Ans. C.

1094. Blood group substances consist of

A. Lactose B. Maltose

C. Fructose D. Mucose

Ans. C.

1095. The component of cartilage and cornea is

A. Keratosulphate B. Chondroitin sulphate

C. Cadmium sulphate D. Antimony sulphate

Ans. A.

1096. Benedict's test is less likely to give weakly positive results with concentrated urine due to the action of

A. Urea
B. Uric acid
C. Ammonium salts
D. Phosphates

Ans. B.

1097. The general test for detection of carbohydrates is

A. Iodine test
B. Molisch test
C. Barfoed test
D. Osazone test

Ans. B.

1098. Cyclic AMP is formed from ATP by the enzyme adenylate cyclase which is activated by the hormone:

A. Insulin
B. Epinephrine
C. Testosterone
D. Progesterone

Ans. B.

1099. The carrier of the citric acid cycle is

A. Succinate
B. Fumarate
C. Malate
D. Oxaloacetate

Ans. D.

1100. The conversion of alanine to glucose is termed

A. Glycolysis
B. Oxidative decarboxylation
C. Specific dynamic action
D. Gluconeogenesis

Ans. D.

1101. The blood sugar raising action of the hormones of suprarenal cortex is due to

A. Gluconeogenesis
B. Glycogenolysis
C. Glucagon-like activity
D. Due to inhibition of glomerular filtration

Ans. A.

1102. Under anaerobic conditions the glycolysis one mole of glucose yields __ moles of ATP.

A. One
B. Two
C. Eight
D. Thirty

Ans. B.

1103. Which of the following metabolite integrates glucose and fatty acid metabolism?

A. Acetyl CoA
B. Pyruvate
C. Citrate
D. Lactate

Ans. A.

1104. Cerebrosides consist mostly of this sugar:

A. Glucose
B. Fructose
C. Galactose
D. Arabinose

Ans. C.

1105. Glucose will be converted into fatty acids if the diet has excess of

A. Carbohydrates
B. Proteins
C. Fat
D. Vitamins

Ans. A.

1106. The purple ring of Molisch reaction is due to

A. Furfural
B. Furfural + α Napthol
C. α Napthol
D. Furfurol + H2SO4 + α –Naphthol

Ans. B.

1107. Specific test for ketohexoses:

A. Seliwanoff's test
B. Osazone test
C. Molisch test
D. None of these

Ans. A.

1108. Cane sugar (Sucrose) injected into blood is

A. Changed to fructose
B. Changed to glucose
C. Undergoes no significant change
D. Changed to glucose and fructose

Ans. C.

1109. Conversion of glucose to glucose-6- phosphate in human liver is by

A. Hexokinase only
B. Glucokinase only
C. Hexokinase and glucokinase
D. Glucose-6-phosphate dehydrogenase

Ans. C.

1110. The following is an enzyme required for glycolysis:

A. Pyruvate kinase
B. Pyruvate carboxylase
C. Glucose-6-phosphatose
D. Glycerokinase

Ans. A.

1111. The normal glucose tolerance curve reaches peak is

A. 15 min
B. 1 hr
C. 2 hrs
D. 2 ½ hrs

Ans. B.

1112. Glucose tolerance is increased in

A. Diabetes mellitus
B. Adrenalectomy
C. Acromegaly
D. Thyrotoxicosis

Ans. B.

1113. Glucose tolerance is decreased in

A. Diabetes mellitus
B. Hypopituitarism
C. Addison's disease
D. Hypothyroidism

Ans. A.

1114. Under anaerobic conditions the glycolysis of one mole of glucose yields ——— moles of ATP.

A. One
B. Two
C. Eight
D. Thirty

Ans. B.

1115. Glycogen is converted to glucose-1- phosphate by

A. UDPG transferase
B. Branching enzyme
C. Phosphorylase
D. Phosphatase

Ans. C.

1116. Which of the following is not an enzyme involved in glycolysis?

A. Euolase
B. Aldolose
C. Hexokinase
D. Glucose oxidase

Ans. D.

1117. Tricarboxylic acid cycle to be continuous requires the regeneration of

A. Pyruvic acid
B. oxaloacetic acid
C. α-oxoglutaric acid
D. Malic acid

Ans. B.

1118. The tissues with the highest total glycogen content are

A. Muscle and kidneys
B. Kidneys and liver
C. Liver and muscle
D. Brain and Liver

Ans. C.

1119. Rothera test is not given by

A. β-hydroxy butyrate
B. bile salts
C. Glucose
D. None of these

Ans. A.

1120. Gluconeogenesis is increased in the following condition:

A. Diabetes insipidus B. Diabetes Mellitus

C. Hypothyroidism D. Liver diseases

Ans. B.

1121. The oxidation of lactic acid to pyruvic acid requires the following vitamin derivative as the hydrogen carrier.

A. Lithium pyrophosphate B. Coenyzme A

C. NAD+ D. FMN

Ans. C.

1122. Physiological glycosuria is met with in

A. Renal glycosuria B. Alimentary glycosuria

C. Diabetes Mellitus D. Alloxan diabetes

Ans. B.

1123. The number of molecules of ATP produced by the total oxidation of acetyl CoA in TCA cycle is

A. 6 B. 8

C. 10 D. 12

Ans. D.

1124. Fatty acids cannot be converted into carbohydrates in the body as the following reaction is not possible.

A. Conversion of glucose-6-phosphate into glucose

B. Fructose 1, 6-bisphosphate to fructose-6-phosphate

C. Transformation of acetyl CoA to pyruvate

D. Formation of acetyl CoA from fatty acids

Ans. C.

1125. Tissues form lactic acid from glucose. This phenomenon is termed as

A. Aerobic glycolysis B. Oxidation

C. Oxidative phosphorylation D. Anaerobic glycolysis

Ans. D.

1126. One molecule of glucose gives ———— molecules of CO2 in EM-TCA cycle.

A. 6 B. 3

C. 1 D. 2

Ans. A.

1127. For glycogenesis, Glucose should be converted to

A. Glucuronic acid
B. Pyruvic acid
C. UDP glucose
D. Sorbitol

Ans. C.

1128. Amylo 1, 6 glucosidase is called

A. Branching enzyme
B. debranching enzyme
C. Glucantransferase
D. Phosphorylase

Ans. B.

1129. Glucose enters the cells by

A. insulin independent transport
B. insulin dependent transport
C. enzyme mediated transport
D. Both (A) and (B)

Ans. D.

1130. When O2 supply is inadequate, pyruvate is converted to

A. Phosphopyruvate
B. Acetyl CoA
C. Lactate
D. Alanine

Ans. C.

1131. Reactivation of inactive liver phosphorylase is normally favoured by

A. Insulin
B. Epinephrine
C. ACTH
D. Glucagon

Ans. D.

1132. Before pyruvic acid enters the TCA cycle it must be converted to

A. Acetyl CoA
B. Lactate
C. α-ketoglutarate
D. Citrate

Ans. A.

1133. The hydrolysis of Glucose-6-phosphate is catalysed by a specific phosphatase which is found only in

A. Liver, intestines and kidneys
B. Brain, spleen and adrenals
C. Striated muscle
D. Plasma

Ans. A.

1134. The formation of citrate from oxaloacetate and acetyl CoA is

A. Oxidation
B. Reduction
C. Condensation
D. Hydrolysis

Ans. C.

1135. Which one of the following is a rate limiting enzyme of gluconeogenesis?

A. Hexokinase B. Phsophofructokinase

C. Pyruvate carboxylase D. Pyruvate kinase

Ans. C.

1136. UDP Glucuronic acid is required for the biosynthesis of

A. Chondroitin sulphates B. Glycogen

C. Lactose D. Starch

Ans. A.

1137. Which one of the following can convert glucose to vitamin C ?

A. Albino rats B. Humans

C. Monkeys D. Guinea pigs

Ans. A.

1138. Which one of the following cannot convert glucose to Vitamin C ?

A. Albino rats B. Dogs

C. Monkeys D. Cows

Ans. C.

1139. Two conditions in which gluconeogenesis is increased are

A. Diabetes mellitus and atherosclerosis

B. Fed condition and thyrotoxicosis

C. Diabetes mellitus and Starvation

D. Alcohol intake and cigarette smoking

Ans. C.

1140. Acetyl CoA is not used for the synthesis of

A. Fatty acid B. Cholesterol

C. Pyruvic acid D. Citric acid

Ans. C.

1141. The total glycogen content of the body is about ———— gms.

A. 100 B. 200

C. 300 D. 500

Ans. C.

1142. The total glucose in the body is ———— gms.

A. 10–15 B. 20–30

C. 40–50 D. 60–80

Ans. B.

1143. Pyruvate kinase requires ——— ions for maximum activity.

A. Na+ B. K+

C. Ca2+ D. Mg2+

Ans. B.

1144. ATP is 'wasted' in Rapoport-Lueberring cycle in RBCs as otherwise it will inhibit

A. Phosphoglucomutase B. Phosphohexo isomerase

C. Phosphofructo kinase D. Phosphoenol pyruvate carboxy kinase

Ans. C.

1145. The following co-enzyme is needed for the oxidative decarboxylation of ketoacids:

A. NADP+ B. TPP

C. Folate coenzyme D. Biotin coenzyme

Ans. B.

1146. Synthesis of Glucose from amino acids is termed as

A. Glycolysis B. Gluconeogenesis

C. Glycogenesis D. Lipogenesis

Ans. B.

1147. The following examples are important heteropolysaccharides except

A. Amylopectin B. Heparin

C. Peptidoglycan D. Hyaluronic acid

Ans. A.

1148. Which of the following features are common to monosaccharides?

A. Contain asymmetric centres

B. Are of 2 types – aldoses and ketoses

C. Tend to exist as ring structures in solution

D. Include glucose, galactose and raffinose

Ans. C.

1149. Polysaccharides

A. Contain many monosaccharide units which may or may not be of the same kind

B. Function mainly a storage or structural compounds

C. Are present in large amounts in connective tissue

D. All of these

Ans. D.

1150. The absorption of glucose in the digestive tract

A. Occurs in the small intestine

B. Is stimulated by the hormone Glucagon

C. Occurs more rapidly than the absorption of any other sugar

D. Is impaired in cases of diabetes mellitus

Ans. A.

1151. UDP-Glucose is converted to UDP Glucuronic acid by

A. ATP B. GTP

C. NADP+ D. NAD+

Ans. B.

1152. The enzymes involved in Phosphorylation of glucose to glucose 6- phosphate are

A. Hexokinase B. Glucokinase

C. Phosphofructokinase D. Both (A) and (B)

Ans. D.

1153. In conversion of Lactic acid to Glucose, three reactions of Glycolytic pathway are circumvented, which of the following enzymes do not participate?

A. Pyruvate Carboxylase B. Phosphoenol pyruvate carboxy kinase

C. Pyruvate kinase D. Glucose-6-phosphatase

Ans. C.

1154. The normal resting state of humans, most of the blood glucose burnt as "fuel" is consumed by

A. Liver B. Brain

C. Kidneys D. Adipose tissue

Ans. B.

1155. A regulator of the enzyme Glycogen synthase is

A. Citric acid B. 2, 3 bisphosphoglycerate

C. Pyruvate D. GTP

Ans. C.

1156. Most of the metabolic pathways are either anabolic or catabolic. Which of the following pathways is considered as "amphibolic" in nature?

A. Glycogenesis B. Glycolytic pathway

C. Lipolysis D. TCA cycle

Ans. D.

1157. Transketolase activity is affected in

A. Biotin deficiency
B. Pyridoxine deficiency
C. PABA deficiency
D. Thiamine deficiency

Ans. B.

1158. The following metabolic abnormalities occur in Diabetes mellitus except

A. Increased plasma FFA
B. Increased pyruvate carboxylase activate
C. Decreased lipogenesis
D. Decreased gluconeogenesis

Ans. B.

1159. A substance that is not an intermediate in the formation of D-glucuronic acid from glucose is

A. Glucoss-1-p
B. 6-Phosphogluconate
C. Glucose-6-p
D. UDP-Glucose

Ans. B.

1160. The hydrolysis of Glucose-6-P is catalysed by a phosphatase that is not formed in which of the following?

A. Liver
B. Kidney
C. Muscle
D. Small intestine

Ans. C.

1161. An essential for converting Glucose to Glycogen in Liver is

A. Lactic acid
B. GTP
C. CTP
D. UTP

Ans. D.

1162. The ratio that approximates the number of net molecule of ATP formed per mole of Glucose oxidized in presence of O2 to the net number formed in absence of O2 is

A. 4 : 1
B. 10 : 2
C. 12 : 1
D. 18 : 1

Ans. B.

1163. The "Primaquin sensitivity types of haemolytic anaemia" has been found to relate to reduced R.B.C activity of which enzyme?

A. Pyruvate kinase deficiency
B. Glucose-6-phosphatase deficiency
C. Glucose-6-p dehydrogenase deficiency
D. Hexokinase deficiency

Ans. C.

1164. Which of the following hormones is not involved in carbohydrate metabolism?

A. Cortisol B. ACTH

C. Glucogen D. Vasopressin

Ans. D.

1165. Which of the following statements regarding T.C.A cycle is true?

A. It is an anaerobic process

B. It occurs in cytosol

C. It contains no intermediates for Gluconeogenesis

D. It is amphibolic in nature

Ans. D.

1166. The glycolysis is regulated by

A. Hexokinase B. Phosphofructokinase

C. Pyruvate kinase D. All of these

Ans. D.

1167. How many ATP molecules will be required for conversion of 2-molecules of Lactic acid to Glucose?

A. 2 B. 4

C. 8 D. 6

Ans. D.

1168. In presence of the following cofactor, pyruvate carboxylase converts pyruvate to oxaloacetate

A. ATP, Protein and CO2 B. CO2 and ATP

C. CO2 D. Protein

Ans. A.

1169. For conversion of oxaloacetate to phosphoenol pyruvate, high energy molecule is required in the form of

A. GTP only B. ITP only

C. GTP (or) ITP D. None of these

Ans. C.

1170. If the more negative standard reduction potential of a redox pair, the greater the tendency to

A. To lose electrons B. To gain electrons

C. To lose/gain electrons D. To lose and gain electrons

Ans. A.

1171. Electron transport and phosphorylation can be uncoupled by compounds that increase the permeability of the inner mitochondrial membrane to

A. Electrons B. Protons

C. Uncouplers D. All of these

Ans. B.

1172. The standard free energy of hydrolysis of terminal phosphate group of ATP is

A. –7,300 cal/mol B. –8,300 cal/mol

C. 10,000 cal/mol D. +7,300 cal/mol

Ans. A.

1173. The synthesis of glucose from pyruvate by gluconeogenesis

A. Requires the participation of biotin

B. Occurs exclusively in the cytosol

C. Is inhibited by elevated level of insulin

D. Requires oxidation/reduction of FAD

Ans. A.

1174. The conversion of pyruvate to acetyl CoA and CO2

A. Is reversible B. Involves the participation of lipoic acid

C. Depends on the coenzyme biotin D. Occurs in the cytosol

Ans. B.

1175. Phenylalanine is the precursor of

A. L-DOPA B. Histamine

C. Tyrosine D. Throxine

Ans. C.

1176. D-Mannose is present in some plant products like

A. Resins B. Pectins

C. Mucilage D. Gums

Ans. D.

1177. Galactose is a main constituent of

A. Milk sugar B. Honey

C. Cane sugar D. Chitin

Ans. A.

1178. Glucosamine is an important constituent of

A. Homopolysaccharide B. Heteropolysaccharide

C. Mucopolysaccharide D. Dextran

Ans. C.

1179. Glycogen is present in all body tissues except

A. Liver B. Brain

C. Kidney D. Stomach

Ans. B.

1180. Iodine test is positive for starch, dextrin and

A. Mucoproteins B. Agar

C. Glycogen D. Cellulose

Ans. C.

1181. The general formula for polysaccharide is

A. (C6H10O5)n B. (C6H12C6)n

C. (C6H12O5)n D. (C5H10O5)n

Ans. A.

1182. Epimers of glucose is

A. Fructose B. Galactose

C. Ribose D. Deoxyribose

Ans. B.

1183. Human heart muscle contains

A. D-Arabinose B. D-Ribose

C. D-Xylose D. L-Xylose

Ans. C.

1184. On boiling Benedict's solution is not reduced by

A. Sucrose B. Lactose

C. Maltose D. Fructose

Ans. A.

1185. The distinguishing test between monosaccharides and dissaccharide is

A. Bial's test B. Seliwanoff's test

C. Barfoed's test D. Hydrolysis test

Ans. C.

1186. Barfoed's solution is not reduced by

A. Glucose B. Mannose

C. Sucrose D. Ribose

Ans. C.

1187. Cori cycle is

A. Synthesis of glucose
B. reuse of glucose
C. uptake of glycose
D. Both (A) & (B)

Ans. D.

1188. Cane sugar is known as

A. Galactose
B. Sucrose
C. Fructose
D. Maltose

Ans. B.

1189. α”D-Glucose and β”D-glucose are related by

A. Epimers
B. Anomers
C. Multirotation
D. Ketoenol pair

Ans. B.

1190. The stable ring formation in D-Glucose involves

A. C-1 and C-4
B. C-1 and C-2
C. C-1 and C-5
D. C-2 and C-5

Ans. C.

1191. Reduction of Glucose with Ca++ in water produces

A. Sorbitol
B. Dulcitol
C. Mannitol
D. Glucuronic acid

Ans. A.

1192. Starch and glycogen are polymers of

A. Fructose
B. Mannose
C. α”D-Glucose
D. Galactose

Ans. C.

1193. Reducing ability of carbohydrates is due to

A. Carboxyl group
B. Hydroxyl group
C. Enediol formation
D. Ring structure

Ans. A.

1194. Which of the following is not a polymer of glucose?

A. Amylose
B. Inulin
C. Cellulose
D. Dextrin

Ans. B.

1195. Invert sugar is

A. Lactose B. Mannose

C. Fructose D. Hydrolytic product of sucrose

Ans. D.

1196. The carbohydrate reserved in human body is

A. Starch B. Glucose

C. Glycogen D. Inulin

Ans. C.

1197. A dissaccharide linked by α-1-4 Glycosidic linkages is

A. Lactose B. Sucrose

C. Cellulose D. Maltose

Ans. D.

1198. All proteins contain the

A. Same 20 amino acids

B. Different amino acids

C. 300 Amino acids occurring in nature

D. Only a few amino acids

Ans. A.

1199. Proteins contain

A. Only L- α - amino acids B. Only D-amino acids

C. DL-Amino acids D. Both (A) and (B)

Ans. A.

1200. The optically inactive amino acid is

A. Glycine B. Serine

C. Threonine D. Valine

Ans. A.

1201. At neutral pH, a mixture of amino acids in solution would be predominantly:

A. Dipolar ions B. Nonpolar molecules

C. Positive and monovalent D. Hydrophobic

Ans. A.

1202. The true statement about solutions of amino acids at physiological pH is

A. All amino acids contain both positive and negative charges

B. All amino acids contain positively charged side chains

C. Some amino acids contain only positive charge

D. All amino acids contain negatively charged side chains

Ans. A.

1203. Since the pK values for aspartic acid are 2.0, 3.9 and 10.0, it follows that the isoelectric (pH) is

A. 3.0 B. 3.9

C. 5.9 D. 6.0

Ans. A.

1204. Sulphur containing amino acid is

A. Methionine B. Leucine

C. Valine D. Asparagine

Ans. A.

1205. An example of sulphur containing amino acid is

A. 2-Amino-3-mercaptopropanoic acid

B. 2-Amino-3-methylbutanoic acid

C. 2-Amino-3-hydroxypropanoic acid

D. Amino acetic acid

Ans. A.

1206. All the following are sulphur containing amino acids found in proteins except

A. Cysteine B. Cystine

C. Methionine D. Threonine

Ans. D.

1207. An aromatic amino acid is

A. Lysine B. Tyrosine

C. Taurine D. Arginine

Ans. B.

1208. The functions of plasma albumin are

A. Osmosis B. Transport

C. Immunity D. Both (A)and (B)

Ans. A.

1209. An example of α-amino acid not present in proteins but essential in mammalian metabolism is

A. 3-Amino 3-hydroxypropanoic acid

B. 2-Amino 3-hydroxybutanoic acid

C. 2-Amino 4-mercaptobutanoic acid

D. 2-Amino 3-mercaptopropanoic acid

Ans. C.

1210. An essential amino acid in man is

A. Aspartate
B. Tyrosine
C. Methionine
D. Serine

Ans. C.

1211. Non essential amino acids

A. Are not components of tissue proteins
B. May be synthesized in the body from essential amino acids
C. Have no role in the metabolism
D. May be synthesized in the body in diseased states

Ans. B.

1212. Which one of the following is semiessential amino acid for humans?

A. Valine
B. Arginine
C. Lysine
D. Tyrosine

Ans. B.

1213. An example of polar amino acid is

A. Alanine
B. Leucine
C. Arginine
D. Valine

Ans. C.

1214. The amino acid with a nonpolar side chain is

A. Serine
B. Valine
C. Asparagine
D. Threonine

Ans. B.

1215. A ketogenic amino acid is

A. Valine
B. Cysteine
C. Leucine
D. Threonine

Ans. C.

1216. An amino acid that does not form an α-helix is

A. Valine
B. Proline
C. Tyrosine
D. Tryptophan

Ans. B.

1217. An amino acid not found in proteins is

A. β-Alanine
B. Proline
C. Lysine
D. Histidine

Ans. A.

1218. In mammalian tissues serine can be a biosynthetic precursor of

A. Methionine B. Glycine

C. Tryptophan D. Phenylalanine

Ans. B.

1219. A vasodilating compound is produced by the decarboxylation of the amino acid:

A. Arginine B. Aspartic acid

C. Glutamine D. Histidine

Ans. D.

1220. Biuret reaction is specific for

A. –CONH-linkages B. –CSNH2 group

C. –(NH)NH2 group D. All of these

Ans. A.

1221. Sakaguchi's reaction is specific for

A. Tyrosine B. Proline

C. Arginine D. Cysteine

Ans. C.

1222. Million-Nasse's reaction is specific for the amino acid:

A. Tryptophan B. Tyrosine

C. Phenylalanine D. Arginine

Ans. B.

1223. Ninhydrin with evolution of CO2 forms a blue complex with

A. Peptide bond B. α -Amino acids

C. Serotonin D. Histamine

Ans. B.

1224. The most of the ultraviolet absorption of proteins above 240 nm is due to their content of

A. Tryptophan B. Aspartate

C. Glutamate D. Alanine

Ans. A.

1225. Which of the following is a dipeptide?

A. Anserine B. Glutathione

C. Glucagon D. β–Lipoprotein

Ans. A.

1226. Which of the following is a tripeptide?

A. Anserine
B. Oxytocin
C. Glutathione
D. Kallidin

Ans. C.

1227. An example of metalloprotein is

A. Casein
B. Ceruloplasmin
C. Gelatin
D. Salmine

Ans. B.

1228. An example of chromoprotein is

A. Hemoglobin
B. Sturine
C. Nuclein
D. Gliadin

Ans. A.

1229. An example of scleroprotein is

A. Zein
B. Keratin
C. Glutenin
D. Ovoglobulin

Ans. B.

1230. Casein, the milk protein is

A. Nucleoprotein
B. Chromoprotein
C. Phosphoprotein
D. Glycoprotein

Ans. C.

1231. An example of phosphoprotein present in egg yolk is

A. Ovoalbumin
B. Ovoglobulin
C. Ovovitellin
D. Avidin

Ans. C.

1232. A simple protein found in the nucleoproteins of the sperm is

A. Prolamine
B. Protamine
C. Glutelin
D. Globulin

Ans. B.

1233. Histones are

A. Identical to protamine
B. Proteins rich in lysine and arginine
C. Proteins with high molecular weight
D. Insoluble in water and very dilute acids

Ans. B.

1234. The protein present in hair is

A. Keratin B. Elastin

C. Myosin D. Tropocollagen

Ans. A.

1235. The amino acid from which synthesis of the hair keratin takes place is

A. Alanine B. Methionine

C. Proline D. Hydroxyproline

Ans. B.

1236. The number of amino acids present in one molecule of albumin

A. 510 B. 590

C. 610 D. 650

Ans. C.

1237. Plasma proteins which contain more than 4% hexosamine are

A. Microglobulins B. Glycoproteins

C. Mucoproteins D. Orosomucoids

Ans. C.

1238. After releasing O2 at the tissues, hemoglobin transports

A. CO2 and protons to the lungs B. O2 to the lungs

C. CO2 and protons to the tissue D. Nutrients

Ans. A.

1239. Ehlers-Danlos syndrome characterized by hypermobile joints and skin abnormalities is due to

A. Abnormality in gene for procollagen

B. Deficiency of lysyl oxidase

C. Deficiency of prolyl hydroxylase

D. Deficiency of lysyl hydroxylase

Ans. A.

1240. Proteins are soluble in

A. Anhydrous acetone B. Aqueous alcohol

C. Anhydrous alcohol D. Benzene

Ans. B.

1241. Many globular proteins are stable in solution in spite they lack in

A. Disulphide bonds B. Hydrogen bonds

C. Salt bonds D. Non polar bonds

Ans. D.

1242. The hydrogen bonds between peptide linkages of a protein molecules are interfered by

A. Guanidine
B. Uric acid
C. Oxalic acid
D. Salicylic acid

Ans. A.

1243. Globular proteins have completely folded, coiled polypeptide chain and the axial ratio (ratio of length to breadth) is

A. Less than 10 and generally not greater than 3–4
B. Generally 10
C. Greater than 10 and generally 20
D. Greater than 10

Ans. A.

1244. Fibrous proteins have axial ratio

A. Less than 10
B. Less than 10 and generally not greater than 3–4
C. Generally 10
D. Greater than 10

Ans. D.

1245. Each turn of α-helix contains the amino acid residues (number)

A. 3.6
B. 3.0
C. 4.2
D. 4.5

Ans. A.

1246. Distance traveled per turn of α-helix (amino acid) in nm is

A. 0.53
B. 0.54
C. 0.44
D. 0.48

Ans. B.

1247. Along the α-helix each amino acid residue advances in nm by

A. 0.15
B. 0.10
C. 0.12
D. 0.20

Ans. A.

1248. The number of helices present in a collagen molecule is

A. 1
B. 2
C. 3
D. 4

Ans. C.

1249. In proteins the α-helix and β-pleated sheet are examples of

A. Primary structure
B. Secondary structure
C. Tertiary structure
D. Quaternary structure

Ans. B.

1250. At the lowest energy level α-helix of polypeptide chain is stabilised

A. By hydrogen bonds formed between the H of peptide N and the carbonyl O of the residue
B. Disulphide bonds
C. Non polar bonds
D. Ester bonds

Ans. A.

1251. Both α-helix and β-pleated sheet conformation of proteins were proposed by

A. Watson and Crick
B. Pauling and Corey
C. Waugh and King
D. Y.S.Rao

Ans. B.

1252. The primary structure of fibroin, the principal protein of silk worm fibres consists almost entirely of

A. Glycine
B. Aspartate
C. Keratin
D. Tryptophan

Ans. A.

1253. Tertiary structure of a protein describes

A. The order of amino acids
B. Location of disulphide bonds
C. Loop regions of proteins
D. The ways of protein folding

Ans. D.

1254. In a protein molecule the disulphide bond is not broken by

A. Reduction
B. Oxidation
C. Denaturation
D. X-ray diffraction

Ans. C.

1255. The technique for purification of proteins that can be made specific for a given protein is

A. Gel filtration chromotography
B. Ion exchange chromatography
C. Electrophoresis
D. Affinity chromatography

Ans. D.

1256. Denaturation of proteins results in

A. Disruption of primary structure B. Breakdown of peptide bonds

C. Destruction of hydrogen bonds D. Irreversible changes in the molecule

Ans. C.

1257. Ceruloplasmin is

A. α1-globulin B. α2-globulin

C. β-globulin D. None of these

Ans. A.

1258. The lipoprotein with the fastest electrophoretic mobility and the lowest triglyceride content is

A. Chylomicron B. VLDL

C. IDL D. HDL

Ans. D.

1259. The lipoprotein associated with activation of LCAT is

A. HDL B. LDL

C. VLDL D. IDL

Ans. A.

1260. Serum LDL has been found to be increased in

A. Obstructive jaundice B. Hepatic jaundice

C. Hemolytic jaundice D. Malabsorption syndrome

Ans. A.

1261. A lipoprotein associated with high incidence of coronary atherosclerosis is

A. LDL B. VLDL

C. IDL D. HDL

Ans. A.

1262. A lipoprotein inversely related to the incidence of coronary artherosclerosis is

A. VLDL B. IDL

C. LDL D. HDL

Ans. D.

1263. For synthesis of prostaglandins, the essential fatty acids give rise to a fatty acid containing

A. 12 carbon atoms B. 16 carbon atoms

C. 20 carbon atoms D. 24 carbon atoms

Ans. C.

1264. Normal range of plasma total phospholipids is

A. 0.2–0.6 mmol/L
B. 0.9–2.0 mmol/L
C. 1.8–5.8 mmol/L
D. 2.8–5.3 mmol/L

Ans. C.

1265. Aspirin inhibits the activity of the enzyme:

A. Lipoxygenase
B. Cyclooxygenase
C. Phospholipae A1
D. Phospholipase A2

Ans. B.

1266. A 'suicide enzyme' is

A. Cycloxygenase
B. Lipooxygenase
C. Phospholipase A1
D. Phospholipase A2

Ans. A.

1267. In adipose tissue prostaglandins decrease

A. Lipogenesis
B. Lipolysis
C. Gluconeogenesis
D. Glycogenolysis

Ans. A.

1268. The optimal pH for the enzyme pepsin is

A. 1.0–2.0
B. 4.0–5.0
C. 5.2–6.0
D. 5.8–6.2

Ans. A.

1269. Pepsinogen is converted to active pepsin by

A. HCl
B. Bile salts
C. Ca++
D. Enterokinase

Ans. A.

1270. The optimal pH for the enzyme rennin is

A. 2.0
B. 4.0
C. 8.0
D. 6.0

Ans. B.

1271. The optimal pH for the enzyme trypsin is

A. 1.0–2.0
B. 2.0–4.0
C. 5.2–6.2
D. 5.8–6.2

Ans. C.

1272. The optimal pH for the enzyme chymotrypsin is

A. 2.0
B. 4.0
C. 6.0
D. 8.0

Ans. D.

1273. Trypsinogen is converted to active trypsin by

A. Enterokinase
B. Bile salts
C. HCl
D. Mg^{++}

Ans. A.

1274. Pepsin acts on denatured proteins to produce

A. Proteoses and peptones
B. Polypeptides
C. Peptides
D. Dipeptides

Ans. A.

1275. Renin converts casein to paracasein in presence of

A. Ca^{++}
B. Mg^{++}
C. Na^{+}
D. K^{+}

Ans. A.

1276. The enzyme trypsin is specific for peptide bonds of

A. Basic amino acids
B. Acidic amino acids
C. Aromatic amino acids
D. Next to small amino acid residues

Ans. A.

1277. Chymotrypsin is specific for peptide bonds containing

A. Uncharged amino acid residues
B. Acidic amino acids
C. Basic amino acid
D. Small amino acid residues

Ans. A.

1278. The end product of protein digestion in G.I.T. is

A. Dipeptide
B. Tripeptide
C. Polypeptide
D. Amino acid

Ans. D.

1279. Natural L-isomers of amino acids are absorbed from intestine by

A. Passive diffusion
B. Simple diffusion
C. Faciliated diffusion
D. Active process

Ans. D.

1280. Abnormalities of blood clotting are

A. Haemophilia
B. Christmas disease
C. Gout
D. Both (A) and (B)

Ans. D.

1281. An important reaction for the synthesis of amino acid from carbohydrate intermediates is transamination which requires the cofactor:

A. Thiamin
B. Riboflavin
C. Niacin
D. Pyridoxal phosphate

Ans. D.

1282. The main sites for oxidative deamination are

A. Liver and kidney
B. Skin and pancreas
C. Intestine and mammary gland
D. Lung and spleen

Ans. A.

1283. A positive nitrogen balance occurs

A. In growing infant
B. Following surgery
C. In advanced cancer
D. In kwashiorkor

Ans. A.

1284. The main site of urea synthesis in mammals is

A. Liver
B. Skin
C. Intestine
D. Kidney

Ans. A.

1285. The enzymes of urea synthesis are found in

A. Mitochondria only
B. Cytosol only
C. Both mitochondria and cytosol
D. Nucleus

Ans. C.

1286. The number of ATP required for urea synthesis is

A. 0
B. 1
C. 2
D. 3

Ans. D.

1287. A compound serving a link between citric acid cycle and urea cycle is

A. Malate
B. Citrate
C. Succinate
D. Fumarate

Ans. D.

1288. The 2 nitrogen atoms in urea are contributed by

A. Ammonia and glutamate
B. Glutamine and glutamate
C. Ammonia and aspartate
D. Ammonia and alanine

Ans. C.

1289. Tryptophan could be considered as precursor of

A. Melanotonin
B. Thyroid hormones
C. Melanin
D. Epinephrine

Ans. A.

1290. The enzyme dopamine β-oxidase which catalyses conversion of dopamine to norepinephrine requires

A. Vitamin A
B. Vitamin C
C. Vitamin E
D. Vitamin B12

Ans. B.

1291. In humans the sulphur of methionine and cysteine is excreted mainly as

A. Ethereal sulphate
B. Inorganic sulphate
C. Sulphites
D. Thioorganic compound

Ans. B.

1292. Small amount of urinary oxalates is contributed by the amino acid:

A. Glycine
B. Tyrosine
C. Alanine
D. Serine

Ans. A.

1293. The amino acid which detoxicated benzoic acid to form hippuric acid is

A. Glycine
B. Alanine
C. Serine
D. Glutamic acid

Ans. A.

1294. Chemical score of egg proteins is considered to be

A. 100
B. 60
C. 50
D. 40

Ans. A.

1295. Chemical score of milk proteins is

A. 70
B. 65
C. 60
D. 40

Ans. B.

1296. Chemical score of proteins of bengal gram is

A. 70 B. 60

C. 44 D. 42

Ans. C.

1297. Chemical score of protein gelatin is

A. 0 B. 44

C. 57 D. 60

Ans. A.

1298. Biological value of egg white protein is

A. 94 B. 83

C. 85 D. 77

Ans. B.

1299. Net protein utilisation of egg protein is

A. 75% B. 80%

C. 91% D. 72%

Ans. C.

1300. Net protein utilization of milk protein is

A. 75% B. 80%

C. 86% D. 91%

Ans. A.

1301. A limiting amino acid is an essential amino acid

A. That is most deficient in proteins B. That is most excess in proteins

C. That which increases the growth D. That which increases the weight gain

Ans. A.

1302. The limiting amino acid of rice is

A. Lysine B. Tryptophan

C. Phenylalanine D. Tyrosine

Ans. A.

1303. The limiting amino acid of fish proteins is

A. Tryptophan B. Cysteine

C. Lysine D. Threonine

Ans. A.

1304. Pulses are deficient in

A. Lysine
B. Threonine
C. Methionine
D. Tryptophan

Ans. C.

1305. A trace element deficient in the milk is

A. Magnesium
B. Copper
C. Zinc
D. Chloride

Ans. A.

1306. A conjugated protein present in the egg yolk is

A. Vitellin
B. Livetin
C. Albuminoids
D. Ovo-mucoid

Ans. A.

1307. The chief protein of cow's milk is

A. Albumin
B. Vitellin
C. Livetin
D. Casein

Ans. D.

1308. A water soluble vitamin deficient in egg is

A. Thiamin
B. Ribofalvin
C. Ascrobic acid
D. Cobalamin

Ans. C.

1309. Pulses are rich in

A. Lysine
B. Methionine
C. Tryptophan
D. Phenylalanine

Ans. A.

1310. Milk is deficient in

A. Vitamin B1
B. Vitamin B2
C. Sodium
D. Potassium

Ans. C.

1311. Milk is deficient in

A. Calcium
B. Iron
C. Sodium
D. Potassium

Ans. B.

1312. When net protein utilization (NPU) is low, the requirements for proteins are

A. High
B. Moderate
C. Low
D. Supplementary

Ans. A.

1313. Protein content of human milk is about

A. 1.4%
B. 2.4%
C. 3.4%
D. 4.4%

Ans. B.

1314. Protein content of cow's milk is about

A. 2.5%
B. 3.5%
C. 4.5%
D. 5.5%

Ans. B.

1315. Protein content of soyabean is about

A. 30%
B. 40%
C. 50%
D. 60%

Ans. B.

1316. Lipid content of egg white is

A. 12%
B. 33%
C. 10–11%
D. Traces

Ans. D.

1317. The recommended daily allowance (RDA) of proteins for an adult man is

A. 70 gms
B. 50 gms
C. 40 gms
D. 30 gms

Ans. A.

1318. The basic amino acids are

A. Lysine
B. Bile acids
C. Glycine
D. Alanine

Ans. A.

1319. The daily caloric requirement for the normal adult female is about

A. 1500
B. 2100
C. 2500
D. 2900

Ans. B.

1320. In the total proteins, the percentage of albumin is about

A. 20–40 B. 30–45

C. 50–70 D. 80–90

Ans. C.

1321. In the total proteins percentage of α1 globulin is about

A. 0.2–1.2% B. 1.2–2.0%

C. 2.4–4.4% D. 5.0–10.0%

Ans. C.

1322. In the total proteins the percentage of γ globulin is about

A. 2.4–4.4% B. 10.0–21.0%

C. 6.1–10.1% D. 1.2–2.0%

Ans. B.

1323. Most frequently the normal albumin globulin ratio (A : G) is

A. 1.0 : 0.8 B. 1.5 : 1.0

C. 2.0 : 1.0 D. 2.4 : 1.0

Ans. C.

1324. In Thymol turbidity test the protein involved is mainly

A. Albumin B. α1-Globulin

C. α2-Globulin D. β Globulin

Ans. D.

1325. In quaternary structure, subunits are linked by

A. Peptide bonds B. Disulphide bonds

C. Covalent bonds D. Non-covalent bonds

Ans. D.

1326. Molecular weight of human albumin is about

A. 156,000 B. 90,000

C. 69,000 D. 54,000

Ans. C.

1327. A disulphide bond can be formed between

A. Two methionine residues

B. Two cysteine residues

C. A methionine and a cysteine residue

D. All of these

Ans. B.

1328. A coagulated protein is

A. Insoluble
B. Biologically non-functional
C. Unfolded
D. All of the above

Ans. D.

1329. At a pH below the isoelectric point, an amino acid exists as

A. Cation
B. Anion
C. Zwitterion
D. Undissociated molecule

Ans. A.

1330. An amino acid having a hydrophilic side chain is

A. Alanine
B. Proline
C. Methionine
D. Serine

Ans. D.

1331. An amino acid that does not take part in α helix formation is

A. Histidine
B. Tyrosine
C. Proline
D. Tryptophan

Ans. C.

1332. A protein rich in cysteine is

A. Collagen
B. Keratin
C. Haemoglobin
D. Gelatin

Ans. B.

1333. Primary structure of proteins can be determined by the use of

A. Electrophoresis
B. Chromatography
C. Ninhydrin
D. Sanger's reagent

Ans. D.

1334. Electrostatic bonds can be formed between the side chains of

A. Alanine and leucine
B. Leucine and valine
C. Asparate and glutamate
D. Lysine and aspartate

Ans. D.

1335. Sanger's reagent contains

A. Phenylisothiocyanate
B. Dansyl chloride
C. 1-Fluoro-2, 4-dinitrobenzene
D. Ninhydrin

Ans. C.

1336. The most abundant protein in mammals is

A. Albumin
B. Haemoglobin
C. Collagen
D. Elastin

Ans. C.

1337. Folding of newly synthesized proteins is accelerated by

A. Protein disulphide isomerase
B. Prolyl cis-trans isomerase
C. Chaperonins
D. All of these

Ans. D.

1338. Primary structure of a protein is formed by

A. Hydrogen bonds
B. Peptide bonds
C. Disulphide bonds
D. All of these

Ans. B.

1339. α-Helix is formed by

A. Hydrogen bonds
B. Hydrophobic bonds
C. Electrostatic bonds
D. Disulphide bonds

Ans. A.

1340. Glutelins are present in

A. Milk
B. Eggs
C. Meat
D. Cereals

Ans. D.

1341. Aromatic amino acids can be detected by

A. Sakaguchi reaction
B. Millon-Nasse reaction
C. Hopkins-Cole reaction
D. Xanthoproteic reaction

Ans. D.

1342. Two amino groups are present in

A. Leucine
B. Glutamate
C. Lysine
D. Threonine

Ans. C.

1343. During denaturation of proteins, all of the following are disrupted except

A. Primary structure
B. Secondary structure
C. Tertiary structure
D. Quaternary structure

Ans. B.

1344. All the following are branched chain amino acids except

A. Isoleucine
B. Alanine
C. Leucine
D. Valine

Ans. B.

1345. An –OH group is present in the side chain of

A. Serine
B. Arginine
C. Lysine
D. Proline

Ans. A.

1346. Edman's reagent contains

A. Phenylisothiocyanate
B. 1-Fluoro-2, 4-dinitrobenzene
C. Dansyl Chloride
D. tBOC azide

Ans. A.

1347. Edman's reaction can be used to

A. Determine the number of tyrosine residues in a protein
B. Determine the number of aromatic amino acid residues in a protein
C. Determine the amino acid sequence of a protein
D. Hydrolyse the peptide bonds in a protein

Ans. C.

1348. A pentose found in nucleotide is

A. D-ribose
B. L-ribose
C. D-ribulose
D. L-ribulose

Ans. A.

1349. The following causes laevorotation

A. D-Fructose
B. L-glucose
C. L-ribose
D. All the above

Ans. D.

1350. In straight chain structure of D-glucose, -OH group is present on left hand side of carbon number

A. 2
B. 3
C. 4
D.5

Ans. B.

1351. In straight chain structure of D-ribose, -OH group is present on right hand side of carbon number

A. 2
B. 3
C. 4
D. All the above

Ans. D.

1352. The smallest monosaccharide having furanose ring structure is

A. Erythrose B. Ribose

C. Glucose D. Fructose

Ans. B.

1353. The following is an epimeric pair

A. Glucose and fructose B. Glucose and galactose

C. Galactose and mannose D. Lactose and maltose

Ans. B.

1354. Similar osazones are formed by

A. Glucose and mannose B. Mannose and galactose

C. Glucose and galactose D. None of the above

Ans. A.

1355. α glycosidic bond is present in

A. Lactose B. Maltose

C. Sucrose D. All of the above

Ans. B.

1356. Branching occurs in glycogen approximately after every

A. 5 glucose units B. 10 glucose units

C. 15 glucose units D. 20 glucose units

Ans. B.

1357. Mucopolysaccharides are also known as

A. Mucoproteins B. Glycoproteins

C. Glycosaminoglycans D. Homopolysaccharides

Ans. C.

1358. N-acetylglucosamine is present in

A. Hyaluronic acid B. Chondroitin sulphate

C. Heparin D. All of the above

Ans. A.

1359. α Iduronic acid is present in

A. Hyaluronic acid B. Chondroitin sulphate

C. Dermatan sulphate D. Keratan sulphate

Ans. C.

1360. Iodine gives a red color with

A. Starch B. Dextrin

C. Glycogen D. Inulin

Ans. C.

1361. Amylose is a constituent of

A. Starch B. Cellulose

C. Glycogen D. None of the above

Ans. A.

1362. A homopolymer of glucose is

A. Starch B. Dextrin

C. Glycogen D. All of the above

Ans. D.

1363. What is the main damaging effect of UV radiation on DNA?

A. Formation of thymine dimers B. Depurination

C. Dehydration D. Single strand break

Ans. A.

1364. Telomeres are usually rich in which nucleotide?

A. Guanine B. Adenine

C. Cytosine D. Thymine

Ans. A.

1365. Which histone(s) are associated with the linker DNA of a nucleosome?

A. Histones H2A and H2B B. Histone H1

C. Histone H4 D. Histone H3

Ans. B.

1366. A caesium chloride will separate DNA molecules by

A. Resorption B. Absorption

C. Adhesion D. Density

Ans. D.

1367. The most common liquid volumes in molecular biology are measured in

A. μl B. ml

C. L D. nl

Ans. A.

1368. DNA gyrase in E. coli

A. Can be inhibited with antibiotics

B. Adds positive supercoils to chromosomal DNA

C. Performs the same function as helicase in eukaryotes

D. Is required onlyat the oriC site

Ans. A.

1369. The nucleosome consists of histone

A. Tetramer and 146 bp of DNA

B. Octamer and 146 bp of DNA

C. None of the above

D. Hexamer and 146 bp of DNA

Ans. B.

1370. DNA can be sequenced by the

A. Chain termination method

B. Chemical method

C. Physical method

D. Both A and B

Ans. D.

1371. The chromosomal DNA complexes with

A. 5 types of histones as H1, H2A, H2B, H3 and H4

B. 3 types of histone as H1, H2A and H4

C. 2 types of histone as H1 and H4

D. 4 types of histone as H1, H2A, H3 and H4

Ans. A.

1372. The higher order structure of DNA shows symmetry, whereas the higher order structures of most proteins do not. Why isn't protein shape more regular like DNA?

A. The many different amino acid R groups on proteins confer many different shapes

B. DNA has one main function in cells whereas proteins have many.

C. All of the above

D. None of the above

Ans. C.

1373. If one cell has AT contents 40%, what will be the percentage of Guanine residue?

A. 0.15

B. 0.6

C. Guanine residue can not be calculated

D. 0.3

Ans. D.

1374. When DNA polymerase is in contact with guanine in the parental strand, what does it add to the growing daughter strand?

A. Cytosine
B. Phosphate
C. Guanine
D. Uracil

Ans. A.

1375. The 5' and 3' numbers are related to the

A. Carbon number in sugar
B. Length of the DNA strand
C. The base pair rule
D. The number of phosphates

Ans. A.

1376. Inherited deficiency of β-glucosidase causes

A. Tay-Sachs disease
B. Metachromatic leukodystrophy
C. Gaucher's disease
D. Multiple sclerosis

Ans. C.

1377. Identical osazones are formed by

A. Glucose and fructose
B. Glucose and mannose
C. Mannose and fructose
D. All of the above

Ans. D.

1378. Maltose can be formed by hydrolysis of

A. Starch
B. Dextrin
C. Glycogen
D. All of the above

Ans. D.

1379. α-1, 6 glycosidic bond is not present in

A. Glycogen
B. Dextrin
C. Amylase
D. Amylopectin

Ans. C.

1380. Sulphated iduronic acid is present in

A. Hyaluronic acid
B. Chondroitin sulphate
C. Heparin
D. All of the above

Ans. C.

1381. Monosaccharides can be separated by

A. Electrophoresis
B. Chromatography
C. Salting out
D. None of the above

Ans. B.

1382. Fructose is present in hydrolysate of

A. Sucrose B. Inulin

C. Both of the above D. None of the above

Ans. C.

1383. N-acetylgalactosamine sulphate is present in

A. Hyaluronic acid B. Heparin

C. Chondroitin sulphate D. None of the above

Ans. C.

1384. Invertase catalyses the hydrolysis of

A. Maltose B. Lactose

C. Sucrose D. None of the above

Ans. C.

1385. In fructofuranose, anomeric carbon atom is

A. Carbon 1 B. Carbon 2

C. Carbon 3 D. Carbon 4

Ans. B.

1386. A carbohydrate found in DNA is

A. Ribose B. Deoxyribose

C. Ribulose D. All of the above

Ans. B.

1387. Ribulose is a

A. Ketotetrose B. Aldotetrose

C. Ketopentose D. Aldopentose

Ans. C.

1388. A disaccharide made up of two glucose units is

A. Sucrose B. Maltose

C. Lactose D. Dextrin

Ans. B.

1389. A carbohydrate commonly known as dextrose is

A. Dextrin B. D-Fructose

C. D-glucose D. Glycogen

Ans. C.

1390. Amino sugars are present in

A. Hyaluronic acid
B. Chondroitin sulphate
C. Erythromycin
D. All the above

Ans. D.

1391. A carbohydrate found only in milk is

A. Glucose
B. Galactose
C. Lactose
D. Maltose

Ans. C.

1392. A carbohydrate commonly known as invert sugar

A. Fructose
B. Sucrose
C. Glucose
D. Lactose

Ans. B.

1393. A homopolysaccharide among the following is

A. Heparin
B. Hyaluronic acid
C. Dermatan sulphate
D. Cellulose

Ans. D.

1394. A heteropolysaccharide among the following is

A. Inulin
B. Cellulose
C. Heparin
D. Dextrin

Ans. C.

1395. The predominant form of glucose in solution is

A. Acyclic form
B. Hydrated acyclic form
C. Glucofuranose
D. Glucopyranose

Ans. D.

1396. Optical isomerism is denoted by

A. D- and L-
B. d- and l-
C. (+) and (-)
D. Any of the above

Ans. C.

1397. An L-isomer of monosaccharide formed in human body is

A. L-Fructose
B. L-Erythrose
C. L-Xylose
D. L-Xylulose

Ans. D.

1398. Number of stereoisomers of glucose is

A. 4
B. 8
C. 16
D. None of the above

Ans. C.

1399. A homopolysaccharide made up of fructose is

A. Glycogen
B. Dextrin
C. Cellulose
D. Inulin

Ans. D.

1400. Tay-Sachs disease results from inherited deficiency of

A. Arylsulphatase A
B. Hexosaminidase A
C. Sphingomyelinase
D. Ceramidase

Ans. B.

1401. The largest apolipoprotein is

A. Apo E
B. Apo B-48
C. Apo B-100
D. Apo A-I

Ans. C.

1402. Apolipoprotein B-100 is synthesised in

A. Adipose tissue
B. Liver
C. Intestine
D. Liver and intestine

Ans. B.

1403. Apolipoprotein B-48 is synthesized in

A. Adipose tissue
B. Liver
C. Intestine
D. Liver and intestine

Ans. C.

1404. Apolipoproteins A-I and A-II are present in

A. LDL only
B. LDL and VLDL
C. HDL only
D. HDL and chylomicrons

Ans. D.

1405. Apolipoprotein B-48 is present in

A. Chylomicrons
B. VLDL
C. LDL
D. HDL

Ans. A.

1406. Apolipoprotein B-100 is present in

A. Chylomicrons
B. VLDL only
C. LDL only
D. VLDL and LDL

Ans. B.

1407. Apolipoproteins C-I, C-II and C-III are present in

A. Chylomicrons
B. VLDL
C. HDL
D. All of these

Ans. D.

1408. Apolipoprotiens C-I, C-II and C-III are present in all of the following except

A. Chylomicrons
B. VLDL
C. LDL
D. HDL

Ans. C.

1409. Apolipoprotein A-I acts as

A. Enzyme activator
B. Ligand for receptor
C. Both (A) and (B)
D. None of these

Ans. C.

1410. Apolipoprotien B-100 acts as

A. Enzyme activator
B. Ligand for receptor
C. Both (A) and (B)
D. None of these

Ans. B.

1411. Apolipoprotein C-II is an activator of

A. Lecithin cholesterola acyl transferase
B. Phospholipase C
C. Extrahepatic lipoprotein lipase
D. Hepatic lipoprotein lipase

Ans. C.

1412. Nascent chylomicron receives apolipoproteins C and E from

A. VLDL remnant
B. VLDL
C. LDL
D. HDL

Ans. D.

1413. S1 nuclease hydrolyses

A. DNA of somatic cells
B. DNA of sperms
C. Any double stranded DNA
D. Any single stranded DNA

Ans. D.

1414. Positive nitrogen balance is seen in

A. Starvation
B. Wasting diseases
C. Growing age
D. Intestinal malabsorption

Ans. C.

1415. All of the following statements about aspartate are true except

A. It is non-essential amino acid
B. It is a dicarboxylic amino acid
C. It can be synthesized from pyruvate and glutamate
D. It can be converted into asparagines

Ans. C.

1416. Glycine can be synthesized from

A. Serine
B. Choline
C. Betaine
D. All of these

Ans. D.

1417. All of the following statements about proline are true except

A. It is an imino acid
B. It can be synthesized from glutamate
C. It can be catabolised to glutamate
D. Free proline can be hydroxylated to hydroxyproline

Ans. D.

1418. A protein rich in hydroxyproline is

A. Prolamin
B. Procollagen
C. Collagen
D. Proinsulin

Ans. C.

1419. All the following statement about hydroxyproline are true except

A. There is no codon for hydroxyproline
B. It is present in large amounts in collagen
C. Free proline cannot be hydroxylated to hydroxyproline
D. Hydroxylation of proline residues is catalysed by a dioxygenase

Ans. D.

1420. All of the following are required for hydroxylation of proline residues except

A. Ascorbic acid
B. Glutamate
C. Ferrous ions
D. Molecular oxygen

Ans. B.

1421. Cysteine can be synthesized from methionine and

A. Serine
B. Homoserine
C. Homocysteine
D. Threonine

Ans. A.

1422. Methionine is synthesized in human body from

A. Cysteine and homoserine
B. Homocysteine and serine
C. Cysteine and serine
D. None of these

Ans. D.

1423. Non-Protein amino acids are

A. Ornithine
B. β-alanine
C. γ-amino butyric acid
D. All of these

Ans. A.

1424. The amino acid that undergoes oxidative deamination at significant rate is

A. Alanine
B. Aspartate
C. Glutamate
D. Glutamine

Ans. C.

1425. Allosteric inhibitor of glutamate dehydrogenase is

A. ATP
B. ADP
C. AMP
D. GMP

Ans. A.

1426. Allsoteric activator of glutamate dehydrogenase is

A. ATP
B. GTP
C. ADP and GDP
D. AMP and GMP

Ans. C.

1427. Free ammonia is released during

A. Oxidative deamination of glutamate
B. Catabolism of purines
C. Catabolism of pyrimidines
D. All of these

Ans. D.

1428. An organ which is extremely sensitive to ammonia toxicity is

A. Liver
B. Brain
C. Kidney
D. Heart

Ans. B.

1429. Ammonia is transported from muscles to liver mainly in the form of

A. Free ammonia B. Glutamine

C. Asparagine D. Alanine

Ans. D.

1430. The major site of urea synthesis is

A. Brain B. Kidneys

C. Liver D. Muscles

Ans. B.

1431. Carbamoyl phosphate required for urea synthesis is formed in

A. Cytosol B. Mitochondria

C. Both (A) and (B) D. None of these

Ans. B.

1432. The following enzyme of urea cycle is present in cytosol:

A. Argininosuccinic acid synthetase B. Argininosuccinase

C. Arginase D. All of these

Ans. D.

1433. Daily excretion of nitrogen by an adult man is about

A. 15–20 mg B. 1.5–2 gm

C. 5–10 gm D. 15–20 gm

Ans. C.

1434. Maple syrup urine diseases is an inborn error of metabolism of

A. Sulphur-containing amino acids B. Aromatic amino acids

C. Branched chain amino acids D. Dicarboxylic amino acids

Ans. C.

1435. Cystinuria results from inability to

A. Metabolise cysteine B. Convert cystine into cysteine

C. Incorporate cysteine into proteins D. Reabsorb cystine in renal tubules

Ans. D.

1436. The defective enzyme in histidinemia is

A. Histidine carboxylase B. Histidine decarboxylase

C. Histidase D. Histidine oxidase

Ans. C.

1437. All the following statements about phenylketonuria are correct except

A. Phenylalanine cannot be converted into tyrosine

B. Urinary excretion of phenylpyruvate and phenyllactate is increased

C. It can be controlled by giving a low phenylalanine diet

D. It leads to decreased synthesis of thyroid hormones, catecholamines and melanin

Ans. D.

1438. All the following statements about albinism are correct except

A. Tyrosine hydroxylase (tyrosinase) is absent or deficient in melanocytes

B. Skin is hypopigmented

C. It results in mental retardation

D. Eyes are hypopigmented

Ans. C.

1439. Glycine is not required for the formation of

A. Taurocholic acid B. Creatine

C. Purines D. Pyrimidines

Ans. A.

1440. Histamine is formed from histidine by

A. Deamination B. Dehydrogenation

C. Decarboxylation D. Carboxylation

Ans. C.

1441. DOPA is an intermediate in the synthesis of

A. Thyroid hormones B. Catecholamines

C. Melanin D. Catecholamines and melanin

Ans. D.

1442. All the following statements about pepsin are correct except

A. It is smaller than pepsinogen

B. It is formed by the action of HCl on its precursor

C. Its optimum pH is 1.0–2.0

D. It hydrolyses the C-terminal and N-terminal peptide bonds of proteins

Ans. D.

1443. Pancreatic juice contains the precursors of all of the following except

A. Trypsin B. Chymotrypsin

C. Carboxypeptidase D. Aminopeptidase

Ans. D.

1444. The only correct statement about chymotrypsin is

A. It is formed from trypsin

B. Carboxypeptidase converts trypsin into chymotrypsin

C. Its optimum pH is around 7

D. It hydrolyses peptide bonds involving basic amino acids

Ans. C.

1445. A Zwitterion is

A. Positive ion B. Negative ion

C. Both (A) and (B) D. None of these

Ans. C.

1446. After accounting for SDA, the net gain of energy from 25 gm of proteins is about

A. 70 kcal B. 100 kcal

C. 130 kcal D. 200 kcal

Ans. A.

1447. After accounting for SDA, the net gain of energy from 25 gm of carbohydrates is about

A. 70 kcal B. 95 kcal

C. 100 kcal D. 105 kcal

Ans. B.

1448. After accounting for SDA, the net gain of energy from 100 gm of fat is about

A. 600 kcal B. 780 kcal

C. 900 kcal D. 1020 kcal

Ans. B.

1449. If proteins, carbohydrates and fats are consumed together:

A. The total SDA is the sum of individual SDAs of proteins, carbohydrates and fats

B. The total SDA is more than the sum of individual SDAs of proteins, carbohydrates and fats

C. Carbohydrates and fats lower the SDA of proteins

D. Proteins raise the SDA of carbohydrates and fats

Ans. C.

1450. After calculating the energy requirement of a person:

A. 10% kcal are subtracted on account of SDA

B. 10% kcal are added on account of SDA

C. 20% kcal are subtracted on account of SDA

D. 20% kcal are subtracted on account of SDA

Ans. B.

1451. The recommended energy intake for an adult sedentary Indian man is

A. 1,900 kcal/day
B. 2,400 kcal/day
C. 2,700 kcal/day
D. 3,000 kcal/day

Ans. B.

1452. The recommended energy intake for an adult sedentary Indian woman is

A. 1,900 kcal/day
B. 2,200 kcal/day
C. 2,400 kcal/day
D. 2,700 kcal/day

Ans. A.

1453. During pregnancy, the following should be added to the calculated energy requirement:

A. 300 kcal/day
B. 500 kcal/day
C. 700 kcal/day
D. 900 kcal/day

Ans. A.

1454. During first six months of lactation, the following increment in energy intake is recommended:

A. 200 kcal/day
B. 300 kcal/day
C. 550 kcal/day
D. 1,000 kcal/day

Ans. C.

1455. The proximate principles of diet are

A. Vitamins and minerals
B. Proteins
C. Carbohydrates and fats
D. Carbohydrates, fats and proteins

Ans. D.

1456. The limiting amino acid in wheat is

A. Leucine
B. Lysine
C. Cysteine
D. Methionine

Ans. B.

1457. The limiting amino acid in pulses is

A. Leucine
B. Lysine
C. Tryptophan
D. Methionine

Ans. D.

1458. Maize is poor in

A. Lysine
B. Methionine
C. Tryptophan
D. Lysine and tryptophan

Ans. D.

1459. The percentage of ingested protein/ nitrogen absorbed into blood stream is known as

A. Net protein utilisation
B. Protein efficiency ratio
C. Digestibility coefficient
D. Biological value of protein

Ans. C.

1460. Biological value of a protein is

A. The percentage of ingested protein/nitrogen absorbed into circulation
B. The percentage of ingested protein/nitrogen in the body
C. The percentage of ingested protein utilized for protein synthesis in the body
D. The gain in body weight (gm) per gm of protein ingested

Ans. B.

1461. Net protein utilisation depends upon

A. Protein efficiency ratio
B. Digestibility coefficient
C. Digestibility coefficient and protein efficiency ratio
D. Digestibility coefficient and biological value

Ans. D.

1462. The gain in body weight (gm) per gm of protein ingested is known as

A. Net protein utilisation
B. Protein efficiency ratio
C. Digestibility coefficient
D. Biological value of protein

Ans. B.

1463. The following is considered as reference standard for comparing the nutritional quality of proteins:

A. Milk proteins
B. Egg proteins
C. Meat proteins
D. Fish proteins

Ans. B.

1464. Biological value of egg proteins is about

A. 70 %
B. 80 %
C. 86 %
D. 94 %

Ans. D.

1465. The following has the highest protein efficiency ratio:

A. Milk proteins
B. Egg proteins
C. Meat proteins
D. Fish proteins

Ans. B.

1466. The following has the lowest protein efficiency ratio:

A. Maize proteins
B. Wheat proteins
C. Milk proteins
D. Rice proteins

Ans. A.

1467. Protein content of egg is about

A. 10%
B. 13%
C. 16%
D. 20%

Ans. B.

1468. Protein content of meat is about

A. 10%
B. 13%
C. 16%
D. 20%

Ans. D.

1469. Protein content of rice is about

A. 7%
B. 12%
C. 15%
D. 20%

Ans. A.

1470. The calorific value of wheat is about

A. 2.5 kcal/gm
B. 3.5 kcal/gm
C. 4.5 kcal/gm
D. 5.5 kcal/gm

Ans. B.

1471. For vegetarians, pulses are an important source of

A. Carbohydrates
B. Proteins
C. Fat
D. Iron

Ans. B.

1472. The amino acids present in pulses can supplement the limiting amino acids of

A. Cereals
B. Milk
C. Fish
D. Nuts and beans

Ans. A.

1473. Milk is a good source of

A. Proteins, calcium and iron
B. Proteins, calcium and ascorbic acid
C. Proteins, lactose and retinol
D. Proteins, lactose and essential fatty acids

Ans. C.

1474. Milk is a good source of all of the following except

A. Essential amino acids
B. Vitamin C
C. Galactose
D. Calcium and phosphorous

Ans. B.

1475. Milk is poor in

A. Cholesterol
B. Retinol
C. Calcium
D. Iron

Ans. D.

1476. Egg is rich in all of the following except

A. Cholesterol
B. Saturated fatty acids
C. Ascorbic acid
D. Calcium

Ans. C.

1477. A phosphoprotein present in egg is

A. Casein
B. Albumin
C. Ovoglobulin
D. Ovovitellin

Ans. D.

1478. Consumption of raw eggs can cause deficiency of

A. Calcium
B. Lipoic acid
C. Biotin
D. Vitamin A

Ans. C.

1479. Egg is poor in

A. Essential amino acids
B. Carbohydrates
C. Avidin
D. Biotin

Ans. B.

1480. Cholesterol is present in all the following except

A. Milk
B. Fish
C. Egg white
D. Egg yolk

Ans. C.

1481. Meat is rich in all of the following except

A. Iron
B. Fluorine
C. Copper
D. Zinc

Ans. B.

1482. Kwashiorkor occurs when the diet is severely deficient in

A. Iron
B. Calories
C. Proteins
D. Essential fatty acids

Ans. C.

1483. Clinical features of Kwashiorkor include all of the following except

A. Mental retardation
B. Muscle wasting
C. Oedema
D. Anaemia

Ans. A.

1484. Kwashiorkor usually occurs in

A. The post-weaning period
B. Pregnancy
C. Lactation
D. Old age

Ans. A.

1485. Marasmus occurs from deficient intake of

A. Essential amino acids
B. Essential fatty acids
C. Calories
D. Zinc

Ans. C.

1486. Marasmus differs from Kwashiorkor

A. Mental retardation occurs in kwashiorkor but not in marasmus
B. Growth is retarded in kwashiorkor but not in Marasmus
C. Muscle wasting occurs in marasmus but not kwashiorkor
D. Subcutaneous fat disappears in marasmus but not in kwashiorkor

Ans. D.

1487. Energy reserves of an average well-fed adult man are about

A. 50,000 kcal
B. 100,000 kcal
C. 200,000 kcal
D. 300,000 kcal

Ans. B.

1488. During starvation, the first reserve nutrient to be depleted is

A. Glycogen
B. Proteins
C. Triglycerides
D. Cholesterol

Ans. A.

1489. Synthesis of the following enzymes is increased during starvation.

A. Digestive enzymes
B. Gluconeogenic enzymes
C. Urea cycle enzymes
D. Glucokinase

Ans. B.

1490. In hypoparathyroidism

A. Plasma calcium and inorganic phosphorous are low

B. Plasma calcium and inorganic phosphorous are high

C. Plasma calcium is low and inorganic phosphorous high

D. Plasma calcium is high and inorganic phosphorous low

Ans. C.

1491. The number of amino acid residues in calcitonin in

A. 9 B. 32

C. 51 D. 84

Ans. B.

1492. Calcitonin is synthesised in

A. Parathyroid glands B. Thyroid gland

C. Pars intermedia of pituitary D. Adrenal cortex

Ans. B.

1493. Plasma calcium is lowered by

A. Parathormone B. Calcitonin

C. Aldosterone D. Deoxycorticosterone

Ans. B.

1494. α Cells of Islets of Langerhans secrete

A. Insulin B. Glucagon

C. Somatostatin D. Cholecystokinin

Ans. B.

1495. A/G ratio is

A. Strength of proteins B. ratio of serum proteins

C. ratio of ceruloplasmin D. None of these

Ans. B.

1496. Insulin is made up of

A. A single polypeptide chain having 51 amino acid residues

B. A single polypeptide chain having 84 amino acid residues

C. A-chain having 21 and B-chain having 30 amino acid residues

D. A-chain having 30 and B-chain having 21 amino acid residues

Ans. C.

1497. The number of amino acid residues in pre-proinsulin is

A. 51 B. 84

C. 109 D. 119

Ans. C.

1498. Pre-proinsulin contains a signal sequence having

A. 9 amino acid residues B. 19 amino acid residues

C. 27 amino acid residues D. 33 amino acid residues

Ans. B.

1499. The number of intra-chain disulphide bonds in pro-insulin:

A. One B. Two

C. Three D. Four

Ans. C.

1500. Pentagastrin is a

A. Naturally occurring form of gastrin

B. Inactive metabolite of gastrin

C. Active metabolite of gastrin

D. Synthetic form of gastrin

Ans. D.

1501. Secretion of gastrin is evoked by

A. Entry of food into stomach B. Vagal stimulation

C. Lower aliphatic alcohols D. All of these

Ans. D.

1502. Gastrin stimulates

A. Gastric motility B. Gastric secretion

C. Both (A) and (B) D. None of these

Ans. C.

1503. Secretin is made up of

A. 17 amino acids B. 27 amino acids

C. 37 amino acids D. 47 amino acids

Ans. B.

1504. Secretin causes all of the following except

A. Secretion of pancreatic juice B. Secretion of bile

C. Inhibition of gastric secretion D. Stimulation of intestinal motility

Ans. D.

1505. All of the following statements about cholecystokinin pancreozymin are true except

A. It is secreted by mucosa of small intestine

B. It stimulates secretion of pancreatic juice rich in enzymes

C. It stimulates contraction of gall bladder

D. It inhibits gastric motility

Ans. D.

1506. All of the following statements about pancreatic somatostain are true except

A. It is secreted by δ cells of islets of Langerhans

B. It stimulates the secretion of gastrin

C. It inhibits the secretion of secretin

D. It inhibits the secretion of cholecystokinin pancreozymin

Ans. B.

1507. Histidine is converted into histamine by

A. Carboxylation B. Decarboxylation

C. Methylation D. Hydroxylation

Ans. B.

1508. Histamine is synthesized in

A. Brain B. Mast cells

C. Basophils D. All of these

Ans. D.

1509. Histamine causes all the following except

A. Stimulation of gastric secretion B. Vasoconstriction

C. Pruritus D. Increase in capillary permeability

Ans. B.

1510. H2-receptors are blocked by

A. Diphenhydramine B. Mepayramine

C. Pyrilamine D. Cimetidine

Ans. D.

1511. Serotonin is synthesized from

A. Serine B. Phenylalanine

C. Tyrosine D. Tryptophan

Ans. D.

1512. All the following statements about serotonin are true except

A. It causes vasolidatation

B. It causes bronchoconstriction

C. It is metabolized by monoamine oxidase

D. Its metabolite is 5-hydroxyindole acetic acid

Ans. A.

1513. All the following statements about angiotensin are true except

A. Its precursor is an α2-globulin

B. Its active form is an octapeptide

C. It is a vasodilator

D. It increases the secretion of aldosterone

Ans. C.

1514. Methyl dopa decreases blood pressure by

A. Inhibiting the synthesis of catecholamines

B. Antagonising the action of aldosterone

C. Stimulating the release of renin

D. Inhibiting the breakdown of angiotensin

Ans. A.

1515. Binding of gamma-aminobutyric acid to its receptors in brain increases the permeability of cell membrane to

A. Cl–   B. Na+

C. K+   D. Ca++

Ans. A.

1516. Binding of acetylcholine to its receptors increases the permeability of cell membrane to

A. Ca++   B. Na+

C. K+   D. Na+ and K+

Ans. D.

1517. All of the following are glycoproteins except

A. Collagen   B. Albumin

C. Transferrin   D. IgM

Ans. B.

1518. Sialic acids are present in

A. Proteoglycans B. Glycoproteins
C. Both (A) and (B) D. None of these

Ans. B.

1519. Hyaluronidase hydrolyses

A. Hyaluronic acid
B. Chondroitin sulphate
C. Heparin
D. Hyaluronic acid and chondroitin sulphate

Ans. D.

1520. The most abundant protein in bones is

A. Collagen type I B. Collagen type II
C. Collagen type III D. Non-collagen proteins

Ans. A.

1521. The most abundant collagen in cartilages is

A. Type I B. Type II
C. Type III D. Type IV

Ans. B.

1522. Collagen and elastin have the following similarity:

A. Both are triple helices B. Both have hydroxyproline residues
C. Both have hydrolysine residues D. Both are glycoproteins

Ans. A.

1523. Abnormal collagen structure is seen in all of the following except

A. I-cell disease B. Osteogenesis imperfecta
C. Menke's disease D. Ehlers-Danlos sydrome

Ans. B.

1524. I-cell disease results from absence of the following from lysosomal enzymes:

A. Signal sequence B. Mannose-6-phosphate
C. Sialic acid D. A serine residue

Ans. D.

1525. In I-cell disease, lysosomal enzymes

A. Are not synthesised B. Are inactive
C. Lack signal sequence D. Cannot reach lysosomes

Ans. B.

1526. Renal glycosuria occurs due to

A. Increased filtration of glucose in glomeruli

B. Increased secretion of glucose by renal tubular cells

C. Decreased reabsorption of glucose by renal tubular cells

D. Increased conversion of glycogen into glucose in tubular cells

Ans. D.

1527. Haematuria can occur in

A. Haemolytic anaemia
B. Mismatched blood transfusion
C. Yellow fever
D. Stone in urinary tract

Ans. D.

1528. Haematuria can occur in all of the following except

A. Acute glomerulonephritis
B. Cancer of urinary tract
C. Stone in urinary tract
D. Mismatched blood transfusion

Ans. D.

1529. Chyluria can be detected by addition of the following to the urine:

A. Sulphosalicylic acid
B. Nitric acid
C. Acetic anhydride
D. Chloroform

Ans. D.

1530. Normal range of serum urea is

A. 0.6–1.5 mg/dl
B. 9–11 mg/dl
C. 20–45 mg/dl
D. 60–100 mg/dl

Ans. C.

1531. Normal range of serum creatinine is

A. 0.6–1.5 mg/dl
B. 9–11 mg/dl
C. 20–45 mg/dl
D. 60–100 mg/dl

Ans. A.

1532. Standard urea clearance is

A. 54 ml/min
B. 75 ml/min
C. 110 ml/min
D. 130 ml/min

Ans. A.

1533. Maximum urea clearance is

A. 54 ml/min
B. 75 ml/min
C. 110 ml/min
D. 130 ml/min

Ans. B.

1534. Average creatinine clearance in an adult man is about

A. 54 ml/min B. 75 ml/min

C. 110 ml/min D. 130 ml/min

Ans. C.

1535. Inulin clearance in an average adult man is about

A. 54 ml/min B. 75 ml/min

C. 110 ml/min D. 130 ml/min

Ans. D.

1536. Among the following, a test of tubular function is

A. Creatinine clearance B. Inulin clearance

C. PAH clearance D. PSP excretion test

Ans. D.

1537. A simple way to assess tubular function is to withhold food and water for 12hours and, then, measure

A. Serum urea B. Serum creatinine

C. Urine output in one hour D. Specific gravity of urine

Ans. D.

1538. Among the following, the most sensitive indicator of glomerular function is

A. Serum urea B. Serum creatinine

C. Urea clearance D. Creatinine clearance

Ans. D.

1539. All the following statements about inulin are correct except

A. It is completely non-toxic

B. It is completely filtered by glomeruli

C. It is not reabsorbed by tubular cells

D. It is secreted by tubular cells

Ans. D.

1540. Non-protein nitrogenous substances in blood include all of the following except

A. Urea B. Uric acid

C. Creatinine D. Inositol

Ans. C.

1541. Non-protein nitrogenous substances in blood are raised in

A. Starvation B. Liver damage

C. Renal failure D. All of these

Ans. B.

1542. Creatinine clearance is decreased in

A. Acute tubular necrosis
B. Acute glomerulonephritis
C. Hypertension
D. Myopathies

Ans. D.

1543. Serum amylase is increased in

A. Acute parotitis
B. Acute pancreatitis
C. Pancreatic cancer
D. All of these

Ans. B.

1544. Serum lipase is increased in

A. Acute parotitis
B. Acute pancreatitis
C. Infective hepatitis
D. Biliary obstruction

Ans. A.

1545. The phenomenon of inhibition of glycolysis by O2 is termed as

A. Red drop
B. Pasteur effect
C. Michaelis effect
D. Fischer's effect

Ans. B.

1546. Which amino acid is a lipotropic factor?

A. Lysine
B. Leucine
C. Tryptophan
D. Methionine

Ans. D.

1547. Which among the following is a nutritionally essential amino acid for man ?

A. Alanine
B. Glycine
C. Tyrosine
D. Tryptophan

Ans. D.

1548. The essential amino acids

A. Must be supplied in the diet because the organism has lost the capacity to aminate the corresponding ketoacids

B. Must be supplied in the diet because the human has an impaired ability to synthesize the carbon chain of the corresponding ketoacids

C. Are identical in all species studied

D. Are defined as those amino acids which cannot be synthesized by the organism at a rate adequate to meet metabolic requirements

Ans. B.

1549. Which among the following is an essential amino acid?

A. Cysteine B. Leucine

C. Tyrosine D. Aspartic acid

Ans. B.

1550. Which among the following is a basic amino acid?

A. Aspargine B. Arginine

C. Proline D. Alanine

Ans. B.

1551. This amino acid cannot have optical isomers:

A. Alanine B. Histidine

C. Threonine D. Glycine

Ans. D.

1552. The amino acid which contains a guanidine group is

A. Histidine B. Arginine

C. Citrulline D. Ornithine

Ans. B.

1553. GABA(gama amino butyric acid) is

A. Post-synaptic excitatory transmitter

B. Post-synaptic inhibitor transmitter

C. Activator of glia-cell function

D. Inhibitor of glia-cell function

Ans. B.

1554. Sulphur-containing amino acid is

A. Glutathione B. Chondroitin sulphate

C. Homocysteine D. Tryptophan

Ans. C.

1555. The useful reagent for detection of amino acids is

A. Molisch reagent B. Dichlorophenol Indophenol

C. Ninhydrin D. Biuret

Ans. C.

1556. The amino acid which contains an indole group is

A. Histidine B. Arginine

C. Glycine D. Tryptophan

Ans. D.

1557. Sakaguchi reaction is done for detection of

A. Lysine
B. Ornithine
C. Arginine
D. Arginino succinic acid

Ans. C.

1558. The pH of an amino acid depends

A. Optical rotation
B. Dissociation constant
C. Diffusion coefficient
D. Chain length

Ans. D.

1559. When amino acids are treated with neutral formaldehyde, the pH of the mixture

A. Is not altered
B. Increases
C. Decreases
D. First increases then decreases

Ans. C.

1560. Which among the following has an imidazole group?

A. Histidine
B. Tryptophan
C. Proline
D. Hydroxy proline

Ans. A.

1561. The amino acid exist as Zwitter ions when they are in

A. Solid state
B. Acidic solution
C. Alkaline solution
D. Neutral solution

Ans. D.

1562. Plasma proteins are isolated by

A. Salting out
B. Electrophoresis
C. Flourimetry
D. Both (A) and (B)

Ans. D.

1563. After digestion amino acids

A. Are absorbed into portal circulation
B. Are absorbed into lymph
C. Are excreted to the extent of 50%
D. Converted into glucose in the intestine

Ans. A.

1564. An amino acid which contains a disulphide bond is

A. Lysine
B. Methionine
C. Homocysteine
D. Cystine

Ans. D.

1565. One of the following has a phenolic group:

A. Histidine B. Hydroxy lysine

C. Serotonin D. Hydroxy proline

Ans. C.

1566. An amino acid not containing the usual ——— COOH group is

A. Alanine B. Tryptophan

C. Methionine D. Taurine

Ans. D.

1567. Branched chain amino acids are

A. Cysteine and cystine B. Tyrosine and Tryptophan

C. Glycine and Serine D. Valine, Leucine and Isoleucine

Ans. D.

1568. A Zwitter ion is one which has in aqueous solution:

A. One positive charge and one negative charge

B. Two positive charges and one negative charge

C. Two negative charges and one positive charge

D. No electrical charges at all

Ans. A.

1569. The amino acid which gives yellow colour with Ninhydrin in paper chromatography is

A. Tyrosine B. Proline

C. Tryptophan D. Alanine

Ans. B.

1570. Hydroxylation of Proline and Lysine in a protein is effected by

A. Vitamin B1 B. Vitamin B2

C. Vitamin B6 D. Vitamin C

Ans. D.

1571. Millon's test is for identification of

A. Tyrosine B. Tryptophan

C. Proline D. Arginine

Ans. A.

1572. Hopkins-Cole test is for identification of

A. Tyrosine B. Tryptophan

C. Arginine D. Cysteine

Ans. B.

1573. Collagen is very rich in

A. Glycine B. Serine

C. Aspartic acid D. Glutamic acid

Ans. A.

1574. All amino acids are optically active except

A. Glycine B. Serine

C. Threonine D. Tryptophan

Ans. A.

1575. Out of 200 different amino acids form in nature the number of amino acids present in protein:

A. 20 B. 25

C. 40 D. 35

Ans. A.

1576. Enzyme catalyzed hydrolysis of proteins produces amino acids of the form:

A. D B. L

C. DL D. All of these

Ans. B.

1577. The ionizable groups of amino acids are at least.

A. 1 B. 2

C. 3 D. 4

Ans. B.

1578. The neutral amino acid is

A. Lysine B. Proline

C. Leucine D. Histidine

Ans. C.

1579. The amino acid containing hydroxyl group:

A. Alanine B. Isoleucine

C. Arginine D. Threonine

Ans. D.

1580. The sulphur containing amino acid:

A. Homoserine B. Serine

C. Methionine D. Valine

Ans. C.

1581. The basic amino acid:

A. Glycine
B. Leucine
C. Histidine
D. Proline

Ans. C.

1582. The amino acid which synthesizes many hormones:

A. Valine
B. Phenylalanine
C. Alanine
D. Histidine

Ans. B.

1583. Amino acids are insoluble in

A. Acetic acid
B. Chloroform
C. Ethanol
D. Benzene

Ans. D.

1584. The major end product of protein nitrogen metabolism in man is

A. Glycine
B. Uric acid
C. Urea
D. NH3

Ans. C.

1585. An amino acid not involved in urea cycle is

A. Arginine
B. Histidine
C. Ornithine
D. Citrulline

Ans. B.

1586. NH3 is detoxified in brain chiefly as

A. Urea
B. Uric acid
C. Creatinine
D. Glutamine

Ans. D.

1587. In humans, NH3 is detoxified in liver as

A. Creatinine
B. Uric acid
C. Urea
D. Uronic acid

Ans. C.

1588. The body protein after eighteen years

A. Remains unchanged
B. Is decomposed only slightly at intervals of one month
C. Is in a constant state of flux
D. Is used only for energy requirement

Ans. C.

1589. The only known physiological methylating agents in the animal organism are

A. Choline and betaine

B. Choline and δ-adenosyl methionine

C. Betaine and δ-adenyosyl methionine

D. Dimehtyl glycine and betaine

Ans. C.

1590. In the synthesis of 1 molecule of urea in the Kreb's Hanseleit cycle, the number of ATPs required is

A. 1 B. 2

C. 3 D. 4

Ans. C.

1591. For biosynthesis of proteins

A. Amino acids only are required

B. Amino acids and nucleic acids only are required

C. Amino acid, nucleic acids and ATP only are required

D. Amino acids, nucleic acids, ATP, GTP, enzymes and activators are required

Ans. D.

1592. The 2 energy rich compounds needed for protein biosynthesis are

A. ATP and GTP B. ATP and UTP

C. ATP and CTP D. ATP and TTP

Ans. A.

1593. The following ketoacid is involved in fixing dietary NH3 into amino acid:

A. Pyruvate B. Oxalo acetate

C. Oxalo succinate D. α-keto glutarate

Ans. B.

1594. The metabolite which sustains urea cycle is

A. Ornithine B. Citrulline

C. Carbamoyl phosphate D. n-acetyl glutamate

Ans. C.

1595. More creatinine is excreted by

A. Adult males B. Adult females

C. Children D. Pregnant women

Ans. A.

1596. A growing peptide in a ribosome can not be shifted to the adjacent ribosome because

A. It is firmly attached
B. It will get the amino acid cleaved
C. The gap between the ribosomes is too big for a shift
D. The adjacent ribosomes have different composition

Ans. C.

1597. The first amino acid incorporated in a polypeptide in a ribosome of a human is

A. N formyl methionine
B. Methionine
C. Phenyl alanine
D. Hydroxy lysine

Ans. B.

1598. The first amino acid incorporated in a polypeptide in a ribosome of a bacterium is

A. N formyl methionine
B. Methionine
C. Alamine
D. Glycine

Ans. A.

1599. The integrator between the TCA cycle and urea cycle is

A. Fumarate
B. Malate
C. Pyruvate
D. Citrate

Ans. A.

1600. Bence jones proteinuria characterized by

A. Non-heat coagulability
B. Heat coagulability at 100°C
C. Heat coagulability at 45 to 60°C
D. Precipitation at 25°C

Ans. C.

1601. Bence Jones proteins may be excreted in urine of patients suffering from

A. Tuberculosis
B. Diabetes mellitus
C. Multiple myeloma
D. Hyperthyroidism

Ans. C.

1602. Xanthuric acid is an abnormal metabolite of

A. Xanthine
B. Uric acid
C. Tyrosine
D. Tryptophan

Ans. D.

1603. Two nitrogen atoms of Urea in the urea cycle come from

A. NH3
B. One from NH3 and one from aspartate
C. One from NH3 and one from glutamate
D. One from NH3 and one from alanine

Ans. B.

1604. In the synthesis of 1 molecule of urea in the Kreb's Henseleit cycle the number of AMPs formed is

A. 1
B. 2
C. 3
D. 4

Ans. A.

1605. Formation of melanin from tyrosine requires the action of

A. Dopa decarboxylation
B. Diamine oxidase
C. Peroxidase
D. Tyrosinase

Ans. D.

1606. In one of the following the quality of the protein synthesized is affected:

A. Diabetes mellitus
B. Gout
C. Multiple myeloma
D. Primaquine sensitivity

Ans. C.

1607. Citrulline is an intermediate of

A. TCA cycle
B. Urea cycle
C. Pentose cycle
D. Calvin cycle

Ans. B.

1608. The semialdehydes are formed under the action of enzymes characterized as

A. Aldolases
B. Peptidyl lysyl oxidases
C. Collagenases
D. Elastases

Ans. A.

1609. Which of the following statement about the peptide bond is true ?

A. It is a carbon-carbon bond
B. It has cis hydrogen and oxygen groups
C. It is planar
D. It has rotational freedom

Ans. B.

1610. Isoenzymes for a given reaction

A. Have different specificities
B. Have identical affinities for the same substrate
C. Exhibit different electrophoretic motilities
D. Contain similar ratios of different polypeptide chains

Ans. B.

1611. The highest concentration of cystine can be found in

A. Melanin
B. Chondroitin sulphate
C. Myosin
D. Keratin

Ans. D.

1612. Which of the following techniques is used to separate proteins based upon differences in their mass?

A. Isoelectric focusing
B. Dialysis
C. SDS-gel Electrophoresis
D. Western blotting

Ans. C.

1613. The greatest buffering capacity at physiologic pH would be provided by a protein rich in which of the following amino acids ?

A. Lysine
B. Histidine
C. Aspartic acid
D. Valine

Ans. B.

1614. The lone pair of electrons at one of the ring nitrogens in the given amino acid makes a potential ligand, which is important in binding the iron atoms in hemoglobin:

A. Tryptophan
B. Threonine
C. Histidine
D. Serine

Ans. C.

1615. Optically active compounds are capable of

A. Different reactions
B. Rotating plane of polarized light
C. Showing same chemical properties
D. None of these

Ans. B.

1616. The reference compound for absolute configuration of optically active compound is

A. Alanine
B. Lactic acid
C. Glyceraldehyde
D. Dihydroxy acetone

Ans. C.

1617. All the standard amino acids except the following have one chiral 'c' atom:

A. Threonine, Isoleucine
B. Isoleucine, Alanine
C. Threonine, Alanine
D. Alanine, Glutamine

Ans. C.

1618. The role of complement proteins:

A. Defense
B. Helps immunity of the body
C. Not predictable
D. None of these

Ans. B.

1619. Optical isomers that are mirror images and non superimposable are called

A. Diastereomers B. Enantiomers

C. dl isomers D. Stereomers

Ans. B.

1620. Living cells have the unique ability to synthesize only——— the form of optical isomer due to ————.

A. 'D' form, stereospecific enzymes B. 'L' form, stereospecific enzymes

C. 'D' form, DNA D. 'L' form, DNA

Ans. B.

1621. Isoelectric pH of an amino acid is that pH at which it has a

A. Positive charge B. Negative charge

C. No net charge D. All of these

Ans. C.

1622. Albuminoids are similar to

A. Albumin B. Globulin

C. Both A and B D. None of these

Ans. C.

1623. Abnormal chain of amino acids in sickle cells anaemia is

A. Alpha chain B. Beta chain

C. Gama chain D. Delta chain

Ans. B.

1624. In prehepatic jaundice, protein flocculation test is

A. Normal/weakly positive B. Usually positive

C. Negative D. None of these

Ans. A.

1625. Side chains of all amino acids contain aromatic rings except

A. Pheynlalanine B. Alanine

C. Tyrosine D. Tryptophan

Ans. B.

1626. In Nitroprusside test, amino acid cysteine produces

A. Blue colour complex B. Red colour

C. Yellow colour D. Purple colour

Ans. B.

1627. Bonds that are formed between two cysteine residues is

A. Disulphide
B. Peptide
C. Electrostatic
D. Hydrophobic

Ans. A.

1628. The acid amide of Aspartic acid is

A. Glutamine
B. Arginine
C. Aspargine
D. Ornithine

Ans. C.

1629. It is the only amino acid having an ionizing 'R' group with a pK' near 7 and is important in the active site of some enzymes:

A. Arginine
B. Cystein
C. Cystine
D. Histidine

Ans. D.

1630. Hemoglobin has a high content of this amino acid:

A. Proline
B. Leucine
C. Arginine
D. Histidine

Ans. D.

1631. A hexa peptide with 5 aspartic acid would have a net charge at pH 7:

A. Neutral
B. Positive
C. Negative
D. Not predictable

Ans. C.

1632. In the genetic disorder of cystinuria, the patient excretes large quantities of cystine in their urine and its low solubility causes crystalline cystine to precipitate as stones in kidneys. The remedy involves ingesting Na HCO3. Reaction of this treatment is

A. NaHCO2 combines with cystine
B. NaHCO3 raises the pH above the isoelectric point of cystine
C. NaHCO3 prevents stone formation by hydrolysis of cystine to cysteine
D. None of these

Ans. C.

1633. Amino acids excepting histidine are not good buffering agents in cell because

A. They exist as zwitter ions
B. Their pK not in the physiological pH of a cell
C. Only histidine has pK of its R group at 6.0 unlike the others which have at a different pH
D. None of these

Ans. C.

1634. The amino acids in which the R groups have a net positive charge at pH 7.0 are

A. Lysine, Arginine, Histidine
B. Lysine, Aspargine
C. Histidine, Aspargine
D. Glutamine, Arginine

Ans. A.

1635. Apolipoproteins are

A. A
B. B
C. C
D. All of these

Ans. D.

1636. The amino acid which has a pK near 4 and thus is negatively charged at pH 7 is

A. Alanine
B. Glutamic acid
C. Glutamine
D. Aspargine

Ans. B.

1637. The side chain of which of the following amino acid contain sulphur atom?

A. Methionine
B. Threonine
C. Leucine
D. Tryptophan

Ans. A.

1638. Which of the followings gives a positive test for Ninhydrin?

A. Reducing sugars
B. Triglycerides
C. Alpha aminoacids
D. Esterified Fats

Ans. C.

1639. In glutathione (a tripeptide) ——— is present apart from Glutamic acid and cysteine:

A. Serine
B. Glycine
C. Leucine
D. Phenyl alanine

Ans. B.

1640. 2-Amino 3-OH propanoic acid is

A. Glycine
B. Alanine
C. Valine
D. Serine

Ans. D.

1641. All amino acids have one asymmetric carbon atom, except

A. Arginine
B. Aspargine
C. Histidine
D. Glycine

Ans. D.

1642. Number of amino acids present in the plant, animal and microbial proteins:

A. 20 B. 80

C. 150 D. 200

Ans. A.

1643. The bond in proteins that is not hydrolysed under usual conditions of denaturation.

A. Hydrophobic bond B. Hydrogen bond

C. Disulphide bond D. Peptide bonds

Ans. C.

1644. If the amino group and a carboxylic group of the amino acid are attached to same carbon atom, the amino acid is called

A. Alpha B. Beta

C. Gamma D. Delta

Ans. A.

1645. Zymogen is

A. An intracellular enzyme B. Serum enzyme

C. A complete extracellular enzyme D. An inactivated enzyme

Ans. D.

1646. SGOT level in a adult is

A. 5–40 units/dl B. 1–4 units/dl

C. 5–15 units/dl D. 50–100 units/dl

Ans. A.

1647. Activity of ceruloplasmin shown in vitro:

A. Reductase B. Hydrolase

C. Ligase D. Oxidase

Ans. D.

1648. Increased serum alanine during fasting is due to

A. Breakdown of muscle proteins

B. Decreased utilization of non essential amino acids

C. Leakage of amino acids to plasma

D. Impaired renal function

Ans. A.

1649. The following amino acids are required for completion of urea cycle except

A. Aspartic acid B. Arginine

C. Ornithine D. Glycine

Ans. D.

1650. Number of amino acids present in the dietary proteins:

A. 22 B. 23

C. 20 D. 19

Ans. C.

1651. Urea synthesis takes place in

A. Blood B. Liver

C. Kidney D. Heart

Ans. B.

1652. All followings are ketogenic amino acids except

A. Leucine B. Isoleucine

C. Phenyl alanine D. Glycine

Ans. D.

1653. The amino acid containing an indole ring:

A. Tryptophan B. Arginine

C. Threonine D. Phenylalanine

Ans. A.

1654. Histidine is converted to histamine through the process of

A. Transamination B. Decarboxylation

C. Oxidative deamination D. Urea cycle

Ans. B.

1655. Physiologically active configuration of amino acids:

A. L

B. D

C. For some amino acids it is either of two

D. Neither L nor D

Ans. A.

1656. Cystine is synthesized from

A. Cysteine B. Methionine

C. Arginine D. Leucine

Ans. A.

1657. The major constituent of the proteins of hair and keratin of skin:

A. Arginine B. Cysteine

C. Glycine D. Leucine

Ans. B.

1658. NH3 is removed from brain mainly by

A. Creatinine formation
B. Uric acid production
C. Urea formation
D. Glutamine formation

Ans. D.

1659. Mechanism by which NH3 is removed from the kidneys is

A. Urea formation
B. Uric acid formation
C. Creatinine formation
D. None of these

Ans. D.

1660. Low density plasma proteins are rich in

A. Chylomicrons
B. Cholesterol
C. Triglycerides
D. Phospholipids

Ans. B.

1661. Transcortins are

A. Mucoproteins
B. Glycoproteins
C. Metalloproteins
D. Lipoproteins

Ans. A.

1662. Proteins that carries Iron into different tissues is

A. Ceruloplasmin
B. Transcortin
C. Mucoproteins
D. Glycoproteins

Ans. B.

1663. A dietary deficiency of tryptophan and nicotinate leads to

A. Beri Beri
B. Xerophthalmia
C. Anemia
D. Pellegra

Ans. D.

1664. Which one of the following is an essential amino acid?

A. Arginine
B. Tyrosine
C. Phenylalanine
D. Proline

Ans. C.

1665. One of the following amino acid is solely ketogenic:

A. Lysine
B. Alanine
C. Valine
D. Glutamate

Ans. A.

1666. Along with CO_2, NH_3 and ATP, the amino acid that is needed in urea cycle is

A. Alanine
B. Isoleucine
C. Aspartate
D. Glycine

Ans. C.

1667. Which of the following contributes nitrogen atoms to both purine and pyrimidine rings?

A. Aspartate
B. Carbamoyl phosphate
C. CO_2
D. Glutamine

Ans. A.

1668. Which amino acid is present at 6th position of β-chain of Hbs instead of glutamate in HbA?

A. Cysteine
B. Valine
C. Aspartate
D. Glutamate

Ans. B.

1669. From two amino acids peptide bond formation involves removal of one molecule of

A. Water
B. Ammonia
C. Carbon dioxide
D. Carboxylic acid

Ans. A.

1670. Polymers of more than 100 amino acids are termed

A. Proteins
B. Polypeptides
C. Both (A) and (B)
D. None of these

Ans. A.

1671. The example of scleroproteins:

A. Glutamin
B. Giladin
C. Salmine
D. Elastin

Ans. D.

1672. The example of metalloproteins:

A. Siderophilin
B. OREES mucoid
C. Elastin
D. All of these

Ans. A.

1673. The example of chromoprotein:

A. Salmine
B. Catalase
C. Zein
D. Gliadin

Ans. B.

1674. Deamination is ______ of amino group.

A. Removal
B. Addition
C. Supplementation
D. None of these

Ans. A.

1675. Proteins produce polypeptides from proteins by

A. Oxidizing
B. Reducing
C. Hydrolyzing
D. None of these

Ans. C.

1676. Proteins react with Biuret reagent which is suggestive of 2 or more

A. Hydrogen bonds
B. Peptide bonds
C. Disulphide bonds
D. Hydrophobic bonds

Ans. B.

1677. The disulphide bond is not broken under the usual conditions of

A. Filtration
B. Reduction
C. Oxidation
D. Denaturation

Ans. D.

1678. Insulin is oxidized to separate the protein molecule into its constituent polypeptide chains without affecting the other part of the molecule by the use of

A. Performic acid
B. Oxalic acid
C. Citric acid
D. Malic acid

Ans. A.

1679. Each hydrogen bond is quite

A. Weak
B. Strong
C. Both (A) and (B)
D. None of these

Ans. A.

1680. A coiled structure in which peptide bonds are folded in regular manner by

A. Globular proteins
B. Fibrous proteins
C. Both (A) and (B)
D. None of these

Ans. A.

1681. In many proteins the hydrogen bonding produces a regular coiled arrangement called

A. α-helix
B. β-helix
C. Both (A) and (B)
D. None of these

Ans. A.

1682. Many globular proteins are stable in solution although they lack in

A. Hydrogen bonds
B. Salt bonds
C. Non-polar bonds
D. Disulphide bonds

Ans. D.

1683. Each turn of α-helix contains the number of amino acids

A. 2.8
B. 3.2
C. 3.4
D. 3.6

Ans. D.

1684. The distance travelled per turn of α-helix in nm is

A. 0.34
B. 0.44
C. 0.54
D. 0.64

Ans. C.

1685. α-helix is disrupted by certain amino acids like

A. Proline
B. Arginine
C. Histidine
D. Lysine

Ans. A.

1686. α-helix is stabilized by

A. Hydrogen bonds
B. Disulphide bonds
C. Salt bonds
D. Non-polar bonds

Ans. A.

1687. Foetal haemoglobin contains

A. Two α and two γ chains
B. Two β and two γ chains
C. Both (A) and (B)
D. None of these

Ans. A.

1688. When haemoglobin takes up oxygen there is a change in the structure due to the moving closer together of

A. β-chains
B. β-chains
C. γ-chains
D. α and γ chains

Ans. A.

1689. The hydrogen bonds in the secondary and tertiary structure of proteins are directly attacked by

A. Salts
B. Alkalies
C. Detergents
D. All of these

Ans. B.

1690. The digestibility of certain denatured proteins by proteolytic enzymes

A. Decreases
B. Increases
C. Normal
D. None of these

Ans. A.

1691. The antigenic antibody functions of proteins by denaturation are frequently

A. Not changed
B. Changed
C. Both (A) and (B)
D. None of these

Ans. B.

1692. In case of severe denaturation of protein, there is

A. Reversible denaturation
B. Moderate reversible denaturation
C. Irreversible denaturation
D. None of these

Ans. C.

1693. When egg albumin is heated till it is coagulated, the secondary and tertiary structures of the proteins are completely lost resulting in a mixture of randomly arranged

A. Dipeptide chains
B. Tripeptide chains
C. Polypeptide chains
D. All of these

Ans. C.

1694. In glycoproteins the carbohydrate is in the form of disaccharide units, the number of units are

A. 50–100
B. 200–300
C. 400–500
D. 600–700

Ans. D.

1695. The milk protein in the stomach of the infants is digested by

A. Pepsin
B. Trypsin
C. Chymotrypsin
D. Rennin

Ans. D.

1696. *Achylia gastrica* is said to be when absence of

A. Pepsin only
B. Both pepsin and HCl
C. HCl only
D. All of these

Ans. B.

1697. The pH of gastric juice become low in

A. Hemolytic anemia
B. Pernicious anemia
C. Both (A) and (B)
D. None of these

Ans. B.

1698. In small intestine trypsin hydrolyzes peptide linkages containing

A. Arginine
B. Histidine
C. Serine
D. Aspartate

Ans. A.

1699. Chymotrypsin in the small intestine hydrolyzes peptide linkages containing

A. Alanine
B. Pheynlalanine
C. Valine
D. Methionine

Ans. B.

1700. Carboxy peptidase B in the small intestine hydrolyzes peptides containing

A. Leucine
B. Isoleucine
C. Arginine
D. Cysteine

Ans. C.

1701. The transport of amino acids regulated by active processes of different numbers:

A. 1
B. 2
C. 3
D. 4

Ans. C.

1702. . The third active process for amino acids transport involves

A. Acidic amino acids
B. Basic amino acids
C. Neutral amino acids
D. Sulphur containing amino acids

Ans. C.

1703. If one amino acid is fed excess, the absorption of another is

A. Slightly accelerated
B. Moderately accelerated
C. Highly accelerated
D. Retarded

Ans. D.

1704. Under normal conditions, food proteins are generally readily digested upto the present

A. 67 to 73
B. 74 to 81
C. 82 to 89
D. 90 to 97

Ans. D.

1705. By overheating the nutritional value of cereal proteins is

A. Increased
B. Decreased
C. Unchanged
D. None of these

Ans. B.

1706. More than half of the protein of the liver and intestinal mucosa are broken down and resynthesized in

A. 10 days B. 12 days

C. 15 days D. 18 days

Ans. A.

1707. Protein anabolism is stimulated by

A. ACTH B. Testosterone

C. Glucagon D. Epinephrine

Ans. B.

1708. The metabolism of protein is integrated with that of carbohydrate and fat through

A. Oxaloacetate B. Citrate

C. Isocitrate D. Malate

Ans. A.

1709. The building up and breaking down of protoplasm are concerned with the metabolism of

A. Carbohydrate B. Lipid

C. Protein D. Minerals

Ans. C.

1710. The amino acids abstracted from the liver are not utilized for repair or special synthesis but are broken down to

A. Keto acids B. Sulphur dioxide

C. Water D. Ammonia

Ans. D.

1711. The unwanted amino acids abstracted from the tissues are either used up by the tissue or in the liver converted into

A. Ammonia B. Urea

C. Ammonium salts D. Uric acid

Ans. B.

1712. Amino acids provide the nitrogen for the synthesis of

A. The bases of the phospholipids B. Uric acid

C. Glycolipids D. Chondroitin sulphates

Ans. A.

1713. The metabolism of all proteins ingested over and above the essential requirements is called

A. Exogenous metabolism B. Endogenous metabolism

C. Both (A) and (B) D. None of these

Ans. A.

1714. Sulphur containing amino acids after catabolism produces a substance which is excreted as

A. SO2 B. HNO3

C. H2SO4 D. H3PO4

Ans. C.

1715. The amino acids required for creatine formation:

A. Glycine B. Arginine

C. Methionine D. All of these

Ans. D.

1716. In human and other ureotelic organisms, the end product of amino acid nitrogen metabolism:

A. Bile acids B. Ketone bodies

C. Urea D. Barium sulphate

Ans. C.

1717. Transamination is a

A. Irreversible process B. Reversible process

C. Both (A) and (B) D. None of these

Ans. B.

1718. Most amino acids are substrates for transamination except

A. Alanine B. Threonine

C. Serine D. Valine

Ans. B.

1719. Oxidative conversion of many amino acids to their corresponding –ketoacids occurs in mammalian ——.

A. Liver and kidney B. Adipose tissue

C. Pancreas D. Intestine

Ans. A.

1720. From dietary protein as well as from the urea present in fluids secreted into the gastrointestinal tract intestinal bacteria produce

A. Carbon dioxide B. Ammonia

C. Ammonium sulphate D. Creatine

Ans. B.

1721. The symptom of ammonia intoxication includes

A. Blurring of vision B. Constipation

C. Mental confusion D. Diarrhoea

Ans. A.

1722. Ammonia intoxication symptoms occur when brain ammonia levels are

A. Slightly diminished
B. Highly diminished
C. Increased
D. All of these

Ans. C.

1723. Ammonia production by the kidney is depressed in

A. Acidosis
B. Alkalosis
C. Both (A) and (B)
D. None of these

Ans. B.

1724. Ammonia is excreted as ammonium salts during metabolic acidosis but the majority is excreted as

A. Phosphates
B. Creatine
C. Uric acid
D. Urea

Ans. D.

1725. In brain, the major metabolism for removal of ammonia is the formation of

A. Glutamate
B. Aspartate
C. Asparagine
D. Glutamine

Ans. D.

1726. The biosynthesis of Urea occurs mainly in the liver:

A. Cytosol
B. Microsomes
C. Nucleus
D. Mitochondria

Ans. D.

1727. One mol. of Urea is synthesized at the expense of the _______ molecules of ATP.

A. 2
B. 3
C. 4
D. 5

Ans. B.

1728. Urea biosynthesis occurs mainly in the liver involving the number of amino acids:

A. 3
B. 4
C. 5
D. 6

Ans. D.

1729. The normal daily output of urea through urine in grams:

A. 10 to 20
B. 15 to 25
C. 20 to 30
D. 25 to 35

Ans. C.

1730. In severe acidosis, the output of urea is

A. Decreased
B. Slightly increased
C. Highly increased
D. Moderately increased

Ans. A.

1731. Uremia occurs in

A. Cirrhosis of the liver
B. Nephritis
C. Diabetes mellitus
D. Coronary thrombosis

Ans. B.

1732. Clinical symptom in urea cycle disorder is

A. Mental retardation
B. Drowsiness
C. Diarrhoea
D. Oedema

Ans. A.

1733. Glutathione is a

A. Dipeptide
B. Tripeptide
C. Polypeptide
D. None of these

Ans. B.

1734. All following are conjugated proteins except

A. Nucleoproteins
B. Proteases
C. Metalloproteins
D. Flavoproteins

Ans. B.

1735. Hydrated density of (HD) lipoproteins is

A. 0.94 gm/ml
B. 0.94-1.006 gm/ml
C. 1.006-1.063 gm/ml
D. 1.063-1.21 gm/l

Ans. B.

1736. The bond in proteins that is not broken under usual conditions of denaturation:

A. Hydrophobic bond
B. Hydrogen bond
C. Disulphide bond
D. Peptide bonds

Ans. D.

1737. Plasma proteins act as

A. Buffers
B. Immunoglobulins
C. Reserve proteins
D. All of these

Ans. D.

1738. Group that reacts in the Biuret test:

A. Peptide
B. Amino group
C. Carboxylic group
D. Aldehyde group

Ans. A.

1739. Protein present in hemoglobin has the structure known as

A. Primary
B. Secondary
C. Tertiary
D. Quarternary

Ans. D.

1740. Proteins that constitute keratin, collagen and elastin in body are

A. Protamines
B. Phosphol proteins
C. Scleroproteins
D. Metaproteins

Ans. C.

1741. Systematic name of lysine is

A. Amino acetic acid
B. 2,6 diaminohexanoic acid
C. Aminosuccinic acid
D. 2-Aminopropanoic acid

Ans. B.

1742. Side chains of all following amino acids contain aromatic rings except

A. Phenyl alanine
B. Alanine
C. Tyrosine
D. Tryptophan

Ans. B.

1743. Number of chains in globin part of normal Hb:

A. 1
B. 2
C. 3
D. 4

Ans. D.

1744. The pH of albumin is

A. 3.6
B. 4.7
C. 5.0
D. 6.1

Ans. B.

1745. Ninhydrin reaction gives a purple colour and evolves CO2 with

A. Peptide bonds
B. Histamine
C. Ergothioneine
D. Aspargine

Ans. D.

1746. Denaturation of proteins involves breakdown of

A. Secondary structure
B. Tertiary structure
C. Quarternary structure
D. All of these

Ans. D.

1747. The purity of an isolated protein can be tested by employing various methods.

A. Solubility curve
B. Molecular weight
C. Ultra Centrifugation
D. Immuno Reactivity
E. All of these

Ans. C.

1748. More than one break in the line or in saturation curve indicates the following quality of protein.

A. Non homogenity
B. Purity
C. Homogeneity
D. None of these

Ans. A.

1749. The antibodies raised against a pure protein will show only one sharp spike on this technique:

A. Solubility curve
B. Solvent precipitation
C. Molecular weight determination
D. Immuno electrophoresis

Ans. D.

1750. This technique takes the advantage of the fact that each protein has different pH at which it is electrically neutral i.e., its isoelectric pH:

A. Isoelectric focusing
B. Immunoelectrophoresis
C. Chromatography
D. HPLC

Ans. A.

1751. The following technique makes use of the difference in net charges of proteins at a given pH:

A. Thin layer chromatography
B. Ion exchange chromatography
C. High performance liquid chromatography
D. Paper chromatography

Ans. B.

1752. The ratio of the distance moved by a compound to the distance moved by the solvent front is known as its

A. PI value
B. Linking number
C. Rf value
D. Gold number

Ans. C.

1753. The movement of charged particles towards one of the electrodes under the influence of electrical current is

A. Gel filtration
B. Molecular sieving
C. Gas liquid chromatography
D. Electrophoresis

Ans. D.

1754. An anion exchange resin linked to cellulose backbone is

A. DEAE cellulose
B. CM cellulose
C. Sephadex
D. None of these

Ans. A.

1755. A cation exchange resin linked to cellulose backbone is

A. CM-cellulose
B. DEAE cellulose
C. Starch
D. Biogel

Ans. A.

1756. The sorting out of protein molecules according to size and shape may be carried out by

A. Adsorption chromatography
B. Gel filtration chromatography
C. Paper chromatography
D. None of these

Ans. B.

1757. The solubility of most proteins is lowered at high salt concentrations is called as

A. Salting in process
B. Salting out process
C. Isoelectric focusing
D. None of these

Ans. B.

1758. All the following diuretics inhibit the carbonic anhydrase except

A. Acetazolamide
B. Bumetanide
C. Furosemide
D. Ethacrynic acid

Ans. D.

1759. Proteinous substances which catalyze biochemical reactions are known as

A. Activators
B. Catalysts
C. Enzymes
D. Hormones

Ans. C.

1760. Insulin is a protein which controls

A. Blood clotting
B. Metabolic pathway
C. Digestion
D. Kreb's cycle

Ans. B.

1761. β 1-4 glycosidic bond is present in

A. Maltose
B. Lactose
C. Sucrose
D. None of the above

Ans. B.

1762. Proteins which are responsible for defense mechanism are called

A. Antimetabolites
B. Antibodies
C. Antimycins
D. Apoproteins

Ans. B.

1763. When the net charge on an amino acid is zero, the pH is maintained as?

A. 4.5
B. 11.2
C. 7.0
D. 9.1

Ans. C.

1764. Isoelectric point of amino acids is used for

A. Crystallisation
B. Precipitation
C. Solubility
D. Reactivity

Ans. B.

1765. Xanthoproteic test is positive in proteins containing

A. Sulphur amino acids
B. α-Amino acids
C. Aromatic amino acids
D. Aliphatic amino acids

Ans. C.

1766. All α-amino acids give positive

A. Million's test
B. Biuret test
C. Xanthproteic test
D. Ninhydrine test

Ans. D.

1767. N-terminal amino acids of a polypeptide are estimated by

A. Edmann reaction
B. Sanger's reagent
C. Formaldehyde test
D. Ninhydrine reaction

Ans. A.

1768. Million's test is positive for

A. Phenylalanine
B. Glycine
C. Tyrosine
D. Proline

Ans. C.

1769. Indole group of tryptophan responses positively to

A. Glyoxylic acid B. Schiff's reagent

C. Biuret test D. Resorcinol test

Ans. A.

1770. Guanidine group of arginine gives positive test with

A. Lead acetate B. Sakaguchi reagent

C. Tricholoroacetic acid D. Molisch's reagent

Ans. B.

1771. Thiol group of cysteine gives red colour with

A. Sodium acetate B. Lead acetate

C. Sodium nitroprusside D. Barfoed's reagent

Ans. C.

1772. Protein deficiency disease is known as

A. Cushing's disease B. Fabry's disease

C. Parkinson's disease D. Kwashiorkor and marasmus

Ans. D.

1773. A vegetable source of protein is

A. Egg plant B. Soyabean

C. Tree of the Heaven D. Devil's dung

Ans. B.

1774. Oxaloacetate is converted to aspartic acid by

A. Reductase B. Oxidase

C. Transaminase D. Catalase

Ans. C.

1775. Deficiency of biotin results in decrease in

A. Amino acid synthesis B. Lipid synthesis

C. Kidney function D. Fatty acid synthesis

Ans. D.

1776. The precursor of bile salts, sex hormones and vitamin D is

A. Diosgenin B. Cholesterol

C. Campesterol D. Ergosterol

Ans. B.

1777. Unsaturated fatty acids is known as

A. Non-essential fatty acids
B. Essential fatty acids
C. Cerebrosides
D. Phospholipids

Ans. B.

1778. Biuret test is specific for

A. Two peptide linkage
B. Phenolic group
C. Imidazole ring
D. None of these

Ans. A.

1779. Most of calcium is present in bone, but 2% present in soft tissue and the blood is called

A. Calcinated blood
B. Solidified blood
C. Physiological blood
D. Colloidal blood

Ans. C.

1780. Calcium present with protein is known as free while in salt form is called as

A. Bound
B. Precipitated
C. Solid
D. Polymorphs

Ans. A.

1781. The following ions help in enzymatic transfer of phosphate from ATP to pyruvic acid:

A. Sodium
B. Calcium
C. Magnesium
D. Potassium

Ans. D.

1782. International enzyme commission classifies enzymes into

A. Three classes
B. Six classes
C. Four classess
D. Ten classes

Ans. B.

1783. Michaelis – Menten equation is used to explain the effect of substrate concentration on

A. Carbohydrate
B. Enzyme
C. Lipid
D. Protein

Ans. B.

1784. The pH at which an enzyme has maximum activity is known as

A. Isoelectric pH
B. Optimum pH
C. Low pH
D. High pH

Ans. B.

1785. Degradation of proteins to amino acids, glucose from carbohydrates and fatty acids from lipids is known as

A. Anabolism
B. Metabolism
C. Catabolism
D. Cretinism

Ans. C.

1786. During glycolysis of glucose the energy liberated in the absence of oxygen is known as

A. Oxygenesis
B. Glyconeogenesis
C. Glycogenolysis
D. Anaerobic fermentation

Ans. D.

1787. Accumulation of trytophan in blood is known as

A. Pompe's disease
B. Wilson's disease
C. Wolman's disease
D. Hartnup's disease

Ans. D.

1788. Treatment of pentoses with a concentrated mineral acid yields a cyclic aldehyde known as

A. Pentaldehyde
B. Cyclopental
C. Hexaldehyde
D. Furfural

Ans. D.

1789. About 6.25 g of haemoglobin is produced and destroyed in the body each day and the total amount of haemoglobin in a normal healthy 70 kg weighing male adult is

A. 250 g
B. 150 g
C. 100 g
D. 70 g

Ans. D.

1790. Pancreatic juice contains all of the following except

A. Trypsinogen
B. Lipase
C. Cholecystokinin
D. Chymotrypsinogen

Ans. C.

1791. The milk protein in the stomach in an adult is digested by

A. Pepsin
B. Rennin
C. HCl
D. Chymotrypsinogen

Ans. A.

1792. Carboxypeptidase, an enzyme of pancreatic juice, contains

A. Cu
B. Zinc
C. Magnesium
D. Manganese

Ans. B.

1793. The zymogen from trypsinogen of pancreatic juice is converted to active trypsin by

A. Pepsin
B. Enterocrinin
C. Enterokinase
D. Rennin

Ans. C.

1794. Inactive zymogens are precursors of all the following gastrointestinal enzymes except

A. Carboxypeptidase
B. Pepsin
C. Amino peptidase
D. Chymotrypsin

Ans. C.

1795. Rennin acts on casein of milk in infants in presence of

A. Mg++
B. Zn++
C. Co++
D. Ca++

Ans. D.

1796. All the following are true about phenylketonuria except

A. Deficiency of phenylalanine hydroxylase
B. Mental retardation
C. Increased urinary excretion of p-hydroxyphenyl pyruvic acid
D. Decrease serotonin formation

Ans. C.

1797. Which of the amino acid produces a vasodilator on decarboxylation?

A. Glutamic acid
B. Histidine
C. Ornithine
D. Cysteine

Ans. B.

1798. Neutral amino acid is

A. Leucine
B. Lysine
C. Aspartic acid
D. Histidine

Ans. A.

1799. The amino acid containing hydroxyl group:

A. Glycine
B. Isoleucine
C. Arginine
D. Thereonine

Ans. D.

1800. The amino acid which synthesizes many hormornes:

A. Valine
B. Phenylalanine
C. Alanine
D. Histidine

Ans. B.

1801. In many proteins the hydrogen bonding produces a regular coiled arrangement which is called as

A. β-Helix
B. α-Helix
C. Both (A) and (B)
D. Spiral

Ans. B.

1802. Protein anabolism is stimulated by

A. ACTH
B. Testosterone
C. Glucagon
D. Epinephrine

Ans. B.

1803. The number of helices present in a collagen molecule is

A. 1
B. 2
C. 3
D. 4

Ans. C.

1804. Which bond is present in the primary structure of protein?

A. Ester
B. Hydrogen
C. Ionic bond
D. Peptide

Ans. D.

1805. With the exception of glycine all amino acids found in protein are

A. Isocitrate dehydrogenase
B. Fumarase
C. Succinate thiokinase
D. ATPase

Ans. B.

1806. In protein structure the α-helix and β-pleated sheets are example of

A. Primary structure
B. Secondary structure
C. Tertiary structure
D. Quaternary structure

Ans. B.

1807. An essential amino acid in man is

A. Proline
B. Threonine
C. Asparagine
D. Tyrosine

Ans. B.

1808. An amino acid that does not form an α-helix is

A. Asparagine
B. Tyrosine
C. Tryptophan
D. Proline

Ans. D.

1809. The protein present in hair is

A. Elastin
B. Prolamine
C. Keratin
D. Gliadin

Ans. C.

1810. Which co-enzyme is not involved in oxidative decarboxylation of pyruvic acid?

A. TPP
B. Mg++
C. Biotin
D. CoA-SH

Ans. C.

1811. A polymeric unit of starch which has a branched structure is

A. Glucose
B. Amylopectin
C. Isomaltose
D. Amylose

Ans. B.

1812. The repeating unit in hyaluronic acid is

A. Glucuronic acid and Galactosamine
B. Glucuronic acid are glucosamine
C. Glucuronic acid and N-acetyl glucosamine
D. Glucuronic acid and N-acetyl galactosamine

Ans. C.

1813. The repeating disaccharide unit in cellulose is

A. Sucrose
B. Maltose
C. Dextrose
D. Cellobiose

Ans. D.

1814. An example of a hydroxy fatty acid is

A. Ricinoleic acid
B. Crotonic acid
C. Butyric acid
D. Oleic acid

Ans. A.

1815. An example of a saturated fatty acid is

A. Palmitic acid
B. Oleic acid
C. Linoleic acid
D. Erucic acid

Ans. A.

1816. If the fatty acid is esterified with an alcohol of high molecular weight instead of glycerol, the resulting compound is

A. Lipositol B. Plasmalogen

C. Wax D. Cephalin

Ans. C.

1817. A fatty acid which is not synthesized in the body and has to be supplied in the diet is

A. Palmitic acid B. Lauric acid

C. Linolenic acid D. Palmitoleic acid

Ans. C.

1818. Essential fatty acid:

A. Linoleic acid B. Linolenic acid

C. Arachidonic acid D. All these

Ans. D.

1819. The fatty acid present in cerebrosides is

A. Lignoceric acid B. Valeric acid

C. Caprylic acid D. Behenic acid

Ans. A.

1820. The number of double bonds in arachidonic acid is

A. 1 B. 2

C. 4 D. 6

Ans. C.

1821. A lipid containing alcoholic amine residue is

A. Phosphatidic acid B. Ganglioside

C. Glucocerebroside D. Sphingomyelin

Ans. D.

1822. Cephalin consists of

A. Glycerol, fatty acids, phosphoric acid and choline

B. Glycerol, fatty acids, phosphoric acid and ethanolamine

C. Glycerol, fatty acids, phosphoric acid and inositol

D. Glycerol, fatty acids, phosphoric acid and serine

Ans. B.

1823. In mammals, the major fat in adipose tissues is

A. Phospholipid
B. Cholesterol
C. Sphingolipids
D. Triacylglycerol

Ans. D.

1824. Glycosphingolipids are a combination of

A. Ceramide with one or more sugar residues
B. Glycerol with galactose
C. Sphingosine with galactose
D. Sphingosine with phosphoric acid

Ans. A.

1825. The importance of phospholipids as constituent of cell membrane is because they possess

A. Fatty acids
B. Both polar and nonpolar groups
C. Glycerol
D. Phosphoric acid

Ans. B.

1826. In neutral fats, the unsaponificable matter includes

A. Hydrocarbons
B. Triacylglycerol
C. Phospholipids
D. Cholsesterol

Ans. A.

1827. Higher alcohol present in waxes is

A. Benzyl
B. Methyl
C. Ethyl
D. Cetyl

Ans. D.

1828. Gangliosides are complex glycosphingolipids found in

A. Liver
B. Brain
C. Kidney
D. Muscle

Ans. B.

1829. Unsaturated fatty acid found in the cod liver oil and containing 5 double bonds is

A. Clupanodonic acid
B. Cervonic acid
C. Elaidic acid
D. Timnodonic acid

Ans. D.

1830. Phospholipid acting as surfactant is

A. Cephalin
B. Phosphatidyl inositol
C. Lecithin
D. Phosphatidyl serine

Ans. C.

1831. An oil which contains cyclic fatty acids and once used in the treatment of leprosy is

A. Elaidic oil
B. Rapeseed oil
C. Lanoline
D. Chaulmoogric oil

Ans. D.

1832. Unpleasant odours and taste in a fat (rancidity) can be delayed or prevented by the addition of

A. Lead
B. Copper
C. Tocopherol
D. Ergosterol

Ans. C.

1833. Gangliosides derived from glucosylceramide contain in addition one or more molecules of

A. Sialic acid
B. Glycerol
C. Diacylglycerol
D. Hyaluronic acid

Ans. A.

1834. 'Drying oil', oxidized spontaneously by atmospheric oxygen at ordinary temperature and forms a hard water proof material is

A. Coconut oil
B. Peanut oil
C. Rape seed oil
D. Linseed oil

Ans. D.

1835. Deterioration of food (rancidity) is due to presence of

A. Cholesterol
B. Vitamin E
C. Peroxidation of lipids
D. Phenolic compounds

Ans. C.

1836. The number of ml of N/10 KOH required to neutralize the fatty acids in the distillate from 5 gm of fat is called

A. Reichert-Meissel number
B. Polenske number
C. Acetyl number
D. Non volatile fatty acid number

Ans. A.

1837. Molecular formula of cholesterol is

A. $C_{27}H_{45}OH$
B. $C_{29}H_{47}OH$
C. $C_{29}H_{45}OH$
D. $C_{23}H_{41}OH$

Ans. A.

1838. The cholesterol molecule is

A. Benzene derivative
B. Quinoline derivative
C. Steroid
D. Straight chain acid

Ans. C.

1839. Salkowski test is performed to detect

A. Glycerol
B. Cholesterol
C. Fatty acids
D. Vitamin D

Ans. B.

1840. Palmitic, oleic or stearic acid ester of cholesterol used in manufacture of cosmetic creams is

A. Elaidic oil
B. Lanoline
C. Spermaceti
D. Chaulmoogric oil

Ans. B.

1841. Dietary fats after absorption appear in the circulation as

A. HDL
B. VLDL
C. LDL
D. Chylomicron

Ans. D.

1842. Free fatty acids are transported in the blood

A. Combined with albumin
B. Combined with fatty acid binding protein
C. Combined with β -lipoprotein
D. In unbound free salts

Ans. A.

1843. Long chain fatty acids are first activated to acetyl-CoA in

A. Cytosol
B. Microsomes
C. Nucleus
D. Mitochondria

Ans. A.

1844. The enzymes of β-oxidation are found in

A. Mitochondria
B. Cytosol
C. Golgi apparatus
D. Nucleus

Ans. A.

1845. Long chain fatty acids penetrate the inner mitochondrial membrane

A. Freely
B. As acyl-CoA derivative
C. As carnitine derivative
D. Requiring Na dependent carrier

Ans. C.

1846. An important finding of Fabry's disease is

A. Skin rash
B. Exophthalmos
C. Hemolytic anemia
D. Mental retardation

Ans. A.

1847. An important finding in Neimann-Pick disease is

A. Leukopenia
B. Cardiac enlargement
C. Corneal opacity
D. Hepatosplenomegaly

Ans. D.

1848. Neonatal tyrosinemia improves on administration of

A. Thiamin
B. Riboflavin
C. Pyridoxine
D. Ascorbic acid

Ans. A.

1849. Absence of phenylalanine hydroxylase causes

A. Neonatal tyrosinemia
B. Phenylketonuria
C. Primary hyperoxaluria
D. Albinism

Ans. D.

1850. Richner-Hanhart syndrome is due to defect in

A. Tyrosinase
B. Phenylalanine hydroxylase
C. Hepatic tyrosine transaminase
D. Fumarylacetoacetate hydrolase

Ans. B.

1851. Plasma tyrosine level in Richner-Hanhart syndrome is

A. 1–2 mg/dL
B. 2–3 mg/dL
C. 4–5 mg/dL
D. 8–10 mg/dL

Ans. C.

1852. Amount of phenylacetic acid excreted in the urine in phenylketonuria is

A. 100–200 mg/dL
B. 200–280 mg/dL
C. 290–550 mg/dL
D. 600–750 mg/dL

Ans. C.

1853. An important finding in Histidinemia is

A. Impairment of conversion of α-Glutamate to α-ketoglutarate
B. Speech defect
C. Decreased urinary histidine level
D. Patients can not be treated by diet

Ans. B.

1854. An important finding in glycinuria is

A. Excess excretion of oxalate in the urine

B. Deficiency of enzyme glycinase

C. Significantly increased serum glycine level

D. Defect in renal tubular reabsorption of glycine

Ans. D.

1855. Increased urinary indole acetic acid is diagnostic of

A. Maple syrup urine disease
B. Hartnup disease
C. Homocystinuia
D. Phenylketonuria

Ans. B.

1856. In glycinuria daily urinary excretion of glycine ranges from

A. 100–200 mg
B. 300–500 mg
C. 600–1000 mg
D. 1100–1400 mg

Ans. C.

1857. An inborn error, maple syrup urine disease is due to deficiency of the enzyme:

A. Isovaleryl-CoAhydrogenase
B. Phenylalnine hydroxylase
C. Adenosyl transferase
D. α-Ketoacid decarboxylase

Ans. D.

1858. An important feature of maple syrup urine disease is

A. Patient can not be treated by dietary regulation

B. Without treatment death, of patient may occur by the end of second year of life

C. Blood levels of leucine, isoleucine and serine are increased

D. Excessive brain damage

Ans. D.

1859. Ochronosis is an important finding of

A. Tyrosinemia
B. Tyrosinosis
C. Alkaptonuria
D. Richner Hanhart syndrome

Ans. C.

1860. Phrynoderma is a deficiency of

A. Essential fatty acids
B. Proteins
C. Amino acids
D. None of these

Ans. A.

1861. The percentage of linoleic acid in safflower oil is

A. 73 B. 57

C. 40 D. 15

Ans. A.

1862. The percentage of polyunsaturated fatty acids in soyabean oil is

A. 62 B. 10

C. 3 D. 2

Ans. A.

1863. The percentage of polyunsaturated fatty acids in butter is

A. 60 B. 37

C. 25 D. 3

Ans. D.

1864. Dietary fibre denotes

A. Undigested proteins

B. Plant cell components that cannot be digested by own enzymes

C. All plant cell wall components

D. All non digestible water insoluble polysaccharide

Ans. B.

1865. A high fibre diet is associated with reduced incidence of

A. Cardiovascular disease B. C.N.S. disease

C. Liver disease D. Skin disease

Ans. A.

1866. Dietary fibres are rich in

A. Cellulose B. Glycogen

C. Starch D. Proteoglycans

Ans. A.

1867. Minimum dietary fibre is found in

A. Dried apricot B. Peas

C. Bran D. Cornflakes

Ans. B.

1868. A bland diet is recommended in

A. Peptic ulcer B. Atherosclerosis

C. Diabetes D. Liver disease

Ans. A.

1869. A dietary deficiency in both the quantity and the quality of protein results in

A. Kwashiorkar
B. Marasmus
C. Xerophtalmia
D. Liver diseases

Ans. A.

1870. The deficiency of both energy and protein causes

A. Marasmus
B. Kwashiorkar
C. Diabetes
D. Beri-beri

Ans. A.

1871. Kwashiorkar is characterized by

A. Night blindness
B. Edema
C. Easy fracturability
D. Xerophthalmia

Ans. B.

1872. A characteristic feature of Kwashiorkar is

A. Fatty liver
B. Emaciation
C. Low insulin level
D. Occurrence in less than 1 year infant

Ans. A.

1873. The normal range of total serum bilirubin is

A. 0.2–1.2 mg/100 ml
B. 1.5–1.8 mg/100 ml
C. 2.0–4.0 mg/100 ml
D. Above 7.0 mg/100 ml

Ans. A.

1874. The normal range of direct reacting (conjugated) serum bilirubin is

A. 0–0.1 mg/100 ml
B. 0.1–0.4 mg/100 ml
C. 0.4–06 mg/100 ml
D. 0.5–1 mg/100 ml

Ans. B.

1875. The normal range of indirect (unconjugated) bilirubin in serum is

A. 0–0.1 mg/100 ml
B. 0.1–0.2 mg/100 ml
C. 0.2–0.7 mg/100 ml
D. 0.8–1.0 mg/100 ml

Ans. C.

1876. Jaundice is visible when serum bilirubin exceeds

A. 0.5 mg/100 ml
B. 0.8 mg/100 ml
C. 1 mg/100 ml
D. 2.4 mg/100 ml

Ans. C.

1877. An increase in serum unconjugated bilirubin occurs in

A. Hemolytic jaundice
B. Obstructive jaundice
C. Nephritis
D. Glomerulonephritis

Ans. A.

1878. Increased urobilinogen in urine and absence of bilirubin in the urine suggests

A. Obstructive jaundice
B. Hemolytic jaundice
C. Viral hepatitis
D. Toxic jaundice

Ans. A.

1879. A jaundice in which serum alanine transaminase and alkaline phosphatase are normal is

A. Hepatic jaundice
B. Hemolytic jaundice
C. Parenchymatous jaundice
D. Obstructive Jaundice

Ans. B.

1880. Fecal stercobilinogen is increased in

A. Hemolytic jaundice
B. Hepatic jaundice
C. Viral hepatitis
D. Obstructive jaundice

Ans. B.

1881. Fecal urobilinogen is increased in

A. Hemolytic jaundice
B. Obstruction of biliary duct
C. Extrahepatic gall stones
D. Enlarged lymph nodes

Ans. A.

1882. A mixture of conjugated and unconjugated bilirubin is found in the circulation in

A. Hemolytic jaundice
B. Hepatic jaundice
C. Obstructive jaundice
D. Post hepatic jaundice

Ans. B.

1883. Hepatocellular jaundice as compared to pure obstructive type of jaundice is characterized by

A. Increased serum alkaline phosphate, LDH and ALT
B. Decreased serum alkaline phosphatase, LDH and ALT
C. Increased serum alkaline phosphatase and decreased levels of LDH and ALT
D. Decreased serum alkaline phosphatase and increased serum LDH and ALT

Ans. D.

1884. Icteric index of an normal adult varies between

A. 1–2
B. 2–4
C. 4–6
D. 10–15

Ans. C.

1885. Clinical jaundice is present with an icteric index above

A. 4
B. 8
C. 10
D. 15

Ans. D.

1886. Normal quantity of urobilinogen excreted in the feces per day is about

A. 10–25 mg
B. 50–250 mg
C. 300–500 mg
D. 700–800 mg

Ans. B.

1887. Fecal urobilinogen is decreased in

A. Obstruction of biliary duct
B. Hemolytic jaundice
C. Excess fat intake
D. Low fat intake

Ans. A.

1888. A complete absence of fecal urobilinogen is strongly suggestive of

A. Obstruction of bile duct
B. Hemolytic jaundice
C. Intrahepatic cholestasis
D. Malignant obstructive disease

Ans. D.

1889. Immediate direct Vanden Bergh reaction indicates

A. Hemolytic jaundice
B. Hepatic jaundice
C. Obstructive jaundice
D. Megalobastic anemia

Ans. B.

1890. The presence of bilirubin in the urine without urobilinogen suggests

A. Obstructive jaundice
B. Hemolytic jaundice
C. Pernicious anemia
D. Damage to the hepatic parenchyma

Ans. A.

1891. Impaired galactose tolerance test suggests

A. Defect in glucose utilisation
B. Liver cell injury
C. Renal defect
D. Muscle injury

Ans. B.

1892. Increased serum ornithine carabamoyl transferase activity is diagnostic of

A. Myocardial infarction
B. Hemolytic jaundice
C. Bone disease
D. Acute viral hepatitis

Ans. D.

1893. The best known and most frequently used test of the detoxicating functions of liver is

A. Hippuric acid test
B. Galactose tolerance test
C. Epinephrine tolerance test
D. Rose Bengal dye test

Ans. A.

1894. The ability of liver to remove a dye like BSP from the blood suggests a normal

A. Excretory function
B. Detoxification function
C. Metabolic function
D. Circulatory function

Ans. A.

1895. Removal of BSP dye by the liver involves conjugation with

A. Thiosulphate
B. Glutamine
C. Cystein component of glutathione
D. UDP glucuronate

Ans. C.

1896. Normal value of plasma total proteins varies between

A. 3–4 gm/100ml
B. 6–8 gm/100ml
C. 10–12 gm/100ml
D. 14–16 gm/100ml

Ans. B.

1897. A decrease in albumin with increased production of other unidentified proteins which migrate in β, γ region suggests

A. Cirrhosis of liver
B. Nephrotic syndrome
C. Infection
D. Chronic lymphatic leukemia

Ans. A.

1898. In increase in α2-Globulin with loss of albumin in urine suggests

A. Primary immune deficiency
B. Nephrotic syndrome
C. Cirrhosis of liver
D. Multiple myeloma

Ans. B.

1899. The normal levels of prothrombin time is about

A. 2 sec
B. 4 sec
C. 14 sec
D. 10–16 sec

Ans. C.

1900. In obstructive jaundice prothrombin time

A. Remains normal
B. Decreases
C. Responds to Vit K and becomes normal
D. Responds to Vit K and increases

Ans. C.

1901. In parenhymatous liver disease the prothrombin time

A. Remains normal
B. Increases
C. Decreases
D. Responds to Vit K

Ans. B.

1902. Urea clearance test is used to determine the

A. Glomerular filtration rate
B. Renal plasma flow
C. Ability of kidney to concentrate the urine
D. Measurement of tubular mass

Ans. A.

1903. Average maximum urea clearance is

A. 30 ml
B. 50 ml
C. 75 ml
D. 90 ml

Ans. C.

1904. The average normal value for standard urea clearance is

A. 20 ml
B. 30 ml
C. 40 ml
D. 54 ml

Ans. D.

1905. Urea clearance is lowered in

A. Acute nephritis
B. Pneumonia
C. Early stage of nephritic syndrome
D. Benign hypertension

Ans. A.

1906. Glomerular filtration rate can be measured by

A. Endogenous creatinine clearance B. Para-aminohippurate test

C. Addis test D. Mosenthal test

Ans. A.

1907. At normal levels of creatinine in the blood, this metabolite is

A. Filtered at the glomerulus but not secreted nor reabsorbed by the tubule

B. Secreted by the tubule

C. Reabsorbed by the tubule

D. Secreted and reabsorbed by tubule

Ans. A.

1908. The normal values for creatinine clearance varies from

A. 20–40 ml/min B. 40–60 ml/min

C. 70–85 ml/min D. 95–105 ml/min

Ans. D.

1909. Measurement of insulin clearance test is a measure of

A. Glomerular filtration rate B. Filtration factor

C. Renal plasma flow D. Tubular secretory mass

Ans. A.

1910. The polysaccharide insulin is

A. Filtered at the glomerulus but neither secreted nor reabsorbed by the tubule

B. Filtered at the glomerulus and secreted by the tubule

C. Filtered at the glomerulus and reabsorbed by the tubule

D. Filtered at the glomerulus, secreted and reabsorbed by the tubule

Ans. A.

1911. Creatinine EDTA clearance is a test to measure

A. Renal plasma flow B. Filtration fraction

C. Glomerular filtration rate D. Tubular function

Ans. C.

1912. The end products of saponification:

A. glycerol B. acid

C. soap D. Both (A) and (C)

Ans. D.

1913. Para amino hippurate is

A. Filtered at glomeruli and secreted by the tubules

B. Filtered at glomeruli and not secreted by the tubules

C. Filtered at glomeruli and reabsorbed completely

D. Not removed completely during a single circulation of the blood through the kidney.

Ans. A.

1914. Which of the following is a polyunsaturated fatty acid?

A. Palmitic acid
B. Palmitoleic acid
C. Linoleic acid
D. Oleic acid

Ans. C.

1915. Which of the following is omega-3 polyunsaturated fatty acid?

A. Linoleic acid
B. α-Linolenic acid
C. γ-Linolenic acid
D. Arachidonic acid

Ans. B.

1916. Triglycerides are

A. Heavier than water
B. Major constituents of membranes
C. Non-polar
D. Hydrophilic

Ans. C.

1917. Cerebronic acid is present in

A. Glycerophospholipids
B. Sphingophospholipids
C. Galactosyl ceramide
D. Gangliosides

Ans. C.

1918. Acylsphingosine is also known as

A. Sphingomyelin
B. Ceramide
C. Cerebroside
D. Sulphatide

Ans. B.

1919. The highest phospholipids content is found in

A. Chylomicrons
B. VLDL
C. LDL
D. HDL

Ans. D.

1920. The major lipid in chylomicrons is

A. Triglycerides
B. Phospholipids
C. Cholesterol
D. Free fatty acids

Ans. A.

1921. Number of carbon atoms in cholesterol is

A. 17 B. 19

C. 27 D. 30

Ans. C.

1922. The lipoprotein richest in cholesterol is

A. Chylomicrons B. VLDL

C. LDL D. HDL

Ans. C.

1923. The major storage form of lipids is

A. Esterified cholesterol B. Glycerophospholipids

C. Triglycerides D. Sphingolipids

Ans. C.

1924. Cerebonic acid is present in

A. Triglycerides B. Cerebrosides

C. Esterified cholestrol D. Sphingomyelin

Ans. B.

1925. The nitrogenous base in lecithin is

A. Ethanolamine B. Choline

C. Serine D. Betaine

Ans. B.

1926. All the following are omega-6-fatty acids except

A. Linoleic acid B. α-Linolenic acid

C. γ-Linolenic acid D. Arachidonic acid

Ans. B.

1927. All the following have 18 carbon atoms except

A. Linoleic acid B. Linolenic acid

C. Arachidonic acid D. Stearic acid

Ans. C.

1928. A 20-carbon fatty acid among the following is

A. Linoleic acid B. α -Linolenic acid

C. β -Linolenic acid D. Arachidonic acid

Ans. D.

1929. Triglycerides are transported from liver to extrahepatic tissues by

A. Chylomicrons B. VLDL
C. HDL D. LDL

Ans. B.

1930. Cholesterol is transported from liver to extrahepatic tissues by

A. Chylomicrons B. VLDL
C. HDL D. LDL

Ans. D.

1931. Elevated plasma level of the following protects against atherosclerosis:

A. Chylomicrons B. VLDL
C. HDL D. LDL

Ans. C.

1932. All the following amino acids are nonessential except

A. Alanine B. Histidine
C. Cysteine D. Proline

Ans. B.

1933. Sulphydryl group is present in

A. Cysteine B. Methionine
C. Both (A) and (B) D. None of these

Ans. A.

1934. Oligosaccharide-pyrophosphoryl dolichol is required for the synthesis of

A. N-linked glycoproteins B. O-linked glycoproteins
C. GPI-linked glycoproteins D. All of these

Ans. A.

1935. In N-linked glycoproteins, oligosaccharide is attached to protein through its

A. Asparagine residue B. Glutamine residue
C. Arginine residue D. Lysine residue

Ans. A.

1936. de novo synthesis of fatty acids occurs in

A. Cytosol B. Mitochondria
C. Microsomes D. All of these

Ans. A.

1937. Acyl Carrier Protein contains the vitamin:

A. Biotin B. Lipoic acid

C. Pantothenic acid D. Folic acid

Ans. C.

1938. de novo synthesis of fatty acids requires all of the following except

A. Biotin B. NADH

C. Panthothenic acid D. ATP

Ans. D.

1939. β-Oxidation of fatty acids requires all the following coenzymes except

A. CoA B. FAD

C. NAD D. NADP

Ans. D.

1940. Which of the following can be oxidized by β-oxidation pathway?

A. Saturated fatty acids B. Monosaturated fatty acids

C. Polyunsaturated fatty acids D. All of these

Ans. D.

1941. An enzyme required for the synthesis of ketone bodies as well as cholesterol is

A. Acetyl CoA carboxylase B. HMG CoA synthetase

C. HMG CoA reductase D. HMG CoA lyase

Ans. B.

1942. Ketone bodies are synthesized in

A. Adipose tissue B. Liver

C. Muscles D. Brain

Ans. B.

1943. All the following statements about ketone bodies are true except

A. Their synthesis increases in diabetes mellitus

B. They are synthesized in mitchondria

C. They can deplete the alkali reserve

D. They can be oxidized in the liver

Ans. D.

1944. All the following statements about carnitine are true except

A. It can be synthesized in the human body

B. It can be synthesized from methionine and lysine

C. It is required for transport of short chain fatty acids into mitochondria

D. Its deficiency can occur due to haemodialysis

Ans. C.

1945. Which of the following can be synthesized in the human body if precursors are available?

A. Oleic acid
B. Palmitoleic acid
C. Arachidonic acid
D. All of these

Ans. D.

1946. All the following can be oxidized by β- oxidation except

A. Palmitic acid
B. Phytanic acid
C. Linoleic acid
D. Fatty acids having an odd number of carbon atoms

Ans. B.

1947. Anti-inflammatory corticosteroids inhibit the synthesis of

A. Leukotrienes
B. Prostaglandins
C. Thromboxanes
D. All of these

Ans. D.

1948. Diets having a high ratio of polyunsaturated : saturated fatty acids can cause

A. Increase in serum triglycerides
B. Decrease in serum cholesterol
C. Decrease in serum HDL
D. Skin lesions

Ans. B.

1949. Thromboxanes cause

A. Vasodilation
B. Bronchoconstriction
C. Platelet aggregation
D. All of these

Ans. C.

1950. Slow reacting substance of anaphylaxis is a mixture of

A. Prostaglandins
B. Prostacyclins
C. Thromboxanes
D. Leukotrienes

Ans. D.

1951. In glycerophospholipids, a polyunsaturated fatty acid is commonly attached to which of the following carbon atom of glycerol?

A. Carbon 1
B. Carbon 2
C. Both (A) and (B)
D. None of these

Ans. B.

1952. Lysolecithin is formed from lecithin by removal of

A. Fatty acid from position 1
B. Fatty acid from position 2
C. Phosphorylcholine
D. Choline

Ans. B.

1953. Cerebrosides contain all the following except

A. Galactose
B. Sulphate
C. Sphingosine
D. Fatty acid

Ans. B.

1954. Chylomicron remnants are catabolised in

A. Intestine
B. Adipose tissue
C. Liver
D. Liver and intestine

Ans. C.

1955. VLDL remnant may be converted into

A. VLDL
B. LDL
C. HDL
D. Chylomicrons

Ans. C.

1956. Receptors for chylomicron remnants are

A. Apo A specific
B. Apo B-48 specific
C. Apo C specific
D. Apo E specific

Ans. B.

1957. LDL receptor is specific for

A. Apo B-48 and Apo B 100
B. Apo B-48 and Apo E
C. Apo B-100 and Apo D
D. Apo B-100 and Apo D

Ans. C.

1958. Nascent HDL of intestinal origin lacks

A. Apo A
B. Apo C
C. Apo E
D. Apo C and Apo E

Ans. D.

1959. HDL is synthesized in

A. Adipose tissue
B. Liver
C. Intestine
D. Liver and intestine

Ans. D.

1960. Nascent HDL of intestinal origin acquires Apo C and Apo E from

A. Chylomicrons B. VLDL

C. LDL D. HDL of the hepatic origin

Ans. D.

1961. Activated lecithin cholesterol acyl transferase is essential for the conversion of

A. VLDL remnants into LDL B. Nascent HDL into HDL

C. HDL2 into HDL3 D. HDL3 into HDL2

Ans. B.

1962. Fatty liver may be caused by

A. Deficiency of methionine B. Puromycin

C. Chronic alcoholism D. All of these

Ans. D.

1963. Alcohol dehydrogenase converts ethanol into

A. Acetyl CoA B. Acetaldehyde

C. Acetate D. CO_2 and H_2O

Ans. B.

1964. Lipids are stored in the body mainly in the form of

A. Phospholipids B. Glycolipids

C. Triglycerides D. Fatty acids

Ans. C.

1965. Lipid stores are mainly present in

A. Liver B. Brain

C. Muscles D. Adipose tissue

Ans. D.

1966. Glycerol released from adipose tissue by hydrolysis of triglycerides is mainly

A. Taken up by liver B. Taken up by extrahepatic tissues

C. Reutilised in adipose tissue D. Excreted from the body

Ans. A.

1967. Free glycerol cannot be used for triglyceride synthesis in

A. Liver B. Kidney

C. Intestine D. Adipose tissue

Ans. D.

1968. A digestive secretion that does not contain any digestive enzyme is

A. Saliva
B. Gastric juice
C. Pancreatic juice
D. Bile

Ans. D.

1969. Saliva contains a lipase which acts on triglycerides having

A. Short chain fatty acids
B. Medium chain fatty acids
C. Long chain fatty acids
D. All of these

Ans. A.

1970. Salivary lipase hydrolyses the ester bond at

A. Position 1 of triglycerides
B. Position 2 of triglycerides
C. Position 3 of triglycerides
D. All of these

Ans. C.

1971. Salivary lipase converts dietary triglycerides into

A. Diglycerides and fatty acids
B. Monoglycerides and fatty acids
C. Glycerol and fatty acids
D. All of these

Ans. A.

1972. Pancreatic lipase requires for its activity:

A. Co-lipase
B. Bile salts
C. Phospholipids
D. All of these

Ans. D.

1973. Pancreatic lipase converts triacylglycerols into

A. 2, 3-Diacylglycerol
B. 1-Monoacylglycerol
C. 2-Monoacylglycerol
D. 3-Monoacylglycerol

Ans. C.

1974. Oxidation of fatty acids occurs

A. In the cytosol
B. In the matrix of mitochondria
C. On inner mitochondrial membrane
D. On the microsomes

Ans. B.

1975. Activation of fatty acids requires all the following except

A. ATP
B. Coenzyme A
C. Thiokinase
D. Carnitine

Ans. D.

1976. Mitochondrial thiokinase acts on

A. Short chain of fatty acids
B. Medium chain fatty acids
C. Long chain fatty acids
D. All of these

Ans. A.

1977. Carnitine is required for the transport of

A. Triglycerides out of liver
B. Triglycerides into mitochondria
C. Short chain fatty acids into mitochondria
D. Long chain fatty acids into mitochondria

Ans. D.

1978. Net ATP generation on complete oxidation of stearic acid is

A. 129
B. 131
C. 146
D. 148

Ans. C.

1979. α-Oxidation of fatty acids occurs mainly in

A. Liver
B. Brain
C. Muscles
D. Adipose tissue

Ans. B.

1980. Refsum's disease results from a defect in the following pathway except

A. Alpha-oxidation of fatty acids
B. Beta-oxidation of fatty acids
C. Gamma-oxidation of fatty acids
D. Omega-oxidation of fatty acids

Ans. A.

1981. de novo synthesis of fatty acids is catalysed by a multi-enzyme complex which contains

A. One-SH group
B. Two-SH groups
C. Three-SH groups
D. Four-SH groups

Ans. D.

1982. Fat depots are located in

A. Intermuscular connective tissue
B. Mesentary
C. Omentum
D. All of these

Ans. D.

1983. Salivary lipase is secreted by

A. Parotid glands
B. Sub-maxillary glands
C. Dorsal surface of tongue
D. None of these

Ans. C.

1984. Co-lipase is a

A. Bile salt
B. Vitamin
C. Protein
D. Phospholipid

Ans. C.

1985. Plasma becomes milky

A. Due to high level of HDL
B. Due to high level of LDL
C. During fasting
D. After a meal

Ans. D.

1986. Mitochondrial membrane is permeable to

A. Short chain fatty acids
B. Medium chain fatty acids
C. Long chain fatty acids
D. All of these

Ans. A.

1987. During each cycle of β-oxidation

A. One carbon atom is removed from the carboxyl end of the fatty acid
B. One carbon atom is removed from the methyl end of the fatty acid
C. Two carbon atoms are removed from the carboxyl end of the fatty acid
D. Two carbon atoms are removed from the methyl end of the fatty acid

Ans. C.

1988. Net generation of energy on complete oxidation of palmitic acid is

A. 129 ATP equivalents
B. 131 ATP equivalents
C. 146 ATP equivalents
D. 148 ATP equivalents

Ans. D.

1989. Net generation of energy on complete oxidation of a 17-carbon fatty acid is

A. Equal to the energy generation from a 16-carbon fatty acid
B. Equal to the energy generation from an 18-carbon fatty acid
C. Less than the energy generation from a 16-carbon fatty acid
D. In between the energy generation from a 16-carbon fatty acid and an 18-carbon fatty acid

Ans. C.

1990. Net energy generation on complete oxidation of linoleic acid is

A. 148 ATP equivalents
B. 146 ATP equivalents
C. 144 ATP equivalents
D. 142 ATP equivalents

Ans. D.

1991. Extramitochondrial synthesis of fatty acids occurs in

A. Mammary glands
B. Lungs
C. Brain
D. All of these

Ans. D.

1992. One functional sub-unit of multi-enzyme complex for de novo synthesis of fatty acids contains

A. One —SH group
B. Two —SH groups
C. Three —SH groups
D. Four —SH groups

Ans. B.

1993. Fatty liver may be prevented by all of the following except

A. Choline
B. Betaine
C. Methionine
D. Ethionine

Ans. D.

1994. Human desaturase enzyme system cannot introduce a double bond in a fatty acid beyond

A. Carbon 9
B. Carbon 6
C. Carbon 5
D. Carbon 3

Ans. A.

1995. Which of the following lipid is absorbed actively from intestines?

A. Glycerol
B. Cholesterol
C. Monoacylglycerol
D. None of these

Ans. D.

1996. Sphingomyelins:

A. Phospholipids
B. Nitrolipids
C. Alcohols
D. None of these

Ans. A.

1997. All of the following statements about hypoglycin are true except

A. It is a plant toxin
B. It causes hypoglycaemia
C. It inhibits oxidation of short chain fatty acids
D. It inhibits oxidation of long chain fatty acids

Ans. A.

1998. Synthesis of prostaglandins is inhibited by

A. Glucocorticoids
B. Aspirin
C. Indomethacin
D. All of these

Ans. D.

1999. Lipo-oxygenase is required for the synthesis of

A. Prostaglandins
B. Leukotrienes
C. Thromboxanes
D. All of these

Ans. B.

2000. All of the following statements about multiple sclerosis are true except

A. There is loss of phospholipids from white matter
B. There is loss of sphingolipids from white matter
C. There is loss of esterified cholesterol from white matter
D. White matter resembles gray matter in composition

Ans. C.

2001. After entering cytosol, free fatty acids are bound to

A. Albumin
B. Globulin
C. Z-protein
D. None of these

Ans. C.

2002. Release of free fatty acids from adipose tissue is increased by all of the following except

A. Glucagon
B. Epinephrine
C. Growth hormone
D. Insulin

Ans. D.

2003. Lovastatin and mevastatin lower

A. Serum triglycerides
B. Serum cholesterol
C. Serum phospholipids
D. All of these

Ans. B.

2004. Lovastatin is a

A. Competitive inhibitor of acetyl CoA carboxylase
B. Competitive inhibitor of HMG CoA synthetase
C. Non-competitive inhibitor of HMG CoA reductase
D. Competitive inhibitor of HMG CoA reductase

Ans. D.

2005. Abetalipoproteinaemia occurs due to a block in the synthesis of

A. Apoprotein A
B. Apoprotein B
C. Apoprotein C
D. Cholesterol

Ans. B.

2006. All of the following statements about Tangier disease are true except

A. It is a disorder of HDL metabolism
B. Its inheritance is autosomal recessive
C. Apoproteins A-I and A-II are not synthesized
D. Plasma HDL is increased

Ans. D.

2007. Phenylbutazone and indomethacin inhibit

A. Phospholipase A1
B. Phospholipase A2
C. Cyclo-oxygenase
D. Lipo-oxygenase

Ans. C.

2008. Prostaglandins stimulate

A. Aggregation of platelets
B. Lipolysis in adipose tissue
C. Bronchodilatation
D. Gastric acid secretion

Ans. C.

2009. For extramitochondrial fatty acid synthesis, acetyl CoA may be obtained from

A. Citrate
B. Isocitrate
C. Oxaloacetate
D. Succinate

Ans. A.

2010. Fluidity of membranes is increased by the following constituent except

A. Polyunsaturated fatty acids
B. Saturated fatty acids
C. Integral proteins
D. Cholesterol

Ans. A.

2011. Acetyl CoA formed from pyruvate can be used for the synthesis of all the following except

A. Glucose
B. Fatty acids
C. Cholesterol
D. Steroid hormones

Ans. A.

2012. Anti-inflammatory corticosteroids inhibit

A. Phospholipase A1
B. Phospholipase A2
C. Cyclo-oxygenase
D. Lipo-oxygenase

Ans. B.

2013. Cyclo-oxygenase is involved in the synthesis of

A. Prostaglandins
B. Thromboxanes
C. Both (A) and (B)
D. None of these

Ans. C.

2014. Leukotrienes cause

A. Increase in capillary permeability
B. Aggregation of platelets
C. Bronchodilatation
D. None of these

Ans. A.

2015. Prostaglandins decrease all of the following except

A. Gastric acid secretion
B. Blood pressure
C. Uterine contraction
D. Platelet aggregation

Ans. C.

2016. Hypocholesterolaemia can occur in

A. Hyperthyroidism
B. Nephrotic syndrome
C. Obstructive jaundice
D. Diabetes mellitus

Ans. A.

2017. De novo synthesis and oxidation of fatty acids differ in the following respect:

A. Synthesis occurs in cytosol and oxidation in mitochondria
B. Synthesis is decreased and oxidation increased by insulin
C. NADH is required in synthesis and FAD in oxidation
D. Malonyl CoA is formed during oxidation but not during synthesis

Ans. A.

2018. Free fatty acids released from adipose tissue are transported in blood by

A. Albumin
B. VLDL
C. LDL
D. HDL

Ans. A.

2019. β -Galactosidase is deficient in

A. Fabry's disease
B. Krabbe's disease
C. Gaucher's disease
D. Metachromatic leukodystrophy

Ans. B.

2020. Hexosaminidase A is deficient in

A. Tay-Sachs disease
B. Gaucher's disease
C. Niemann-Pick disease
D. Fabry's disease

Ans. A.

2021. Mental retardation occurs in

A. Tay-Sachs disease B. Gaucher's disease

C. Niemann-Pick disease D. All of these

Ans. D.

2022. The enzyme deficient in Fabry's disease is

A. α-Galactosidase B. β-Galactosidase

C. α-Glucosidase D. β-Glucosidase

Ans. A.

2023. Highest protein content amongst the following is present in

A. Wheat B. Rice

C. Pulses D. Soyabean

Ans. D.

2024. Daily protein requirement of an adult man is

A. 0.5 gm/kg of body weight B. 0.8 gm/kg of body weight

C. 1.0 gm/kg of body weight D. 1.5 gm/kg of body weight

Ans. C.

2025. Daily protein requirement of an adult woman is

A. 0.5 gm/kg of body weight B. 0.8 gm/kg of body weight

C. 1.0 gm/kg of body weight D. 1.5 gm/kg of body weight

Ans. C.

2026. Cysteine can partially meet the requirement of

A. Phenylalanine B. Threonine

C. Methionine D. None of these

Ans. C.

2027. Invisible fat is present in

A. Milk B. Coconut oil

C. Groundnut oil D. Hydrogenated oils

Ans. A.

2028. Visible fat is present in

A. Milk B. Pulses

C. Coconut oil D. Egg yolk

Ans. C.

2029. Fat content of eggs is about

A. 7%
B. 10%
C. 13%
D. 16%

Ans. C.

2030. Fat content of pulses is about

A. 5%
B. 10%
C. 15%
D. 20%

Ans. A.

2031. Predominant fatty acids in meat are

A. Saturated
B. Monounsaturated
C. Polyunsaturated
D. Mono and poly-unsaturated

Ans. A.

2032. Oils having more than 50 % polyunsaturated fatty acids include all of the following except

A. Groundnut oil
B. Soyabean oil
C. Sunflower oil
D. Safflower oil

Ans. A.

2033. Cholesterol is present in all of the following except

A. Egg
B. Fish
C. Milk
D. Pulses

Ans. D.

2034. Which of the following has the highest cholesterol content?

A. Meat
B. Fish
C. Butter
D. Milk

Ans. C.

2035. Which of the following has the highest cholesterol content?

A. Egg yolk
B. Egg white
C. Meat
D. Fish

Ans. A.

2036. The following contains the least cholesterol:

A. Milk
B. Meat
C. Butter
D. Cheese

Ans. A.

2037. Which of the following constitutes fibre or roughage in food?

A. Cellulose B. Pectin

C. Inulin D. All of these

Ans. D.

2038. The starch content of wheat is about

A. 50% B. 60%

C. 70% D. 80%

Ans. C.

2039. The starch content of pulses is about

A. 50% B. 60%

C. 70% D. 80%

Ans. B.

2040. A significant source of starch among vegetables is

A. Radish B. Spinach

C. Potato D. Cauliflower

Ans. C.

2041. In Ames' assay, addition of a carcinogen to the culture medium allows *S. typhimurium* to grow

A. In the presence of histidine B. In the presence of arginine

C. In the absence of histidine D. In the absence of arginine

Ans. C.

2042. In Ames' assay, liver homogenate is included in the culture medium because

A. It converts pro-carcinogens into carcinogens

B. Liver can metabolise histidine

C. Salmonella mainly infects liver

D. Liver is very susceptible to cancer

Ans. A.

2043. Bile pigments are present and urobilinogen absent in urine in

A. Haemolytic jaundice B. Hepatocellular jaundice

C. Obstructive jaundice D. Crigler-Najjar syndrome

Ans. C.

2044. Bile pigments are absent and urobilinogen increased in urine in

A. Haemolytic jaundice B. Hepatocellular jaundice

C. Obstructive jaundice D. Rotor's syndrome

Ans. A.

2045. In obstructive jaundice, urine shows

A. Absence of bile pigments and urobilinogen

B. Presence of bile pigments and urobilinogen

C. Absence of bile pigments and presence of urobilinogen

D. Presence of bile pigments and absence of urobilinogen

Ans. D.

2046. In haemolytic jaundice, urine shows

A. Absence of bile pigments and urobilinogen

B. Presence of bile pigments and urobilinogen

C. Absence of bile pigments and presence of urobilinogen

D. Presence of bile pigments and absence of urobilinogen

Ans. C.

2047. Serum albumin may be decreased in

A. Haemolytic jaundice
B. Hepatocellular jaundice
C. Obstructive jaundice
D. All of these

Ans. B.

2048. Normal range of serum albumin is

A. 2.0–3.6 gm/dl
B. 2.0–3.6 mg/dl
C. 3.5–5.5 gm/dl
D. 3.5–5.5 mg/dl

Ans. C.

2049. Normal range of serum globulin is

A. 2.0–3.6 mg/dl
B. 2.0–3.6 gm/dl
C. 3.5–5.5 mg/dl
D. 3.5–5.5 gm/dl

Ans. B.

2050. Serum albumin: globulin ratio is altered in

A. Gilbert's disease
B. Haemolytic jaundice
C. Viral hepatitis
D. Stones in bile duct

Ans. C.

2051. Esterification of cholesterol occurs mainly in

A. Adipose tissue
B. Liver
C. Muscles
D. Kidneys

Ans. B.

2052. Galactose intolerance can occur in

A. Haemolytic jaundice
B. Hepatocellular jaundice
C. Obstructive jaundice
D. None of these

Ans. B.

2053. Prothrombin is synthesised in

A. Erythrocytes
B. Reticulo-endothelial cells
C. Liver
D. Kidneys

Ans. C.

2054. Prothrombin time remains prolonged even after parenteral administration of vitamin K in

A. Haemolytic jaundice
B. Liver damage
C. Biliary obstruction
D. Steatorrhoea

Ans. B.

2055. All the following statements about obstructive jaundice are true except

A. Conjugated bilirubin in serum is normal
B. Total bilirubin in serum is raised
C. Bile salts are present in urine
D. Serum alkaline phosphatase is raised

Ans. A.

2056. A test to evaluate detoxifying function of liver is

A. Serum albumin: globulin ratio
B. Galactose tolerance test
C. Hippuric acid test
D. Prothrombin time

Ans. C.

2057. Hippuric acid is formed from

A. Benzoic acid and alanine
B. Benzoic acid and glycine
C. Glucuronic acid and alanine
D. Glucuronic acid and glycine

Ans. B.

2058. An enzyme which is excreted in urine is

A. Lactase dehydrogenase
B. Amylase
C. Ornithine transcarbamoylase
D. None of these

Ans. C.

2059. Serum gamma glutamyl transpeptidase is raised in

A. Haemolytic jaundice
B. Myocardial infarction
C. Alcoholic hepatitis
D. Acute cholecystitis

Ans. C.

2060. Oliguria can occur in

A. Diabetes mellitus
B. Diabetes insipidus
C. Acute glomerulonephritis
D. Chronic glomerulonephritis

Ans. A.

2061. Urea clearance is the

A. Amount of urea excreted per minute
B. Amount of urea present in 100 ml of urine
C. Volume of blood cleared of urea in one minute
D. Amount of urea filtered by glomeruli in one minute

Ans. A.

2062. Inulin clearance is a measure of

A. Glomerular filtration rate
B. Tubular secretion flow
C. Tubular reabsorption rate
D. Renal plasma flow

Ans. B.

2063. Phenolsulphonephthalein excretion test is an indicator of

A. Glomerular filtration
B. Tubular secretion
C. Tubular reabsorption
D. Renal blood low

Ans. D.

2064. Para-amino hippurate excretion test is an indicator of

A. Glomerular filtration
B. Tubular secretion
C. Tubular reabsorption
D. Renal plasma flow

Ans. D.

2065. Renal plasma flow of an average adult man is

A. 120–130 ml/minute
B. 325–350 ml/minute
C. 480–52 ml/minute
D. 560–830 ml/minute

Ans. D.

2066. Among the following, a test of glomerular function is

A. Urea clearance
B. PSP excretion test
C. PAH clearance
D. Hippuric acid excretion test

Ans. D.

2067. Esters of fatty acids with higher alcohols other than glycerol are said to be

A. Waxes
B. Fats
C. Both (A) and (B)
D. None of these

Ans. A.

2068. The combination of an amino alcohol, fatty acid and sialic acid form

A. Phospholipids
B. Sulpholipids
C. Glycolipids
D. Aminolipids

Ans. C.

2069. Hydrolysis of fats by alkali is called

A. Saponification number
B. Saponification
C. Both (A) and (B)
D. None of these

Ans. B.

2070. The number of milliliters of 0.1 N KOH required to neutralize the insoluble fatty acids from 5 gms of fat is called

A. Acid number
B. Acetyl number
C. Halogenation
D. Polenske number

Ans. D.

2071. The rate of fatty acid oxidation is increased by

A. Phospholipids
B. Glycolipids
C. Aminolipids
D. All of these

Ans. A.

2072. Lecithin contains a nitrogenous base named as

A. Ethanolamine
B. Choline
C. Inositol
D. All of these

Ans. B.

2073. Lecithins contain an unsaturated fatty acid at position:

A. α
B. α and β
C. β
D. None of these

Ans. C.

2074. Lecithins are soluble in ordinary solvents except

A. Benzene
B. Ethyl alcohol
C. Methyl alcohol
D. Acetone

Ans. D.

2075. Lecithins combine with protein to form

A. Phosphoprotein
B. Mucoprotein
C. Lipoprotein
D. Glycoprotein

Ans. C.

2076. The concentration of sphingomyelins are increased in

A. Gaucher's disease | B. Fabry's disease
C. Fabrile disease | D. Niemann-Pick disease

Ans. B.

2077. Sphingomyelins contain a complex amino alcohol named as

A. Serine | B. Lysolecithin
C. Sphingosine | D. Glycol

Ans. C.

2078. The types of sphingomyelins are

A. 1 | B. 3
C. 4 | D. 5

Ans. B.

2079. Glycolipids contain an amino alcohol:

A. Sphingosine | B. Iso-sphingosine
C. Both (A) and (B) | D. None of these

Ans. C.

2080. Cerebrosides may also be classified as

A. Sphingolipids | B. Sulpholipids
C. Aminolipids | D. Glycolipids

Ans. A.

2081. Gaucher's disease is characterized specially by the increase in

A. Lignoceric acid | B. Nervonic acid
C. Cerebomic acid | D. Hydroxynervonic acid

Ans. C.

2082. Gangliosides are the glycolipids occurring in

A. Brain | B. Liver
C. Kidney | D. Muscle

Ans. A.

2083. Lipoprotein present in cell membrane is by nature:

A. Hydrophilic | B. Hydrophobic
C. Both (A) and (B) | D. None of these

Ans. A.

2084. The density of lipoproteins increases as the protein content

A. Increases
B. Decreases
C. Highly decreases
D. Slightly and promptly decreases

Ans. A.

2085. Lipoprotiens may be identified more accurately by means of

A. Electrophoresis
B. Ultra centrifugation
C. Centrifugation
D. Immunoelectrophoresis

Ans. D.

2086. Very low density lipoproteins are also known as

A. β-lipoproteins
B. Pre β—lipoproteins
C. α-lipoproteins
D. None of these

Ans. B.

2087. The protein moiety of lipoprotein is known as

A. Apoprotein
B. Pre-protein
C. Post-protein
D. Pseudoprotein

Ans. A.

2088. The β-lipoprotein fraction increases in severe

A. Diabetes Mellitus
B. Uremia
C. Nephritis
D. Muscular dystrophy

Ans. A.

2089. The prostaglandins are synthesized from

A. Arachidonic acid
B. Oleic acid
C. Linoleic acid
D. Linolenic acid

Ans. A.

2090. The Iodine number of essential fatty acids of vegetable oils:

A. High
B. Very high
C. Very low
D. Low

Ans. D.

2091. Waxes contain higher alcohols named as

A. Methyl
B. Ethyl
C. Phytyl
D. Cetyl

Ans. D.

2092. Lieberman-Burchard reaction is performed to detect

A. Cholesterol
B. Glycerol
C. Fatty acid
D. Vitamin D

Ans. A.

2093. Lipase present in the stomach cannot hydrolyze fats owing to

A. Alkalinity
B. Acidity
C. High acidity
D. Neutrality

Ans. C.

2094. Fatty acids are oxidized by

A. α-oxidation
B. β-oxidation
C. ω–oxidation
D. All of these

Ans. D.

2095. The fatty acids containing even number and odd number of carbon atoms as well as the unsaturated fatty acids are oxidized by

A. α-oxidation
B. β-oxidation
C. ω-oxidation
D. All of these

Ans. B.

2096. Long chain fatty acids are first activated to acyl CoA in the

A. Cytosol
B. Mitochondria
C. Ribosomes
D. Microsome

Ans. A.

2097. Long chain acyl CoA penetrates mitochondria in the presence of

A. Palmitate
B. Carnitine
C. Sorbitol
D. DNP

Ans. B.

2098. For the activation of long chain fatty acids the enzyme thiokinase requires the cofactor:

A. Mg^{++}
B. Ca^{++}
C. Mn^{++}
D. K^{+}

Ans. B.

2099. ω-oxidation takes place by the hydroxylase in microsomes involving

A. Cytochrome b
B. Cytochrome c
C. Cytochrome p-4500
D. Cytochrome a3

Ans. C.

2100. Prostaglandins are liberated in the circulation by the stimulation of

A. Anterior pituitary glands B. Posterior pituitary glands

C. Adrenal gland D. Thyroid gland

Ans. C.

2101. All active prostaglandins have atleast one double bond between positions:

A. 7 and 8 B. 9 and 10

C. 11 and 12 D. 13 and 14

Ans. A.

2102. The enzyme systems for lengthening and shortening for saturating and desaturating of fatty acids occur in

A. Intestine B. Muscle

C. Kidney D. Liver

Ans. D.

2103. Which of the following are classified as essential fatty acids?

A. Arachidonic acid B. Oleic acid

C. Acetic acid D. Butyric acid

Ans. A.

2104. Biological functions of lipids include

A. Source of energy B. Insulating material

C. Maintenance of cellular integrity D. All of these

Ans. D.

2105. Saponification number is

A. mg of KOH required to saponify one gm of fat or oil

B. mg of KOH required to neutralize free fatty acids of one gm of fat

C. mg of KOH required to neutralize the acetic acid obtained by saponification of one gm of fat after it has been acetylated

D. None of these

Ans. C.

2106. Lipids have the following properties:

A. Insoluble in water and soluble in fat solvent

B. High energy content

C. Structural component of cell membrane

D. All of these

Ans. D.

2107. Carbohydrate moiety in cerebrosides is

A. Glucose
B. Sucrose
C. Galactose
D. Maltose

Ans. B.

2108. Which of the following is not an unsaturated fatty acid?

A. Oleic acid
B. Stearic acid
C. Linoleic acid
D. Palmitic acid

Ans. B.

2109. All the following are functions of prostaglandins except

A. Lowering of B.P
B. Introduction of labour
C. Anti inflammatory
D. Prevention of myocardial infraction

Ans. D.

2110. Calorific value of lipids per gm is

A. 4 Kcal
B. 8 Kcal
C. 9 Kcal
D. None of these

Ans. C.

2111. All the following are ketones except

A. Xylulose
B. Ribolose
C. Erythrose
D. Fructose

Ans. C.

2112. Saponification:

A. Hydrolysis of fats by alkali
B. Hydrolysis of glycerol by liposes
C. Esterification
D. Reduction

Ans. A.

2113. Number of ml of 0.1 N KOH required to neutralize fatty acids from 5 gms of fat:

A. Iodine number
B. Polenske number
C. Reichert-Miessl number
D. None of these

Ans. B.

2114. Hydrated density of HD lipoproteins is

A. 0.94 gm/ml
B. 0.94–1.006 gm/ml
C. 1.006–1.063 gm/ml
D. 1.063–1.21 gm/ml

Ans. D.

2115. Acrolein Test is positive for
A. Glycerol
B. Prostaglandins
C. Carbohydrates
D. Proteins

Ans. A.

2116. Maximum energy produced by
A. Fats
B. Carbohydrates
C. Proteins
D. Nucleic acids

Ans. A.

2117. Lecithins are composed of
A. Glycerol + Fatty acids + Phosphoric acid +Choline
B. Glycerol + Fatty acids + Phosphoric acid +Ethanolamine
C. Glycerol + Fatty acids + Phosphoric acid +Serine
D. Glycerol + Fatty acids + Phosphoric acid +Betaine

Ans. A.

2118. Sphingomyelins are composed of fatty acids, phosphoric acid and
A. Sphingosine and choline
B. Glycerol and sphingosine
C. Glycerol and Serine
D. Glycerol and Choline

Ans. A.

2119. Depot fats of mammalian cells comprise mostly of
A. Cholesterol
B. Cholesterol esters
C. Triacyl glycerol
D. Phospholipids

Ans. C.

2120. Acrolein test is answered by
A. Cholesterol
B. Glycerol
C. Glycosides
D. Sphingol

Ans. B.

2121. The smell of fat turned rancid is due to
A. Presence of vit E
B. Presence of quinones
C. Phenols
D. Volatile fatty acids

Ans. D.

2122. Phospholipids are important cell membrane components because
A. They have glycerol
B. They can form bilayers in water
C. They have both polar and non polar components
D. They combine covalently with proteins

Ans. C.

2123. Which one of the following is not a phospholipid ?

A. Lecithin B. Plasmalogen

C. Lysolecithin D. Gangliosides

Ans. D.

2124. A fatty acid which is not synthesized in human body and has to be supplied in the diet

A. Palmitic acid B. Oleic acid

C. Linoleic acid D. Stearic acid

Ans. C.

2125. Amphiphatic lipids are

A. Hydrophilic B. Hydrophobic

C. Both (A) and (B) D. Lipophilic

Ans. C.

2126. Which of the following is not essential fatty acid?

A. Oleic acid B. Linoleic acid

C. Arachidonic acid D. Linolenic acid

Ans. A.

2127. The calorific value of lipid is

A. 4.0 Kcal/gm B. 6.0 Kcal/gm

C. 9.0 Kcal/gm D. 15 Kcal/gm

Ans. C.

2128. Rancidity of butter is prevented by the addition of

A. Vitamin D B. Tocopherols

C. Presence of priotin D. Presence of 'Cu'

Ans. B.

2129. Sphingomyelins on hydrolysis yields

A. Glycerol, fatty acids, phosphoric acid and choline

B. Glycerol, sphingosine, choline and fatty acids

C. Sphingosine, phosphoric acid, Glycerol and inositol

D. Sphingosine, fatty acids, phosphoric acid and choline

Ans. D.

2130. Inherited deficiency of enzyme cerebrosidase produces

A. Fabry's disease B. Niemann pick disease

C. Gaucher's disease D. Tay-sach's disease

Ans. C.

2131. The maximum number of double bonds present in essential fatty acid is

A. 1 B. 2

C. 3 D. 4

Ans. D.

2132. Cerebrosides are composed of

A. Sphingosine, fatty acids, glycerol and phosphoric acid

B. Sphingosine, fatty acids, galactose

C. Glycerol, fatty acids, galactose

D. Glycerol, fatty acids, galactose, sphingol

Ans. B.

2133. Which amino acid is a lipotropic factor?

A. Lysine B. Leucine

C. Tryptophan D. Methionine

Ans. D.

2134. The class of lipoproteins having a beneficial effect in atherosclerosis is

A. Low density of lipoproteins B. very low density lipoproteins

C. High density lipoproteins D. Chylomicrons

Ans. C.

2135. Cholesterol is the precursor for the biosynthesis of

A. fatty acid B. prostaglandins

C. bile acids D. sphingmyelin

Ans. C.

2136. Which of the following condition is characterized by ketonuria but without glycosuria?

A. Diabetes mellitus B. Diabetes insipidus

C. Prolonged starvation D. Addison's disease

Ans. C.

2137. Ketone bodies are formed in

A. Kidney B. Liver

C. Heart D. Intestines

Ans. B.

2138. Changes in serum high density lipoproteins (HDL) are more truly reflected by those of

A. HDL-1 B. HDL-2

C. HDL-3 D. HDLC

Ans. B.

2139. Most animal tissues contain appreciable amounts of lipid, when in the form of depot fat it consists largely of

A. Cholesterol ester
B. Phosphatides
C. Chylomicrons
D. Triacylglycerol

Ans. D.

2140. The 'free fatty acids' (FFA) of plasma:

A. metabolically inert
B. mainly bound to β-lipoproteins
C. stored in the fat
D. mainly bound to serum albumin

Ans. D.

2141. Main metabolic end product of cholesterol:

A. Coprosterol
B. 5-pregnenolone
C. Bile acid
D. Glycine

Ans. C.

2142. Normal fat content of liver is about ———— gms %.

A. 5
B. 8
C. 10
D. 15

Ans. A.

2143. Obesity is accumulation of———— in the body.

A. Water
B. NaCl
C. Fat
D. Proteins

Ans. C.

2144. The first lipoprotein to be secreted by the liver is

A. VLDL
B. nascent VLDL
C. LDL
D. IDL

Ans. B.

2145. This lipoprotein removes cholesterol from the body

A. HDL
B. VLDL
C. IDL
D. Chylomicrons

Ans. A.

2146. When the stired triacylglycerol is lipolysed in the adipose tissue blood levels of—
——— increased.

A. FFA only
B. Glycerol only
C. Free fatty acids (FFA) and Glycerol
D. Triacyl glycerol

Ans. C.

2147. All long chain fatty acids with even number of carbon atoms are oxidized to a pool of———— by β-oxidation.

A. CO2

B. Propionic acid

C. Acetic acid

D. Acetyl CoA

Ans. D.

2148. The level of free fatty acids in plasma is increased by

A. Insulin

B. Caffeine

C. Glucose

D. Niacin

Ans. B.

2149. Cholesterol is excreted as such into ————.

A. Urine

B. Faeces

C. Bile

D. Tears

Ans. C.

2150. Cholesterol molecule has ——— carbon atoms.

A. 27

B. 21

C. 15

D. 12

Ans. A.

2151. Avidin is antagonistic to

A. Niacin

B. PABA

C. Biotin

D. Pantothenic acid

Ans. C.

2152. CTP is required for the synthesis of

A. Fatty acids

B. Proteins

C. Phospholipids

D. Cholesterol

Ans. C.

2153. Cholesterol circulates in blood stream chiefly as

A. Free cholesterol

B. Ester cholesterol

C. Low density lipoproteins

D. Low density lipoproteins and high density lipoproteins

Ans. D.

2154. What is the sub cellular site for the β- oxidation of fatty acids?

A. Nucleus

B. Mitochondria

C. Lysosome

D. Cytosol

Ans. B.

2155. A diet containing this fat is helpful in lowering the blood cholesterol level.

A. Unsaturated B. Saturated

C. Vitamin enriched D. Refined

Ans. A.

2156. Pancreatic lipase is an enzyme which hydrolyzes fats. It acts as a/an

A. peptidase B. hydrolase

C. carbohydrates D. dehydrogenase

Ans. B.

2157. Acyl carrier protein is involved in the synthesis of

A. Protein

B. Glycogen

C. Fatty acid outside the mitochondria

D. Fatty acid in the mitochondria

Ans. C.

2158. Liposomes are

A. Lipid bilayered B. Water in the middle

C. Carriers of drugs D. All of these

Ans. D.

2159. The acetyl CoA formed on β-oxidation of all long chain fatty acids is metabolized under normal circumstances to

A. CO2 and water B. Cholesterol

C. Fatty acids D. Ketone bodies

Ans. A.

2160. Very low density lipoproteins are relatively rich in

A. Cholesterol B. Triacyl glycerol

C. Free fatty acids D. Phospholipids

Ans. B.

2161. Neutral fat is stored in

A. Liver B. Pancreas

C. Adipose tissue D. Brain

Ans. C.

2162. In β-Oxidation of fatty acids, which of the following are utilized as coenzymes?

A. NAD+ and NADP+ B. FADH2 and NADH + H+

C. FAD and FMN D. FAD and NAD+

Ans. D.

2163. All of the following tissue are capable of using ketone bodies except

A. Brain
B. Renal cortex
C. R.B.C.
D. Cardiac muscle

Ans. C.

2164. The major source of cholesterol in arterial smooth muscle cells is from

A. IDL
B. LDL
C. HDL
D. Chylomicrons

Ans. B.

2165. Ketone bodies are synthesized from fatty acid oxidation products by which of the following organs?

A. Liver
B. Skeletal muscles
C. Kidney
D. Brain

Ans. A.

2166. Chain elongation of fatty acids occurring in mammalian liver takes place in which of the following subcellular fractions of the cell?

A. Nucleus
B. Ribosomes
C. Lysosomes
D. Microsomes

Ans. D.

2167. Which of the following lipoproteins would contribute to a measurement of plasma cholesterol in a normal individual following a 12 hr fast?

A. Chylomicrons
B. VLDL
C. Both VLDL and LDL
D. LDL

Ans. D.

2168. All the following statements regarding ketone bodies are true except

A. They may result from starvation
B. They are formed in kidneys
C. They include acetoacetic acid and acetone
D. They may be excreted in urine

Ans. B.

2169. β-Oxidation of odd-carbon fatty acid chain produces

A. Succinyl CoA
B. Propionyl CoA
C. Acetyl CoA
D. Malonyl CoA

Ans. D.

2170. Brown adipose tissue is characterized by which of the following?

A. Present in large quantities in adult humans

B. Mitochondrial content higher than white adipose tissue

C. Oxidation and phosphorylation are tightly coupled

D. Absent in hibernating animals

Ans. B.

2171. Ketosis is partly ascribed to

A. Over production and Glucose B. Under production of Glucose

C. Increased carbohydrate utilization D. Increased fat utilization

Ans. D.

2172. Carnitine is synthesized from

A. Lysine B. Serine

C. Choline D. Arginine

Ans. A.

2173. All the following are constituents of ganglioside molecule except

A. Glycerol B. Sialic acid

C. Hexose sugar D. Sphingosine

Ans. A.

2174. Chylomicron, intermediate density lipoproteins (IDL), low density lipoproteins (LDL) and very low density lipoproteins (VLDL) all are serum lipoproteins. What is the correct ordering of these particles from the lowest to the greatest density?

A. LDL, IDL, VLDL, Chylomicron B. Chylomicron, VLDL, IDL, LDL

C. VLDL, IDL, LDL, Chylomicron D. Chylomicron, IDL, VLDL, LDL

Ans. B.

2175. A compound normally used to conjugate bile acids is

A. Serine B. Glycine

C. Glucoronic acid D. Fatty acid

Ans. B.

2176. Cholesterol, bile salts, vitamin D and sex hormones are

A. Mucolipids B. Glycolipids

C. Phospholipids D. Isoprenoid lipids

Ans. D.

2177. Water soluble molecular aggregates of lipids are known as

A. Micelle B. Colloids

C. Sphingol D. Mucin

Ans. A.

2178. Hypoglycemia depresses insulin secretion and thus increases the rate of

A. Hydrolysis B. Reduction

C. Gluconeogenesis D. Respiratory acidosis

Ans. C.

2179. The process of breakdown of glycogen to glucose in the liver and pyruvate and lactate in the muscle is known as

A. Glyogenesis B. Glycogenolysis

C. Gluconeogenesis D. Cellular degradation

Ans. B.

2180. Osteomalacia can be prevented by the administration of calcium and a vitamin:

A. A B. B

C. C D. D

Ans. D.

2181. Milk sugar is known as

A. Fructose B. Glucose

C. Sucrose D. Lactose

Ans. D.

2182. The Intrinsic Factor (HCl and mucoproteins) present in the gastric juice help in the absorption of

A. Vitamin B2 B. Tocopherols

C. Folic acid D. Vitmain B12

Ans. D.

2183. Lipase can act only at pH:

A. 2.5–4 B. 3.5–5

C. 4 to 5 D. 5–7

Ans. D.

2184. Bile is produced by

A. Liver B. Gall-bladder

C. Pancreas D. Intestine

Ans. A.

2185. Non-protein part of rhodopsin is

A. Retinal B. Retinol

C. Carotene D. Repsin

Ans. A.

2186. The lipoprotein with the fastest electrophoretic mobility and lowest TG content are

A. VLDL B. LDL

C. HDL D. Chylomicrons

Ans. C.

2187. The essential fatty acids retard

A. Atherosclerosis B. Diabetes mellitus

C. Nepritis D. Oedema

Ans. A.

2188. The majority of absorbed fat appears in the forms of

A. HDL B. Chylomicron

C. VLDL D. LDL

Ans. B.

2189. Daily output of urea in grams is

A. 10 to 20 B. 15 to 25

C. 20 to 30 D. 35 to 45

Ans. C.

2190. Uremia occurs in

A. Cirrohsis of liver B. Nephritis

C. Diabetes mellitus D. Coronary thrombosis

Ans. B.

2191. Carboxyhemoglobin is formed by

A. CO B. CO2

C. HCO3 D. HCN

Ans. A.

2192. Methemoglobin is formed as a result of the oxidation of haemoglobin by oxidation agent:

A. Oxygen of Air B. H2O2

C. K4Fe(CN)6 D. KMnO4

Ans. C.

2193. Methemoglobin can be reduced to haemoglobin by

A. Removal of hydrogen
B. Vitamin C
C. Glutathione
D. Creatinine

Ans. B.

2194. Fats are solids at

A. 10°C
B. 20°C
C. 30°C
D. 40°C

Ans. B.

2195. Esters of fatty acids with higher alcohol other than glycerol are called as

A. Oils
B. Polyesters
C. Waxes
D. Terpenoids

Ans. C.

2196. The main physiological buffer in the blood is

A. Haemoglobin buffer
B. Acetate
C. Phosphate
D. Bicarbonate

Ans. D.

2197. Urine turbidity may be caused by any of the following except

A. Phosphates
B. Protein
C. RBC
D. WBC

Ans. B.

2198. In obstructive jaundice, urinary bilirubin is

A. Absent
B. Increased
C. Present
D. Present in small amount

Ans. B.

2199. The pH of gastric juice of infants is

A. 2.0
B. 4.0
C. 4.5
D. 5.0

Ans. D.

2200. The pH of blood is about 7.4 when the ratio between ($NaHCO_3$) and (H_2CO_3) is

A. 10 : 1
B. 20 : 1
C. 25 : 1
D. 30 : 1

Ans. B.

2201. The absorption of glucose is decreased by the deficiency of

A. Vitamin A
B. Vitamin D
C. Thiamine
D. Vitamin B12

Ans. C.

2202. Which of the following hormone increases the absorption of glucose from G.I.T?

A. Insulin
B. Thyroid hormones
C. Glucagon
D. FSH

Ans. B.

2203. Predominant form of storage:

A. Carbohydrates
B. Fats
C. Lipids
D. Both (B) and (C)

Ans. D.

2204. Degradations of Hb takes place in

A. Mitochondrion
B. Erythrocytes
C. Cytosol of cell
D. R.E. cells

Ans. D.

2205. Biliverdin is converted to bilirubin by the process of

A. Oxidation
B. Reduction
C. Conjugation
D. Decarboxylation

Ans. B.

2206. Amylase present in saliva is

A. α-Amylase
B. β-Amylase
C. γ -Amylase
D. All of these

Ans. A.

2207. Phospholipids occur in

A. Myelin sheath
B. Chylomicrons
C. Erythrocyte membrane
D. All of these

Ans. D.

2208. The maximum number of double bonds present in essential fatty acid is

A. 2
B. 3
C. 4
D. 5

Ans. C.

2209. Selwanof's test is positive in

A. Glucose
B. Fructose
C. Galactose
D. Mannose

Ans. B.

2210. Spermatozoa in seminal fluid utilizes the following sugar for metabolism:

A. Galactose
B. Glucose
C. Sucrose
D. Fructose

Ans. D.

2211. Acroleic test is given by

A. Cholesterol
B. Glycerol
C. Glycosides
D. Sphingol

Ans. B.

2212. Vitamins are

A. Accessory food factors
B. Generally synthesized in the body
C. Produced in endocrine glands
D. Proteins in nature

Ans. A.

2213. Vitamin A or retinal is a

A. Steroid
B. Polyisoprenoid compound containing a cyclohexenyl ring
C. Benzoquinone derivative
D. 6-Hydroxychromane

Ans. B.

2214. Preformed Vitamin A is supplied by

A. Milk, fat and liver
B. All yellow vegetables
C. All yellow fruits
D. Leafy green vegetables

Ans. A.

2215. Fat soluble vitamins are

A. Soluble in alcohol
B. One or more Propene units
C. Stored in liver
D. All these

Ans. D.

2216. The international unit of vitamin A is equivalent to the activity caused by

A. 0.3 μg of Vitamin A alcohol
B. 0.344 μg of Vitamin A alcohol
C. 0.6 μg of Vitamin A alcohol
D. 1.0 μg of Vitamin A alcohol

Ans. A.

2217. Retinol is transported in blood bound to

A. Aporetinol binding protein B. α2-Globulin

C. β-Globulin D. Albumin

Ans. A.

2218. The normal serum concentration of vitamin A in mg/100 ml is

A. 5–10 B. 15–60

C. 100–150 D. 0–5

Ans. B.

2219. One manifestation of vitamin A deficiency is

A. Painful joints B. Night blindness

C. Loss of hair D. Thickening of long bones

Ans. B.

2220. Deficiency of Vitamin A causes

A. Xeropthalmia B. Hypoprothrombinemia

C. Megaloblastic anemia D. Pernicious anemia

Ans. A.

2221. An important function of vitamin A is

A. To act as coenzyme for a few enzymes

B. To play an integral role in protein synthesis

C. To prevent hemorrhages

D. To maintain the integrity of epithelial tissue

Ans. D.

2222. Carr-Price reaction is used to detect

A. Vitamin A B. Vitamin D

C. Ascorbic acid D. Vitamin E

Ans. A.

2223. Vitamin D absorption is increased in

A. Acid pH of intestine B. Alkaline pH of intestine

C. Impaired fat absorption D. Contents of diet

Ans. A.

2224. The most potent Vitamin D metabolite is

A. 25-Hydroxycholecalciferol B. 1,25-Dihydroxycholecalciferol

C. 24, 25-Dihydroxycholecalciferol D. 7-Dehydrocholesterol

Ans. B.

2225. The normal serum concentration of 1,25-dihydroxycholecalciferol in pg/ml is

A. 26–65
B. 1–5
C. 5–20
D. 80–100

Ans. A.

2226. A poor source of Vitamin D is

A. Egg
B. Butter
C. Milk
D. Liver

Ans. C.

2227. Richest source of Vitamin D is

A. Fish liver oils
B. Margarine
C. Egg yolk
D. Butter

Ans. A.

2228. Deficiency of vitamin D causes

A. Ricket and osteomalacia
B. Tuberculosis of bone
C. Hypthyroidism
D. Skin cancer

Ans. A.

2229. One international unit (I.U) of vitamin D is defined as the biological activity of

A. 0.025 μg of cholecalciferol
B. 0.025 μg of 7-dehydrocholecalciferol
C. 0.025 μg of ergosterol
D. 0.025 μg of ergocalciferol

Ans. A.

2230. The β-ring of 7-dehydrocholesterol is cleaved to form cholecalciferol by

A. Infrared light
B. Dim light
C. Ultraviolet irradiation with sunlight
D. Light of the tube lights

Ans. C.

2231. Insignificant amount of Vitamin E is present in

A. Wheat germ oil
B. Sunflower seed oil
C. Safflower seed oil
D. Fish liver oil

Ans. D.

2232. The activity of tocopherols is destroyed by

A. Commercial cooking
B. Reduction
C. Conjugation
D. All of these

Ans. A.

2233. The requirement of vitamin E is increased with greater intake of

A. Carbohydrates
B. Proteins
C. Polyunsaturated fat
D. Saturated fat

Ans. C.

2234. Vitamin E reduces the requirement of

A. Iron
B. Zinc
C. Selenium
D. Magnesium

Ans. C.

2235. The most important natural antioxidant is

A. Vitamin D
B. Vitamin E
C. Vitamin B12
D. Vitamin K

Ans. B.

2236. Tocopherols prevent the oxidation of

A. Vitamin A
B. Vitamin D
C. Vitamin K
D. Vitamin C

Ans. A.

2237. Creatinuria is caused due to the deficiency of vitamin

A. A
B. K
C. E
D. D

Ans. C.

2238. All the following conditions produce a real or functional deficiency of vitamin K except

A. Prolonged oral, broad spectrum antibiotic therapy
B. Total lack of red meat in the diet
C. The total lack of green leafy vegetables in the diet
D. Being a new born infant

Ans. B.

2239. Vitamin K is found in

A. Green leafy plants
B. Meat
C. Fish
D. Milk

Ans. A.

2240. Function of Vitamin A:

A. Healing epithelial tissues
B. Protein synthesis regulation
C. Cell growth
D. All of these

Ans. D.

2241. Vitamin K2 was originally isolated from

A. Soyabean B. Wheat gram

C. Alfa Alfa D. Putrid fish meal

Ans. D.

2242. Vitamin synthesized by bacteria in the intestine is

A. A B. C

C. D D. K

Ans. D.

2243. Vitamin K is involved in posttranslational modification of the blood clotting factors by acting as cofactor for the enzyme:

A. Carboxylase B. Decarboxylase

C. Hydroxylase D. Oxidase

Ans. A.

2244. Hypervitaminosis K in neonates may cause

A. Porphyria B. Jaundice

C. Pellagra D. Prolonged bleeding

Ans. B.

2245. In the individuals who are given liberal quantities of vitamin C, the serum ascorbic acid level is

A. 1–1.4 μg/100 ml B. 2–4 μg /100 ml

C. 1–10 μg /100 ml D. 10–20 μg /100 ml

Ans. A.

2246. The vitamin which would most likely become deficient in an individual who develop a completely carnivorous life style is

A. Thiamin B. Niacin

C. Vitamin C D. Cobalamin

Ans. C.

2247. In human body highest concentration of ascorbic acid is found in

A. Liver B. Adrenal cortex

C. Adrenal medulla D. Spleen

Ans. B.

2248. The vitamin required for the formation of hydroxyproline (in collagen) is

A. Vitamin C B. Vitamin A

C. Vitamin D D. Vitamin E

Ans. A.

2249. Vitamin required in conversion of folic acid to folinic acid is

A. Biotin B. Cobalamin

C. Ascorbic acid D. Niacin

Ans. C.

2250. Sterilised milk lacks in

A. Vitamin A B. Vitamin D

C. Vitamin C D. Thiamin

Ans. C.

2251. Scurvy is caused due to the deficiency of

A. Vitamin A B. Vitamin D

C. Vitamin K D. Vitamin C

Ans. D.

2252. Both Wernicke's disease and beriberi can be reversed by administrating

A. Retinol B. Thiamine

C. Pyridoxine D. Vitamin B12

Ans. B.

2253. The Vitamin B1 deficiency causes

A. Ricket B. Nyctalopia

C. Beriberi D. Pellagra

Ans. C.

2254. Concentration of pyruvic acid and lactic acid in blood is increased due to deficiency of the vitamin

A. Thiamine B. Riboflavin

C. Niacin D. Pantothenic acid

Ans. A.

2255. Increased glucose consumption increases the dietary requirement for

A. Pyridoxine B. Niacin

C. Biotin D. Thiamine

Ans. D.

2256. Riboflavin is a coenzyme in the reaction catalysed by the enzyme

A. Acyl CoA synthetase B. Acyl CoA dehydrogenase

C. β-Hydroxy acyl CoA D. Enoyl CoA dehydrogenase

Ans. B.

2257. The daily requirement of riboflavin for adult in mg is

A. 0–1.0
B. 1.2–1.7
C. 2.0–3.5
D. 4.0–8.0

Ans. B.

2258. In new born infants phototherapy may cause hyperbilirubinemia with deficiency of

A. Thiamin
B. Riboflavin
C. Ascorbic acid
D. Pantothenic acid

Ans. B.

2259. Riboflavin deficiency causes

A. Cheilosis
B. Loss of weight
C. Mental deterioration
D. Dermatitis

Ans. A.

2260. Magenta tongue is found in the deficiency of the vitamin

A. Riboflavin
B. Thiamin
C. Nicotinic acid
D. Pyridoxine

Ans. A.

2261. Corneal vascularisation is found in deficiency of the vitamin:

A. B1
B. B2
C. B3
D. B6

Ans. B.

2262. Pellagra is caused due to the deficiency of

A. Ascorbic acid
B. Pantothenic acid
C. Pyridoxine
D. Niacin

Ans. D.

2263. Niacin or nicotinic acid is a monocarboxylic acid derivative of

A. Pyridine
B. Pyrimidine
C. Flavin
D. Adenine

Ans. A.

2264. Niacin is synthesized in the body from

A. Tryptophan
B. Tyrosine
C. Glutamate
D. Aspartate

Ans. A.

2265. The proteins present in maize are deficient in

A. Lysine B. Threonine

C. Tryptophan D. Tyrosine

Ans. C.

2266. Niacin is present in maize in the form of

A. Niatin B. Nicotin

C. Niacytin D. Nicyn

Ans. C.

2267. In the body 1 mg of niacin can be produced from

A. 60 mg of pyridoxine B. 60 mg of tryptophan

C. 30 mg of tryptophan D. 30 mg of pantothenic acid

Ans. B.

2268. Dietary requirement of Vitamin D:

A. 400 I.U. B. 1000 I.U.

C. 6000 I.U. D. 700 I.U.

Ans. A.

2269. The Vitamin which does not contain a ring in the structure is

A. Pantothenic acid B. Vitamin D

C. Riboflavin D. Thiamine

Ans. A.

2270. The precursor of CoA is

A. Riboflavin B. Pyridoxamine

C. Thiamine D. Pantothenate

Ans. D.

2271. 'Burning foot syndrome' has been ascribed to the deficiency of

A. Pantothenic acid B. Thiamine

C. Cobalamin D. Pyridoxine

Ans. A.

2272. Vitamin B6 deficiency may occur during therapy with

A. Isoniazid B. Terramycin

C. Sulpha drugs D. Aspirin

Ans. A.

2273. Deficiency of vitamin B6 may occur in

A. Obese person B. Thin person

C. Alcoholics D. Diabetics

Ans. C.

2274. Epileptiform convulsion in human infants have been attributed to the deficiency of the vitamin

A. B1 B. B2

C. B6 D. B12

Ans. C.

2275. The coenzyme required for conversion of pyruvate to oxaloacetate is

A. FAD B. NAD

C. TPP D. Biotin

Ans. D.

2276. Consumption of raw eggs can cause deficiency of

A. Biotin B. Pantothenic acid

C. Riboflavin D. Thiamine

Ans. A.

2277. The central ring structure of Vit B12 consists of

A. Cobalt B. Manganese

C. Magnesium D. Iron

Ans. A.

2278. The central heavy metal cobalt of vitamin B12 is coordinately bound to

A. Cyanide group B. Amino group

C. Carboxyl group D. Sulphide group

Ans. A.

2279. Vitamin B12 has a complex ring structure (corrin ring) consisting of four

A. Purine rings B. Pyrimidine rings

C. Pyrrole rings D. Pteridine rings

Ans. C.

2280. A deficiency of vitamin B12 causes

A. Beri-Beri B. Scurvy

C. Perniciuos anemia D. Ricket

Ans. C.

2281. Vitamin B12 deficiency can be diagnosed by urinary excretion of

A. Pyruvate
B. Methylmalonate
C. Malate
D. Lactate

Ans. B.

2282. Subacute combined degeneration of cord is caused due to deficiency of

A. Niacin
B. Cobalamin
C. Biotin
D. Thiamine

Ans. B.

2283. Sulpha drugs interfere with bacterial synthesis of

A. Lipoate
B. Vitamin E
C. Tetrahydrofolate
D. Ascorbic acid

Ans. C.

2284. Folate deficiency causes

A. Microcytic anemia
B. Hemolytic anemia
C. Iron deficiency anemia
D. Megaloblastic anemia

Ans. D.

2285. Thiamin deficiency includes

A. Mental depression
B. Fatigue
C. Beriberi
D. All of these

Ans. D.

2286. Loss of thiamin can be decreased by using

A. Unpolished rice
B. Parboiled rice
C. Whole wheat flour
D. All of these

Ans. D.

2287. Daily requirement of thiamin is

A. 0.1 mg/1,000 Calories
B. 0.5 mg/1,000 Calories
C. 0.8 mg/1,000 Calories
D. 1.0 mg/1,000 Calories

Ans. B.

2288. Thiamin requirement is greater in

A. Non-vegetarians
B. Alcoholics
C. Pregnant women
D. Both B and C

Ans. D.

2289. People consuming polished rice as their staple food are prone to

A. Beriberi
B. Pellagra
C. Both (A) and (B)
D. None of these

Ans. A.

2290. Riboflavin deficiency can cause

A. Peripheral neuritis
B. Diarrhoea
C. Angular stomatitis
D. None of these

Ans. C.

2291. NAD is required as a coenzyme in

A. Citric acid cycle
B. HMP shunt
C. β-Oxidation of fatty acids
D. Both (A) and (C)

Ans. D.

2292. Daily requirement of niacin is

A. 5 mg
B. 10 mg
C. 20 mg
D. 30 mg

Ans. C.

2293. Niacin deficiency is common in people whose staple food is

A. Wheat
B. Polished rice
C. Maize and /or sorghum
D. None of these

Ans. C.

2294. In pellagra, dermatitis usually affects

A. Exposed parts of body
B. Covered parts of body
C. Trunk only
D. All parts of the body

Ans. A.

2295. Niacin deficiency can occur in

A. Hartnup disease
B. Phenylketonuria
C. Alkaptonuria
D. None of these

Ans. A.

2296. Pantothenic acid contains an amino acid which is

A. Aspartic acid
B. Glutamic acid
C. β-Alanine
D. β-Aminoisobutyric acid

Ans. C.

2297. Coenzyme A contains a nitrogenous base which is

A. Adenine
B. Guanine
C. Choline
D. Ethanolamine

Ans. A.

2298. The following is required for the formation of coenyzme A:

A. ATP
B. GTP
C. CTP
D. None of these

Ans. A.

2299. Deficiency of pantothenic acid in human beings can affect

A. Nervous system
B. Digestive system
C. Both (A) and (B)
D. None of these

Ans. C.

2300. Pyridoxine deficiency can be diagnosed by measuring urinary excretion of

A. Pyruvic acid
B. Oxaloacetic acid
C. Xanthurenic acid
D. None of these

Ans. C.

2301. Pyridoxine deficiency can be diagnosed by measuring the urinary excretion of xanthurenic acid following a test dose of

A. Glycine
B. Histidine
C. Tryptophan
D. Pyridoxine

Ans. C.

2302. Pyridoxine requirement depends upon the intake of

A. Carbohydrates
B. Proteins
C. Fats
D. None of these

Ans. B.

2303. Anti-egg white injury factor is

A. Pyridoxine
B. Biotin
C. Thiamin
D. Lipoic acid

Ans. B.

2304. When eggs are cooked

A. Biotin is destroyed but avidin remains unaffected
B. Avidin is inactivated but biotin remains unaffected
C. Both avidin and biotin are inactivated
D. Both avidin and biotin remain unaffected

Ans. B.

2305. Chemically, lipoic acid is

A. Saturated fatty acid
B. Unsaturated fatty acid
C. Amino acid
D. Sulphur containing fatty acid

Ans. D.

2306. Riboflavin deficiency symptoms are

A. Glossitis
B. Stomatitis
C. Vomitting
D. Both (A) and (B)

Ans. D.

2307. Vitamin B12 forms coenzymes known as

A. Cobamide
B. Transcobalamin I
C. Transcobalamin II
D. Both (B) and (C)

Ans. A.

2308. Absorption of Vitamin B12 requires the presence of

A. Pepsin
B. Hydrochloric acid
C. Intrinsic factor
D. Both (B) and (C)

Ans. D.

2309. Vitamin B12 is

A. Not stored in the body
B. Stored in bone marrow
C. Stored in liver
D. Stored in RE cells

Ans. C.

2310. Vitamin B12 is transported in blood by

A. Albumin
B. Transcortin
C. Transcobalamin I
D. Transcobalamin II

Ans. D.

2311. Vitamin B12 is synthesized by

A. Bacteria only
B. Plants only
C. Animals only
D. Both (A) and (C)

Ans. A.

2312. Deficiency of vitamin B12 can occur because of

A. Decreased intake of vitamin B12
B. Atrophy of gastric mucosa
C. Intestinal malabsorption
D. All of these

Ans. D.

2313. Deficiency of vitamin B12 can be diagnosed by

A. Carr-Price reaction B. Ames assay

C. Watson-Schwartz test D. Schilling test

Ans. D.

2314. Ascorbic acid is required to synthesize all of the following except

A. Collagen B. Bile acids

C. Bile pigments D. Epinephrine

Ans. C.

2315. Vitamin C enhances the intestinal absorption of

A. Potassium B. Iodine

C. Iron D. None of these

Ans. C.

2316. Vitamin C activity is present in

A. D-Ascorbic acid B. D-Dehydroascorbic acid

C. L-Ascorbic acid D. Both A and B

Ans. C.

2317. Deficiency of vitamin C causes

A. Beriberi B. Pellagra

C. Pernicious anaemia D. Scurvy

Ans. D.

2318. An early diagnosis of vitamin C deficiency can be made by

A. Measuring plasma ascorbic acid B. Measuring urinary ascorbic acid

C. Ascorbic acid saturation test D. All of these

Ans. C.

2319. Daily requirement of vitamin C in adults is about

A. 10 mg B. 25 mg

C. 70 mg D. 100 mg

Ans. C.

2320. The vitamin having the highest daily requirement among the following is

A. Thiamine B. Riboflavin

C. Pyridoxine D. Ascorbic acid

Ans. D.

2321. Anaemia can occur due to the deficiency of all the following except

A. Thiamine
B. Pyridoxine
C. Folic acid
D. Cyanocobalamin

Ans. A.

2322. A vitamin which can be synthesized by human beings is

A. Thiamine
B. Niacin
C. Folic acid
D. Cyanocobalamin

Ans. B.

2323. Laboratory diagnosis of vitamin B12 deficiency can be made by measuring the urinary excretion of

A. Xanthurenic acid
B. Formiminoglutamic acid
C. Methylmalonic acid
D. Homogentisic acid

Ans. C.

2324. Precursor of Vitamin A is

A. α-Carotene
B. β-Carotene
C. γ-Carotene
D. All of these

Ans. D.

2325. Two molecules of vitamin A can be formed from 1 molecule of

A. α-Carotene
B. β-Carotene
C. γ-Carotene
D. All of these

Ans. B.

2326. Vitamin A is stored in the body in

A. Liver
B. Adipose tissue
C. Reticuloendothelial cells
D. All of these

Ans. A.

2327. When light falls on rod cells

A. All-cis-retinal is converted into all-trans-retinal
B. 11-cis-retinal is converted into 11-trans-retinal
C. 11-trans-retinal is converted into all-transretinal
D. 11-cis-retinal is converted into all-trans-retinal

Ans. D.

2328. Retinol isomerase is present in

A. Retina
B. Liver
C. Both (A) and (B)
D. None of these

Ans. B.

2329. Anti-oxidant activity is present in

A. β-Carotene
B. Retinol
C. Retinoic acid
D. All of these

Ans. A.

2330. One international Unit of vitamin A is the activity present in

A. 0.3 μg of β-Carotene
B. 0.3 μg of retinol
C. 0.6 μg of retinoic acid
D. All of these

Ans. B.

2331. Daily requirement of vitamin A in an adult man can be expressed as

A. 400 IU
B. 1,000 IU
C. 5,000 IU
D. 10,000 IU

Ans. C.

2332. Vitamin B6 includes

A. Pyridoxal
B. Pyridoxamine
C. Pyridoxine
D. All of these

Ans. D.

2333. An early effect of vitamin A deficiency is

A. Xerophthalmia
B. Keratomalacia
C. Prolonged dark adaptation time
D. Follicular hyperkeratosis

Ans. C.

2334. Nyctalopia is

A. Drying of eyes
B. Destruction of cornea
C. Blindness
D. Inability to see in dim light

Ans. D.

2335. Rod cells possess a trans-membrane protein which is

A. Adenylate cyclase
B. Transducin
C. Rhodopsin
D. B as well as C

Ans. C.

2336. Provitamins A include

A. Retinal
B. Retionic acid
C. Carotenes
D. All of these

Ans. C.

2337. Provitamin D3 is

A. Cholecalciferol B. Ergosterol

C. 7-Dehydrocholesterol D. Ergocaliferol

Ans. C.

2338. Ergosterol is found in

A. Animals B. Plants

C. Bacteria D. All of these

Ans. B.

2339. A provitamin D synthesized in human beings is

A. Ergosterol B. 7-Dehydrocholesterol

C. Cholecalciferol D. 25-Hydroxycholecalciferol

Ans. B.

2340. 25-Hydroxylation of vitamin D occurs in

A. Skin B. Liver

C. Kidneys D. Intestinal mucosa

Ans. B.

2341. Tubular reabsorption of calcium is increased by

A. Cholecalciferol B. 25-Hydroxycholecalciferol

C. Calcitriol D. All of these

Ans. C.

2342. Calcification of soft tissues can occur in

A. Osteomalacia B. Rickets

C. Hypervitaminosis D D. None of these

Ans. C.

2343. Levels of serum calcium and inorganic phosphorus are increased in

A. Hypervitaminosis D B. Hypoparathyroidism

C. Hypovitaminosis D D. None of these

Ans. A.

2344. Requirement of vitamin E increases with the increasing intake of

A. Calories B. Proteins

C. PUFA D. Cholesterol

Ans. C.

2345. A water soluble form of vitamin K is

A. Phylloquinone B. Farnoquinone

C. Menadione D. None of these

Ans. C.

2346. Prothrombin time is prolonged in

A. Vitamin K deficiency B. Liver damage

C. Both (A) and (B) D. None of these

Ans. C.

2347. A synthetic form of vitamin K is

A. Menadione B. Farnoquinone

C. Phylloquinone D. None of these

Ans. A.

2348. Carotenes are transported with the

A. Minerals B. Proteins

C. Lipids D. Lipoproteins

Ans. D.

2349. The percentage of Vitamin A in the form of esters is stored in the liver:

A. 80 B. 85

C. 90 D. 95

Ans. D.

2350. The performed Vitamin A is supplied by foods such as

A. Butter B. Eggs

C. Fish liver oil D. All of these

Ans. D.

2351. The non-protein part of rhodopsin is

A. Retinal B. Retinol

C. Carotene D. Repsin

Ans. A.

2352. The normal concentration of vitamin A in blood in I.U/dl:

A. 20–55 B. 24–60

C. 30–65 D. 35–70

Ans. B.

2353. Continued intake of excessive amounts of vitamin A especially in children produces

A. Irritability B. Anorexia

C. Headache D. All of these

Ans. D.

2354. The poor sources of vitamin D:

A. Eggs B. Butter

C. Milk D. Liver

Ans. C.

2355. The activity of tocopherols is destroyed by

A. Oxidation B. Reduction

C. Conjugation D. All of these

Ans. A.

2356. Vitamin E stored in

A. Mitochondria B. Microsomes

C. Both (A) and (B) D. None of these

Ans. C.

2357. The tocopherols prevent the oxidation of

A. Vitamin A B. Vitamin D

C. Vitamin K D. Vitamin C

Ans. A.

2358. Vitamin E protects enzymes from destruction in

A. Muscles B. Nerves

C. Gonads D. All of these

Ans. D.

2359. Vitamin K regulates the synthesis of blood clotting factors:

A. VII B. IX

C. X D. All of these

Ans. D.

2360. Sterilized milk is devoid of

A. Vitamin A B. Vitamin B1

C. Vitamin C D. Vitamin D

Ans. C.

2361. The symptoms of scurvy are

A. Poor healing of wounds
B. Loosening of teeth
C. Anaemia
D. All of these

Ans. B.

2362. Kwashiorkor results from

A. Vitamin A deficiency
B. Vitamin D deficiency
C. Deficiency of minerals in diet
D. Protein and caloric deficiency in diet

Ans. D.

2363. The number of nutritionally essential amino acids for man is

A. 6
B. 8
C. 10
D. 12

Ans. B.

2364. Avidin is present in

A. Cow's milk
B. Raw egg
C. Green leafy vegetables
D. Carrots

Ans. B.

2365. Marasmus is due to malnutrition of

A. Proteins
B. Proteins and calories
C. Proteins and vitamins
D. Proteins and minerals

Ans. B.

2366. Energy value in kilocalorie per gram of fat in the body is

A. 1
B. 4
C. 9
D. 18

Ans. C.

2367. Which among the following is an essential amino acid for man?

A. Alanine
B. Serine
C. Valine
D. Glutamic acid

Ans. C.

2368. Under what condition to basal metabolic rate goes up?

A. Cold environment
B. Hot environment
C. Intake of base forming foods
D. Hypothyroidism

Ans. A.

2369. What is the major form of caloric storage in human body?

A. ATP
B. Glycogen
C. Creatine phosphate
D. triacylglycerol

Ans. C.

2370. The phosphoprotein of milk is

A. Lactalbumin
B. Lactoglobulin
C. Vitellin
D. Casein

Ans. D.

2371. Dietary deficiency of this vitamin leads to night blindness:

A. Retinol
B. Niacin
C. Ascorbic acid
D. Cholecalciferol

Ans. A.

2372. A non essential amino acid is not

A. Absorbed in the intestines
B. Required in the diet
C. Incorporated into the protein
D. Metabolized by the body

Ans. B.

2373. The deficiency of Vitamin B12 leads to

A. Pernicious anaemia
B. Megaloblastic anaemia
C. Both (A) and (B)
D. None of these

Ans. C.

2374. Which among the following is a nutritionally essential amino acid for man?

A. Alanine
B. Glycine
C. Tyrosine
D. Isoleucine

Ans. D.

2375. The maximum specific dynamic action of food stuff is exerted by

A. Carbohydrates
B. Fats
C. Proteins
D. Vitamins

Ans. C.

2376. The essential amino acids

A. Must be supplied in the diet because the organism has lost the capacity to aminate the corresponding ketoacids
B. Must be supplied in the diet because the human has an impaired ability to synthesize the carbon chain of the corresponding ketoacids
C. Are identical in all species studied
D. Are defined as these amino acids which cannot be synthesized by the organism at a rate adequate to meet metabolic requirements

Ans. B.

2377. Fibre in the diet is beneficial in

A. Hyper glycemia
B. Hyper cholseteremia
C. Colon cancer
D. All of these

Ans. D.

2378. Sucrose intolerance leads to

A. Hyper glycemia
B. Glycosuria
C. Diarrhoea
D. Hypoglycemia

Ans. C.

2379. There can be intolerance with respect to the following sugar:

A. Glucose
B. Lactose
C. Maltose
D. Xylose

Ans. B.

2380. Milk contains very poor amounts of

A. Calcium
B. Phosphate
C. Iron
D. Riboflavin

Ans. C.

2381. Egg contains very little

A. Fat
B. Proteins
C. Carbohydrates
D. Calcium and phosphorus

Ans. C.

2382. BMR (Basal Metabolic rate) is elevated in

A. Hyper thyroidism
B. Under nutrition
C. Starvation
D. Hypothyroidism

Ans. A.

2383. Soyabean proteins are rich in

A. Lysine
B. Alanine
C. Glcyine
D. Aspartic acid

Ans. B.

2384. Corn and gliadin are low in

A. Lysine
B. Alanine
C. Glycine
D. Aspartic acid

Ans. D.

2385. What is the disease caused by thiamine deficiency?

A. Nycalopia B. Scurvy

C. Rickets D. Beriberi

Ans. D.

2386. Retinol and retinol –binding protein (RBP) bound with this protein:

A. Albumin B. Prealbumin

C. α2-globulin D. β-globulin

Ans. B.

2387. This vitamin acts as anti-oxidant:

A. Vitamin A B. Vitamin D

C. Vitamin E D. Vitamin K

Ans. C.

2388. The egg injury factor in raw egg white is

A. Biotin B. Avidin

C. Albumin D. Calcium salts

Ans. B.

2389. The following has cyanide:

A. Vitamin B12 B. Adenyl cobamide

C. Benzimidazole cobamide D. Methyl cobamide

Ans. A.

2390. The human species can biosynthesize

A. Vitamin C B. Vitamin B12

C. Thiamine D. Niacin

Ans. D.

2391. Retina contains this photosensitive pigment:

A. Rhodopsin B. Opsin

C. Retinol D. Melanin

Ans. A.

2392. Anti xerophthalmic vitamin is

A. Vitamin B1 B. Vitamin B2

C. Vitamin B6 D. Vitamin A

Ans. A.

2393. One of the following is not a symptom of addison's disease.

A. Hypoglycemia
B. Hyponatremia
C. Hypokalemia
D. Hypochloremia

Ans. C.

2394. Gammaxane is an antimetabolite of

A. Thiamine
B. Riboflavin
C. Pyridoxin
D. Inositol

Ans. D.

2395. Pyridoxin deficiency may lead to convulsions as it is needed for the synthesis of

A. GABA
B. PABA
C. EFA
D. SAM

Ans. A.

2396. Sulpha drugs are antimetabolities of

A. Vitamin K
B. Pyridoxin
C. Folic acid
D. Vitamin B2

Ans. C.

2397. This abnormal metabolite may be responsible for the neurological manifestation of pernicious anemia:

A. Taurine
B. Methyl malonic acid
C. Xantherunic acid
D. Phenyl pyruvic acid

Ans. A.

2398. The vitamin in leafy vegetables:

A. D
B. K
C. A
D. Both (B) and (C)

Ans. D.

2399. Isonicotinic acid hydrazide given in the treatment of tuberculosis may lead to a deficiency of

A. Vitamin A
B. Pyridoxine
C. Folate
D. Inositol

Ans. B.

2400. Biotin is required for the reaction of CO2 with

A. Water
B. Acetyl CoA
C. NH3
D. Incorporation of carbon 6 in purine

Ans. B.

2401. A deficiency of folate leads to

A. Megaloblastic anemia
B. Aplastic anemia
C. Pernicious anemia
D. Hypochromic microcytic anemia

Ans. B.

2402. A deficiency of Iron leads to

A. Megaloblastic anemia
B. Aplastic anemia
C. Pernicious anemia
D. Hypochromic microcytic anemia

Ans. A.

2403. Vitamin B12 initially binds to the proteins known as

A. Transcobalamin I
B. R-Proteins
C. Transcobalamin II
D. Intrinsic factor of castle

Ans. B.

2404. Extrinsic factor of castle is

A. Vitamin B12
B. Glycoprotein
C. R-Proteins
D. Sigma protein

Ans. B.

2405. Intrinsic factor of castle is

A. Vitamin B12
B. Glycoprotein
C. R-Proteins
D. Sigma protein

Ans. A.

2406. Pernicious means

A. Prolonged
B. Dangerous
C. Intermittent
D. Idiopathic

Ans. B.

2407. Reduction of D-ribonucleotides to D-deoxy ribonucleotides in prokaryotes requires

A. 5, 6 dimethyl benzimidazole cobamide
B. Thioredoxin
C. Tetra hydrobiopterin
D. Tetra hydrofolate

Ans. B.

2408. Biotin is also known as

A. Anti egg white injury factor
B. Rutin
C. Both (A) and (B)
D. None of these

Ans. A.

2409. Prothrombin time is prolonged by administering

A. Vitamin K B. Dicoumarol

C. Calcium D. Prothrombin

Ans. A.

2410. This is a photo-labile vitamin.

A. Thiamine B. Riboflavin

C. Niacin D. Cholecalciferol

Ans. C.

2411. Convulsive episodes occur when there is a severe deficiency of

A. Pyridoxine B. Folic acid

C. Thiamine D. Riboflavin

Ans. B.

2412. Metastatic classification is seen in hypervitaminosis:

A. A B. K

C. D D. E

Ans. A.

2413. Several pantothenic acid deficiency in man has been reported to cause

A. Burning feet syndrome B. Scurvy

C. Cataract D. Xerophthalmia

Ans. C.

2414. Cholesterol is a precursor in the biogenesis of

A. Vitamin A B. Vitamin D

C. Vitamin E D. None of these

Ans. A.

2415. This vitamin is a potent antioxidant of vitamin A:

A. Vitamin C B. Vitamin E

C. Vitamin K D. Vitamin D

Ans. B.

2416. Convulsions and delirium could be caused by a severe deficiency of

A. Thiamine B. Glutamate

C. Niacin D. Magnesium

Ans. D.

2417. Rice polishings contain this vitamin:

A. Riboflavin B. Niacin

C. Thiamine D. Vitamin B12

Ans. D.

2418. In beri beri there will be accumulation of _______ in blood.

A. Aceto acetic acid B. β-OH butyric acid

C. Pyruvic acid D. Methyl malonic acid

Ans. C.

2419. Symptoms of pellagra are

A. Dermatitis and diarrhea only B. Dermatitis and dementia only

C. Diarrhea, dermatitis and dementia D. Diarrhea only

Ans. C.

2420. Pyridoxine deficiency leads to

A. Megaloblastic anemia B. Aplastic anemia

C. Hypochromic microcytic anemia D. Permicious anemia

Ans. C.

2421. Irradiation of foods raises the content of

A. Vitamin A B. Vitamin D

C. Vitamin E D. Vitamin K

Ans. C.

2422. An anti-vitamin for folic acid is

A. Amethoptesin B. Dicoumarol

C. Pyrithoamine D. Isoniazid

Ans. A.

2423. Thymine is

A. Water soluble vitamin B. Fat soluble vitamin

C. Purine base D. Pyrimidine base

Ans. D.

2424. The sulphur-containing vitamins among the following B-Vitamin is

A. Thiamine B. Riboflavin

C. Niacin D. Pyridoxine

Ans. A.

2425. Taurinuria may be encountered in

A. Permicious anemia
B. Beriberi
C. Pellegra
D. Folate deficiency

Ans. A.

2426. The three vitamins which are specially required for proper nerve functions are acid:

A. Thiamine, niacin and riboflavin
B. Thiamine, folic acid, choline
C. Thiamine, riboflavin, patothenic acid
D. Thiamine, pyridoxin, vitamin B12

Ans. D.

2427. This is a rich source for vitamin C.

A. Rice
B. Milk
C. Egg
D. Lemon

Ans. D.

2428. Antisterility vitamin is

A. Vitamin B1
B. Vitamin B2
C. Vitamin E
D. Vitamin K

Ans. C.

2429. All the following vitamins give rise to cofactors that are phosphorylated in the active form except

A. Vitamin A
B. Vitamin B1
C. Vitamin D
D. Vitamin E

Ans. B.

2430. Molecular Iron, Fe, is

A. Stored in the body in combination with Ferritin
B. Stored primarily in the spleen
C. Excreted in the urine as Fe2+
D. absorbed in the intestine by albumin

Ans. A.

2431. Humans most easily tolerate a lack of which of the following nutrients?

A. Protein
B. Iodine
C. Carbohydrate
D. Lipid

Ans. C.

2432. A deficiency of vitamin B12 causes

A. Cheliosis B. Beriberi

C. Pernicious anemia D. Scurvy

Ans. C.

2433. In adults a severe deficiency of vitamin D causes

A. Night blindness B. Osteomalacia

C. Rickets D. Skin cancer

Ans. B.

2434. Which of the following vitamins would most likely become deficient in a person who develops a completely carnivorous life style?

A. Thiamine B. Niacin

C. Cobalamine D. Vitamin C

Ans. D.

2435. Which of the following statements regarding Vitamin A is true?

A. It is not an essential Vitamin B. It is related to tocopherol

C. It is a component of rhodopsin D. It is also known as Opsin

Ans. C.

2436. Biotin is involved in which of the following types of reactions?

A. Hydroxylation B. Carboxylation

C. Decarboxylation D. Deamination

Ans. B.

2437. Which of the following vitamins is the precursor of CoA?

A. Riboflavin B. Pantothenate

C. Thiamine D. Cobamide

Ans. B.

2438. Vitamins that function as dinucleotide derivatives include all the following except

A. Thiamine B. Niacin

C. Nicotinate D. Vitamin B2

Ans. A.

2439. What is the disease caused by thiamine deficiency?

A. Nyctalopia B. Scurvy

C. Rickets D. Beriberi

Ans. D.

2440. Retinol and Retinol binding protein are bound with this protein:

A. Albumin | B. Prealbumin
C. α-globulin | D. β-globulin

Ans. B.

2441. Megaloblastic anemia is caused by the deficiency of

A. Folic acid | B. Vitamin B6
C. Iron | D. Protein

Ans. A.

2442. The human species can biosynthesize

A. Vitamin C | B. Vitamin B12
C. Thiamine | D. Niacin

Ans. D.

2443. Retina contains this photo sensitive pigment.

A. Rhodopsin | B. Opsin
C. Retinol | D. Malanin

Ans. A.

2444. Antixerophthalmic vitamin is

A. Vitamin B1 | B. Vitamin B2
C. Vitamin B6 | D. Vitamin A

Ans. D.

2445. Sulpha drugs are antimetabolites of

A. PABA | B. Pyridoxin
C. Vitamin B2 | D. Pantothenic acid

Ans. A.

2446. This abnormal metabolite may be responsible for the neurological manifestation of pernicious anemia.

A. Taurine | B. Methyl malonic acid
C. Xanthurenic acid | D. Phenyl pyruvic acid

Ans. B.

2447. Choline is not required for the formation of

A. Lecithins | B. Acetyl choline
C. Sphingomyelin | D. Cholic acid

Ans. D.

2448. Isonicotinic acid hydrazide given in the treatment of tuberculosis may lead to a deficiency of

A. Vitamin A
B. Pyridoxine
C. Folate
D. Inositol

Ans. B.

2449. Steroidal prohormone is

A. Vitamin A
B. Vitamin C
C. Vitamin D
D. None of these

Ans. C.

2450. Deficiency of Iron leads to

A. Megaloblastic anemia
B. Aplastic anemia
C. Pernicious anemia
D. Hypochromic microcytic anemia

Ans. D.

2451. Corrinoid coenzymes are coenzymes of

A. Vitamin B6
B. Vitamin B12
C. Vitamin B2
D. Vitamin B1

Ans. B.

2452. Extrinsic factor of castle is

A. Vitamin B12
B. Glycoprotein
C. R-proteins
D. Sigma protein

Ans. A.

2453. Intrinsic factor of castle is

A. Vitamin B12
B. Glycoprotein
C. R-proteins
D. Sigma protein

Ans. B.

2454. Angular stomatitis is due to

A. Ariboflavinosis
B. Deficiency of Vitamin C
C. Deficiency of Vitamin B1
D. Deficiency of folate

Ans. A.

2455. Prothrombin time is prolonged by administering

A. Vitamin K
B. Dicoumarol
C. Calcium
D. Prothrombin

Ans. B.

2456. Cholesterol is a precursor in the biogenesis of

A. Vitamin A
B. Vitamin D
C. Vitamin E
D. None of these

Ans. B.

2457. Rice-polishing contain which of the following Vitamin?

A. Riboflavin
B. Niacin
C. Thiamine
D. Vitamin B12

Ans. C.

2458. The significant ocular lesion in a riboflavinosis is

A. Keratomalacia
B. Bitot's spots
C. Vascularisation of the cornea
D. Lachrynal metaplasia

Ans. C.

2459. An anti-vitamin for folic acid is

A. Aminopterin
B. Dicoumarol
C. Pyrithiamine
D. Isoniazid

Ans. A.

2460. The vitamin that is useful in cancer is

A. A
B. B complex
C. C
D. E

Ans. A.

2461. Vitamin A over dosage causes injury to

A. Mitochondria
B. Microtubules
C. Lysosomes
D. E.R

Ans. C.

2462. The vitamin required for carboxylation reaction is

A. Vitamin B2
B. Vitamin B6
C. Biotin
D. Vitamin B12

Ans. C.

2463. Biological activity of tocopherols has been attributed in part to their action as

A. Antioxidant
B. Anticoagulants
C. Provitamin
D. Carriers in electron transport system

Ans. B.

2464. Which of the following vitamin act as a respiratory catalyst?

A. B2
B. Pyridoxine
C. B12
D. C

Ans. A.

2465. Whole wheat is an excellent source of

A. Vitamin D
B. Vitamin C
C. Vitamin A
D. Thiamine

Ans. D.

2466. The most active form of Vitamin D is

A. 25-Hydroxycholecalciferol
B. 1, 25-dihydroxycholecalciferol
C. 25-dihydroxyergocalciferol
D. None of these

Ans. A.

2467. The conversion of carotenoids to Vitamin A takes place in

A. Intestine
B. Liver
C. Kidney
D. Skin

Ans. A.

2468. Excessive vitamin A in children produces

A. Irritability
B. Anorexia
C. Headache
D. All of these

Ans. D.

2469. Tocopherols prevent the oxidation of

A. Vitamin A
B. Vitamin D
C. Vitamin K
D. Vitamin C

Ans. A.

2470. Vitamin K regulates the synthesis of blood clotting factors.

A. VII
B. IX
C. X
D. All of these

Ans. D.

2471. The colour of cyanomethemoglobin is

A. Pale yellow
B. Pink
C. Brown
D. Bright red

Ans. D.

2472. Vitamin K2 was originally isolated from

A. Soyabean
B. Putrid fishmeal
C. Alfa alfa
D. Oysters

Ans. B.

2473. Increased carbohydrate consumption increases the dietary requirement for

A. Thiamine
B. Riboflavin
C. Pyridoxine
D. Folic acid

Ans. A.

2474. Increased protein intake is accompanied by an increased dietary requirement for

A. Thiamine
B. Riboflavin
C. Folic acid
D. Nicotininic acid

Ans. A.

2475. The deficiency of which one of the following vitamin causes creatinuria?

A. Vitamin E
B. Vitamin K
C. Vitamin A
D. Vitamin B6

Ans. A.

2476. Non steroidal anti inflammatory drugs, such as aspirin act by inhibiting the activity of the enzyme:

A. Lipoxygenase
B. Cyclooxygenase
C. Phospholipase A2
D. Lipoprotein lipase

Ans. B.

2477. A Holoenzyme is

A. Functional unit
B. Apo enzyme
C. Coenzyme
D. All of these

Ans. D.

2478. Gaucher's disease is due to the deficiency of the enzyme:

A. α-Fucosidase
B. β-Galactosidase
C. β-Glucosidase
D. Sphingomyelinase

Ans. C.

2479. Neimann-Pick disease is due to the deficiency of the enzyme:

A. Hexosaminidase A and B
B. Ceramidase
C. Ceramide lactosidase
D. Sphingomyelinase

Ans. D.

2480. Krabbe's disease is due to the deficiency of the enzyme:

A. Ceramide lactosidase
B. Ceramidase
C. β-Galactosidase
D. GM1 β-Galactosidase

Ans. C.

2481. Fabry's disease is due to the deficiency of the enzyme:

A. Ceramide trihexosidase
B. Galactocerebrosidase
C. Phytanic acid oxidase
D. Sphingomyelinase

Ans. A.

2482. Farber's disease is due to the deficiency of the enzyme:

A. α-Galactosidase
B. Ceramidase
C. β-Glucocerebrosidase
D. Arylsulphatase A

Ans. B.

2483. A synthetic nucleotide analogue, used in organ transplantation as a suppressor of immunologic rejection of grafts is

A. Theophylline
B. Cytarabine
C. 4-Hydroxypyrazolopyrimidine
D. 6-Mercaptopurine

Ans. D.

2484. Example of an extracellular enzyme is

A. Lactate dehydrogenase
B. Cytochrome oxidase
C. Pancreatic lipase
D. Hexokinase

Ans. C.

2485. Enzymes, which are produced in inactive form in the living cells, are called

A. Papain
B. Lysozymes
C. Apoenzymes
D. Proenzymes

Ans. D.

2486. An example of lyases is

A. Glutamine synthetase
B. Fumarase
C. Cholinesterase
D. Amylase

Ans. B.

2487. Activation or inactivation of certain key regulatory enzymes is accomplished by covalent modification of the amino acid:

A. Tyrosine
B. Phenylalanine
C. Lysine
D. Serine

Ans. D.

2488. The enzyme which can add water to a carbon-carbon double bond or remove water to create a double bond without breaking the bond is

A. Hydratase
B. Hydroxylase
C. Hydrolase
D. Esterase

Ans. A.

2489. Fischer's 'lock and key' model of the enzyme action implies that

A. The active site is complementary in shape to that of substance only after interaction.
B. The active site is complementary in shape to that of substance
C. Substrates change conformation prior to active site interaction
D. The active site is flexible and adjusts to Substrate

Ans. B.

2490. An inducer is absent in the type of enzyme:

A. Allosteric enzyme
B. Constitutive enzyme
C. Co-operative enzyme
D. Isoenzymic enzyme

Ans. B.

2491. A demonstrable inducer is absent in

A. Allosteric enzyme
B. Constitutive enzyme
C. Inhibited enzyme
D. Co-operative enzyme

Ans. B.

2492. Enzyme involved in joining together two substrates is

A. Glutamine synthetase
B. Aldolase
C. Gunaine deaminase
D. Arginase

Ans. A.

2493. The pH optima of most of the enzymes is

A. Between 2 and 4
B. Between 5 and 9
C. Between 8 and 12
D. Above 12

Ans. B.

2494. Coenzymes are

A. Heat stable, dialyzable, non protein organic molecules
B. Soluble, colloidal, protein molecules
C. Structural analogue of enzymes
D. Different forms of enzymes

Ans. A.

2495. Isoenzymes are

A. Chemically, immunologically and electrophoretically different forms of an enzyme

B. Different forms of an enzyme similar in all properties

C. Catalysing different reactions

D. Having the same quaternary structures like the enzymes

Ans. A.

2496. Isoenzymes can be characterized by

A. Proteins lacking enzymatic activity that are necessary for the activation of enzymes

B. Proteolytic enzymes activated by hydrolysis

C. Enzymes with identical primary structure

D. Similar enzymes that catalyse different reaction

Ans. B.

2497. Factors affecting enzyme activity:

A. Concentration
B. pH
C. Temperature
D. All of these

Ans. D.

2498. Serum acid phosphatase level increases in

A. Metastatic carcinoma of prostate
B. Myocardial infarction
C. Wilson's disease
D. Liver diseases

Ans. A.

2499. Serum alkaline phosphatase level increases in

A. Hypothyroidism
B. Carcinoma of prostate
C. Hyperparathyroidism
D. Myocardial ischemia

Ans. C.

2500. Serum lipase level increases in

A. Paget's disease
B. Gaucher's disease
C. Acute pancreatitis
D. Diabetes mellitus

Ans. C.

2501. Serum ferroxidase level decreases in

A. Gaucher's disease
B. Cirrhosis of liver
C. Acute pancreatitis
D. Wilson's disease

Ans. D.

2502. The isoenzymes LDH5 is elevated in

A. Myocardial infarction
B. Peptic ulcer
C. Liver disease
D. Infectious diseases

Ans. C.

2503. On the third day of onset of acute myocardial infarction the enzyme elevated is

A. Serum AST
B. Serum CK
C. Serum LDH
D. Serum ALT

Ans. C.

2504. LDH1 and LDH2 are elevated in

A. Myocardial infarction
B. Liver disease
C. Kidney disease
D. Brain disease

Ans. A.

2505. In acute pancreatitis, the enzyme raised in first five days is

A. Serum amylase
B. Serum lactic dehydrogenase
C. Urinary lipase
D. Urinary amylase

Ans. A.

2506. Acute pancreatitis is characterized by

A. Lack of synthesis of zymogen enzymes
B. Continuous release of zymogen enzymes into the gut
C. Premature activation of zymogen enzymes
D. Inactivation of zymogen enzymes

Ans. C.

2507. The pH optima for sucrase is

A. 5.0–7.0
B. 5.8–6.2
C. 5.4–6.0
D. 8.6

Ans. A.

2508. The pH optima for maltase is

A. 1.0–2.0
B. 5.2–6.0
C. 5.8–6.2
D. 5.4–6.0

Ans. C.

2509. The pH optima for lactase is

A. 1.0-2.0
B. 5.4–6.0
C. 5.0–7.0
D. 5.8–6.2

Ans. B.

2510. The substrate for amylase is

A. Cane sugar
B. Starch
C. Lactose
D. Ribose

Ans. B.

2511. The ion which activates salivary amylase activity is

A. Chloride
B. Bicarbonate
C. Sodium
D. Potassium

Ans. A.

2512. The pancreatic amylase activity is increased in the presence of

A. Hydrochloric acid
B. Bile salts
C. Thiocyanate ions
D. Calcium ions

Ans. B.

2513. A carbohydrate which can not be digested in human gut is

A. Cellulose
B. Starch
C. Glycogen
D. Maltose

Ans. A.

2514. In the intestine the rate of absorption is highest for

A. Glucose and galactose
B. Fructose and mannose
C. Fructose and pentose
D. Mannose and pentose

Ans. A.

2515. Glucose absorption is promoted by

A. Vitamin A
B. Thiamine
C. Vitamin C
D. Vitamin K

Ans. B.

2516. The hormone acting directly on intestinal mucosa and stimulating glucose absorption is

A. Insulin
B. Glucagon
C. Thyroxine
D. Vasopressin

Ans. C.

2517. Erythrocytes under normal conditions and microorganisms under anaerobic conditions may accumulate

A. NADPH
B. Pyruvate
C. Phosphoenolpyruvate
D. Lactate

Ans. D.

2518. Hexokinase is inhibited in an allosteric manner by

A. Glucose-6-Phosphate
B. Glucose-1-Phosphate
C. Fructose-6-phosphate
D. Fructose-1, 6-biphosphate

Ans. A.

2519. The net number of ATP formed per mole of glucose in anaerobic glycolysis is

A. 1
B. 2
C. 6
D. 8

Ans. B.

2520. Pyruvate dehydrogenase a multienzyme complex is required for the production of

A. Acetyl-CoA
B. Lactate
C. Phosphoenolpyruvate
D. Enolpyruvate

Ans. A.

2521. Dietary deficiency of thiamine inhibits the activity of the enzyme:

A. Pyruvate kinase
B. Pyruvate dehydrogenase
C. Phosphofructokinase
D. Enolase

Ans. B.

2522. Pyruvate dehydrogenase activity is inhibited by

A. Mercury
B. Zinc
C. Calcium
D. Sodium

Ans. A.

2523. In the normal resting state of humans, most of the blood glucose burned as fuel is consumed by

A. Liver
B. Adipose tissue
C. Muscle
D. Brain

Ans. A.

2524. All the enzymes of glycolysis pathway are found in

A. Extramitochondrial soluble fraction of the cell
B. Mitochondria
C. Nucleus
D. Endoplasmic reticulum

Ans. A.

2525. Most major metabolic pathways are considered mainly either anabolic or catabolic. Which of the following pathway is most correctly considered to be amphibolic?

A. Citric acid cycle
B. Gluconeogenesis
C. Lipolysis
D. Glycolysis

Ans. A.

2526. The enzymes of the citric acid cycle are located in

A. Mitochondrial matrix

B. Extramitochondrial soluble fraction of the cell

C. Nucleus

D. Endoplasmic reticulum

Ans. A.

2527. The substance which may be considered to play a catalytic role in citric acid cycle is

A. Oxaloacetate B. Isocitrate

C. Malate D. Fumarate

Ans. A.

2528. The number of ATP molecules generated for each turn of the citric acid cycle is

A. 8 B. 12

C. 24 D. 38

Ans. B.

2529. Oxidation of one molecule of glucose yields

A. 12 ATP B. 24 ATP

C. 38 ATP D. 38 ATP

Ans. D.

2530. Which of the following intermediates of metabolism can be both a precursor and a product of glucose?

A. Lactate B. Pyruvate

C. Alanine D. Acetyl-CoA

Ans. A.

2531. Mitochondrial membrane is freely preamble to

A. Pyruvate B. Malate

C. Oxaloacetate D. Fumarate

Ans. B.

2532. The glycogen content of the liver is upto

A. 6% B. 8%

C. 10% D. 12%

Ans. A.

2533. Action of glycogen synthase is inhibited by

A. Insulin B. Glucose

C. $Mg2+$ D. Cyclic AMP

Ans. C.

2534. The hormone activating the glycogen synthase activity is

A. Insulin B. Glucagon

C. Epinephrine D. ACTH

Ans. A.

2535. Cori disease (Limit dextrinosis) is caused due to absence of

A. Branching enzyme B. Debranching enzyme

C. Glycogen synthase D. Phosphorylase

Ans. B.

2536. Pompe's disease is caused due to deficiency of

A. Lysosomal α-1$\rightarrow$4 and 1$\rightarrow$6-glucosidase

B. Glucose-6-phosphatase

C. Glycogen synthase

D. Phosphofructokinase

Ans. A.

2537. Amylopectinosis is caused due to absence of

A. Debranching enzyme B. Branching enzyme

C. Acid maltase D. Glucose-6-phosphatase

Ans. B.

2538. Her's disease is characterized by deficiency of

A. Muscle phosphorylase B. Liver phosphorylase

C. Debranching enzyme D. Glycogen synthase

Ans. B.

2539. Tarui disease is characterized by the deficiency of the enzyme:

A. Liver phosphorylase

B. Muscle phosphorylase

C. Muscle and erythrocyte phosphofructokinase

D. Lysosomal acid maltase

Ans. C.

2540. The enzymes of the pentose phosphate pathway are found in the

A. Cytosol B. Mitochondria

C. Nucleus D. Endoplasmic reticulum

Ans. A.

2541. The pentose phosphate pathway protects erythrocytes against hemolysis by assisting the enzyme:

A. Superoxide dismutase B. Catalase

C. Glutathionic peroxidase D. Cytochrome oxidase

Ans. C.

2542. Hemolytic anemia is caused by the deficiency of certain enzymes of the pentose phosphate pathway, the principal enzyme involved is

A. Glucose-6-phosphate dehydrogenase

B. Aldolase

C. Fructose 1, 6-bisphosphatase

D. Phosphohexose isomerase

Ans. A.

2543. The sites for gluconeogenesis are

A. Liver and kidney B. Skin and pancreas

C. Lung and brain D. Intestine and lens of eye

Ans. A.

2544. An enzyme involved in gluconeogenesis is

A. Pyruvate kinase B. Pyruvate carboxylase

C. Hexokinase D. Phosphohexose isomerase

Ans. B.

2545. The enzyme pyruvate carboxylase is present in

A. Cytosol B. Mitochondria

C. Nucleus D. Golgi bodies

Ans. B.

2546. The enzyme glucose 6-phosphatase is present in

A. Liver B. Muscle

C. Adipose tissue D. Brain

Ans. A.

2547. The number of ATP molecules required to convert 2 molecules of lactate into glucose in mammalian liver is

A. 2 B. 4

C. 5 D. 6

Ans. D.

2548. Pentosuria is a rare hereditary disease is characterized by increased urinary excretion of

A. L-xylulose B. Xylitol

C. Xylulose 5-phosphate D. Ribose 5-phosphate

Ans. A.

2549. Galactose is synthesized from glucose in

A. Mammary gland B. Intestine

C. Kidney D. Adipose tissue

Ans. A.

2550. Galactose is readily converted to glucose in

A. Liver B. Intestine

C. Kidney D. Adipose tissue

Ans. A.

2551. Insulin has no effect on the activity of the enzyme:

A. Glycogen synthetase B. Fructokinase

C. Pyruvate kinase D. Pyruvate dehydrogenase

Ans. B.

2552. The pathogenesis of diabetic cataract involves accumulation of

A. Galactose B. Mannitol

C. Sorbitol D. Pyruvate

Ans. C.

2553. Hereditary fructose intolerance involves the absence of the enzyme:

A. Aldalose B B. Fructokinase

C. Triokinase D. Phosphotriose isomerase

Ans. A.

2554. Essential fructosuria is characterized by the lack of the hepatic enzyme:

A. Phosphohexose isomerase B. Aldalose A

C. Aldolase B D. Fructokinase

Ans. D.

2555. In normal individuals glycosuria occurs when the venous blood glucose concentration exceeds

A. 5–6 mmol/L
B. 7–8 mmol/L
C. 8.5–9 mmol/L
D. 9.5–10 mmol/L

Ans. D.

2556. Phlorizin inhibits

A. Renal tubular reabsorption of glucose
B. Glycolysis
C. Gluconeogenesis
D. Glycogenolysis

Ans. A.

2557. Renal glycosuria is characterized by

A. Hyperglycemia
B. Hyperglycemia with glycosuria
C. Normal blood glucose level with glycosuria
D. Hyperglycemia with ketosis

Ans. C.

2558. Acute hemolytic episode after administration of antimalarial, primaquin, is due to deficiency of the enzyme:

A. 6-Phosphogluconate dehydrogenase
B. Glucose-6-phosphate dehydrogenase
C. Epimerase
D. Transketolase

Ans. B.

2559. The pH optima of gastric lipase is

A. 3.0–6.0
B. 1.0–2.0
C. 8.0
D. 8.6

Ans. A.

2560. The optimum pH of pancreatic lipase is

A. 2.0
B. 4.0
C. 6.0
D. 8.0

Ans. C.

2561. ω-oxidation is normally a very minor pathway and is brought by hydroxylase enzymes involving

A. Cytochrome A
B. Cytochrome B
C. Cytochrome C
D. Cytochrome P-450

Ans. C.

2562. α-Oxidation i.e., the removal of one carbon at a time from the carboxyl end of the molecule has been detected in

A. Brain tissue
B. Liver
C. Adipose tissue
D. Intestine

Ans. A.

2563. The concentration of ketone bodies in the blood does not normally exceed

A. 0.2 mmol/L
B. 0.4 mmol/L
C. 1 mmol/L
D. 2 mmol/L

Ans. A.

2564. In humans under normal conditions loss of ketone bodies via urine is usually less than

A. 1 mg/24 hr
B. 4 mg/24 hr
C. 8 mg/24 hr
D. 10 mg/24 hr

Ans. A.

2565. The structure which appears to be the only organ to add significant quantities of ketone bodies to the blood is

A. Brain
B. Erythrocytes
C. Liver
D. Skeletal muscle

Ans. C.

2566. The starting material for ketogenesis is

A. Acyl-CoA
B. Acetyl-CoA
C. Acetoacetyl-CoA
D. Malonyl-CoA

Ans. C.

2567. Enzymes responsible for ketone body formation are associated mainly with the

A. Mitochondria
B. Endoplasmic reticulum
C. Nucleus
D. Golgi apparatus

Ans. A.

2568. Ketone bodies serve as a fuel for

A. Extrahepatic tissues
B. Hepatic tissues
C. Erythrocytes
D. Mitochondria

Ans. A.

2569. Ketosis reflects

A. Increased hepatic glucose liberation

B. Increased fatty acid oxidation

C. Increased carbohydrate utilisation

D. Incresed gluconeogenesis

Ans. B.

2570. Ketosis is associated with the disease:

A. Nephritis
B. Diabetes mellitus
C. Edema
D. Coronary artery diseases

Ans. B.

2571. The main pathway for denovo synthesis of fatty acids occur in

A. Cytosol
B. Mitochondria
C. Microsomes
D. Nucleus

Ans. A.

2572. Chain elongation of fatty acids in mammalian liver occurs in

A. Nucleus
B. Ribosomes
C. Lysosomes
D. Microsomes

Ans. D.

2573. The fatty acid synthase complex catalyses

A. 4 sequential enzymatic steps
B. 6 sequential enzymatic steps
C. 7 sequential enzymatic steps
D. 8 sequential enzymatic steps

Ans. B.

2574. In fatty acids synthase of both bacteria and mammals, ACP (acyl carrier protein) contain the vitamin:

A. Thiamin
B. Pyridoxine
C. Riboflavin
D. Pantothenic acid

Ans. D.

2575. The glycerol for fatty acid esterification in adipocytes is

A. For the most part, derived from glucose

B. Obtained primarily from phosphorylation of glycerol by glycerol kinase

C. Formed from gluconeogenesis

D. Formed from glycogenolysis

Ans. A.

2576. The desaturation and chain elongation system of polyunsaturated fatty acid are enhanced by

A. Insulin B. Glucagon

C. Epinephrine D. Thyroxine

Ans. A.

2577. Higher rate of lipogenesis is associated with

A. High proportion of carbohydrate in diet

B. Restricted caloric intake

C. High fat diet

D. Deficiency of insulin

Ans. A.

2578. Brown adipose tissue is

A. Prominent tissue in human

B. Characterised by high content of mitochondria

C. Associated with high activity of ATP synthase

D. Characterised by low content of cytochromes

Ans. B.

2579. Fatty liver is caused due to accumulation of

A. Fatty acids B. Cholesterol

C. Phospholipids D. Triacylglycerol

Ans. D.

2580. A lipotropic factor is

A. Choline B. Palmitic acid

C. Calcium D. Vitamin C

Ans. A.

2581. Fatty liver is also caused by

A. CH3Cl B. CCl4

C. Na2SO4 D. Riboflavin

Ans. B.

2582. All the enzymes involved in the synthesis of cholesterol are found in

A. Mitochondria B. Golgi apparatus

C. Nucleus D. Endoplasmic reticulum and cytosol

Ans. D.

2583. Hypolipidemic drugs reduce serum cholesterol and triacylglycerol. The effect of clofibrate is attributed to

A. Block in absorption from G.I.T.

B. Decrease in secretion of triacylglycerol and cholesterol containing VLDL by liver

C. Block in the reabsorption of bile acids

D. Decreased synthesis of cholesterol

Ans. B.

2584. The principal sterol excreted in feces is

A. Coprostanol B. Zymosterol

C. Lanosterol D. Desmosterol

Ans. A.

2585. Hypercholesterolemia is found in

A. Xanthomatosis B. Thyrotoxicosis

C. Hemolytic jaundice D. Malabsorption syndrome

Ans. A.

2586. Hypocholesterolemia is found in

A. Thyrotoxicosis B. Diabetes mellitus

C. Obstructive jaundice D. Nephrotic syndrome

Ans. A.

2587. The major source of extracellular cholesterol for human tissue is

A. Very low density lipoprotein B. High density lipoprotein

C. Low density lipoprotein D. Albumin

Ans. C.

2588. Correct ordering of lipoprotein molecules from lowest to the greater density is

A. LDL, IDL, VLDL, chylomicron B. Chylomicron, VLDL, IDL, LDL

C. VLDL, IDL, LDL, chylomicron D. LDL, VLDL, IDL, chylomicron

Ans. B.

2589. In Hurler's syndrome, urine shows the presence of

A. Keratan sulphate I

B. Chondroitin sulphate

C. Dermatan sulphate and heparan sulphate

D. Keratan sulphate II

Ans. D.

2590. Defective enzyme in Hunter's syndrome is

A. α-L-iduronidase
B. Iduronate sulphatase
C. Arylsulphatase B
D. C-acetyl transferase

Ans. B.

2591. In Hunter's syndrome

A. There is progressive corneal opacity
B. Keratan sulphate is excreted in the urine
C. Enzyme defective is arylsulphatase B
D. Hearing loss is perceptive

Ans. D.

2592. An important feature of Von-Gierke's disease is

A. Muscle cramps
B. Cardiac failure
C. Hypoglycemia
D. Respiratory alkalosis

Ans. C.

2593. The affected organ in Mc Ardle's syndrome is

A. Liver
B. Kidney
C. Liver and Heart
D. Skeletal muscle

Ans. D.

2594. Refsum's disease is due to deficiency of the enzyme:

A. Pytantate-α-oxidase
B. Glucocerebrosidase
C. Galactocerebrosidase
D. Ceramide trihexosidase

Ans. A.

2595. An important finding in Refsum's disease is

A. Accumulation of ceramide trihexoside in the kidney
B. Accumulation of phytanic acid in the blood and tissues
C. Accumulation of gangliosides in brain and spleen
D. Skin eruptions

Ans. B.

2596. α-Galactosidase enzyme is defective in

A. Tay-sach's disease
B. Refsum's disease
C. Sandhoff's disease
D. Fabry's disease

Ans. D.

2597. An important finding in Tay-sach's disease is

A. Renal failure

B. Accumulation of gangliosides in brain and spleen

C. Cardiac failure

D. Anemia

Ans. B.

2598. The enzyme deficient in Krabbe's disease is

A. Hexosaminidase A
B. Arylsuphatase A
C. β-Galactosidase
D. α-Fucosidase

Ans. C.

2599. The enzyme ceramidase is deficient in

A. Farber's disease
B. Fabry's disease
C. Sandhoff's disease
D. Refsum's disease

Ans. A.

2600. Niemann-Pick disease is due to deficiency of the enzyme

A. Ceramidase
B. Glucocerebrosidase
C. Galactocerebrosidase
D. Sphingomyelinase

Ans. D.

2601. Wolman's disease is due to deficiency of

A. Cholesteryl ester hydrolase
B. Hexosaminidase A
C. α-Fucosidase
D. Arylsulphatase A

Ans. A.

2602. The enzyme deficient in Sandhoff's disease is

A. α-Fucosidase
B. Hexosaminidase A and B
C. β-Galactosidase
D. β-Glucosidase

Ans. B.

2603. Jamaican vomiting sickness is due to inactivation of the enzyme

A. Pyruvate carboxylase
B. Acyl-Co-A synthetase
C. Acyl-Co-A dehydrogense
D. Thiolase

Ans. C.

2604. Zellweger's syndrome is due to inherited absence of

A. Peroxisomes
B. Phospholipase A1
C. Acyl-Co-A dehydrogenase
D. Thiolase

Ans. A.

2605. Bassen-Kornzweig syndrome is due to

A. Absence of Apo-C-II
B. Defect in Apo-B synthesis
C. Absence of Apo-E
D. Absence of Apo-D

Ans. B.

2606. Albinism is due to deficiency of the enzyme:

A. Phenylalanine hydroxylase
B. Tyrosinase
C. p-Hydroxyphenylpyruvic acid oxidase
D. Tyrosine dehydrogenase

Ans. C.

2607. Which of the following is a substrate specific enzyme?

A. Hexokinase
B. Thiokinase
C. Lactase
D. Aminopeptidase

Ans. C.

2608. Coenzymes combine with

A. Proenzymes
B. Apoenzymes
C. Holoenzymes
D. Antienzymes

Ans. B.

2609. Coenzyme A contains a vitamin which is

A. Thiamin
B. Ascorbic acid
C. Pantothenic acid
D. Niacinamide

Ans. C.

2610. A coenzyme required in carboxylation reactions is

A. Lipoic acid
B. Coenzyme A
C. Biotin
D. All of these

Ans. C.

2611. Which of the following coenzyme takes part in tissue respiration?

A. Coenzyme Q
B. Coenzyme A
C. NADP
D. Cobamide

Ans. A.

2612. The enzyme hexokinase is a

A. Hydrolase
B. Oxidoreductase
C. Transferase
D. Ligase

Ans. C.

2613. Which of the following is a proteolytic enzyme?

A. Pepsin B. Trypsin

C. Chymotrypsin D. All of these

Ans. D.

2614. Enzymes which catalyse binding of two substrates by covalent bonds are known as

A. Lyases B. Hydrolases

C. Ligases D. Oxidoreductases

Ans. C.

2615. The induced fit model of enzyme action was proposed by

A. Fischer B. Koshland

C. Mitchell D. Markert

Ans. B.

2616. Allosteric inhibition is also known as

A. Competitive inhibition B. Non-competitive inhibition

C. Feedback inhibition D. None of these

Ans. C.

2617. Competitive inhibition can be relieved by raising the

A. Enzyme concentration B. Substrate concentration

C. Inhibitor concentration D. None of these

Ans. B.

2618. Carbonic anhydrase is competitively inhibited by

A. Allopurinol B. Acetazolamide

C. Aminopterin D. Neostigmine

Ans. B.

2619. Serum lactate dehydrogenase rises in

A. Viral hepatitis B. Myocardial infarction

C. Carcinomatosis D. All of these

Ans. D.

2620. Which of the following serum enzyme rises in myocardial infarction:

A. Creatine kinase B. GOT

C. LDH D. All of these

Ans. D.

2621. From the following myocardial infarction, the earliest serum enzyme to rise is

A. Creatine Kinase B. GOT
C. GPT D. LDH

Ans. A.

2622. Proenzymes:

A. Chymotrysinogen B. Pepsinogen
C. Both (A) and (B) D. None of these

Ans. B.

2623. Alkaline phosphatase is present in

A. Liver B. Bones
C. Placenta D. All of these

Ans. D.

2624. Which of the following isoenzyme of lactate dehydrogenase is raised in serum in myocardial infarction:

A. LD1 B. LD2
C. LD1 and LD2 D. LD5

Ans. C.

2625. Enzymes which are always present in an organism are known as

A. Inducible enzymes B. Constitutive enzymes
C. Functional enzymes D. Apoenzymes

Ans. B.

2626. Inactive precursors of enzymes are known as

A. Apoenzymes B. Coenzymes
C. Proenzymes D. Holoenzymes

Ans. C.

2627. Whcih of the following is a proenzyme?

A. Carboxypeptidase B. Aminopeptidase
C. Chymotrypsin D. Pepsinogen

Ans. D.

2628. The first enzyme found to have isoenzymes was

A. Alkaline Phosphatase B. Lactate dehydrogenase
C. Acid Phosphatase D. Creatine kinase

Ans. B.

2629. Lactate dehydrogenase is located in

A. Lysosomes
B. Mitochondria
C. Cytosol
D. Microsomes

Ans. C.

2630. Lactate dehydrogenase is a

A. Monomer
B. Dimer
C. Tetramer
D. Hexamer

Ans. C.

2631. Ceruloplasmin is absent in

A. Cirrhosis of liver
B. Wilson's disease
C. Menke's disease
D. Copper deficiency

Ans. B.

2632. Ceruloplasmin oxidizes

A. Copper
B. Iron
C. Both (A) and (B)
D. None of these

Ans. B.

2633. Creatine kinase is present in all of the following except

A. Liver
B. Myocardium
C. Muscles
D. Brain

Ans. A.

2634. Alkaline phosphatase is present in

A. Liver
B. Bones
C. Intestinal mucosa
D. All of these

Ans. D.

2635. All of the following are zinc-containing enzymes except

A. Acid Phosphatase
B. Alkaline Phosphatase
C. Carbonic anhydrase
D. RNA polymerase

Ans. A.

2636. All of the following are iron-containing enzymes except

A. Carbonic anhydrase
B. Catalase
C. Peroxidase
D. Cytochrome oxidase

Ans. A.

2637. Kinetics of an allosteric enzyme are explained by

A. Michaelis-Menten equation
B. Lineweaver-Burk plot
C. Hill plot
D. All of these

Ans. C.

2638. Covalent modification of an enzyme usually involves phosphorylation / dephosphorylation of

A. Serine residue
B. Proline residue
C. Hydroxylysine residue
D. Hydroxyproline residue

Ans. A.

2639. In enzyme assays, all the following are kept constant except

A. Substrate concentration
B. Enzyme concentration
C. pH
D. Temperature

Ans. B.

2640. Different isoenzymes of an enzyme have the same

A. Amino acid sequence
B. Michaelis constant
C. Catalytic activity
D. All of these

Ans. C.

2641. From the pentapeptide, phe-ala-leu-lys-arg, phenylalanine residue is split off by

A. Trypsin
B. Chymotrypsin
C. Aminopeptidase
D. Carboxypeptidase

Ans. C.

2642. Daily urinary urobilinogen excretion in adult men is

A. 0–4 mg
B. 5–8 mg
C. 9–12 mg
D. 13–20 mg

Ans. A.

2643. In obstructive jaundice, faecal urobilinogen is

A. Absent
B. Decreased
C. Increased
D. Normal

Ans. A.

2644. Acetyl-CoA can be formed from

A. Pyruvate
B. Fatty acids
C. Ketone bodies
D. All of these

Ans. D.

2645. Pyruvate dehydrogenase complex is located in

A. Cytosol
B. Lysosomes
C. Mitochondria
D. Endoplasmic reticulum

Ans. C.

2646. Ribozymes:

A. RNA enzyme
B. Non-protein enzymes
C. Catalyst function
D. All of these

Ans. D.

2647. All of the following are allosteric enzymes except

A. Citrate synthetase
B. a-Ketoglutarate dehdrogenase
C. Succinate thiokinase
D. Succinate dehydrogenase

Ans. C.

2648. All of the following intermediates of citric acid cycle can be formed from amino acids except

A. α-Ketoglutarate
B. Fumarate
C. Malate
D. Oxaloacetate

Ans. C.

2649. Glycolytic pathway is located in

A. Mitochondria
B. Cytosol
C. Microsomes
D. Nucleus

Ans. B.

2650. During fasting, glucose is phosphorylated mainly by

A. Hexokinase
B. Glucokinase
C. Both (A) and (B)
D. None of these

Ans. A.

2651. Glucokinase is found in

A. Muscles
B. Brain
C. Liver
D. All of these

Ans. C.

2652. In anaerobic glycolysis, energy yield from each molecule of glucose is

A. 2 ATP equivalents
B. 8 ATP equivalents
C. 30 ATP equivalents
D. 38 ATP equivalents

Ans. A.

2653. Which of the following is an allosteric enzyme?

A. Phosphohexose isomerase
B. Phosphotriose isomerase
C. Lactate dehydrogenase
D. Phosphofructokinase

Ans. D.

2654. Glycolysis is anaerobic in

A. Liver
B. Brain
C. Kidneys
D. Erythrocytes

Ans. D.

2655. Complete oxidation of one molecule of glucose into CO2 and H2O yields

A. 8 ATP equivalents
B. 15 ATP equivalents
C. 30 ATP equivalents
D. 38 ATP equivalents

Ans. D.

2656. Rapoport-Luebering cycle is located in

A. Liver
B. Muscles
C. Brain
D. Erythrocytes

Ans. D.

2657. HMP shunt is present in

A. Erythrocytes
B. Liver
C. Testes
D. All of these

Ans. D.

2658. Glycogenesis requires

A. GTP
B. CTP
C. UTP
D. None of these

Ans. C.

2659. Glycogenoloysis is increased by

A. Glucagon
B. Insulin
C. Epinephrine
D. cAMP

Ans. B.

2660. Hepatic glycogenoloysis is increased by

A. Insulin
B. Glucagon
C. Epinephrine
D. Glucocorticoids

Ans. B.

2661. Glucose is the only source of energy for

A. Myocardium B. Kidneys
C. Erythrocytes D. Thrombocytes

Ans. C.

2662. Gluconeogenesis does not occur in

A. Brain B. Kidneys
C. Muscles D. Liver

Ans. C.

2663. Glucose cannot be synthesized from

A. Glycerol B. Lactate
C. Alanine D. Leucine

Ans. D.

2664. Therapeutic enzymes:

A. Streptokinase B. Asparaginase
C. Riboflavinase D. Both (A) and (B)

Ans. D.

2665. The maximum possible chain length of fatty acids formed in the pathway of de novo synthesis is

A. 16 Carbon atoms B. 18 Carbon atoms
C. 20 Carbon atoms D. 24 Carbon atoms

Ans. A.

2666. Acetyl CoA required for de novo synthesis of fatty acids is obtained from

A. Breakdown of existing fatty acids B. Ketone bodies
C. Acetate D. Pyruvate

Ans. D.

2667. Formation of acetyl CoA from pyruvate for de novo synthesis of fatty acids requires

A. Pyruvate dehydrogenase complex B. Citrate synthetase
C. ATP citrate lyase D. All of these

Ans. D.

2668. The major site for elongation of medium chain fatty acids is

A. Mitochondria B. Cytosol
C. Microsomes D. All of these

Ans. C.

2669. Which of the following is not a cofactor?

A. Mg
B. Iron
C. Cu
D. Methylcobalamine

Ans. D.

2670. Thiamine is essential for

A. Pyruvate dehydrogenase
B. Isocitrate dehydrogenase
C. Succinate dehydrogenase
D. Acetyl CoA synthetase

Ans. B.

2671. Maximum enzyme activity is observed at

A. Acidic pH
B. Neutral pH
C. Basic pH
D. Optimum pH

Ans. D.

2672. Which of the following is known as bone forming enzyme?

A. Alkaline phosphatase
B. Acid phosphatase
C. Leucine aminopeptidase
D. γ-glutamyl transpeptidase

Ans. A.

2673. Conversion of pepsinogen to pepsin is

A. Intra molecular rearrangement
B. Breaking of hydrogen bonds
C. Covalent modification
D. Polymerisation

Ans. C.

2674. Which of the following is not having an apoenzyme and coenzyme?

A. Lactate dehydrogenase
B. Succinate dehydrogenase
C. Malate dehydrogenase
D. Pepsin

Ans. D.

2675. Coenzyme A contains the vitamin:

A. Riboflavin
B. Pantothenic acid
C. Pyridoxine
D. Thiamine

Ans. B.

2676. Urea is produced physiologically by the action of the enzyme:

A. Urease
B. Glutaminase
C. Arginase
D. None of these

Ans. C.

2677. Urease is a

A. Lyase
B. Ligase
C. Isomerase
D. Hydrolase

Ans. D.

2678. Cobamide coenzymes are

A. Vitamin B1
B. Riboflavin
C. Pyridoxine
D. Vitamin B12

Ans. D.

2679. Pepsin is

A. Exo-peptidase
B. Endo-peptidase
C. Carboxy peptidase
D. Amino peptidase

Ans. B.

2680. An enzyme in saliva which hydrolyzes starch is

A. Pepsinogen
B. Chymotrysin
C. α-Amylase
D. Malate

Ans. C.

2681. Schardinger's enzyme is

A. Lactate dehydrogenase
B. Xanthine dehydrogenase
C. Uric oxidase
D. L amino acid dehydrogenase

Ans. B.

2682. An enzyme which brings about lysis of bacterial cell wall is

A. Amylase
B. Lysozyme
C. Trypsin
D. Lipase

Ans. B.

2683. Trypsin has no action on

A. Hemoglobin
B. Albumin
C. Histone
D. DNA

Ans. D.

2684. Multiple forms of the same enzymes are known as

A. Zymogens
B. Isoenzymes
C. Proenzymes
D. Pre-enzymes

Ans. B.

2685. An allosteric enzyme influences the enzyme activity by

A. Competiting for the catalytic site with the substrate

B. Changing the specificity of the enzyme for the substrate

C. Changing the conformation of the enzyme by binding to a site other than catalytic site

D. Changing the nature of the products formed

Ans. C.

2686. Which of the following regulatory reactions involves a reversible covalent modification of an enzyme?

A. Phosphorylation of serine OH on the enzyme

B. Allosteric modulation

C. Competitive inhibition

D. Non-competitive inhibition

Ans. A.

2687. Vitamin deficiency that causes fatty liver includes all except

A. Vitamin E

B. Pyridoxine

C. Retionic acid

D. Pantothenic acid

Ans. C.

2688. In which of the following types of enzymes an inducer is not required?

A. Inhibited enzyme

B. Cooperative enzyme

C. Allosteric enzyme

D. Constitutive enzyme

Ans. D.

2689. ‘Lock’ and ‘Key’ model of enzyme action proposed by Fisher implies that

A. The active site is flexible and adjusts to substrate

B. The active site requires removal of PO4 group

C. The active site is complementary in shape to that of the substrate

D. Substrates change conformation prior to active site interaction

Ans. C.

2690. The most useful test for the diagnosis of acute hemorrhagic pancreatitis during the first few days is

A. Urinary lipase test

B. Serum calcium

C. Urinary amylase

D. Serum amylase

Ans. D.

2691. The best test for acute pancreatitis in the presence of mumps is

A. A serological test for mumps
B. Serum amylase
C. Urinary amylase
D. Serum lipase

Ans. D.

2692. The slow moving fraction of LDH is typically increased in pancreas with

A. Cerebrovascular accidents
B. Acute myocardial infarction
C. Acute pancreatitis
D. Acute viral hepatitis

Ans. D.

2693. Which of the following enzyme typically elevated in alcoholism?

A. Serum ALP
B. Serum GOT
C. Serum γ-GT
D. Serum acid phosphatase

Ans. C.

2694. Patients with hepatocellular jaundice, as compared to those with purely obstructive jaundice tend to have

A. Lower serum ALP, LDH and AST activity
B. Lower serum ALP, Higher LDH and AST activity
C. Higher serum ALP, LDH and AST activity
D. Higher serum ALP, Lower LDH and AST activity

Ans. B.

2695. Which enzyme estimation will be helpful in differentiating the elevated serum ALP found in obstructive jaundice as well as bone disorders?

A. Serum AST
B. Serum ALT
C. Serum LDH
D. Serum γ-GT

Ans. D.

2696. On the third day following onset of acute myocardial infarction, which enzyme estimation will have the best predictive value?

A. Serum AST
B. Serum CK
C. Serum ALT
D. Serum LDH

Ans. D.

2697. Serum AST activity is not characteristically elevated as the result of

A. Myocardial infarction
B. Passive congestion of liver
C. Muscular dystrophies
D. Peptic ulcer

Ans. D.

2698. On which day following acute myocardial infarction the estimation of serum AST will be of greatest significance?

A. First day
B. Second day
C. Third day
D. Fourth day

Ans. B.

2699. In which diseases of the following organs, isoenzymes LDH-1 and LDH-2 will be released in plasma?

A. Kidney, R.B.C and Liver
B. Heart, Kidney and R.B.C
C. Heart, Kidney and Liver
D. Heart, Lungs and Brain

Ans. B.

2700. Diastase can be used for the hydrolysis of

A. Sucrose
B. Starch
C. Cellulose
D. Maltose

Ans. B.

2701. Which of the following statements is true?

A. Enzymes have names ending ase
B. Enzymes are highly specific in their action
C. Enzymes are living organisms
D. Enzymes get activated on heating

Ans. B.

2702. Enzymes activity is controlled by

A. pH of the solution
B. Temperature
C. Concentration of the enzyme
D. Concentration of the substrate
E. All of these

Ans. C.

2703. Which of the following is not true regarding enzymes?

A. They catalyze only a particular type of reaction
B. They remain active even after separation from the source
C. They are destroyed after the completion of the reaction they catalyse
D. They are irreversibly destroyed at high temperature
E. Their activity depends on the pH of the solution

Ans. C.

2704. The number of enzymes known is about

A. 10,000 B. 100

C. 50 D. 26

Ans. C.

2705. Nicotine present in tobacco is a/an

A. Alkaloid B. Terpene

C. Steroid D. Protein

Ans. A.

2706. The poisonous alkaloid present in the oil of hemlock is

A. Cocaine B. Nicotine

C. Quinine D. Morphine

Ans. A.

2707. Alkaloids are usually purified by extraction with

A. Ether B. Dil HCl

C. NaOH D. Chloroform

Ans. B.

2708. LDH assays are most useful in diagnosing diseases of the

A. Heart B. Pancreas

C. Brain D. Kidney

Ans. A.

2709. The chemical forces that bind most coenzymes and substrates to enzymes such as LDH are

A. Hydrogen bonds B. Peptide bonds

C. Coordinate bonds D. Covalent bonds

Ans. D.

2710. How many different proteins may be present in normal LDH?

A. One B. Two

C. Three D. Four

Ans. D.

2711. Which of the following forms part of a coenzyme?

A. Zn2+ B. Lipase

C. Vitamin B2 D. Lysine

Ans. C.

2712. An enzyme is a

A. Carbohydrate B. Lipid

C. Protein D. Nucleic acid

Ans. C.

2713. Allosteric enzymes contain

A. Multiple subunits B. Single chain

C. Two chains D. Three chains

Ans. A.

2714. Isoenzymes of lactate dehydrogenase are useful for the diagnosis of

A. Heart disease B. Kidney disease

C. Liver disease D. Both (A) and (C)

Ans. D.

2715. The first enzyme isolated, purified and crystallied from Jackbean (Canavalia) in 1926 was

A. Urease B. Insulin

C. Ribonuclease D. Zymase

Ans. A.

2716. Who suggested that enzymes are proteinaceous?

A. Buchner B. Kuhne

C. Sumner D. Pasteur

Ans. C.

2717. The enzyme that converts glucose to glucose-6-phosphate is

A. Phosphatase B. Hexokinase

C. Phosphorylase D. Glucose synthetase

Ans. B.

2718. Enzymes are required in traces because they

A. Have high turnover number

B. Remain unused at the end of reaction and are reused

C. Show cascade effect

D. All correct

Ans. D.

2719. An organic substance bound to an enzyme and essential for the activity of enzyme is called

A. Holoenzyme B. Apoenzyme

C. Coenzyme D. Isoenzyme

Ans. D.

2720. Enzyme catalysed reactions occur in

A. Pico seconds B. Micro seconds

C. Milli seconds D. None of these

Ans. C.

2721. An enzyme can accelerate a reaction up to

A. 1010 times B. 101 times

C. 10100 times D. 10 times

Ans. A.

2722. In plants, enzymes occur in

A. Flowers only B. Leaves only

C. All living cells D. Storage organs only

Ans. C.

2723. Zymogen is a

A. Vitamin B. Enzyme precursor

C. Modulator D. Hormone

Ans. B.

2724. Cofactor (Prosthetic group) is a part of holoenzyme, it is

A. Inorganic part loosely attached

B. Accessory non-protein substance attached firmly

C. Organic part attached loosely

D. None of these

Ans. B.

2725. A protein having both structural and enzymatic traits is

A. Myosin B. Collagen

C. Trypsin D. Actin

Ans. A.

2726. Enzymes are different from catalysts in

A. Being proteinaceous B. Not used up in reaction

C. Functional at high temperature D. Having high rate of diffusion

Ans. A.

2727. Enzymes, vitamins and hormones are common in

A. Being proteinaceous

B. Being synthesized in the body of organisms

C. Enhancing oxidative metabolism

D. Regulating metabolism

Ans. D.

2728. Dry seeds endure higher temperature than germinating seeds as

A. Hydration is essential for making enzymes sensitive to temperature

B. Dry seeds have a hard covering

C. Dry seeds have more reserve food

D. Seedlings are tender

Ans. A.

2729. Coenzymes FMN and FAD are derived from vitamin

A. C B. B6

C. B1 D. B2

Ans. D.

2730. Combination of apoenzyme and coenzyme produces

A. Prosthetic group B. Holoenzyme

C. Enzyme substrate complex D. Enzyme product complex

Ans. B.

2731. An enzyme brings about

A. Decrease in reaction time B. Increase in reaction time

C. Increase in activation energy D. Reduction in activation energy

Ans. D.

2732. Coenzyme is

A. Often a vitamin B. Always an inorganic compound

C. Always a protein D. Often a metal

Ans. A.

2733. The ratio of enzyme to substrate molecules can be as low as

A. 1 : 100,000 B. 1 : 500,000

C. 1 : 10,000 D. 1 : 1,000

Ans. A.

2734. Part of enzyme which combines with nonprotein part to form functional enzyme is

A. Apoenzyme B. Coenzyme

C. Prosthetic group D. None of these

Ans. C.

2735. Who got Nobel Prize in 1978 for working on enzymes?

A. Koshland B. Arber and Nathans

C. Nass and Nass D. H.G. Khorana

Ans. A.

2736. Site of enzyme synthesis in a cell is

A. Ribosomes
B. RER
C. Golgi bodies
D. All of these

Ans. B.

2737. The fruit when kept in open, tastes bitter after 2 hours because of

A. Loss of water from juice
B. Decreased concentration of fructose in juice
C. Fermentation by yeast
D. Contamination by bacterial enzymes

Ans. D.

2738. The best example of extracellular enzymes (exoenzyme) is

A. Nucleases
B. Digestive enzymes
C. Succinic dehydrogenase
D. None of these

Ans. C.

2739. Name the enzyme that acts both as carboxylase at one time and oxygenase at another time.

A. PEP carboxylase
B. RuBP carboxylase
C. Carbonic anyhdrase
D. None of these

Ans. B.

2740. The energy required to start an enzymatic reaction is called

A. Chemical energy
B. Metabolic energy
C. Activation energy
D. Potential energy

Ans. C.

2741. Out of the total enzymes present in a cell, a mitochondrion alone has

A. 4%
B. 70%
C. 95%
D. 50%

Ans. B.

2742. Creatine phosphokinase isoenzyme is a marker for

A. Kidney disease
B. Liver disease
C. Myocardial infarction
D. None of these

Ans. C.

2743. Which one is coenzyme?

A. ATP
B. Vitamin B and C
C. CoQ and CoA
D. All of these

Ans. D.

2744. The active site of an enzyme is formed by

A. R group of amino acids
B. NH2 group of amino acids
C. CO group of amino acids
D. Sulphur bonds which are exposed

Ans. A.

2745. Carbonic anhydrase enzyme has maximum turn over number (36 million). Minimum turn over number for an enzyme:

A. DNA polymerase
B. Lysozyme
C. Penicillase
D. Lactase dehydrogenase

Ans. B.

2746. In cell, digestive enzymes are found mainly in

A. Vacuoles
B. Lysosomes
C. Ribosomes
D. Lomasomes

Ans. B.

2747. Which enzyme hydrolyses starch?

A. Invertase
B. Maltase
C. Sucrase
D. Diastase

Ans. D.

2748. Enzymes functional in cell or mitochondria are

A. Endoenzymes
B. Exoenzymes
C. Apoenzymes
D. Holoenzymes

Ans. A.

2749. A mitochondrial marker enzyme is

A. Aldolase
B. Amylase
C. Succinic dehydrogenase
D. Pyruvate dehydrogenase

Ans. C.

2750. The enzyme used in polymerase chain reaction (PCR) is

A. Taq polymerase
B. RNA polymerase
C. Ribonuclease
D. Endonuclease

Ans. A.

2751. The tear secretion contains an antibacterial enzyme known as

A. Zymase
B. Diastase
C. Lysozyme
D. Lipase

Ans. C.

2752. The biosynthesis of urea occurs mainly in the liver:

A. Cytosol B. Mitochondria

C. Microsomes D. Nuclei

Ans. B.

2753. Bile salts make emulsification with fat for the action of

A. Amylose B. Lipase

C. Pepsin D. Trypsin

Ans. B.

2754. In the normal resting state of human most of the blood glucose burnt as fuel is consumed by

A. Liver B. Brain

C. Adipose tissue D. Muscles

Ans. B.

2755. When ATP forms AMP

A. Inorganic pyrophosphate is produced

B. Inorganic phosphorous is produced

C. Phsophagen is produced

D. No energy is produced

Ans. A.

2756. Alcohol dehydrogenase from liver contains

A. Sodium B. Copper

C. Zinc D. Magnesium

Ans. C.

2757. A molybdenum containing oxidase is

A. Cytochrome oxidase B. Xanthine oxidase

C. Glucose oxidase D. L-Amino acid oxidase

Ans. B.

2758. A copper containing oxidase is

A. Cytochrome oxidase B. Flavin mononucleotide

C. Flavin adenine dinucleotide D. Xanthine oxidase

Ans. A.

2759. The mitochondrial superoxide dismutase contains

A. Mg++ B. Mn++

C. Co++ D. Zn++

Ans. B.

2760. Activity of cytochrome oxidase is inhibited by

A. Sulphite
B. Sulphate
C. Arsenite
D. Cyanide

Ans. D.

2761. Chemiosmotic theory for oxidative phosphorylation has been proposed by

A. Chance and Williams
B. Pauling and Corey
C. S. Waugh
D. P. Mitchell

Ans. D.

2762. The number of ATP produced in the oxidation of 1 molecule of NADPH in oxidative phosphorylation is

A. Zero
B. 2
C. 3
D. 4

Ans. A.

2763. The coupling of oxidation and phosphorylation in intact mitochondria:

A. Puromycin
B. Oligomycin
C. Streptomycin
D. Gentamycin

Ans. B.

2764. Porphyrins are synthesized in

A. Cytosol
B. Mitochondria
C. Cytosol and mitochondria
D. Rough endoplasmic reticulum

Ans. C.

2765. Porphyrin synthesis is inhibited in

A. Mercury poisoning
B. Lead poisoning
C. Manganese poisoning
D. Barium poisoning

Ans. B.

2766. During synthesis of porphyrins, synthesis of δ-amino levulinic acid occurs in

A. Mitochondria
B. Cytosol
C. Both in mitochondria and cytosol
D. Ribosomes

Ans. A.

2767. A cofactor required for the activity of the enzyme ALA dehydratase is

A. Cu
B. Mn
C. Mg
D. Fe

Ans. A.

2768. Many xenobiotics

A. Increase hepatic ALA synthase B. Decrease hepatic ALA sythase

C. Increase hepatic ALA dehydrase D. Decrease hepatic ALA dehydrase

Ans. A.

2769. The major symptom of acute intermittent porphyria includes

A. Abdominal pain B. Photosensitivity

C. No neuropsychiatric signs D. Dermatitis

Ans. A.

2770. Main symptoms of congenital erythropoietic porphyria is

A. Yellowish teeth B. Photosensitivity

C. Abdominal pain D. Brownish urine

Ans. B.

2771. Calcium is excreted by

A. Kidney B. Kidney and intestine

C. Kidney and liver D. Kidney and pancreas

Ans. B.

2772. A decrease in the ionized fraction of serum calcium causes

A. Tetany B. Rickets

C. Osteomalacia D. Osteoporosis

Ans. A.

2773. A rise in blood calcium may indicate

A. Paget's disease B. Rickets

C. Osteomalacia D. Hypervitaminosis D

Ans. D.

2774. The normal serum level of phosphorus in human adult is

A. 1–2 mg B. 2–3 mg

C. 3–4.5 mg D. 5–7 mg

Ans. C.

2775. An increase in carbohydrate metabolism is accompanied by temporary decrease in serum

A. Calcium B. Phosphate

C. Iron D. Sodium

Ans. B.

2776. In rickets of the common low-phosphate variety, serum phosphate values may go as low as

A. 1–2 mg/100 ml B. 2–3 mg/100 ml

C. 3–4 mg/100 ml D. 4–5 mg/100 ml

Ans. A.

2777. The normal serum level of phosphorous in children varies from

A. 1–2 mg/100 ml B. 2–3 mg/100 ml

C. 3–4 mg/100 ml D. 4–7 mg/100 ml

Ans. D.

2778. The total magnesium content in gms of human body is about

A. 5 B. 10

C. 15 D. 21

Ans. D.

2779. Iron is a component of

A. Hemoglobin B. Ceruloplasmin

C. Transferase D. Transaminase

Ans. A.

2780. Daily requirement of iron for normal adult male is about

A. 5 mg B. 10 mg

C. 15 mg D. 20 mg

Ans. B.

2781. The normal content of protein bound iron (PBI) in the plasma of males is

A. 120–140 μg/100 ml B. 200–300 μg/100 ml

C. 120–140 μg/100 ml D. 200–300 μg/100 ml

Ans. A.

2782. In iron deficiency anemia

A. The plasma bound iron is low

B. The plasma bound iron is high

C. Total iron binding capacity is low

D. Both the plasma bound iron and total iron binding capacity are low

Ans. A.

2783. The total iron content of the human body is

A. 400–500 mg B. 1–2 g

C. 2–3 g D. 4–5 g

Ans. D.

2784. In hepatic diseases

A. Both the bound iron and total iron binding capacity of the plasma may be low

B. Both the bound iron and total iron binding capacity of the plasma may be high

C. Only bound iron may be high

D. Only the total iron binding capacity may be high

Ans. A.

2785. The recommended daily requirement of iron for women of 18–55 yrs age is

A. 5 mg B. 8 mg

C. 10 mg D. 15 mg

Ans. D.

2786. The percent of total iron in body in hemoglobin is

A. 10–20 B. 20–30

C. 30–40 D. 60–70

Ans. D.

2787. A good source of iron is

A. Spinach B. Milk

C. Tomato D. Potato

Ans. A.

2788. The best source of iron is

A. Organ meats B. Milk

C. Tomato D. Potato

Ans. A.

2789. An increased serum iron and decreased iron binding capacity is found in

A. Fe deficiency anemia B. Sideroblastic anemia

C. Folate deficiency anemia D. Sickle cell anemia

Ans. B.

2790. The absorption of iron is increased 2–10 times of normal in

A. Iron deficiency anemia B. Pregnancy

C. Spherocytosis D. Sickle cell anemia

Ans. A.

2791. Iron is mainly absorbed from

A. Stomach and duodenum B. Ileum

C. Caecum D. Colon

Ans. A.

2792. The iron containing nonporphyrin is

A. Hemosiderin
B. Catalase
C. Cytochrome C
D. Peroxidase

Ans. A.

2793. Molecular iron is

A. Stored primarily in the spleen
B. Exreted in the urine as Fe2+
C. Stored in the body in combination with ferritin
D. Absorbed in the ferric form

Ans. C.

2794. In hemochromatosis, the liver is infiltrated with

A. Iron
B. Copper
C. Molybdenum
D. Fats

Ans. A.

2795. An acquired siderosis-Bantu siderosis is due to

A. Foods cooked in iron pots
B. Diet high in phosphorous
C. Diet high in calcium
D. High fat diet

Ans. A.

2796. The amount of copper in the human body is

A. 50–80 mg
B. 100–150 mg
C. 400–500 mg
D. 500–1000 mg

Ans. B.

2797. The amount of copper in muscles is about

A. 10 mg
B. 30 mg
C. 64 mg
D. 100 mg

Ans. C.

2798. The amount of copper in bones is about

A. 5 mg
B. 10 mg
C. 15 mg
D. 23 mg

Ans. D.

2799. The normal serum concentration of copper in mg/100 ml varies between

A. 0–5
B. 50–100
C. 100–200
D. 200–300

Ans. C.

2800. Recommended daily dietary requirement of copper for adults is

A. 0.5–1 mg B. 1.5–3.0 mg
C. 3.5–4.5 mg D. 4.5–5.5 mg

Ans. C.

2801. The richest source of copper is

A. Liver B. Milk
C. Legumes D. Green leafy vegetables

Ans. A.

2802. The cytosolic superoxide dismutase enzyme contains

A. Cu2+ B. Cu2+ and Zn2+
C. Zn2+ D. Mn2+

Ans. B.

2803. The deficiency of copper decreases the activity of the enzyme:

A. Lysine oxidase B. Lysine hydroxylase
C. Tyrosine oxidase D. Proline hydroxylase

Ans. A.

2804. Wilson's disease is a condition of toxicosis of

A. Iron B. Copper
C. Chromium D. Molybdenum

Ans. B.

2805. In Wilson's disease

A. Copper fails to be excreted in the bile
B. Copper level in plasma is decreased
C. Ceruloplasmin level is increased
D. Intestinal absorption of copper is decreased

Ans. A.

2806. Menke's disease is due to an abnormality in the metabolism of

A. Iron B. Manganese
C. Magnesium D. Copper

Ans. D.

2807. Menke's disease (Kinky or steel hair disease) is a X-linked disease characterized by

A. High levels of plasma copper
B. High levels of ceruloplasmin
C. Low levels of plasma copper and of ceruloplasmin
D. High level of hepatic copper

Ans. C.

2808. The trace element catalyzing hemoglobin synthesis is

A. Manganese B. Magnesium

C. Copper D. Selenium

Ans. C.

2809. The total body content of manganese is about

A. 2 mg B. 4 mg

C. 8 mg D. 10 mg

Ans. D.

2810. In human blood the values of manganese in μg /100 ml varies between

A. 0–4 B. 2–4

C. 3–5 D. 4–20

Ans. D.

2811. The adequate daily dietary requirement of manganese is

A. 1–2 mg B. 2–5 mg

C. 5–10 mg D. 10–20 mg

Ans. B.

2812. Mitochondrial superoxide dismutase contains

A. Zinc B. Copper

C. Magnesium D. Manganese

Ans. D.

2813. The adequate daily dietary requirement of molybdenum for normal human adult is

A. 10–20 μg B. 25–50 μg

C. 50–70 μg D. 75–200 μg

Ans. D.

2814. In human beings molybdenum is mainly absorbed from

A. Liver B. Kidney

C. Intestine D. Pancreas

Ans. C.

2815. In human beings molybdenum is mainly excreted in

A. Feces B. Sweat

C. Urine D. Tears

Ans. C.

2816. Molybdenum is a constituent of

A. Hydroxylases B. Oxidases

C. Transaminases D. Transferases

Ans. B.

2817. Safe and adequate daily dietary intake of chromium in adults in mg is

A. 0.01–0.02 B. 0.02–0.03

C. 0.03–0.04 D. 0.05–0.2

Ans. D.

2818. Richest source of chromium is

A. Brewer's yeast B. Milk and milk products

C. Yellow vegetables D. Green vegetables

Ans. A.

2819. Metallic constituent of "Glucose tolerance factor" is

A. Sulphur B. Cobalt

C. Chromium D. Selenium

Ans. C.

2820. Intestinal absorption of chromium is shared with

A. Mn B. Mg

C. Ca D. Zn

Ans. D.

2821. Serum level of chromium in healthy adult is about

A. 2-5 μg/100 ml B. 6-20 μg/100 ml

C. 30-60 μg/100 ml D. 50-100 μg/100 ml

Ans. B.

2822. Chromium is potentiator of

A. Insulin B. Glucagon

C. Thyroxine D. Parathromone

Ans. A.

2823. Recommended daily dietary allowance of selenium for adult human in μg is

A. 20 B. 40

C. 50 D. 70

Ans. D.

2824. Total body content of selenium is about

A. 1–2 mg B. 2–4 mg

C. 4–10 mg D. 50–100 mg

Ans. C.

2825. Normal serum level of selenium is

A. 5 μg /100 ml B. 8 μg /100 ml

C. 10 μg /100 ml D. 13 μg /100 ml

Ans. D.

2826. Selenium is a constituent of the enzyme:

A. Glutathione peroxidase B. Homogentisate oxidase

C. Tyrosine hydroxylase D. Phenylalanin hydroxylase

Ans. A.

2827. A nonspecific intracellular antioxidant is

A. Chromium B. Magnesium

C. Selenium D. Nickel

Ans. C.

2828. Cobalt forms an integral part of the vitamin:

A. B1 B. B6

C. B12 D. Folate

Ans. C.

2829. Excess intake of cobalt for longer periods leads to

A. Polycythemia B. Megaloblastic anemia

C. Pernicious anemia D. Microcytic anemia

Ans. A.

2830. The total sulphur content of the body is

A. 25–50 gm B. 50–75 gm

C. 100–125 gm D. 150–200 gm

Ans. D.

2831. Sulphur is made available to the body by the amino acids:

A. Cystine and methionine B. Taurine and alanine

C. Proline and hydroxyproline D. Arginine and lysine

Ans. A.

2832. Sulphur containing coenzyme is

A. NAD | B. FAD
C. Pyridoxal phosphate | D. Biotin

Ans. D.

2833. Iodine is stored in

A. Thyroid gland as thyroglobulin | B. Liver
C. Intestine | D. Skin

Ans. A.

2834. Iodine is the constituent of

A. T3 and T4 | B. PTH
C. Insulin | D. Adrenaline

Ans. A.

2835. Goitrogenic substance present in cabbage is

A. 5-vinyl-2 thio oxalzolidone
B. Pyridine-3-carboxylic acid
C. 3-Hydroxy-4, 5-dihydroxymethyl1–2-methyl pyridine
D. δ-ALA dehydratase

Ans. A.

2836. For an adult male daily requirement of iodine is

A. 25–50 μg | B. 50–100 μg
C. 100–150 μg | D. 200–250 μg

Ans. A.

2837. Recommended daily intake of fluoride for a normal adult is

A. 1.5–4.0 mg | B. 0–1 mg
C. 5–10 mg | D. 10–20 mg

Ans. B.

2838. The percentage of fluoride present in normal bone is

A. 0.01–0.03 | B. 0.04–0.08
C. 0.10–0.12 | D. 0.15–0.2

Ans. A.

2839. The percentage of fluoride present in dental enamel is

A. 0.01–0.02 | B. 0.05–0.10
C. 0.15–0.20 | D. 0.20–0.40

Ans. A.

2840. Fluorosis occurs due to

A. Drinking water containing less than 0.2 ppm of fluorine

B. Drinking water containing high calcium

C. Drinking water containing greater than 1.2 ppm of fluroine

D. Drinking water containing heavy metals

Ans. C.

2841. Dental caries occur due to

A. Drinking water containing less than 0.2 ppm of fluorine

B. Drinking water containing greater than 1.2 ppm of fluorine

C. Drinking water containing high calcium

D. Drinking water containing heavy metals

Ans. A.

2842. Total zinc content of human body is about

A. 800 mg B. 1200 mg

C. 2000 mg D. 3200 mg

Ans. C.

2843. Metal required for polymerization of insulin is

A. Copper B. Chromium

C. Cobalt D. Zinc

Ans. D.

2844. An important zinc containing enzyme is

A. Carboxypeptidase A B. Isocitrate dehydrogenase

C. Cholinesterate D. Lipoprotein lipase

Ans. A.

2845. Hypogonadism develops due to deficiency of

A. Sulphur B. Cobalt

C. Zinc D. Manganese

Ans. C.

2846. Psychotic symptoms and parkinsonism like symptoms develop due to inhalation poisoning of

A. Manganese B. Phosphorous

C. Magnesium D. Zinc

Ans. A.

2847. One gram of protein on complete oxidation in the body yields about

A. 2 Kcal
B. 4 Kcal
C. 8 Kcal
D. 12 Kcal

Ans. B.

2848. R.Q. of mixed diet is about

A. 0.70
B. 0.80
C. 0.85
D. 1.0

Ans. C.

2849. R.Q. of proteins is about

A. 0.70
B. 0.75
C. 0.80
D. 0.85

Ans. C.

2850. R.Q. of carbohydrates is about

A. 0.75
B. 0.80
C. 0.85
D. 1.0

Ans. D.

2851. R.Q. of fats is about

A. 0.75
B. 0.80
C. 0.85
D. 1.0

Ans. A.

2852. Proteins have the SDA:

A. 5%
B. 10%
C. 20%
D. 30%

Ans. D.

2853. Humans most easily tolerate a lack of the nutrient:

A. Protein
B. Lipid
C. Iodine
D. Carbohydrate

Ans. D.

2854. The basal metabolic rate (B.M.R.) is measurement of

A. Energy expenditure during sleep
B. Energy expenditure after 100 m walk
C. Energy expenditure after a meal
D. Energy expenditure under certain basal (Standard) conditions

Ans. D.

2855. B.M.R. is raised in

A. Polycythemia
B. Starvation
C. Lipid nephrosis
D. Hypothyroidism

Ans. A.

2856. B.M.R. is lowered in

A. Hypothyroidism
B. Leukemia
C. Cardiac failure
D. Hyperthyroidism

Ans. A.

2857. B.M.R. is subnormal in

A. Addison's disease
B. Adrenal tumour
C. Cushing's syndrome
D. Fever

Ans. A.

2858. The percentage of nitrogen retained in the body after absorption of diet represents

A. Digestibility coefficient of proteins
B. Biological value of proteins
C. Protein efficiency ratio
D. Net protein utilization

Ans. B.

2859. The percentage of food nitrogen that is retained in the body represents

A. Digestibility coefficient
B. Biological value of proteins
C. Protein efficiency ratio
D. Net protein utilization

Ans. D.

2860. The chemical score of different proteins is calculated in terms of

A. Egg proteins
B. Milk proteins
C. Fish proteins
D. Wheat proteins

Ans. A.

2861. Biological value of egg protein is

A. 94
B. 60
C. 51
D. 40

Ans. A.

2862. Biological value of protein of cow's milk is

A. 95
B. 60
C. 71
D. 67

Ans. B.

2863. Biological value of soyabean protein is

A. 86 B. 71

C. 64 D. 54

Ans. C.

2864. Plasma bicarbonate is decreased in

A. Respiratory alkalosis B. Respiratory acidosis

C. Metabolic alkalosis D. Metabolic acidosis

Ans. D.

2865. Plasma bicarbonate is increased in

A. Respiratory alkalosis B. Metabolic alkalosis

C. Respiratory acidosis D. Metabolic acidosis

Ans. B.

2866. Total CO2 is increased in

A. Respiratory acidosis

B. Metabolic alkalosis

C. Both respiratory acidosis and metabolic alkalosis

D. Respiratory alkalosis

Ans. C.

2867. Meningitis and encephalitis cause

A. Metabolic alkalosis B. Respiratory alkalosis

C. Metabolic acidosis D. Respiratory acidosis

Ans. B.

2868. Metabolic acidosis is caused in

A. Uncontrolled diabetes with ketosis

B. Pneumonia

C. Intestinal Obstruction

D. Hepatic coma

Ans. A.

2869. Metabolic acidosis is caused in

A. Pneumonia B. Prolonged starvation

C. Intestinal obstruction D. Bulbar polio

Ans. B.

2870. Respiratory acidosis occurs in
A. Any disease which impairs respiration like emphysema
B. Renal disease
C. Poisoning by an acid
D. Pyloric stenosis

Ans. A.

2871. Morphine poisoning causes
A. Metabolic acidosis
B. Respiratory acidosis
C. Metabolic alkalosis
D. Respiratory alkalosis

Ans. B.

2872. Salicylate poisoning in early stages causes
A. Metabolic acidosis
B. Respiratory acidosis
C. Metabolic alkalosis
D. Respiratory alkalosis

Ans. D.

2873. The compound having the lowest redox potential amongst the following is
A. Hydrogen
B. NAD
C. Cytochrome b
D. Cytochrome a

Ans. A.

2874. All the oxidases contain a metal named as
A. Copper
B. FAD
C. Manganese
D. None of these

Ans. A.

2875. Superoxide radicals can be detoxified by
A. Cytochrome c
B. Cytochrome b
C. Cytochrome a
D. None of these

Ans. A.

2876. A copper containing cytochrome is
A. Cytochrome a
B. Cytochrome P-450
C. Cytochrome a3
D. None of these

Ans. C.

2877. Rate of tissue respiration is raised when the intracellular concentration of
A. ADP increases
B. ATP increases
C. ADP decreases
D. None of these

Ans. A.

2878. In some reactions, energy is captured in the form of

A. GTP
B. UTP
C. CTP
D. None of these

Ans. A.

2879. Superoxide radicals can be detoxified by

A. Cytochrome c
B. Superoxide dismutase
C. Both (A) and (B)
D. None of these

Ans. C.

2880. The porphyrin present in haem is

A. Uroporphyrin
B. Protoporphyrin I
C. Coproporphyrin
D. Protoporphyrin II

Ans. D.

2881. An amino acid required for porphyrin synthesis is

A. Proline
B. Glycine
C. Serine
D. Histidine

Ans. A.

2882. Which of the following coenzyme is required for porphyrin synthesis?

A. Coenzyme A
B. Pyridoxal phosphate
C. Both (A) and (B)
D. None of these

Ans. C.

2883. The regulatory enzyme for haem synthesis is

A. ALA synthetase
B. haem synthetase
C. Both (A) and (B)
D. None of these

Ans. A.

2884. Sigmoidal oxygen dissociation curve is a property of

A. Haemoglobin
B. Carboxyhaemoglobin
C. Myoglobin
D. Methaemoglobin

Ans. A.

2885. Cyanmethaemoglobin can be formed from

A. Oxy Hb
B. Met Hb
C. Carboxy Hb
D. All of these

Ans. B.

2886. In thalassemia, an amino acid is substituted in

A. Alpha chain
B. Beta chain
C. Alpha and beta chains
D. Any chain

Ans. D.

2887. Pre- hepatic jaundice occurs because of

A. Increased haemolysis
B. Liver damage
C. Biliary obstruction
D. None of these

Ans. A.

2888. Kernicterus can occur in

A. Haemolytic jaundice
B. Hepatic jaundice
C. Obstructive jaundice
D. All of these

Ans. A.

2889. Bile pigments are not present in urine in

A. Haemolytic jaundice
B. Hepatic jaundice
C. Obstructive jaundice
D. Rotor's syndrome

Ans. A.

2890. Serum alkaline phosphatase is greatly increased in

A. Haemolytic jaundice
B. Hepatic jaundice
C. Obstructive jaundice
D. None of these

Ans. C.

2891. The active transport system for hepatic uptake of bilirubin is congenitally defective in

A. Gilbert's disease
B. Crigler-Najjar syndrome
C. Rotor's syndrome
D. Dubin-Johnson syndrome

Ans. A.

2892. Unconjugated bilirubin in serum is soluble in

A. Water
B. Alkalis
C. Acids
D. Methanol

Ans. D.

2893. Breakdown of 1gm haemoglobin produces

A. 20 mg of bilirubin
B. 35 mg of bilirubin
C. 50 mg of bilirubin
D. 70 mg of bilirubin

Ans. B.

2894. The total amount of calcium in an average adult man is about

A. 100 gm B. 500 gm

C. 1 kg D. 10 kg

Ans. C.

2895. The percentage of total body calcium is present in bones and teeth:

A. 75% B. 90%

C. 95% D. 99%

Ans. D.

2896. The normal range of plasma calcium is

A. 3-5 mg/dl B. 5-10 mg/dl

C. 9-11 mg/dl D. 11-15 mg/dl

Ans. C.

2897. Tetany can occur in

A. Hypocalcaemia B. Hypercalcaemia

C. Alkalosis D. Hypocalcaemia and alkalosis

Ans. D.

2898. Intestinal absorption of calcium occurs by

A. Active takeup B. Simple diffusion

C. Facilitated diffusion D. Endocytosis

Ans. A.

2899. Intestinal absorption of calcium is hampered by

A. Phosphate B. Phytate

C. Proteins D. Lactose

Ans. B.

2900. Calcitriol facilitates calcium absorption by increasing the synthesis of the following in intestinal mucosa:

A. Calcium Binding Protein B. Alkaline Phosphatase

C. Calcium-dependent ATPase D. All of these

Ans. D.

2901. A high plasma calcium level decreases intestinal absorption of calcium by

A. Stimulating the secretion of parathormone

B. Inhibiting the secretion of parathormone

C. Decreasing the synthesis of cholecalciferol

D. Inhibiting the secretion of thyrocalcitonin

Ans. B.

2902. The daily calcium requirement of an adult man is about

A. 400 mg B. 600 mg
C. 800 mg D. 1,000 mg

Ans. C.

2903. The daily calcium requirement in pregnancy and lactation is about

A. 600 mg B. 800 mg
C. 1,200 mg D. 1,500 mg

Ans. C.

2904. Hypercalcaemia can occur in all the following except

A. Hyperparathyroidism B. Hypervitaminosis D
C. Milk alkali syndrome D. Nephrotic syndrome

Ans. D.

2905. Hypocalcaemia can occur in all the following except

A. Rickets B. Osteomalacia
C. Hyperparathyroidism D. Intestinal malabsorption

Ans. C.

2906. The major calcium salt in bones is

A. Calcium carbonate B. Calcium chloride
C. Calcium hydroxide D. Calcium phosphate

Ans. D.

2907. The correct statement about serum inorganic phosphorous concentration is

A. It is higher in men than in women
B. It is higher in women than in men
C. It is higher in adults than in children
D. It is higher in children than in adults

Ans. D.

2908. The product of serum calcium concentration (mg/dl) and serum inorganic phosphorous concentration (mg/dl) in adults is about

A. 30 B. 40
C. 50 D. 60

Ans. A.

2909. The product of serum calcium concentration (mg/dl) and serum inorganic phosphorous concentration (mg/dl) in children is about

A. 30 B. 40
C. 50 D. 60

Ans. C.

2910. The product of serum calcium concentration (mg/dl) and serum inorganic phosphorous concentration (mg/dl) is decreased in

A. Rickets B. Hypoparathyroidism

C. Hyperparathyroidism D. Renal failure

Ans. A.

2911. Serum inorganic phosphorous rises in all the following conditions except

A. Hypoparathyroidism B. Hypervitaminosis D

C. Chronic renal failure D. After a carbohydrate-rich meal

Ans. D.

2912. Serum inorganic phosphorous decreases in all the following conditions except

A. Hyperparathyroidism B. Intestinal malabsorption

C. Osteomalacia D. Chronic renal failure

Ans. D.

2913. Serum magnesium level ranges between

A. 2–3 mg/dl B. 3–5 mg/dl

C. 6–8 mg/dl D. 9–11 mg/dl

Ans. A.

2914. Normal range of serum sodium is

A. 30–70 mEq/L B. 70–110 mEq/L

C. 117–135 mEq/L D. 136–145 mEq/L

Ans. D.

2915. Sodium is involved in the active uptake of

A. D-Glucose B. D-Galactose

C. L-Amino acids D. All of these

Ans. D.

2916. Aldosterone increases reabsorption of sodium in

A. Proximal convoluted tubules B. Ascending limb of loop of Henle

C. Descending limb of loop of Henle D. Distal convoluted tubules

Ans. D.

2917. Restriction of sodium intake is commonly advised in

A. Addison's disease B. Diarrhoea

C. Hypertension D. None of these

Ans. C.

2918. Serum sodium level rises in all of the following except

A. Renal failure
B. Prolonged steroid therapy
C. Aldosteronism
D. Dehydration

Ans. A.

2919. Hyponatraemia occurs in the following condition:

A. Addison's disease
B. Chronic renal failure
C. Severe diarrhoea
D. All of these

Ans. D.

2920. Serum potassium level decreases in

A. Familial periodic paralysis
B. Addison's disease
C. Renal failure
D. All of these

Ans. A.

2921. Concentration of the following is higher in intracellular fluid than in extracellular fluid

A. Sodium
B. Potassium
C. Chloride
D. Bicarbonate

Ans. B.

2922. Normal range of serum potassium is

A. 2.1-3.4 mEq/L
B. 3.5-5.3 mEq/L
C. 5.4–7.4 mEq/L
D. 7.5–9.5 mEq/L

Ans. B.

2923. Normal range of serum chloride is

A. 24–27 mEq/L
B. 70–80 mEq/L
C. 100–106 mEq/L
D. 120–140 mEq/L

Ans. C.

2924. An extracellular fluid having a higher concentration of chloride than serum is

A. Bile
B. Sweat
C. CSF
D. Pancreatic juice

Ans. C.

2925. Total amount of iron in an adult man is about

A. 1–2 gm
B. 2–3 gm
C. 3–4 gm
D. 6–7 gm

Ans. C.

2926. Haemoglobin contains about

A. 30% of the total body iron
B. 50% of the total body iron
C. 75% of the total body iron
D. 90% of the total body iron

Ans. C.

2927. About 5% of the total body, iron is present in

A. Transferrin
B. Myoglobin
C. Cytochromes
D. Haemosiderin

Ans. B.

2928. Each haemoglobin molecule contains

A. One iron atom
B. Two iron atoms
C. Four iron atoms
D. Six iron atoms

Ans. C.

2929. Each myoglobin molecule contains

A. One iron atom
B. Two iron atoms
C. Four iron atoms
D. Six iron atoms

Ans. A.

2930. Ferritin is present in

A. Intestinal mucosa
B. Liver
C. Spleen
D. All of these

Ans. D.

2931. Iron is stored in the form of

A. Ferritin and transferrin
B. Transferrin and haemosiderin
C. Haemoglobin and myoglobin
D. Ferritin and haemosiderin

Ans. D.

2932. Iron is transported in blood in the form of

A. Ferritin
B. Haemosiderin
C. Transferrin
D. Haemoglobin

Ans. C.

2933. Molecular weight of transferrin is about

A. 40,000
B. 60,000
C. 80,000
D. 1,00,000

Ans. C.

2934. Normal plasma iron level is

A. 50-100 µg/dl B. 100-150 µg/dl

C. 50-175 µg/dl D. 250-400 µg/dl

Ans. C.

2935. Total daily iron loss of an adult man is about

A. 0.1 mg B. 1 mg

C. 5 mg D. 10 mg

Ans. B.

2936. Iron absorption is hampered by

A. Ascorbic acid B. Succinic acid

C. Phytic acid D. Amino acid

Ans. C.

2937. Daily iron requirement of an adult man is about

A. 1 mg B. 5 mg

C. 10 mg D. 18 mg

Ans. C.

2938. Daily iron requirement of a woman of reproductive age is about

A. 1 mg B. 2 mg

C. 10 mg D. 20 mg

Ans. D.

2939. All the following are good sources of iron except

A. Milk B. Meat

C. Liver D. Kidney

Ans. A.

2940. Relatively more iron is absorbed from

A. Green leafy vegetables B. Fruits

C. Whole grain cereals D. Organ meats

Ans. D.

2941. Iron absorption from a mixed diet is about

A. 1–5 % B. 5–10 %

C. 20–25 % D. 25–50 %

Ans. B.

2942. Iron deficiency causes

A. Normocytic anaemia
B. Microcytic anaemia
C. Megaloblastic anaemia
D. Pernicious anaemia

Ans. B.

2943. Prolonged and severe iron deficiency can cause astrophy of epithelium of

A. Oral cavity
B. Oesophagus
C. Stomach
D. All of these

Ans. D.

2944. All of the following statements about bronzed diabetes are true except

A. It is caused by excessive intake of copper
B. Skin becomes pigmented
C. There is damage to β cells of Islets of Langerhans
D. Liver is damaged

Ans. A.

2945. The total amount of iodine in the body of an average adult is

A. 10–15 mg
B. 20–25 mg
C. 45–50 mg
D. 75–100 mg

Ans. C.

2946. Iodine content of thyroid gland in an adult is about

A. 1–3 mg
B. 4–8 mg
C. 10–15 mg
D. 25–30 mg

Ans. C.

2947. Daily iodine requirement of an adult is about

A. 50 μg
B. 100 μg
C. 150 μg
D. 1 mg

Ans. C.

2948. Consumption of iodised salt is recommended in

A. Patients with hyperthyroidism
B. Patients with hypothyroidism
C. Pregnant women
D. Goitre belt areas

Ans. D.

2949. All the following statements about endemic goiter are true except

A. It occurs in areas where soil and water have low iodine content
B. It leads to enlargement of thyroid gland
C. It results ultimately in hyperthyroidism
D. It can be prevented by consumption of iodised salt

Ans. C.

2950. The total amount of copper in the body of an average adult is

A. 1 gm
B. 500 mg
C. 100 mg
D. 10 mg

Ans. C.

2951. The normal range of plasma copper is

A. 25–50 μg/dl
B. 50–100 μg/dl
C. 100–200 μg/dl
D. 200–400 μg/dl

Ans. C.

2952. Copper deficiency can cause

A. Polycythaemia
B. Leukocytopenia
C. Thrombocytopenia
D. Microcytic anaemia

Ans. D.

2953. Daily requirement of copper in adults is about

A. 0.5 mg
B. 1 mg
C. 2.5 mg
D. 5 mg

Ans. C.

2954. All the following statements about ceruloplasmin are correct except

A. It is a copper-containing protein
B. It possesses oxidase activity
C. It is synthesised in intestinal mucosa
D. Its plasma level is decreased inWilson's disease

Ans. C.

2955. All the following statements about Wilson's disease are correct except

A. It is a genetic disease
B. The defect involves copper-dependent P-type ATPase
C. Copper is deposited in liver, basal ganglia and around cornea
D. Plasma copper level is increased in it

Ans. D.

2956. Which of the following statements about Menke's disease are true.

A. It is an inherited disorder of copper metabolism
B. It occurs only in males
C. Plasma copper is increased in it
D. Hair becomes steely and kinky in it

Ans. C.

2957. The total amount of zinc in an average adult is

A. 0.25–0.5 gm
B. 0.5–1.0 gm
C. 1.5–2.0 gm
D. 2.5–5.0 gm

Ans. C.

2958. Plasma zinc level is

A. 10–50 μg/dl
B. 50–150 μg/dl
C. 150–250 μg/dl
D. 250–500 μg/dl

Ans. B.

2959. Zinc is a cofactor for

A. Acid phosphatase
B. Alkaline phosphatase
C. Amylase
D. Lipase

Ans. B.

2960. Zinc is involved in storage and release of

A. Histamine
B. Acetylcholine
C. Epinephrine
D. Insulin

Ans. D.

2961. Intestinal absorption of zinc is retarded by

A. Calcium
B. Cadmium
C. Phytate
D. All of these

Ans. D.

2962. The daily zinc requirement of an average adult is

A. 5 mg
B. 10 mg
C. 15 mg
D. 25 mg

Ans. C.

2963. Zinc deficiency occurs commonly in

A. Acrodermatitis enteropathica
B. Wilson's disease
C. Xeroderma pigmentosum
D. Menke's disease

Ans. D.

2964. Hypogonadism can occur in deficiency of

A. Copper
B. Chromium
C. Zinc
D. Manganese

Ans. C.

2965. Healing of wounds may be impaired in deficiency of

A. Selenium B. Copper

C. Zinc D. Cobalt

Ans. C.

2966. Hypochromic microcytic anaemia can occur in

A. Zinc B. Copper

C. Manganese D. None of these

Ans. B.

2967. The daily requirement for manganese in adults is about

A. 1–2 mg B. 2–5 mg

C. 2–5 μg D. 5–20 μg

Ans. B.

2968. Molybdenum is a cofactor for

A. Xanthine oxidase B. Aldehyde oxidase

C. Sulphite oxidase D. All of these

Ans. D.

2969. A trace element having antioxidant function is

A. Selenium B. Tocopherol

C. Chromium D. Molybdenum

Ans. A.

2970. Selenium is a constituent of

A. Glutathione reductase B. Glutathione peroxidase

C. Catalase D. Superoxide dismutase

Ans. B.

2971. Selenium decreases the requirement of

A. Copper B. Zinc

C. Vitamin D D. Vitamin E

Ans. D.

2972. Upper safe limit of fluorine in water is

A. 0.4 ppm B. 0.8 ppm

C. 1.2 ppm D. 2 ppm

Ans. C.

2973. The daily fluoride intake should not exceed

A. 0.5 mg
B. 1 mg
C. 2 mg
D. 3 mg

Ans. D.

2974. In adults, water constitutes about

A. 50% of body weight
B. 55% of body weight
C. 60% of body weight
D. 75% of body weight

Ans. C.

2975. 1 kcal is roughly equal to

A. 4.2 J
B. 42 J
C. 4.2 KJ
D. 42 KJ

Ans. C.

2976. Calorific value of proteins as determined in a bomb calorimeter is

A. 4 kcal/gm
B. 4.8 kcal/gm
C. 5.4 kcal/gm
D. 5.8 kcal/gm

Ans. C.

2977. Calorific value of proteins in a living person is less than that in a bomb calorimeter because

A. Digestion and absorption of proteins is less than 100%
B. Respiratory quotient of proteins is less than 1
C. Specific dynamic action of proteins is high
D. Proteins are not completely oxidized in living persons

Ans. D.

2978. Calorific value of alcohol is

A. 4 kcal/gm
B. 5.4 kcal/gm
C. 7 kcal/gm
D. 9 kcal/gm

Ans. C.

2979. Energy expenditure of a person can be measured by

A. Bomb calorimetry
B. Direct calorimetry
C. Indirect calorimetry
D. Direct or indirect calorimetry

Ans. D.

2980. Respiratory quotient of carbohydrates is about

A. 0.5
B. 0.7
C. 0.8
D. 1.0

Ans. D.

2981. Respiratory quotient of fats is about

A. 0.5 B. 0.7

C. 0.8 D. 1.0

Ans. B.

2982. Respiratory quotient of proteins is about

A. 0.5 B. 0.7

C. 0.8 D. 1.0

Ans. C.

2983. Respiratory quotient of an average mixed diet is about

A. 0.65 B. 0.7

C. 0.75 D. 0.85

Ans. D.

2984. At a respiratory quotient of 0.85, every litre of oxygen consumed represents an energy expenditure of

A. 5.825 kcal B. 4.825 kcal

C. 3.825 kcal D. 2.825 kcal

Ans. B.

2985. BMR of healthy adult men is about

A. 30 kcal/hour/square metre B. 35 kcal/hour/square metre

C. 40 kcal/hour/square metre D. 45 kcal/hour/square metre

Ans. C.

2986. BMR of healthy adult women is about

A. 32 kcal/hour/square metre B. 36 kcal/hour/square metre

C. 40 kcal/hour/square metre D. 44 kcal/hour/square metre

Ans. B.

2987. BMR is higher in

A. Adults than in children

B. Men than in women

C. Vegetarians than in non-vegetarians

D. Warmer climate than in colder climate

Ans. B.

2988. BMR is decreased in

A. Pregnancy B. Starvation

C. Anaemia D. Fever

Ans. B.

2989. BMR is increased in

A. Starvation B. Hypothyroidism

C. Addison's disease D. Pregnancy

Ans. D.

2990. BMR is decreased in all of the following except

A. Fever B. Addison's disease

C. Starvation D. Hypothyroidism

Ans. A.

2991. BMR is increased in all of the following except

A. Hyperthyroidism B. Anaemia

C. Addison's disease D. Pregnancy

Ans. C.

2992. Specific dynamic action of carbohydrates is about

A. 5% B. 13%

C. 20% D. 30%

Ans. A.

2993. Specific dynamic action of proteins is about

A. 5% B. 13%

C. 20% D. 30%

Ans. D.

2994. All following are essential trace elements except

A. Iron B. Iodine

C. Zinc D. Cadmium

Ans. D.

2995. Maximum quantity of sodium is excreted through

A. Urine B. Faeces

C. Sweat D. None of these

Ans. A.

2996. All followings are rich sources of magnesium, except

A. Milk B. Eggs

C. Meat D. Cabbage

Ans. C.

2997. All followings are poor sources of iron except

A. Milk B. Potatoes

C. Wheat flour D. Liver

Ans. D.

2998. The Iron deficient children, absorption of Iron from GIT is

A. Unaltered B. Double than in normal child

C. Manifold than in normal child D. Lesser than in normal child

Ans. B.

2999. Main source of fluoride for human beings is

A. Milk B. Water

C. Vegetables D. Eggs

Ans. B.

3000. Quantity of copper present in the body of an adult is

A. 0–50 mg B. 50–100 mg

C. 100–150 mg D. 150–250 mg

Ans. C.

3001. A level of 310–340 mg per 1000 ml of blood is normal for the

A. Copper B. Iron

C. Potassium D. Sodium

Ans. D.

3002. Daily requirement of phosphorous for an infant is

A. 240–400 mg B. 1.2 gms

C. 800 mg D. 800–1200 mg

Ans. A.

3003. Maximum quantity of Zinc is present in the body in

A. Prostate B. Choroid

C. Skin D. Bones

Ans. C.

3004. Average concentration of chloride ions in cerebrospinal fluid per 100 ml is

A. 40 mg B. 440 mg

C. 160 mg D. 365 mg

Ans. B.

3005. Total iron content of the normal adult is

A. 1-2 gm B. 3-4 gm

C. 4-5 gm D. 7-10 gm

Ans. C.

3006. Absorption of phosphorous from diet is favoured by

A. Moderate amount of fat B. Acidic environment

C. High calcium content D. High phytic acid

Ans. B.

3007. Daily intake of potassium for a normal person should be

A. 1 gm B. 2 gm

C. 3 gm D. 4 gm

Ans. D.

3008. Absorption of calcium decreases if there is high concentration in the diet of

A. Copper B. Sodium

C. Magnesium D. Cadmium

Ans. C.

3009. Of the following highest concentration of calcium is seen in

A. Blood B. CSF

C. Muscle D. Nerve

Ans. C.

3010. Cobalt is essential component of

A. Vitamin B1 B. Vitamin B6

C. Vitamin B12 D. All of these

Ans. C.

3011. Molecular iron (Fe) is

A. Stored primarily in spleen

B. Absorbed in the intestine

C. Absorbed in the ferric, Fe+++ form

D. Stored in the body in combination with ferritin

Ans. D.

3012. Iron is absorbed from

A. Stomach
B. Duodenum and jejunum
C. Ileum
D. Noen of the above

Ans. B.

3013. The normal route of calcium excretion is

A. Kidney
B. Kidney and Liver
C. Kidney and Intestine
D. Kidney, Intestine and Pancreas

Ans. C.

3014. Hypocalcaemia affects

A. Skeletal muslces
B. Smooth muscles
C. Cardiac muscles
D. Skeletal muscles + smooth muscles + cardiac muscles

Ans. D.

3015. Transferrin is a type of

A. Albumin
B. α-globulin
C. β1 globulin
D. γ-globulin

Ans. B.

3016. The % of 'K' in Extracellular fluid is about

A. 1%
B. 2 to 3%
C. 10%
D. 15%

Ans. A.

3017. The Fe containing pigments is

A. Haematoidin
B. Bilirubin
C. Hemasiderin
D. Urobilinogen

Ans. C.

3018. All of the following are true of Wilson's disease except

A. Low total plasma Cu
B. Elevated urinary copper
C. Arthritis
D. Aminoaciduria

Ans. C.

3019. An increased serum 'Iron' and decreased 'Fe' binding capacity are found in

A. Fe-deficiency anaemia
B. Sideroblastic anaemia
C. Thalassaemia
D. Anaemia of chromic disorders

Ans. B.

3020. Iron therapy is ineffective in which of the following conditions:

A. Chronic blood loss

B. Inadequate Fe intake

C. Hypochromic anaemia of pregnancy

D. Thalassaemia minor

Ans. D.

3021. Cytosolic superoxide dismutase contains

A. Zn only B. Cu only

C. Zn and Cu D. Mn

Ans. C.

3022. A rise in blood 'Ca' may indicate

A. Paget's disease B. Vitamin D deficiency

C. Cushing's disease D. Hypervitaminosis D

Ans. D.

3023. The essential trace element which catalyzes the formation of Hb in the body is

A. Mn B. Se

C. Mg D. Cu

Ans. D.

3024. Zinc is a constituent of the enzyme:

A. Succinate dehydrogenase

B. Carbonic anhydrase

C. Mitochondrial superoxide dismutase

D. Aldolase

Ans. B.

3025. The principal cation of extra cellular fluid:

A. K+ B. Na+

C. H+ D. Ca2+

Ans. B.

3026. What is the principal cation of intracellular fluid?

A. K+ B. Na+

C. Ca2+ D. Mg2+

Ans. A.

3027. What is the normal level of K+ in the serum ?

A. 137–148 mEq/L
B. 120–160 mEq/L
C. 3.9–5.0 mEq/L
D. 0.3–0.59 mEq/L

Ans. C.

3028. The general functions of minerals are

A. The structural components of body tissues
B. In the regulation of body fluids
C. In acid-base balance
D. All of these

Ans. D.

3029. What are the functions of potassium?

A. In muscle contraction
B. Cell membrane function
C. Enzyme action
D. All of these

Ans. D.

3030. The daily requirement of calcium is

A. 200 mg
B. 400 mg
C. 800 mg
D. 600 mg

Ans. C.

3031. The normal serum inorganic phosphorous level is

A. 1.5–2.5 mg/100 ml
B. 2.5–4.5 mg/100 ml
C. 4.5–6.5 mg/100 ml
D. 0.5–1.5 mg/100 ml

Ans. B.

3032. When phosphorous level is lowered ?

A. In hyper thyroidism
B. Cirrosis of liver
C. Leukemia
D. Hypothyroidism

Ans. A.

3033. Ferritin is

A. Coenzyme
B. One of the component of photophosphorylation
C. It is the stored form of iron
D. Non-protein moiety

Ans. C.

3034. What is ceruloplasmin?

A. Plasma protein
B. Stored form of copper
C. Both A and B
D. None of these

Ans. C.

3035. The following are the functions of copper:

A. Constituent of cytochromes
B. Catalase
C. Tyrosinase
D. All of these

Ans. D.

3036. Zn is present as prosthetic group in this enzyme:

A. Carbonic anhydrase
B. Carboxy peptidase
C. Lactate dehydrogenase
D. All of these

Ans. D.

3037. Fluorosis is caused due to

A. Excessive intake of fluorine
B. Low intake of fluorine
C. Discoloration of the teeth due to low intake
D. All of these

Ans. A.

3038. What is the state of iron in transferrin?

A. Ferrous form
B. Ferric form
C. Both A and B
D. None of these

Ans. B.

3039. Haemoglobin formation needs both

A. Iron and Zinc
B. Iron and Calcium
C. Iron and Copper
D. Iron and Magnesium

Ans. C.

3040. Hormones

A. Act as coenzyme
B. Act as enzyme
C. Influence synthesis of enzymes
D. Belong to B-complex group

Ans. C.

3041. Hormone that binds to intracellular receptor is

A. Adrenocorticotropic hormone
B. Thyroxine
C. Follicle stimulating hormone
D. Glucagon

Ans. B.

3042. A hormone secreted from anterior pituitary is

A. Growth hormone
B. Vasopressin
C. Oxytocin
D. Epinephrine

Ans. A.

3043. A hormone secreted from posterior pituitary is

A. Vasopressin
B. Thyrotropic hormone
C. Prolactin
D. Adrenocorticotropic hormone

Ans. A.

3044. The number of amino acids in human growth hormone is

A. 91
B. 151
C. 191
D. 291

Ans. C.

3045. Growth hormone causes hyperglycemia. It is a result of

A. Decreased peripheral utilization of glucose
B. Decreased hepatic production via gluconeogenesis
C. Increased glycolysis in muscle
D. Decrersed lipolysis

Ans. A.

3046. Acromegaly results due to excessive release of

A. Thyroxine
B. Growth hormone
C. Insulin
D. Glucagon

Ans. B.

3047. Growth hormone is released by

A. Somatostatin
B. Growth hormone releasing hormone
C. Prolactin release inhibiting hormone
D. Luteinizing releasing hormone

Ans. B.

3048. The number of amino acids in prolactin is

A. 134
B. 146
C. 172
D. 199

Ans. D.

3049. Adrenocorticotropic hormone (ACTH) is a single polypeptide containing

A. 25 amino acid B. 39 amino acid

C. 49 amino acid D. 52 amino acid

Ans. B.

3050. Biological activity of ACTH requires

A. 10-N-terminal amino acid B. 24-N-terminal amino acid

C. 24-C-terminal amino acid D. 15-C-terminal amino acid

Ans. B.

3051. ACTH stimulates the secretion of

A. Glucocorticoids B. Epinephrine

C. Thyroxine D. Luteinizing hormone

Ans. A.

3052. Excessive secretion of ACTH causes

A. Cushing's syndrome B. Addison's disease

C. Myxoedema D. Thyrotoxicosis

Ans. A.

3053. In Cushing's syndrome-a tumour associated disease of adrenal cortex, there is

A. Decreased epinephrine production

B. Excessive cortisol production

C. Excessive epinephrine production

D. Decreased cortsoil production

Ans. B.

3054. ACTH induces rise in

A. Cyclic AMP B. Cyclic GMP

C. Calcium D. Magnesium

Ans. A.

3055. The predominant glucocorticoid is

A. Cortisol B. Aldosterone

C. Dehydroephiandrosterone D. Androstenedione

Ans. A.

3056. Cortisol is synthesized in

A. Zona fasiculata B. Zona glomerulosa

C. Zona reticularis D. Chromaffin cells

Ans. A.

3057. All mammalian steroid hormones are formed from

A. Purine
B. Pyrimidine
C. Cholesterol
D. Pyrrole

Ans. C.

3058. A very efficient inhibitor of steroid biosynthesis is

A. Aminoglutethimide
B. Aminoimidazole
C. Aminoimidazolesuccinyl carboxamine
D. Aminopterin

Ans. A.

3059. In adrenal gland the cholesterol is stored

A. Mostly in the free form
B. Mostly in esterified form
C. Large amount of free form and less amount of esterified form
D. Equal amounts of free and esterified form

Ans. B.

3060. In the resting state plasma concentration of cortisol is

A. 0.4–2.0 μg/100 ml
B. 2.0–4.0 μg/100 ml
C. 5.0–15.0 μg/100 ml
D. 18.0–25.0 μg/100 ml

Ans. C.

3061. The most important effect of aldosterone is to

A. Increase the rate of tubular reabsorption of sodium
B. Decrease the rate of tubular reabsorption of potassium
C. Decrease the reabsorption of chloride
D. Decrease the renal reabsorption of sodium

Ans. A.

3062. In the rennin-angiotensin system the primary hormone is

A. Angiotensinogen
B. Angiotensin I
C. Angiotensin II
D. Angiotensin III

Ans. C.

3063. Catecholamine hormones are synthesized in the

A. Chromaffin cells of adrenal medulla
B. Zona glomerulosa of adrenal cortex
C. Zona fasciculate of adrenal cortex
D. Zona reticularis of adrenal cortex

Ans. A.

3064. The hormone required for uterine muscle contraction for child birth is

A. Progesterone
B. Estrogen
C. Oxytocin
D. Vasopressin

Ans. C.

3065. The number of amino acids in the hormone oxytocin is

A. 7
B. 9
C. 14
D. 18

Ans. B.

3066. Vasopressin and oxytocin circulate unbound to proteins and have very short plasma half lives, on the order of

A. 1–2 minutes
B. 2–4 minutes
C. 5–8 minutes
D. 10–12 minutes

Ans. B.

3067. The number of amino acids in antidiuretic hormone is

A. 9
B. 18
C. 27
D. 36

Ans. A.

3068. ADH

A. Reabsorbs water from renal tubules
B. Excretes water from renal tubules
C. Excretes hypotonic urine
D. Causes low specific gravity of urine

Ans. A.

3069. Increased reabsorption of water from the kidney is the major consequence of the secretion of the hormone?

A. Cortisol
B. Insulin
C. Vasopressin
D. Aldosterone

Ans. C.

3070. A hormone which cannot cross the blood brain barrier is

A. Epinephrine
B. Aldosterone
C. ACTH
D. TSH

Ans. A.

3071. The plasma level of epinephrine is less than

A. 0.1 ng/ml
B. 0.2 ng/ml
C. 0.4 ng/ml
D. 0.8 ng/ml

Ans. A.

3072. Pheochromocytomas are tumours of

A. Adrenal cortex
B. Adrenal medulla
C. Pancreas
D. Bone

Ans. B.

3073. A characteristic of pheochromocytoma is elevated urinary excretion of

A. Dopamine
B. Tyrosine
C. Vinylmandelic acid
D. Phenylalanine

Ans. C.

3074. Epinephrine stimulates glycogenolysis in

A. Liver
B. Muscle
C. Liver and muscle
D. Kidney

Ans. C.

3075. A cup of strong coffee would be expected to

A. Interfere with the synthesis of prostaglandins
B. Decrease the effect of glucagon
C. Enhance the effect of epinephrine
D. Provide the vitamin nicotinic acid

Ans. C.

3076. Epinephrine is derived from norepinephrine by

A. Decarboxylation
B. Hydroxylation
C. Oxidation
D. N-methylation

Ans. D.

3077. 5- HIAA test is negative if patient is taking

A. Aspirin
B. Colchicine
C. Phenothiazone
D. Methotrexate

Ans. C.

3078. Presence of significant amount of 5-HIAA in urine indicates

A. Carcinoid in liver
B. Carcinoid in appendix
C. Metastasis of carcinoma of liver
D. Hepatoma

Ans. B.

3079. The normal serum level of thyroxine (T4) is

A. 2.0–4.0 μg/100 ml
B. 5.5–13.5 μg/100 ml
C. 14.0–20.3 μg/100 ml
D. 20.0–25.0 μg/100 ml

Ans. B.

3080. Excess secretion of thyroid hormones causes

A. Hyperthyroidism
B. Myxoedema
C. Cretinism
D. Cushing syndrome

Ans. A.

3081. Insufficient free T3 and T4 results in

A. Grave's disease
B. Myxoedema
C. Cushing syndrome
D. Gigantism

Ans. B.

3082. In primary hypothyroidism the useful estimation is of

A. T3
B. T4
C. TBG
D. Autoantibodies

Ans. D.

3083. When iodine supplies are sufficient the T3 and T4 ratio in thyroglobulin is

A. 1 : 2
B. 1 : 4
C. 1 : 7
D. 1 : 10

Ans. C.

3084. A substance which competes with iodide uptake mechanism by thyroid gland is

A. Thiocynate
B. Iodoacetate
C. Fluoride
D. Fluoroacetate

Ans. A.

3085. Thyroperoxidase enzyme contains

A. Heme
B. Copper
C. Zinc
D. Magnesium

Ans. A.

3086. Thyroid stimulating hormone is a dimer. The α-subunits of TSH, LH, FSH are identical. Thus the biological specificity must therefore be β subunit in which the number of amino acids is

A. 78
B. 112
C. 130
D. 199

Ans. B.

3087. Thyroid hormones are synthesized by the iodination of the amino acid:

A. Glycine B. Phenylalanine
C. Alanine D. Tyrosine

Ans. D.

3088. The tyrosine residues per molecule of thyroglobulin is

A. 85 B. 95
C. 115 D. 135

Ans. C.

3089. The number of amino acids in parathormone is

A. 65 B. 84
C. 115 D. 122

Ans. B.

3090. The sequence of amino acid in which the biological value of parathormone is

A. 1–15 B. 1–34
C. 30–50 D. 50–84

Ans. B.

3091. PTH

A. Reduces the renal clearance or excretion of calcium
B. Increases renal phosphate clearance
C. Increases the renal clearance of calcium
D. Decreases the renal phosphate clearance

Ans. A.

3092. The number of amino acids in the peptide hormone calcitonin is

A. 16 B. 24
C. 32 D. 40

Ans. C.

3093. Calcitonin causes

A. Calcinuria and phosphaturia B. Decrease in urinary calcium
C. Decrease in urinary phosphorous D. Increase in blood calcium level

Ans. A.

3094. The characteristic of hyperparathyroidism is

A. Low serum calcium
B. High serum phosphorous
C. Low serum calcium and high serum phosphorous
D. High serum calcium and low serum phosphate

Ans. D.

3095. Parathyroid hormone

A. Is released when serum Ca++ is too high

B. Inactivates vitamin D

C. Is secreted when Ca++ is too low

D. Depends on vitamin K for adequate activity

Ans. C.

3096. δ-Cells of islet of langerhans of pancreas produce

A. Pancreatic polypeptide B. Pancreatic lipase

C. Somatostatin D. Steapsin

Ans. C.

3097. β-cells of islet of langerhans of the pancreas secrete

A. Insulin B. Glucagon

C. Somatostatin D. Pancreatic polypeptide

Ans. A.

3098. Target tissue of insulin is

A. Red blood cells B. Renal tubular cells

C. GI tract epithelial cells D. Liver

Ans. D.

3099. Insulin is a dimmer. The number of amino acids in the A and B chain respectively is

A. 19 and 28 B. 21 and 30

C. 25 and 35 D. 29 and 38

Ans. B.

3100. In A chain of the insulin molecule the N terminal amino acid is

A. Glycine B. Valine

C. Serine D. Phenylalanine

Ans. A.

3101. In the A chain of insulin molecule the Cterminal amino acid is

A. Asparagine B. Threonine

C. Valine D. Tyrosine

Ans. A.

3102. In the B chain of insulin molecule, the N terminal amino acid is

A. Proline B. Threonine

C. Phenylalanine D. Lysine

Ans. C.

3103. In the B chain of insulin molecule, the C-terminal amino acid:

A. Threonine
B. Tyrosine
C. Glutamate
D. Valine

Ans. A.

3104. In the insulin molecule, the number of interchain disulphide brides is

A. 1
B. 2
C. 3
D. 4

Ans. B.

3105. In the insulin molecule, the number of intrachain disulphide bridges is

A. 1
B. 2
C. 3
D. 4

Ans. A.

3106. Insulin exists in polymeric forms, for polymerization it requires

A. Calcium
B. Magnesium
C. Manganese
D. Zinc

Ans. D.

3107. The number of amino acids in pre-proinsulin is

A. 51
B. 86
C. 109
D. 132

Ans. C.

3108. Proinsulin has

A. 74 amino acids
B. 86 amino acids
C. 105 amino acids
D. 109 amino acids

Ans. B.

3109. Daily secretion of insulin in a normal adult man is about

A. 10 units
B. 20 units
C. 30 units
D. 50 units

Ans. D.

3110. The insulin content of pancreas is about

A. 50–70 units
B. 100–150 units
C. 150–180 units
D. 200–250 units

Ans. D.

3111. The half life of insulin is

A. < 3–5 minutes
B. < 8–10 minutes
C. < 15 minutes
D. < 25 minutes

Ans. A.

3112. Insulin stimulates

A. Hepatic glycogenolysis
B. Hepatic glycogenesis
C. Lipolysis
D. Gluconeogenesis

Ans. B.

3113. Action of insulin on lipid metabolism is

A. It increases lipolysis and increases triglyceride synthesis
B. It decreases lipolysis and increases triglyceride synthesis
C. It decreases lipolysis and decreases triglyceride synthesis
D. It increases synthesis of triglyceride and increased ketogenesis

Ans. B.

3114. The human insulin gene located on the short arm of chromosome:

A. 11
B. 17
C. 18
D. 20

Ans. A.

3115. Normal serum insulin level varies between

A. 4–25 μU/ml
B. 25–50 μU/ml
C. 70–90 μU/ml
D. 100–120 μU /ml

Ans. A.

3116. Deficiency of insulin results in

A. Rapid uptake of sugar
B. Low blood glucose level
C. Decrease urine output
D. Presence of glucose in urine

Ans. D.

3117. The α-cells of pancreas islets produce

A. Insulin
B. Glucagon
C. Somatostatin
D. Pancreatic polypeptide

Ans. B.

3118. The number of amino acids in single chain polypeptide glucagons is

A. 21
B. 29
C. 31
D. 39

Ans. B.

3119. Glucagon enhances

A. Hepatic glycogenolysis B. Muscle glycogenolysis

C. Hepatic glycogenesis D. Lipogenesis

Ans. A.

3120. Normal serum glucagons level in fasting state varies between

A. 0—10 pg/ml B. 20–100 pg/ml

C. 200–300 pg/ml D. 400–500 pg/ml

Ans. B.

3121. Glucagon

A. Increases protein synthesis B. Inhibits lipolysis in adipocytes

C. Increases gluconeogenesis in liver D. Stimulates muscle glycogenolysis

Ans. C.

3122. Normal serum free testosterone in adult men varies between

A. 1–5 ng/dl B. 6–9 ng/dl

C. 10–30 ng/dl D. 50–100 ng/dl

Ans. C.

3123. Normal serum free testosterone in adult women varies between

A. 0.0–0.2 ng/dl B. 0.3–2 ng/dl

C. 10–30 ng/dl D. 50–100 ng/dl

Ans. B.

3124. The prepubertal total serum testosterone is

A. <100 ng/100 ml B. < 200 ng/100 ml

C. <300 ng/100 ml D. < 400 ng/100 ml

Ans. A.

3125. The total serum testosterone in adult men is

A. 50–100 ng/100 ml B. 150–250 ng/100 ml

C. 300–1000 ng/100 ml D. 1000–3000 ng/100 ml

Ans. C.

3126. The total serum testosterone in adult women is

A. 0–5 ng/100 ml B. 10–15 ng/100 ml

C. 20–80 ng/100 ml D. 100–200 ng/100 ml

Ans. C.

3127. The serum estradiol level in men is

A. 0–5 pg/ml B. 5–10 pg/ml

C. 24–68 pg/ml D. 40–60 pg/ml

Ans. C.

3128. The serum progesterone level in follicular phase is about

A. 0.2–1.5 ng/100 ml B. 2.0–2.5 ng/100 ml

C. 3.5–4.5 ng/100 ml D. 5.0–6.5 ng/100 ml

Ans. A.

3129. Serum progesterone level during pregnancy is

A. <12 ng/ml B. >12 ng/ml

C. <20 ng/ml D. >24 ng/ml

Ans. D.

3130. Androgens are produced by

A. Cells of sertoli B. Leydig cells

C. Rete testis D. Efferent ductules

Ans. B.

3131. The production of progesterone by corpus luteum cell is stimulated by

A. LH B. TSH

C. ACTH D. MSH

Ans. A.

3132. Conversion of testosterone to estradiol requires the enzyme:

A. Aromatase B. Dehydrogenase

C. Lyase D. Isomerase

Ans. A.

3133. The precursor of testosterone is

A. Aldosterone B. Methyl testosterone

C. Estrone D. Pregnenolone

Ans. D.

3134. The hormone measured in urine to test pregnancy is

A. Anterior pituitary luteinizing hormone

B. Androgen

C. Progesterone

D. Chorinic gonadotropin

Ans. D.

3135. Total number of amino acids in human chorionic gonadotropin is

A. 53 B. 92

C. 145 D. 237

Ans. D.

3136. A hormone produced by corpus luteum and placenta, concerned with relaxation of pelvis tissue is

A. HCG B. Chorionic somatomammotropin

C. Relaxin D. Progestins

Ans. C.

3137. Synthetic progesterone used in oral contraceptive is

A. Norethindrone B. Pregnenolone

C. Androstenodione D. Stilbestrol

Ans. A.

3138. Young women are protected against myocardial infaracation because of the activity of

A. Estrogen B. Progesterone

C. Growth hormone D. Oxytocin

Ans. A.

3139. Insulin receptor is a

A. Monomer B. Dimer

C. Trimer D. Tetramer

Ans. D.

3140. Melatonin is synthesised in

A. Hypothalamus B. Posterior pituitary gland

C. Pineal gland D. Melanocytes

Ans. C.

3141. Melatonin is synthesised from

A. Phenylalanine B. Tyrosine

C. Tryptophan D. None of these

Ans. C.

3142. Melanocyte stimulating hormone is secreted by

A. Pineal gland B. Anterior lobe of pituitary gland

C. Posterior lobe of pituitary gland D. Intermediate lobe of pituitary gland

Ans. D.

3143. A hormone synthesised in the hypothalamus is

A. Melatonin
B. Melanocyte stimulating hormone
C. Vasopressin
D. Prolactin

Ans. C.

3144. Posterior pituitary gland secretes

A. Catecholamines
B. Oxytocin
C. Follicle stimulating hormone
D. Serotonin

Ans. B.

3145. A nonapeptide among the following is

A. Antidiuretic hormone
B. Insulin
C. ACTH
D. Thyrotropin releasing hormone

Ans. A.

3146. Diabetes insipidus is caused by deficient secretion of

A. Insulin
B. Glucagon
C. Vasopressin
D. Oxytocin

Ans. C.

3147. Peripheral vasoconstriction is caused by high concentrations of

A. Antidiuretic hormone
B. Melatonin
C. Glucagon
D. Oxytocin

Ans. A.

3148. Somatotropin is secreted by

A. Hypothalamus
B. Anterior pituitary
C. Posterior pituitary
D. Thyroid gland

Ans. B.

3149. Secretion of Insulin-like Growth Factor-I is promoted by

A. Insulin
B. Glucagon
C. Growth hormone
D. Somatomedin C

Ans. C.

3150. Growth hormone increases

A. Protein synthesis
B. Lipogenesis
C. Glycogenolysis
D. All of these

Ans. A.

3151. Secretion of growth hormone is inhibited by

A. Somatomedin C
B. Somatostatin
C. Feedback inhibition
D. All of these

Ans. B.

3152. Secretion of somatotrophin is promoted by

A. Somatomedin C
B. Somatostatin
C. Growth hormone releasing hormone
D. Hypoglycaemia

Ans. C.

3153. Human growth hormone has

A. One polypeptide chain and one intra-chain disulphide bond
B. One polypeptide chain and two intra-chain disulphide bond
C. Two polypeptide chains joined by one disulphide bond
D. Two polypeptide chains joined by two disulphide bond

Ans. B.

3154. Number of amino acid residues in human growth hormone is

A. 51
B. 84
C. 191
D. 198

Ans. C.

3155. Number of amino acid residues in prolactin is

A. 51
B. 84
C. 191
D. 198

Ans. D.

3156. ACTH is a polypeptide made up of

A. 39 amino acids
B. 41 amino acids
C. 51 amino acids
D. 84 amino acids

Ans. A.

3157. CRH is a polypeptide made up of

A. 39 amino acids
B. 41 amino acids
C. 51 amino acids
D. 84 amino acids

Ans. B.

3158. All the following statements about TSH are true except

A. It is a tropic hormone

B. It acts on para-follicular cells of thyroid glands

C. Its receptors are membrane-bound

D. Its second messenger is cyclic AMP

Ans. B.

3159. In males, luteinising hormone acts on

A. Leydig cells
B. Sertoli cells
C. Prostate gland
D. All of these

Ans. A.

3160. Acromegaly results from overproduction of

A. ACTH during childhood

B. TSH during adult life

C. Growth hormone during childhood

D. Growth hormone during adult life

Ans. D.

3161. Acromegaly results in all the following except

A. Overgrowth of the bones of face, hands and feet

B. Increased stature

C. Enlargements of viscera

D. Impaired glucose tolerance

Ans. B.

3162. Overproduction of growth hormone during childhood causes

A. Acromegaly
B. Gigantism
C. Cushing's disease
D. Simmond's disease

Ans. B.

3163. Decreased secretion of growth hormone during childhood causes

A. Simmond's disease
B. Cushing's disease
C. Dwarfism
D. Cretinism

Ans. C.

3164. Stature is increased in

A. Gigantism
B. Acromegaly
C. Simmond's disease
D. Cushing's disease

Ans. A.

3165. An amino acid used for the synthesis of thyroid hormone is

A. Tyrosine
B. Tryptophan
C. Histidine
D. Proline

Ans. A.

3166. An enzyme required for the synthesis of thyroid hormones is

A. Iodinase
B. Deiodinase
C. Thyroperoxidase
D. Thyroxine synthetase

Ans. C.

3167. Thyroperoxidase iodinates

A. Free tyrosine in thyroid gland
B. Tyrosine residues of thyroglobulin
C. Tyrosine residues of thyroxine binding globulin
D. Tyrosine residues of thyroxine binding prealbumin

Ans. B.

3168. Thyroid hormones are present in blood

A. In free form
B. In association with thyroxine binding globulin (TBG)
C. In association with thyroxine binding prealbumin (TBPA)
D. Mainly in association with TBG, partly in free form and sometimes in association with TBPA also

Ans. D.

3169. When thyroxine binding globulin and thyroxine binding pre-albumin are saturated with thyroxine, the excess hormone is transported by

A. Albumin
B. Gamma globulins
C. Transcortin
D. None of these

Ans. A.

3170. Receptors for thyroid hormones are present

A. On the cell membrane
B. Across the cell membrane
C. Inside the cells
D. In association with G-proteins

Ans. C.

3171. The most powerful thyroid hormone is

A. Reverse T3
B. DIT
C. T3
D. T4

Ans. C.

3172. The most abundant thyroid hormone in blood is

A. Free T3 B. T3 bound to TBG

C. Free T4 D. T4 bound to TBG

Ans. D.

3173. Secretion of thyroid hormones is regulated by

A. Hypothalamus B. Anterior pituitary

C. Feedback regulation D. All of these

Ans. D.

3174. Clinical features of hyperthyroidism include

A. Goitre, heat intolerance, weight loss and tachycardia

B. Goitre, tremors, tachycardia and cold intolerance

C. Exophthalmos, goiter, tachycardia and loss of appetite

D. Exophthalmos, goiter, tremors and obesity

Ans. A.

3175. All the following may occur in hyperthyroidism except

A. Goitre B. Increased appetite

C. Loss of weight D. Low BMR

Ans. D.

3176. All the following may occur in myxoedema except

A. Cold intolerance B. Low BMR

C. Tachycardia D. Dry and coarse skin

Ans. C.

3177. Mental retardation can occur in

A. Cretinism B. Juvenile myxoedema

C. Myxoedema D. Juvenile thyrotoxicosis

Ans. A.

3178. Parathyroid hormone (PTH) is synthesized in

A. Chief cells of parathyroid glands

B. Oxyphil cells of parathyroid glands

C. Para follicular cells of thyroid glands

D. Follicular cells of thyroid gland

Ans. A.

3179. The number of amino acid residues in PTH:

A. 51 B. 84

C. 90 D. 115

Ans. B.

3180. Amino acid residues which are essential for the biological activity of PTH are

A. N-terminal 34 amino acids B. N-terminal 50 amino acids

C. C-terminal 34 amino acids D. C-terminal 50 amino acids

Ans. A.

3181. Half-life of PTH is

A. A few seconds B. A few minutes

C. A few hours D. A few days

Ans. B.

3182. PTH causes all of the following except

A. Increased intestinal absorption of calcium

B. Increased intestinal absorption of phosphate

C. Increased tubular reabsorption of calcium

D. Increased tubular reabsorption of phosphate

Ans. D.

3183. Secretion of PTH is regulated by

A. Hypothalamus B. Anterior pituitary

C. Feedback effect of plasma PTH D. Feedback effect of plasma calcium

Ans. D.

3184. A high concentration of PTH in blood causes

A. Increase in plasma calcium and inorganic phosphorous

B. Decrease in plasma calcium and inorganic phosphorous

C. Increase in plasma calcium and decrease in plasma inorganic phosphorous

D. Decrease in plasma calcium and increase in plasma inorganic phosphorous

Ans. C.

3185. Tetany can occur

A. In primary hyperparathyroidism

B. In secondary hyperparathyroidism

C. In idiopathic hypoparathyroidism

D. After accidental removal of parathyroid glands

Ans. D.

3186. Crystallisation of insulin occurs in the presence of

A. Chromium B. Copper

C. Zinc D. Calcium

Ans. C.

3187. Daily secretion of insulin is about

A. 10–20 mg B. 40–50 mg

C. 10–20 units D. 40–50 units

Ans. D.

3188. Insulin receptors are decreased in number in

A. Obesity B. Starvation

C. Hyperinsulinism D. Kwashiorkor

Ans. A.

3189. Insulin binding sites are present on the

A. α-subunits of insulin receptor B. β-subunits of insulin receptor

C. γ-subunits of insulin receptor D. α-and β”subunits of insulin receptor

Ans. A.

3190. α-Subunits of insulin receptor are present

A. Outside the cell membrane B. In the cell membrane

C. Across the cell membrane D. In the cytosol

Ans. A.

3191. β-Subunits of insulin receptor are present

A. Outside the cell membrane B. In the cell membrane

C. Across the cell membrane D. In the cytosol

Ans. C.

3192. Insulin receptor is made up of

A. One α-and one β-subunit B. Two α-and two β-subunit

C. Two, α two β-and two γ-subunit D. One α, one β-one γ-and one δ-subunit

Ans. B.

3193. Insulin is required for the active uptake of glucose by most of the cells except

A. Muscle cells B. Renal tubular cells

C. Adipocytes D. Liver cells

Ans. D.

3194. Insulin decreases

A. Glycogenesis
B. Glyolysis
C. Gluconeogenesis
D. Tubular reabsorption of glucose

Ans. C.

3195. Insulin increases

A. Glycogenesis
B. Gluconeogenesis
C. Lipolysis
D. Blood glucose

Ans. A.

3196. Insulin increases

A. Protein synthesis
B. Fatty acid synthesis
C. Glycogen synthesis
D. All of these

Ans. D.

3197. Diabetes mellitus can occur due to all of the following except

A. Deficient insulin secretion
B. Tumour of β"cells
C. Decrease in number of insulin receptors
D. Formation of insulin antibodies

Ans. B.

3198. Hypoglycaemic coma can occur

A. In untreated diabetes mellitus
B. In starvation
C. After overdose of oral hypoglycaemic drugs
D. After overdose of insulin

Ans. D.

3199. Number of amino acid residues in glucagons is

A. 29
B. 34
C. 51
D. 84

Ans. A.

3200. Glucagon secretion increases

A. After a carbohydrate-rich meal
B. After a fat-rich meal
C. When blood glucose is high
D. When blood glucose is low

Ans. D.

3201. The main effect of glucagons is to increase
A. Glycolysis in muscles
B. Glycogenolysis in muscles
C. Glycogenolysis in liver
D. Glycogenesis in liver

Ans. C.

3202. Tyrosine is required for the synthesis of all of the following except
A. Melatonin
B. Epinephrine
C. Norepinephrine
D. Thyroxine

Ans. A.

3203. Dopamine is synthesised from
A. Dihydroxyphenylalanine
B. Epinephrine
C. Norepinephrine
D. Metanephrine

Ans. A.

3204. Blood brain barrier can be crossed by
A. Epinephrine
B. Dopamine
C. Dopa
D. All of these

Ans. C.

3205. Epinephrine is synthesised in
A. Chromaffin cells of adrenal medulla
B. Sympathetic ganglia
C. Brain
D. All of these

Ans. D.

3206. Immediate precursor of epinephrine is
A. Metanephrine
B. Norepinephrine
C. Dopa
D. Dopamine

Ans. B.

3207. Epinephrine decreases
A. Glycogenesis
B. Glycogenolysis
C. Gluconeogenesis
D. Lipolysis

Ans. A.

3208. Epinephrine increases the concentration of free fatty acids in plasma by increasing
A. Extramitochondrial fatty acid synthesis
B. Mitochondrial fatty acid chain elongation
C. Microsomal fatty acid chain elongation
D. Lipolysis in adipose tissue

Ans. D.

3209. Epinephrine increases all of the following except

A. Glycogenolysis in muscles
B. Lipolysis in adipose tissue
C. Gluconeogenesis in muscles
D. Glucagon secretion

Ans. C.

3210. Zona glomerulosa of adrenal cortex synthesises

A. Glucocorticoids
B. Mineralocorticoids
C. Androgens
D. Estrogen and progesterone

Ans. A.

3211. Cortisol is a

A. Glucocorticoid
B. Mineralocorticoid
C. Androgen
D. Estrogen

Ans. B.

3212. Steroid hormones are synthesised in all of the following except

A. Testes
B. Ovaries
C. Adrenal medulla
D. Adrenal cortex

Ans. A.

3213. Steroid hormones are synthesised from

A. Cholesterol
B. 7-Dehydrocholesterol
C. Calcitriol
D. 7-Hydroxycholesterol

Ans. A.

3214. A common intermediate in the synthesis of all the steroid hormones is

A. Pregnenolone
B. 17-Hydroxypregnenolone
C. Corticosterone
D. Progesterone

Ans. A.

3215. A common intermediate in the synthesis of cortisol and aldosterone is

A. Progesterone
B. Testosterone
C. Estradiol
D. None of these

Ans. A.

3216. A common intermediate in the synthesis of estrogens is

A. Cortisol
B. Andostenedione
C. Corticosterone
D. 11-Deoxycorticosterone

Ans. B.

3217. Glucocorticoids are transported in blood

A. In association with transcortin chiefly

B. In association with albumin to some extent

C. In free form partly

D. All of these

Ans. D.

3218. The second messenger for glucocorticoids is

A. Cyclic AMP
B. Cyclic GMP
C. Inositol triphosphate
D. No second messenger is required

Ans. D.

3219. Secretion of glucocorticoids is regulated by all the following except

A. Hypothalamus

B. Anterior pituitary

C. Feedback control by blood glucose

D. Feedback control by glucocorticoids

Ans. C.

3220. Excessive secretion of glucocorticoids raises blood glucose by

A. Decreasing glycogenesis
B. Increasing glycogenolysis
C. Increasing gluconeogenesis
D. Inhibiting HMP shunt

Ans. C.

3221. Mineralcorticoids regulate the metabolism of all of the following except

A. Sodium
B. Potassium
C. Calcium
D. Chloride

Ans. C.

3222. Mineralocorticoids increase the tubular reabsorption of

A. Sodium and calcium
B. Sodium and potassium
C. Sodium and chloride
D. Potassium and chloride

Ans. C.

3223. Mineralocorticoids increase the tubular secretion of

A. Sodium
B. Potassium
C. Chloride
D. Bicarbonate

Ans. B.

3224. In Addison's disease, there is excessive retention of

A. Potassium
B. Sodium
C. Chloride
D. Water

Ans. A.

3225. Spironolactone is an antagonist of

A. Cortisol
B. Hydrocortisone
C. Aldosterone
D. Testosterone

Ans. C.

3226. Androgens are synthesised in

A. Leydig cells in testes
B. Sertoli cells in testes
C. Seminiferous tubules
D. Prostate gland

Ans. A.

3227. Testosterone is transported in blood by

A. Transcortin
B. Testosterone binding globulin
C. Testosterone estrogen binding globulin
D. Albumin

Ans. C.

3228. An androgen which is more powerful than testosterone is

A. Androstenedione
B. Dihydrotestosterone
C. Androsterone
D. Epiandrosterone

Ans. B.

3229. Secretion of androgens is increased by

A. LH
B. FSH
C. ACTH
D. Growth hormone

Ans. A.

3230. During late pregnancy, the major source of progesterone is

A. Adrenal cortex
B. Placenta
C. Corpus luteum
D. Graafian follicles

Ans. B.

3231. Progesterone is transported in blood by

A. Transcortin
B. Sex hormone binding globulin
C. Albumin
D. Testosterone estrogen binding globulin

Ans. A.

3232. The major metabolite of progesterone is
A. Pregnenolone
B. Pregnanediol
C. Estradiol
D. Norethindrone

Ans. B.

3233. Secretion of progesterone
A. Is more in first half of menstrual cycle than in second half
B. Is more in second half of menstrual cycle than in first half
C. Remains constant during menstrual cycle
D. Decreases during pregnancy

Ans. B.

3234. Women become susceptible to osteoporosis after menopause due to decreased
A. Secretion of Parathormone
B. Conversion of vitamin D into calcitriol
C. Secretion of estrogen
D. Secretion of progesterone

Ans. C.

3235. A hormone used for detection of pregnancy is
A. Estrogen
B. Progesterone
C. Oxytocin
D. Chorionic gonadotropin

Ans. D.

3236. Placenta secretes all of the following except
A. FSH
B. Progesterone
C. Estrogen
D. Chorionic gonadotropin

Ans. A.

3237. Gastrin is a polypeptide made up of
A. Five amino acids
B. Twelve amino acids
C. Seventeen amino acids
D. Twenty amino acids

Ans. C.

3238. Biological activity of gastrin is present in the
A. Four N-terminal amino acids
B. Four C-terminal amino acids
C. Five N-terminal amino acids
D. Five C-terminal amino acids

Ans. B.

3239. Iodide uptake by thyroid gland is decreased by
A. Thiocyanate
B. Thiouracil
C. Thiourea
D. Methimazole

Ans. A.

3240. Proteoglycans are made up of proteins and

A. Glucosamine
B. Mannosamine
C. Sialic acid
D. Mucopolysaccharides

Ans. D.

3241. Sweat chlorides are increased in

A. Cystic fibrosis
B. Pancreatic cancer
C. Acute pancreatitis
D. None of these

Ans. A.

3242. Radioactive iodine uptake by thyroid gland 24 hours of a test dose is

A. 1.5–15% of the test dose
B. 15–20% of the test dose
C. 20–40% of the test dose
D. 50–70% of the test dose

Ans. C.

3243. Radioactive iodine uptake by thyroid gland is increased in

A. Endemic goitre
B. Hyperthyroidism
C. Myxoedema
D. Creatinism

Ans. B.

3244. Normal range of total thyroxine in serum is

A. 0.8–2.4 ng/dl
B. 0.8–2.4 μg/dl
C. 5–12 ng/dl
D. 5–12 μg/dl

Ans. D.

3245. Administration of TSH increases serum T3 and T4 in

A. Hyperthyroidism of pituitary origin
B. Hyperthyroidism of thyroid origin
C. Hypothyroidism of pituitary origin
D. Hypothyroidism of thyroid origin

Ans. C.

3246. High level of T3 and T4 and low TSH in serum indicates

A. Hyperthyroidism of pituitary origin
B. Hypothyroidism of pituitary origin
C. Hyperthyroidism of thyroid origin
D. Hypothyroidism of thyroid origin

Ans. C.

3247. BMR is increased in

A. Endemic goitre
B. Thyrotoxicosis
C. Myxoedema
D. Cretinism

Ans. B.

3248. Which one of the following causes frame shift mutation?

A. Transition
B. Transversion
C. Deletion
D. Substitution of purine to pyrimidine

Ans. C.

3249. The most potent hormone concerned with the retention of sodium in the body is

A. Cortisone
B. Aldosterone
C. Corticosterone
D. Cortisol

Ans. B.

3250. Aspirin blocks the synthesis of

A. Prostaglandins only
B. Prostacyclins only
C. Thromboxanes only
D. All of these

Ans. D.

3251. Retention of sodium in the body leads to a retention of

A. Potassium
B. Water
C. Potassium and water
D. Neither potassium nor water

Ans. B.

3252. There is polyuria without glycosuria in this disorder

A. Diabetes insipidus
B. Diabetes millitus
C. Bronze diabetes
D. Juvenile diabetes

Ans. A.

3253. In hyperparathyroidism there is

A. Hypocalcemia
B. Hypophophatemia
C. Hypokalemia
D. Hyperkalemia

Ans. B.

3254. Insulin resistance is encountered in

A. Addison's disease
B. Hypothyroidism
C. Hypopitutarism
D. Acromegaly

Ans. D.

3255. Richest source of prostaglandins in a human male is

A. Blood
B. Urine
C. Semen
D. C.S.F.

Ans. C.

3256. This pancreatic hormone increases the blood-sugar level:

A. Insulin
B. Glucagon
C. Pancreozymin
D. Pancreatic polypeptide

Ans. B.

3257. Which one of the following statements is fully correct?

A. Hormones are needed in the diet
B. Hormones can be elaborated only by endocrine glands
C. All the hormones enter the cells and perform their function
D. Hormones are substance synthesized in the body in small quantities and control and regulate metabolic events

Ans. D.

3258. T3 is

A. Thyroxine
B. Triiodothyronine
C. Triodo tyrosine
D. Reverse tri iodo thyronine

Ans. B.

3259. Whcih of the following hormone is a peptide of less than ten amino acids?

A. Insulin
B. Growth hormone
C. Oxytocin
D. Parathyroid hormone

Ans. C.

3260. Whcih of the following hormone does not activate adenylate cyclase?

A. Epinephrine
B. Glucagon
C. Parathyroid hormone
D. Insulin

Ans. D.

3261. Pheochromacytoma is a tumor of

A. Adrenal medulla
B. Bone
C. Head of Pancreas
D. Pituitary

Ans. A.

3262. Which one of the following statements is incorrect?

A. Insulin increases glucose phosphorylation
B. Insulin increases glycolysis
C. Insulin augments HMP shunt
D. Insulin promotes gluconeogenesis

Ans. D.

3263. Which one ring in the structure of the following is aromatic?

A. Androgens
B. Estrogens
C. Cholesterol
D. Bile acids

Ans. B.

3264. Which of one of the following is not GUT hormone?

A. Motiline
B. Secretion
C. Gastrin
D. Calcitonin

Ans. D.

3265. Which of the following hormones are synthesized as prehormones

A. Vasopressin and oxytocin
B. Growth hormone and insulin
C. Insulin and parathyroid hormone
D. Insulin and Glucagon

Ans. C.

3266. This hormone has disulphide group:

A. Glucagon
B. Insulin
C. T4
D. Epinephrine

Ans. B.

3267. The blood sugar raising action of the hormone of supradrenal cortex is due to

A. Glyconeogenesis
B. Glycogenolysis
C. Glucagon like activity
D. Due to inhibition of glomerular filtration of glucose

Ans. A.

3268. Hyper insulinism can cause coma since

A. The chief nutrient for the brain is glucose
B. The chief nutrient for the heart is glucose
C. The glucostatic role of the liver is damaged
D. The kidneys are damaged

Ans. A.

3269. Which of the following property of prostaglandins has been utilized by clinicians in hospital for

A. Inducing fever
B. Causing inflammation
C. Effecting smooth muscle contraction
D. Disaggregation of spermatozoa

Ans. C.

3270. A major structural difference between estrogens and androgens is the fact that

A. The androgens are usually C21 steroids

B. The estrogens are usually digitonin - precipitable

C. The androgens have an aromatic ring

D. The estrogens have an aromatic ring

Ans. D.

3271. Alloxan can experimentally induce diabetes mellitus due to

A. Stimulation of α cells of the islets of langerhans

B. Necrosis of the β cells of the islets

C. Potentiation of insulinase activity

D. Epinephrine like action

Ans. B.

3272. Which of the following alleviates asthma?

A. PGE1 only
B. PGE1 and PGE2
C. PGF2
D. PGA

Ans. B.

3273. Thyroxine is derived from

A. Tyrosine
B. Tyranine
C. Taurine
D. Tryptaine

Ans. A.

3274. Adrneal cortical response is poor in

A. Kwashiorkor
B. Marasmus
C. Fatty liver
D. Atherosclerosis

Ans. A.

3275. Protein bound iodine in blood is present to the extent of———— / dL

A. 3–8 mg
B. 4–8 mg
C. 3–8 gm
D. 4–8 gm

Ans. A.

3276. Prostaglandins are

A. C2 unsaturated acids
B. C27 saturated alcohols
C. C20 saturated acids
D. C27 saturated alcohols

Ans. A.

3277. Which of the following scientists has not worked in the field of prostaglandins?

A. Voneuler B. Sultan Karim

C. Andre robet D. Kendal

Ans. D.

3278. The suffix number in the names of prostaglandins gives the number of

A. OH groups B. Double bonds

C. Acid groups D. Ketoacids

Ans. B.

3279. One of the important functions of prostacyclins is

A. Inhibition of platelet aggregation B. Contraction of uterus

C. Decrease of gastric secretion D. Relieving osthma

Ans. A.

3280. Vasopressin is also known as

A. Antidiabetogenic hormone B. Antidiuretic hormone

C. Somatotropic hormone D. Pitoxin

Ans. A.

3281. Which of the following is used for inducing labour?

A. Prostaglandins B. Prostacyclins

C. Vasopressin D. Thromboxanes

Ans. A.

3282. Which of the following does not have disulphide bond?

A. Oxytocin B. Vasopressin

C. Insulin D. Glucagon

Ans. D.

3283. Which is incorrect ? Epinephrin promotes the glycogenolysis in

A. Muscle B. Liver

C. Heart D. None of these

Ans. C.

3284. Which one of the following is released by hypothalamus?

A. Somatostatin B. Somatotropic hormone

C. Somato medin C D. Luteinising hormone

Ans. A.

3285. Which of the following organ prefers fructose to glucose

A. Liver
B. Testes
C. Pancreas
D. Heart

Ans. B.

3286. Total synthesis of creatine can be done by

A. Liver
B. Kidneys
C. Pancreas
D. Heart

Ans. C.

3287. Thyrotropin releasing hormone is a

A. Dipeptide
B. Tripeptide
C. Octapeptide
D. Decapeptide

Ans. B.

3288. The sequence of amino acids in human growth hormone and the synthesis were done by

A. Sanger
B. Krebs
C. Chah Holi
D. Molisch

Ans. C.

3289. Adrenalin is synthesized from

A. Adenine
B. Adenosine
C. Tyrosine
D. Tryptophan

Ans. C.

3290. Prolactin release inhibiting hormone is believed to be

A. Serotonin
B. Norepinephrine
C. Dopamine
D. Acetyl choline

Ans. C.

3291. Whcih one of the following is not a symptom of cushing's disease?

A. Hyperglycemia
B. Hypernatremia
C. Hirsutism
D. Hyperkalemia

Ans. D.

3292. Somatostatin is produced by

A. Hypothalamus
B. Pancreas
C. Hypothalamus and Pancreas
D. Hypothalamus and Adrenals

Ans. C.

3293. Insulin like growth hormones are produced by

A. Hypophysis
B. Liver
C. Pancreas
D. Thyroid

Ans. B.

3294. One of the following does not bind T3 and T4:

A. Albumin
B. TBG
C. TBPA
D. Haptoglobin

Ans. D.

3295. Epinephrine causes in muscle:

A. Gluconeogenesis
B. Glycogenesis
C. Glycolysis
D. Glycogenolysis

Ans. D.

3296. Reverse T3 is

A. A synthetic compound given counter the effects of T3
B. Formed from T4 but has no hormone function
C. Formed by isomerisation of T3
D. Formed from T4 and has hormone function

Ans. B.

3297. This pancreatic hormone promotes hypogenesis:

A. Insulin
B. Glucagon
C. Stomatostatin
D. Pancreozymine

Ans. A.

3298. It is unique that the following single antidiabetogenic hormone effectively counter acts the several diabetogenic hormones:

A. Glucagon
B. Glucocorticoids
C. Insulin
D. Growth hormone

Ans. C.

3299. Which of the following statements is correct?

A. Thyroxine inhibits utilization of glucose
B. Insulin increases utilization of glucose
C. Glucagon promotes muscle glycogenolysis
D. Insulin inhibits lipogenesis from carbohydrates

Ans. B.

3300. Steroid hormones are synthesized from

A. Adenine
B. Protein
C. Vitamin
D. Cholesterol

Ans. D.

3301. Hormones act only on specific organs or tissues. These are called

A. Active sites
B. Reaction centre
C. Target organ/Tissue
D. Physiological site

Ans. C.

3302. —————— hormone is a single chain polypeptide having 32 amino acids with molecular weight of 3,600.

A. Testosterone
B. Thyroxine
C. Calcitonin
D. Vasopressin

Ans. C.

3303. Which of the following is noted in Cushing's syndrome, a tumor associated disease of the adrenal cortex?

A. Decreased production of epinephrine
B. Excessive production of epinephrine
C. Excessive production of vasopressin
D. Excessive production of cortisol

Ans. D.

3304. A cup of strong coffee would be expected to

A. Interfere with synthesis of prostaglandins
B. Decrease the effects of Glucagon
C. Enhance the effects of epinephrine
D. Provide the vitamin nicotinic acid

Ans. C.

3305. Increased reabsorption of water from the kidney is the major consequence of which of the following hormones?

A. Cortisol
B. Insulin
C. Vasopressin
D. Aldosterone

Ans. C.

3306. ADP ribosylation is the mode of action of

A. Cholera toxin
B. Acetyl choline
C. Muscerinic receptors
D. Cyclic AMP

Ans. A.

3307. Which one of the following hormones is derived most completely from tyrosine?

A. Glucagon B. Thyroxine

C. Insulin D. Prostaglandins

Ans. B.

3308. All the following hormones use cAMP as a second messenger except

A. Estrogen B. FSH

C. Luteinizing D. Glucagon

Ans. A.

3309. All the following hormones promote hyperglycemia except

A. Epinephrine B. Norepinephrine

C. Insulin D. Glucagon

Ans. C.

3310. Glucagon activates the enzyme adenylcyclase which causes the increase of blood sugar level. Hence this hormone is called

A. Hypoglycemic factor B. Hyper glycemic factor

C. Antidiauritic factor D. Thyrotropin-releasing factor

Ans. B.

3311. TSH hormone biochemically is a

A. Protein B. Fat

C. Glycoprotein D. Carbohydrate

Ans. C.

3312. The secondary sexual characters in females is effected by

A. Estrogens B. Gluco corticoids

C. MIS D. None of these

Ans. A.

3313. Gastric Secretion is regulated by the hormone:

A. Glucagon B. Gastrin

C. Epinephrin D. ACTH

Ans. B.

3314. An essential agent for converting glucose to glycogen in liver is

A. Latic acid B. GTP

C. UTP D. Pyruvic acid

Ans. C.

3315. Which of the following hormones is not involved in carbohydrate metabolism?

A. ACTH
B. Glucagon
C. Vasopressin
D. Growth hormone

Ans. C.

3316. In the process of transcription, the flow of genetic information is from

A. DNA to DNA
B. DNA to protein
C. RNA to protein
D. DNA to RNA

Ans. D.

3317. Anticodon region is an important part of the structure of

A. r-RNA
B. t-RNA
C. m-RNA
D. z-DNA

Ans. B.

3318. A nucleoside consists of

A. Nitrogenous base
B. Purine or pyrimidine base + sugar
C. Purine or pyrimidine base + phosphorous
D. Purine + pyrimidine base + sugar +phosphorous

Ans. B.

3319. A nucleotide consists of

A. A nitrogenous base like choline
B. Purine + pyrimidine base + sugar +phosphorous
C. Purine or pyrimidine base + sugar
D. Purine or pyrimidine base + phosphorous

Ans. B.

3320. A purine nucleotide is

A. AMP
B. UMP
C. CMP
D. TMP

Ans. A.

3321. A pyrimidine nucleotide is

A. GMP
B. AMP
C. CMP
D. IMP

Ans. C.

3322. Adenine is

A. 6-Amino purine
B. 2-Amino-6-oxypurine
C. 2-Oxy-4-aminopyrimidine
D. 2, 4-Dioxypyrimidine

Ans. A.

3323. 2, 4-Dioxypyrimidine is

A. Thymine
B. Cystosine
C. Uracil
D. Guanine

Ans. C.

3324. The chemical name of guanine is

A. 2,4-Dioxy-5-methylpyrimidine
B. 2-Amino-6-oxypurine
C. 2-Oxy-4-aminopyrimidine
D. 2, 4-Dioxypyrimidine

Ans. B.

3325. Uracil and ribose form

A. Uridine
B. Cytidine
C. Guanosine
D. Adenosine

Ans. A.

3326. The most abundant free nucleotide in mammalian cells is

A. ATP
B. NAD
C. GTP
D. FAD

Ans. A.

3327. The mean intracellular concentration of ATP in mammalian cell is about

A. 1 mM
B. 2 mM
C. 0.1 mM
D. 0.2 mM

Ans. A.

3328. The nucleic acid base found in mRNA but not in DNA is

A. Adenine
B. Cytosine
C. Guanine
D. Uracil

Ans D.

3329. In RNA molecule 'Caps'

A. Allow tRNA to be processed
B. Are unique to eukaryotic mRNA
C. Occur at the 3' end of tRNA
D. Allow correct translation of prokaryotic mRNA

Ans. B.

3330. In contrast to eukaryotic mRNA, prokaryotic mRNA

A. Can be polycistronic
B. Is synthesized with introns
C. Can only be monocistronic
D. Has a poly A tail

Ans. A.

3331. The size of small stable RNA ranges from

A. 0–40 nucleotides
B. 40–80 nucleotides
C. 90–300 nucleotides
D. More than 320 nucleotides

Ans. C.

3332. The number of small stable RNAs per cell ranges from

A. 10–50,000
B. 50,000–1,00,000
C. 1,00,000–10,00,000
D. More than 10 lakhs

Ans. C.

3333. In RNA molecule guanine content does not necessarily equal to its cytosine content nor does its adenine content necessarily equal its uracil content since it is a

A. Single strand molecule
B. Double stranded molecule
C. Double stranded helical molecule
D. Polymer of purine and pyrimidine ribonucleotides

Ans. A.

3334. The nitrogenous base present in the RNA molecule is

A. Thymine
B. Uracil
C. Xanthine
D. Hypoxanthine

Ans. B.

3335. RNA does not contain

A. Uracil
B. Adenine
C. Thymine
D. Ribose

Ans. C.

3336. The sugar moiety present in RNA is

A. Ribulose
B. Arabinose
C. Ribose
D. Deoxyribose

Ans. C.

3337. In RNA molecule

A. Guanine content equals cytosine

B. Adenine content equals uracil

C. Adenine content equals guanine

D. Guanine content does not necessarily equal its cytosine content

Ans. D.

3338. Methylated purines and pyrimidines are characteristically present in

A. mRNA
B. hnRNA
C. tRNA
D. rRNA

Ans. C.

3339. Thymine is present in

A. tRNA
B. Ribosomal RNA
C. Mammalian mRNA
D. Prokaryotic mRNA

Ans. A.

3340. The approximate number of nucleotides in tRNA molecule is

A. 25
B. 50
C. 75
D. 100

Ans. C.

3341. In every cell, the number of tRNA molecules is at least

A. 10
B. 20
C. 30
D. 40

Ans. B.

3342. The structure of tRNA appears like a

A. Helix
B. Hair pin
C. Clover leaf
D. Coil

Ans. C.

3343. Although each specific tRNA differs from the others in its sequence of nucleotides, all tRNA molecules contain a base paired stem that terminates in the sequence CCA at

A. 3' Termini
B. 5' Termini
C. Anticodon arm
D. 3' 5' Termini

Ans. A.

3344. Transfer RNAs are classified on the basis of the number of base pairs in

A. Acceptor arm B. Anticodon arm

C. D arm D. Extra arm

Ans. D.

3345. In tRNA molecule D arm is named for the presence of the base:

A. Uridine B. Pseudouridine

C. Dihydrouridine D. Thymidine

Ans. A.

3346. The acceptor arm in the tRNA molecule has

A. 5 Base pairs B. 7 Base pairs

C. 10 Base pairs D. 20 Base pairs

Ans. B.

3347. In tRNA molecule, the anticodon arm possesses

A. 5 Base pairs B. 7 Base pairs

C. 8 Base pairs D. 10 Base pairs

Ans. A.

3348. The T ø C arm in the tRNA molecule possesses the sequence

A. T, pseudouridine and C B. T, uridine and C

C. T, dihydrouridine and C D. T, adenine and C

Ans. A.

3349. Double helical structure model of the DNA was proposed by

A. Pauling and Corey B. Peter Mitchell

C. Watson and Crick D. King and Wooten

Ans. C.

3350. DNA does not contain

A. Thymine B. Adenine

C. Uracil D. Deoxyribose

Ans. C.

3351. The sugar moiety present in DNA is

A. Deoxyribose B. Ribose

C. Lyxose D. Ribulose

Ans. A.

3352. DNA rich in A-T pairs have

A. 1 Hydrogen bond
B. 2 Hydrogen bonds
C. 3 Hydrogen bonds
D. 4 Hydrogen bonds

Ans. B.

3353. In DNA molecule

A. Guanine content does not equal cytosine content
B. Adenine content does not equal thymine content
C. Adenine content equals uracil content
D. Guanine content equals cytosine content

Ans. D.

3354. DNA rich in G-C pairs have

A. 1 Hydrogen bond
B. 2 Hydrogen bonds
C. 3 Hydrogen bonds
D. 4 Hydrogen bonds

Ans. C.

3355. The fact that DNA bears the genetic information of an organism implies that

A. Base composition should be identical from species to species
B. DNA base composition should charge with age
C. DNA from different tissues in the same organism should usually have the same base composition
D. DNA base composition is altered with nutritional state of an organism

Ans. C.

3356. The width (helical diameter) of the double helix in B-form DNA in nm is

A. 1
B. 2
C. 3
D. 4

Ans. B.

3357. The number of base pair in a single turn of B-form DNA about the axis of the molecule is

A. 4
B. 8
C. 10
D. 12

Ans. C.

3358. The distance spanned by one turn of B form DNA is

A. 1.0 nm
B. 2.0 nm
C. 3.0 nm
D. 3.4 nm

Ans. D.

3359. In a DNA molecule the thymine concentration is 30%, the guanosine concentration will be

A. 10% B. 20%

C. 30% D. 40%

Ans. B.

3360. In a DNA molecule, the guanosine content is 40%, the adenine content will be

A. 10% B. 20%

C. 30% D. 40%

Ans. A.

3361. An increased melting temperature of duplex DNA results from a high content of

A. Adenine + Guanine B. Thymine + Cytosine

C. Cytosine + Guanine D. Cytosine + Adenine

Ans. C.

3362. A synthetic nucleotide analogue, 4-hydroxypyrazolopyrimidine is used in the treatment of

A. Acute nephritis B. Gout

C. Cystic fibrosis of lung D. Multiple myeloma

Ans. B.

3363. A synthetic nucleotide analogue, used in the chemotherapy of cancer and viral infections is

A. Arabinosyl cytosine B. 4-Hydroxypyrazolopyrimidine

C. 6-Mercaptopurine D. 6-Thioguanine

Ans. A.

3364. Infantile convulsions due to lesser formation of gamma amino butyric acid from glutamic acid is seen in the deficiency of

A. Glutamate-dehydrogenase B. Pyridoxine

C. Folic acid D. Thiamine

Ans. B.

3365. Which of the following amino acids produce a vasoconstrictor on decarboxylation?

A. Histidine B. Tyrosine

C. Threonine D. Arginine

Ans. B.

3366. Purine biosynthesis is inhibited by

A. Aminopterin B. Tetracyclin

C. Methotrexate D. Chloramphenicol

Ans. A.

3367. Pyrimidine and purine nucleoside biosynthesis share a common precursor:

A. PRPP B. Glycine

C. Fumarate D. Alanine

Ans. A.

3368. A substrate for enzymes of pyrimidine nucleotide biosynthesis is

A. Allopurinol B. Tetracylin

C. Chloramphenicol D. Puromycin

Ans. A.

3369. The enzyme aspartate transcarbamoylase of pyrimidine biosynthesis is inhibited by

A. ATP B. ADP

C. AMP D. CTP

Ans. D.

3370. In humans end product of purine catabolism is

A. Uric acid B. Urea

C. Allantoin D. Xanthine

Ans. A.

3371. In humans purine are catabolised to uric acid due to lack of the enzyme:

A. Urease B. Uricase

C. Xanthine oxidase D. Guanase

Ans. B.

3372. In mammals other than higher primates uric acid is converted by

A. Oxidation to allantoin B. Reduction to ammonia

C. Hydrolysis to ammonia D. Hydrolysis to allantoin

Ans. A.

3373. The correct sequence of the reactions of catabolism of adenosine to uric acid is

A. Adenosine→hypoxanthine→xanthine→uric acid

B. Adenosine→xanthine→inosine→uric acid

C. Adenosine→inosine→hypoxanthine→xanthine→uric acid

D. Adenosine→xanthine→inosine→hypoxanthine→uric acid

Ans. C.

3374. Gout is a metabolic disorder of catabolism of

A. Pyrimidine B. Purine

C. Alanine D. Phenylalanine

Ans. B.

3375. Gout is characterized by increased plasma levels of

A. Urea B. Uric acid

C. Creatine D. Creatinine

Ans. B.

3376. The major catabolic product of pyrimidines in human is

A. β-Alanine B. Urea

C. Uric acid D. Guanine

Ans. A.

3377. An autosomal recessive disorder, xanthinuria is due to deficiency of the enzymes:

A. Adenosine deaminase B. Xanthine oxidase

C. HGPRTase D. Transaminase

Ans. B.

3378. Polysomes lack in

A. DNA B. mRNA

C. rRNA D. tRNA

Ans. A.

3379. Genetic code is

A. Collection of codon B. Collection of amino acids

C. Collection of purine nucleotide D. Collection of pyrimidine nucleotide

Ans. A.

3380. Degeneracy of genetic code implies that

A. Codons do not code for specific amino acid

B. Multiple codons must decode the same amino acids

C. No anticodon on tRNA molecule

D. Specific codon decodes many amino acids

Ans. B.

3381. Genetic code is

A. Overlapping B. Non-overlapping

C. Not universal D. Ambiguous

Ans. B.

3382. mRNA is complementary to the nucleotide sequence of

A. Coding strand
B. Ribosomal RNA
C. tRNA
D. Template strand

Ans. A.

3383. In DNA replication the enzyme required in the first step is

A. DNA directed polymerase
B. Unwinding proteins
C. DNA polymerase
D. DNA ligase

Ans. B.

3384. The smallest unit of DNA capable of coding for the synthesis of a polypeptide is

A. Operon
B. Repressor gene
C. Cistron
D. Replicon

Ans. C.

3385. Termination of the synthesis of the RNA molecule is signaled by a sequence in the template strand of the DNA molecule, a signal that is recognized by a termination protein, the

A. Rho (ρ) factor
B. ó factor
C. δ factor
D. ε factor

Ans. A.

3386. In the process of transcription in bacterial cells

A. Initiation requires rho protein
B. RNA polymerase incorporates methylated bases in correct sequence
C. Both the sigma unit and core enzymes of RNA polymerase are required for accurate promotor site binding
D. Primase is necessary for initiation

Ans. C.

3387. The correct statement concerning RNA and DNA polymerases is

A. RNA polymerase use nucleoside diphosphates
B. RNA polymerase require primers and add bases at 5' end of the growing polynucleotide chain
C. DNA polymerases can add nucleotides at both ends of the chain
D. All RNA and DNA polymerases can add nucleotides only at the 3' end of the growing polynucleotide chain

Ans. D.

3388. The eukaryotic nuclear chromosomal DNA

A. Is a linear and unbranched molecule

B. Is not associated with a specific membranous organelle

C. Is not replicated semiconservatively

D. Is about of the same size as each prokaryotic chromoses

Ans. A.

3389. All pribnow boxes are variants of the sequence:

A. 5' – TATAAT – 3' B. 5' – GAGCCA – 3'

C. 5' – UAACAA – 3' D. 5' – TCCTAG – 3'

Ans. A.

3390. 5'-Terminus of mRNA molecule is capped with

A. Guanosine triphosphate B. 7-Methylguanosine triphophate

C. Adenosine triphosphate D. Adenosine diphosphate

Ans. B.

3391. The first codon to be translated on mRNA is

A. AUG B. GGU

C. GGA D. AAA

Ans. A.

3392. AUG, the only identified codon for methionine is important as

A. A releasing factor for peptide chains

B. A chain terminating codon

C. Recognition site on tRNA

D. A chain initiating codon

Ans. D.

3393. In biosynthesis of proteins the chain terminating codons are

A. UAA, UAG and UGA B. UGG, UGU and AGU

C. AAU, AAG and GAU D. GCG, GCA and GCU

Ans. A.

3394. The formation of initiation complex during protein synthesis requires a factor:

A. IF-III B. EF-I

C. EF-II D. IF-I

Ans. A.

3395. The amino terminal of all polypeptide chain at the time of synthesis in E. coli is tagged to the amino acid residue:

A. Methionine
B. Serine
C. N-formyl methinine
D. N-formal serine

Ans. C.

3396. Initiation of protein synthesis begins with binding of

A. 40S ribosomal unit on mRNA
B. 60S ribosomal unit
C. Charging of tRNA with specific amino acid
D. Attachment of aminoacyl tRNA on mRNA

Ans. A.

3397. Initiation of protein synthesis requires

A. ATP
B. AMP
C. GDP
D. GTP

Ans. D.

3398. The enzyme amino acyl tRNA synthetase is involved in

A. Dissociation of discharged tRNA from 80S ribosome
B. Charging of tRNA with specific amino acids
C. Termination of protein synthesis
D. Nucleophilic attack on esterified carboxyl group of peptidyl tRNA

Ans. B.

3399. In the process of activation of amino acids for protein synthesis, the number of high energy phosphate bond equivalent utilised is

A. 0
B. 1
C. 2
D. 4

Ans. C.

3400. Translation results in a product known as

A. Protein
B. tRNA
C. mRNA
D. rRNA

Ans. A.

3401. In eukaryotic cells

A. Formylated tRNA is important for initiation of translation
B. Cyclohexamide blocks elongation during translation
C. Cytosolic ribosomes are smaller than those found in prokaryotes
D. Erythromycin inhibits elongation during translation

Ans. B.

3402. The mushroom poison amanitin is an inhibitor of

A. Protein synthesis
B. mRNA synthesis
C. DNA synthesis
D. Adenosine synthesis

Ans. B.

3403. Tetracylin prevents synthesis of polypeptide by

A. Blocking mRNA formation from DNA
B. Releasing peptides from mRNA-tRNA complex
C. Competing with mRNA for ribosomal binding sites
D. Preventing binding of aminoacyl tRNA

Ans. D.

3404. In prokaryotes, chloramphenicol

A. Causes premature release of the polypeptide chain
B. Causes misreading of the mRNA
C. Depolymerises DNA
D. Inhibits peptidyl transferase activity

Ans. A.

3405. Streptomycin prevents synthesis of polypeptide by

A. Inhibiting initiation process
B. Releasing premature polypeptide
C. Inhibiting peptidyl transferase activity
D. Inhibiting translocation

Ans. A.

3406. Erythromycin acts on ribosomes and inhibit

A. Formation of initiation complex
B. Binding of aminoacyl tRNA
C. Peptidyl transferase activity
D. Translocation

Ans. D.

3407. The binding of prokaryotic DNA dependent RNA polymerase to promoter sites of genes is inhibited by the antibiotic:

A. Puromycin
B. Rifamycin
C. Terramycin
D. Streptomycin

Ans. B.

3408. In the lac operon concept, a protein molecule is

A. Operator
B. Inducer
C. Promoter
D. Repressor

Ans. D.

3409. The enzyme DNA ligase

A. Introduces superhelical twists
B. Connects the end of two DNA chains
C. Unwinds the double helix
D. Synthesises RNA primers

Ans. B.

3410. Restriction endonucleases

A. Cut RNA chains at specific locations
B. Excise introns from hnRNA
C. Remove Okazaki fragments
D. Act as defensive enzymes to protect the host bacterial DNA from DNA of foreign organisms

Ans. D.

3411. The most likely lethal mutation is

A. Substitution of adenine for cytosine
B. Insertion of one nucleotide
C. Deletion of three nucleotides
D. Substitution of cytosine for guanine

Ans. B.

3412. Restriction endonucleases recognize and cut a certain sequence of

A. Single stranded DNA
B. Double stranded DNA
C. RNA
D. Protein

Ans. B.

3413. Interferon

A. Is virus specific
B. Is a bacterial product
C. Is a synthetic antiviral agent
D. Requires expression of cellular genes

Ans. D.

3414. Repressor binds to DNA sequence and regulate the transcription. This sequence is called

A. Attenuator
B. Terminator
C. Anti terminator
D. Operator

Ans. D.

3415. Okazaki fragment is related to

A. DNA synthesis
B. Protein synthesis
C. mRNA formation
D. tRNA formation

Ans. A.

3416. The region of DNA known as TATA BOX is the site for binding of

A. DNA polymerase
B. DNA topoisomerase
C. DNA dependent RNA polymerase
D. Polynucleotide phosphorylase

Ans. C.

3417. Reverse transcriptase is capable of synthesising

A. RNA→DNA
B. DNA→RNA
C. RNA→RNA
D. DNA→DNA

Ans. A.

3418. A retrovirus is

A. Polio virus
B. HIV
C. Herpes virus
D. Tobacco mosaic virus

Ans. B.

3419. Peptidyl transferase activity is located in

A. Elongation factor
B. A charged tRNA molecule
C. Ribosomal protein
D. A soluble cytosolic protein

Ans. C.

3420. Ultraviolet light can damage a DNA strand causing

A. Two adjacent purine residue to form a covalently bounded dimer
B. Two adjacent pyrimidine residues to form covalently bonded dimer
C. Disruption of phosphodiesterase linkage
D. Disruption of non-covalent linkage

Ans. B.

3421. Presence of arginine can be detected by

A. Sakaguchi reaction
B. Million-Nasse reaction
C. Hopkins-Cole reaction
D. Gas chromatography

Ans. A.

3422. In nucleotides, phosphate is attached to sugar by

A. Salt bond
B. Hydrogen bond
C. Ester bond
D. Glycosidic bond

Ans. C.

3423. Cyclic AMP can be formed from

A. AMP
B. ADP
C. ATP
D. All of these

Ans. C.

3424. A substituted pyrimidine base of pharmacological value is

A. 5-Iododeoxyuridine B. Cytisine arabinoside
C. 5-Fluorouracil D. All of these

Ans. C.

3425. The 'transforming factor' discovered by Avery, McLeod and McCarty was later found to be

A. mRNA B. tRNA
C. DNA D. None of these

Ans. C.

3426. In DNA, the complementary base of adenine is

A. Guanine B. Cytosine
C. Uracil D. Thymine

Ans. D.

3427. In DNA, three hydrogen bonds are formed between

A. Adenine and guanine B. Adenine and thymine
C. Guanine and cytosine D. Thymine and cytosine

Ans. C.

3428. Left handed double helix is present in

A. Z-DNA B. A-DNA
C. B-DNA D. None of these

Ans. A.

3429. Nuclear DNA is present in combination with

A. Histones B. Non-histones
C. Both (A) and (B) D. None of these

Ans. C.

3430. Number of guanine and cytosine residues is equal in

A. mRNA B. tRNA
C. DNA D. None of these

Ans. C.

3431. Alkalis cannot hydrolyse

A. mRNA B. tRNA
C. rRNA D. DNA

Ans. D.

3432. Codons are present in

A. Template strand of DNA
B. mRNA
C. tRNA
D. rRNA

Ans. B.

3433. Amino acid is attached to tRNA at

A. 5'-End
B. 3'-End
C. Anticodon
D. DHU loop

Ans. B.

3434. In prokaryotes, the ribosomal subunits are

A. 30 S and 40 S
B. 40 S and 50 S
C. 30 S and 50 S
D. 40 S and 60 S

Ans. C.

3435. Ribozymes are

A. Enzymes present in ribosomes
B. Enzymes which combine the ribosomal subunits
C. Enzymes which dissociate
D. Enzymes made up of RNA

Ans. D.

3436. The smallest RNA among the following is

A. rRNA
B. hnRNA
C. mRNA
D. tRNA

Ans. D.

3437. The number of adenine and thymine bases is equal in

A. DNA
B. mRNA
C. tRNA
D. rRNA

Ans. A.

3438. The number of hydrogen bonds between adenine and thymine in DNA is

A. One
B. Two
C. Three
D. Four

Ans. B.

3439. The complementary base of adenine in RNA is

A. Thymine
B. Cystosine
C. Guanine
D. Uracil

Ans. D.

3440. Extranuclear DNA is present in

A. Ribosomes B. Endoplasmic reticulum

C. Lysosomes D. Mitochondria

Ans. D.

3441. Mitochondrial DNA is present in

A. Bacteria B. Viruses

C. Eukaryotes D. All of these

Ans. C.

3442. Ribothymidine is present in

A. DNA B. tRNA

C. rRNA D. hnRNA

Ans. B.

3443. Ten base pairs are present in one turn of the helix in

A. A-DNA B. B-DNA

C. C-DNA D. Z-DNA

Ans. B.

3444. Transfer RNA transfers

A. Information from DNA to ribosomes

B. Information from mRNA to cytosol

C. Amino acids from cytosol to ribosomes

D. Proteins from ribosomes to cytosol

Ans. C.

3445. Nucleotides required for the synthesis of nucleic acids can be obtained from

A. Dietary nucleic acids and nucleotides

B. De novo synthesis

C. Salvage of pre-existing bases and nucleosides

D. De novo synthesis and salvage

Ans. D.

3446. De novo synthesis of purine nucleotide occurs in

A. Mitochondria B. Cytosol

C. Microsmes D. Ribosomes

Ans. B.

3447. The nitrogen atoms for de novo synthesis of purine nucleotides are provided by

A. Aspartate and glutamate
B. Aspartate and glycine
C. Aspartate, glutamine and glycine
D. Aspartate, glutamate and glycine

Ans. C.

3448. For de novo synthesis of purine nucleotides, glycine provides

A. One nitrogen atom
B. One nitrogen and one carbon atom
C. Two carbon atoms
D. One nitrogen and two carbon atoms

Ans. D.

3449. For de novo synthesis of purine nucleotides, aspartate provides

A. Nitrogen 1
B. Nitrogen 3
C. Nitrogen 7
D. Nitrogen 9

Ans. A.

3450. In the purine nucleus, carbon 6 is contributed by

A. Glycine
B. CO2
C. Aspartate
D. Glutamine

Ans. B.

3451. 5-Phosphoribosyl-1-pyrophosphate is required for the synthesis of

A. Purine nucleotides
B. Pyrimidine nucleotides
C. Both (A) and (B)
D. None of these

Ans. C.

3452. Free purine bases which can be salvaged are

A. Adenine and guanine
B. Adenine and hypoxanthine
C. Guanine and hypoxanthine
D. Adenine, guanine and hypoxanthine

Ans. D.

3453. Uric acid is the end product of purine as well as protein catabolism in

A. Man
B. Fish
C. Birds
D. None of these

Ans. C.

3454. Daily uric acid excretion in adult men is

A. 2–6 mg
B. 20–40 mg
C. 150–250 mg
D. 40–600 mg

Ans. D.

3455. Dietary purines are catabolised in

A. Liver
B. Kidneys
C. Intesitnal mucosa
D. All of these

Ans. C.

3456. De novo synthesis of pyrimidine nucleotides occurs in

A. Mitochondria
B. Cytosol
C. Microsomes
D. Ribosomes

Ans. B.

3457. An enzyme common to de novo synthesis of pyrimidine nucleotides and urea is

A. Urease
B. Carbamoyl phosphate synthetase
C. Aspartate transcarbamoylase
D. Argininosuccinase

Ans. B.

3458. The nitrogen atoms of pyrimidine nucleus are provided by

A. Glutamate
B. Glutamate and aspartate
C. Glutamine
D. Glutamine and aspartate

Ans. D.

3459. The carbon atoms of pyrimidine nucleus are provided by

A. Glycine and aspartate
B. CO2 and aspartate
C. CO2 and glutamate
D. CO2 and glutamine

Ans. B.

3460. The following cannot be salvaged in human beings:

A. Cytidine
B. Deoxycytidine
C. Cytosine
D. Thymidine

Ans. C.

3461. Free ammonia is liberated during the catabolism of

A. Cytosine
B. Uracil
C. Thymine
D. All of these

Ans. D.

3462. β -Alanine is formed from catabolism of

A. Thymine
B. Thymine and cytosine
C. Thymine and uracil
D. Cytosine and uracil

Ans. D.

3463. Inheritance of primary gout is

A. Autosomal recessive
B. Autosomal dominant
C. X-linked recessive
D. X-linked dominant

Ans. C.

3464. All the following statements about primary gout are true except

A. Its inheritance is X-linked recessive
B. It can be due to increased activity of PRPP synthetase
C. It can be due to increased activity of hypoxanthine guanine phosphoribosyl transferase
D. De novo synthesis of purines is increased in it

Ans. C.

3465. All of the following statements about uric acid are true except

A. It is a catabolite of purines
B. It is excreted by the kidneys
C. It is undissociated at pH above 5.8
D. It is less soluble than sodium urate

Ans. C.

3466. All of the following statements about uric acid are true except

A. It can be formed from allantoin
B. Formation of uric acid stones in kidneys can be decreased by alkalinisation of urine
C. Uric acid begins to dissociate at pH above 5.8
D. It is present in plasma mainly as monosodium urate

Ans. A.

3467. All of the following statements about primary gout are true except

A. Uric acid stones may be formed in kidneys
B. Arthritis of small joints occurs commonly
C. Urinary excretion of uric acid is decreased
D. It occurs predominantly in males

Ans. C.

3468. All of the following statements about allopurinol are true except

A. It is a structural analogue of uric acid
B. It can prevent uric acid stones in the kidneys
C. It increases the urinary excretion of xanthine and hypoxanthine
D. It is a competitive inhibitor of xanthine oxidase

Ans. A.

3469. Inherited deficiency of adenosine deaminase causes

A. Hyperuricaemia and gout B. Mental retardation

C. Immunodeficiency D. Dwarfism

Ans. C.

3470. Complete absence of hypoxanthine guanine phospharibosyl transferase causes

A. Primary gout B. Immunodeficiency

C. Uric acid stones D. Lesh-Nyhan syndrome

Ans. D.

3471. All of the following can occur in Lesch- Nyhan syndrome except

A. Gouty arthritis B. Uric acid stones

C. Retarted growth D. Self-mutiliating behavior

Ans. C.

3472. Inherited deficiency of purine nucleoside phosphorylase causes

A. Dwarfism B. Mental retardation

C. Immunodeficiency D. Gout

Ans. C.

3473. Mammals other than higher primates do not suffer from gout because they

A. Lack xanthine oxidase

B. Lack adenosine deaminase

C. Lack purine nucleoside phosphorylase

D. Possess uricase

Ans. D.

3474. Synthesis of DNA is also known as

A. Duplication B. Replication

C. Transcription D. Translation

Ans. B.

3475. Replication of DNA is

A. Conservative B. Semi-conservative

C. Non-conservative D. None of these

Ans. B.

3476. Direction of DNA synthesis is

A. 5' '! 3' B. 3' '! 5'

C. Both (A) and (B) D. None of these

Ans. A.

3477. Okazaki pieces are made up of

A. RNA B. DNA

C. RNA and DNA D. RNA and proteins

Ans. C.

3478. Okazaki pieces are formed during the synthesis of

A. mRNA B. tRNA

C. rRNA D. DNA

Ans. D.

3479. After formation of replication fork

A. Both the new strands are synthesized discontinuously

B. One strand is synthesized continuously and the other discontinuously

C. Both the new strands are synthesized continuously

D. RNA primer is required only for the synthesis of one new strand

Ans. B.

3480. An Okazaki fragment contains about

A. 10 Nucleotides B. 100 Nucleotides

C. 1,000 Nucleotides D. 10,000 Nucleotides

Ans. C.

3481. RNA primer is formed by the enzyme:

A. Ribonuclease B. Primase

C. DNA polymerase I D. DNA polymerase III

Ans. B.

3482. In RNA, the complementary base of adenine is

A. Cytosine B. Guanine

C. Thymine D. Uracil

Ans. D.

3483. During replication, the template DNA is unwound

A. At one of the ends B. At both the ends

C. At multiple sites D. Nowhere

Ans. C.

3484. During replication, unwinding of double helix is initiated by

A. DNA A protein B. DNA B protein

C. DNA C protein D. Rep protein

Ans. B.

3485. For unwinding of double helical DNA,

A. Energy is provided by ATP

B. Energy is provided by GTP

C. Energy can be provided by either ATP or GTP

D. No energy is required

Ans. A.

3486. Helicase and DNA B protein cause

A. Rewinding of DNA and require ATP as a source of energy

B. Rewinding of DNA but do not require any source of energy

C. Unwinding of DNA and require ATP as a source of energy

D. Unwinding of DNA but do not require any source of energy

Ans. C.

3487. The unwound strands of DNA are held apart by

A. Single strand binding protein B. Double strand binding protein

C. Rep protein D. DNA A protein

Ans. A.

3488. Deoxyribonucleotides are added to RNA primer by

A. DNA polymerase I B. DNA polymerase II

C. DNA polymerase III holoenzyme D. All of these

Ans. C.

3489. Ribonucleotides of RNA primer are replaced by deoxyribonucleotides by the enzyme

A. DNA polymerase I B. DNA polymerase II

C. DNA polymerase III holoenzyme D. All of these

Ans. A.

3490. DNA fragments are sealed by

A. DNA polymerase II B. DNA ligase

C. DNA gyrase D. DNA topoisomerase II

Ans. B.

3491. Negative supercoils are introduced in DNA by

A. Helicase B. DNA ligase

C. DNA gyrase D. DNA polymerase III holoenzyme

Ans. C.

3492. Reverse transcriptase activity is present in the eukaryotic

A. DNA polymerase α
B. DNA polymerase γ
C. Telomerase
D. DNA polymerase II

Ans. C.

3493. DNA polymerase III holoenzyme possesses

A. Polymerase activity
B. 3'-5' Exonuclease activity
C. 5'-3' Exonuclease and polymerase activities
D. 3'-5' Exonuclease and polymerase activities

Ans. D.

3494. DNA polymerase I possesses

A. Polymerase activity
B. 3'-5' Exonuclease activity
C. 5'-3' Exonuclease activity
D. All of these

Ans. D.

3495. 3'-5' Exonuclease activity of DNA polymerase I

A. Removes ribonucleotides
B. Adds deoxyribonucleotides
C. Corrects errors in replication
D. Hydrolyses DNA into mononucleotides

Ans. C.

3496. All of the following statements about RNA-dependent DNA polymerase are true except:

A. It synthesizes DNA using RNA as a template
B. It is also known as reverse transcriptase
C. It synthesizes DNA in 5'-3' direction
D. It is present in all the viruses

Ans. D.

3497. Reverse transcriptase catalyses

A. Synthesis of RNA
B. Breakdown of RNA
C. Synthesis of DNA
D. Breakdown of DNA

Ans. C.

3498. DNA A protein can bind only to

A. Positively supercoiled DNA
B. Negatively supercoiled DNA
C. Both (A) and (B)
D. None of these

Ans. B.

3499. DNA topoisomerase I of *E. coli* catalyses

A. Relaxation of negatively supercoiled DNA

B. Relaxation of positively supercoiled DNA

C. Conversion of negatively supercoiled DNA into positively supercoiled DNA

D. Conversion of double helix into supercoiled DNA

Ans. A.

3500. In mammalian cell cycle, synthesis of DNA occurs during

A. S phase B. G1 phase

C. Mitotic Phase D. G2 phase

Ans. A.

3501. Melting temperature of DNA is the temperature at which

A. Solid DNA becomes liquid

B. Liquid DNA evaporates

C. DNA changes from double helix into supercoiled DNA

D. Native double helical DNA is denatured

Ans. D.

3502. Melting temperature of DNA is increased by its

A. A and T content B. G and C content

C. Sugar content D. Phosphate content

Ans. B.

3503. Buoynat density of DNA is increased by its

A. A and T content B. G and C content

C. Sugar content D. None of these

Ans. B.

3504. Relative proportions of G and C versus A and T in DNA can be determined by its

A. Melting temperature B. Buoyant density

C. Both (A) and (B) D. None of these

Ans. C.

3505. Some DNA is present in mitochondria of

A. Prokaryotes B. Eukaryotes

C. Both (A) and (B) D. None of these

Ans. B.

3506. Satellite DNA contains

A. Highly repetitive sequences
B. Moderately repetitive sequences
C. Non-repetitive sequences
D. DNA-RNA hybrids

Ans. A.

3507. Synthesis of RNA and a DNA template is known as

A. Replication
B. Translation
C. Transcription
D. Mutation

Ans. C.

3508. Direction of RNA synthesis is

A. 5'-3'
B. 3'-5'
C. Both (A) and (B)
D. None of these

Ans. A.

3509. DNA-dependent RNA polymerase is a

A. Monomer
B. Dimer
C. Trimer
D. Tetramer

Ans. D.

3510. DNA-dependent RNA polymerase requires the following for its catalytic activity:

A. Mg++
B. Mn++
C. Both (A) and (B)
D. None of these

Ans. C.

3511. The initiation site for transcription is recognized by

A. α"Subunit of DNA-dependent RNA polymerase
B. β"Subunit of DNA-dependent RNA polymerase
C. Sigma factor
D. Rho factor

Ans. C.

3512. The termination site for transcription is recognized by

A. α"Subunit of DNA-dependent RNA polymerase
B. β"Subunit of DNA-dependent RNA polymerase
C. Sigma factor
D. Rho factor

Ans. D.

3513. Mammalian RNA polymerase I synthesises

A. mRNA B. rRNA

C. tRNA D. hnRNA

Ans. B.

3514. Mammalian RNA polymerase III synthesises

A. rRNA B. mRNA

C. tRNA D. hnRNA

Ans. C.

3515. In mammals, synthesis of mRNA is catalysed by

A. RNA polymerase I B. RNA polymerase II

C. RNA polymerase III D. RNA polymerase IV

Ans. B.

3516. Heterogeneous nuclear RNA is the precursor of

A. mRNA B. rRNA

C. tRNA D. None of these

Ans. A.

3517. Post-transcriptional modification of hnRNA involves all of the following except

A. Addition of 7-methylguanosine triphosphate cap

B. Addition of polyadenylate tail

C. Insertion of nucleotides

D. Deletion of introns

Ans. C.

3518. Newly synthesized tRNA undergoes posttranscriptional modifications which include all the following except

A. Reduction in size B. Methylation of some bases

C. Formation of pseudouridine D. Addition of C-C-A terminus at 5' end

Ans. D.

3519. Post-transcriptional modification does not occur in

A. Eukaryotic tRNA B. Prokaryotic tRNA

C. Eukaryotic hnRNA D. Prokaryotic mRNA

Ans. D.

3520. A consensus sequence on DNA, called TATA box, is the site for attachment of

A. RNA-dependent DNA polymerase
B. DNA-dependent RNA polymerase
C. DNA-dependent DNA polymerase
D. DNA topoisomerase II

Ans. B.

3521. Polyadenylate tail is not present in mRNA synthesising

A. Globin
B. Histone
C. Apoferritin
D. Growth hormone

Ans. B.

3522. Introns are present in DNA of

A. Viruses
B. Bacteria
C. Man
D. All of these

Ans. C.

3523. A mammalian DNA polymerase among the following is

A. DNA polymerase α
B. DNA polymerase I
C. DNA polymerase II
D. DNA polymerase IV

Ans. A.

3524. Mammalian DNA polymerase γ is located in

A. Nucleus
B. Nucleolus
C. Mitochondria
D. Cytosol

Ans. C.

3525. Replication of nuclear DNA in mammals is catalysed by

A. DNA polymerase α
B. DNA polymerase β
C. DNA polymerase γ
D. DNA polymerase III

Ans. A.

3526. Primase activity is present in

A. DNA polymerase II
B. DNA polymerase α
C. DNA polymerase β
D. DNA polymerase δ

Ans. B.

3527. The mammalian DNA polymerase involved in error correction is

A. DNA polymerase α
B. DNA polymerase β
C. DNA polymerase γ
D. DNA polymerase δ

Ans. B.

3528. Novobicin inhibits the synthesis of

A. DNA B. mRNA

C. tRNA D. rRNA

Ans. A.

3529. Ciprofloxacin inhibits the synthesis of

A. DNA B. mRNA

C. tRNA D. rRNA

Ans. A.

3530. Ciprofloxacin inhibits

A. DNA topisomerase II B. DNA polymerase I

C. DNA polymerase III D. DNA gyrase

Ans. D.

3531. Rifampicin inhibits

A. Unwinding of DNA B. Initiation of replication

C. Initiation of translation D. Initiation of transcription

Ans. D.

3532. Actinomycin D binds to

A. Double stranded DNA B. Single stranded DNA

C. Single stranded RNA D. DNA-RNA hybrid

Ans. A.

3533. DNA contains some palindromic sequences which

A. Mark the site for the formation of replication forks

B. Direct DNA polymerase to turn back to replicate the other strand

C. Are recognized by restriction enzymes

D. Are found only in bacterial DNA

Ans. C.

3534. Introns in genes

A. Encode the amino acids which are removed during post-translational modification

B. Encode signal sequences which are removed before secretion of the proteins

C. Are the non-coding sequences which are not translated

D. Are the sequences that intervene between two genes

Ans. C.

3535. All of the following statements about post-transcriptional processing of tRNA are true except

A. Introns of some tRNA precursors are removed

B. CCA is added at 3' end

C. 7-Methylguanosine triphosphate cap is added at 5' end

D. Some bases are methylated

Ans. C.

3536. α-Amanitin inhibits

A. DNA polymerase II of prokaryotes

B. DNA polymerase α of eukaryotes

C. RNA polymerase II of eukaryotes

D. RNA-dependent DNA polymerase

Ans. C.

3537. Ciprofloxacin inhibits the synthesis of

A. DNA in prokaryotes

B. DNA in prokaryotes and eukaryotes

C. RNA in prokaryotes

D. RNA in prokaryotes and eukaryotes

Ans. A.

3538. All of the following statements about bacterial promoters are true except

A. They are smaller than eukaryotic promoters

B. They have two consensus sequences upstream from the transcription star site

C. TATA box is the site for attachment of RNA polymerase

D. TATA box has a high melting temperature

Ans. D.

3539. All of the following statements about eukaryotic promoters are true except

A. They may be located upstream or down stream from the structural gene

B. They have two consensus sequences

C. One consensus sequence binds RNA polymerase

D. Mutations in promoter region can decrease the efficiency of transcription of the structural gene

Ans. A.

3540. In sanger's method of DNA sequence determination, DNA synthesis is stopped by using

A. 1', 2' - Dideoxyribonucleoside triphosphates

B. 2', 3' - Dideoxyribonucleoside triphosphates

C. 2', 4' - Dideoxyribonucleoside triphosphates

D. 2', 5' - Dideoxyribonucleoside triphosphates

Ans. B.

3541. tRNA genes have

A. Upstream promoters
B. Downstream promoters
C. Intragenic promoters
D. No promoters

Ans. C.

3542. Anticodons are present on

A. Coding strand of DNA
B. mRNA
C. tRNA
D. rRNA

Ans. C.

3543. Codons are present on

A. Non-coding strand of DNA
B. hnRNA
C. tRNA
D. None of these

Ans. B.

3544. Nonsense codons are present on

A. mRNA
B. tRNA
C. rRNA
D. None of these

Ans. A.

3545. Genetic code is said to be degenerate because

A. It can undergo mutations
B. A large proportion of DNA is non-coding
C. One codon can code for more than one amino acids
D. More than one codons can code for the same amino acids

Ans. D.

3546. All the following statements about genetic code are correct except

A. It is degenerate
B. It is unambigous
C. It is nearly universal
D. It is overlapping

Ans. D.

3547. All of the following statements about nonsense codons are true except

A. They do not code for amino acids
B. They act as chain termination signals
C. They are identical in nuclear and mitochondrial DNA
D. They have no complementary anticodons

Ans. C.

3548. A polycistronic mRNA can be seen in

A. Prokaryotes B. Eukaryotes

C. Mitochondria D. All of these

Ans. A.

3549. Non-coding sequence are present in the genes of

A. Bacteria B. Viruses

C. Eukaryotes D. All of these

Ans. C.

3550. Non-coding sequences in a gene are known as

A. Cistrons B. Nonsense codons

C. Introns D. Exons

Ans. C.

3551. Splice sites are present in

A. Prokaryotic mRNA B. Eukaryotic mRNA

C. Eukaryotic hnRNA D. All of these

Ans. C.

3552. The common features of introns include all the following except

A. The base sequence begins with GU

B. The base sequence ends with AG

C. The terminal AG sequence is preceded by a purine rich tract of ten nucleotides

D. An adenosine residue in branch site participates in splicing

Ans. C.

3553. Self-splicing can occur in

A. Some precursors of rRNA B. Some precursors of tRNA

C. hnRNA D. None of these

Ans. A.

3554. Pribnow box is present in

A. Prokaryotic promoters B. Eukaryotic promoters

C. Both (A) and (B) D. None of these

Ans. A.

3555. Hogness box is present in

A. Prokaryotic promoters B. Eukaryotic promoters

C. Both (A) and (B) D. None of these

Ans. B.

3556. CAAT box is present in

A. Prokaryotic promoters 10 bp upstream of transcription start site

B. Prokaryotic promoters 35 bp upstream of transcription start site

C. Eukaryotic promoters 25 bp upstream of transcription start site

D. Eukaryotic promoters 70–80 bp upstream of transcription start site

Ans. D.

3557. Eukaryotic promoters contain

A. TATA box 25bp upstream of transcription start site

B. CAAT box 70-80 bp upstream of transcription start site

C. Both (A) and (B)

D. None of these

Ans. C.

3558. All the following statements about tRNA are correct except

A. A given tRNA can be charged with only one particular amino acid

B. The amino acid is recognized by the anticodon of tRNA

C. The amino acid is attached to end of tRNA

D. The anticodon of tRNA finds the complementary codon on mRNA

Ans. B.

3559. All the following statements about charging of tRNA are correct except

A. It is catalysed by amino acyl tRNA synthetase

B. ATP is converted into ADP and phosphate in this reaction

C. The enzyme recognizes the tRNA and the amino acid

D. There is a separate enzyme for each tRNA

Ans. B.

3560. All the following statements about recognition of a codon on mRNA by an anticodon on tRNA are correct except

A. The recognition of the third base of the codon is not very precise

B. Imprecise recognition of the third base results in wobble

C. Wobble is partly responsible for the degeneracy of the genetic code

D. Wobble results in incorporation of incorrect amino acids in the protein

Ans. D.

3561. The first amino acyl tRNA which initiates translation in eukaryotes is

A. Methionyl tRNA
B. Formylmethionyl tRNA
C. Tyrosinyl tRNA
D. Alanyl tRNA

Ans. A.

3562. The first amino acyl tRNA which initiates translation in prokaryotes is

A. Mehtionyl tRNA
B. Formylmethionyl tRNA
C. Tyrosinyl tRNA
D. Alanyl tRNA

Ans. B.

3563. In eukaryotes, the 40 S pre-initiation complex contains all the following initiation factors except

A. eIF-1A
B. eIF-2
C. eIF-3
D. eIF-4

Ans. D.

3564. Eukaryotic initiation factors 4A, 4B and 4F bind to

A. 40 S ribosomal subunit
B. 60 S ribosomal subunit
C. mRNA
D. Amino acyl tRNA

Ans. C.

3565. The codon which serves as translation start signal is

A. AUG
B. UAG
C. UGA
D. UAA

Ans. A.

3566. Binding of formylmehtionyl tRNA to 30 S ribosomal subunit of prokaryotes is inhibited by

A. Streptomycin
B. Chloramphenicol
C. Erythromycin
D. Mitomycin

Ans. B.

3567. Tetracyclines inhibit binding of amino acyl tRNAs to

A. 30 S ribosomal subunits
B. 40 S ribosomal subunits
C. 50 S ribosomal subunits
D. 60 S ribosomal subunits

Ans. A.

3568. Peptidyl transferase activity of 50 S ribosomal subunits is inhibited by

A. Rifampicin
B. Cycloheximide
C. Chloramphenicol
D. Erythromycin

Ans. C.

3569. Erythromycin binds to 50 S ribosomal subunit and

A. Inhibits binding of amino acyl tRNA

B. Inhibits Peptidyl transferase activity

C. Inhibits translocation

D. Causes premature chain termination

Ans. C.

3570. Puromycin causes premature chain termination in

A. Prokaryotes B. Eukaryotes

C. Both (A) and (B) D. None of these

Ans. C.

3571. Diphtheria toxin inhibits

A. Prokaryotic EF-1 B. Prokaryotic EF-2

C. Eukaryotic EF-1 D. Eukaryotic EF-2

Ans. D.

3572. The proteins destined to be transported out of the cell have all the following features except

A. They possess a signal sequence

B. Ribosomes synthesizing them are bound to endoplasmic reticulum

C. After synthesis, they are delivered into Golgi apparatus

D. They are tagged with ubiquitin

Ans. D.

3573. SRP receptors involved in protein export are present on

A. Ribosomes B. Endoplasmic reticulum

C. Golgi appartus D. Cell membrane

Ans. B.

3574. The signal sequence of proteins is cleaved off

A. On the ribosomes immediately after synthesis

B. In the endoplasmic reticulum

C. During processing in Golgi apparatus

D. During passage through the cell membrane

Ans. B.

3575. The half-life of a protein depends upon its

A. Signal sequence
B. N-terminus amino acid
C. C-terminus amino acid
D. Prosthetic group

Ans. B.

3576. Besides structural genes that encode proteins, DNA contains some regulatory sequences which are known as

A. Operons
B. Cistrons
C. Cis-acting elements
D. Trans-acting factors

Ans. C.

3577. Inducers and repressors are

A. Enhancer and silencer elements respectively
B. Trans-acting factors
C. Cis-acting elements
D. Regulatory proteins

Ans. B.

3578. cis-acting elements include

A. Steroid hormones
B. Calcitriol
C. Histones
D. Silencers

Ans. D.

3579. Silencer elements

A. Are trans-acting factors
B. Are present between promoters and the structural genes
C. Decrease the expression of some structural genes
D. Encode specific repressor proteins

Ans. C.

3580. trans-acting factors include

A. Promoters
B. Repressors
C. Enhancers
D. Silencers

Ans. B.

3581. Enhancer elements have all the following features except

A. They increase gene expression through a promoter
B. Each enhancer activates a specific promoter
C. They may be located far away from the promoter
D. They may be upstream or downstream from the promoter

Ans. B.

3582. Amplification of dihydrofolate reductase gene may be brought about by

A. High concentrations of folic acid

B. Deficiency of folic acid

C. Low concentration of thymidylate

D. Amethopterin

Ans. D.

3583. Proteins which interact with DNA and affect the rate of transcription possess the following structural motif:

A. Helix-turn-helix motif
B. Zinc finger motif
C. Leucine zipper motif
D. All of these

Ans. D.

3584. Lac operon is a cluster of genes present in

A. Human beings
B. E. coli
C. Lambda phage
D. All of these

Ans. B.

3585. Lac operon is a cluster of

A. Three structural genes

B. Three structural genes and their promoter

C. A regulatory gene, an operator and a promoter

D. A regulatory gene, an operator, a promoter and three structural genes

Ans. D.

3586. The regulatory i gene of lac operon

A. Is inhibited by lacotse

B. Is inhibited by its own product, the repressor protein

C. Forms a regulatory protein which increases the expression of downstream structural genes

D. Is constitutively expressed

Ans. D.

3587. RNA polymerase holoenzyme binds to lac operon at the following site:

A. i gene
B. z gene
C. Operator locus
D. Promoter region

Ans. D.

3588. Trancription of z, y and a genes of lac operon is prevented by

A. Lactose
B. Allo-lactose
C. Repressor
D. cAMP

Ans. C.

3589. Mutations can be caused by

A. Nitrosamine
B. Dimethyl sulphate
C. Acridine
D. All of these

Ans. D.

3590. Nitrosamine can deaminate

A. Cytosine to form uracil
B. Adenine to form xanthine
C. Guanine to form hypoxanthine
D. All of these

Ans. A.

3591. Exposure of DNA to ultraviolet radiation can lead to the formation of

A. Adenine dimmers
B. Guanine dimers
C. Thymine dimmers
D. Uracil dimmers

Ans. C.

3592. Damage to DNA caused by ultraviolet radiation can be repaired by

A. uvr ABC excinuclease
B. DNA polymerase I
C. DNA ligase
D. All of these

Ans. D.

3593. Xeroderma pigmentosum results from a defect in

A. uvr ABC excinuclease
B. DNA polymerase I
C. DNA ligase
D. All of these

Ans. A.

3594. All the following statements about xeroderma pigmentosum are true except

A. It is a genetic disease
B. Its inheritance is autosomal dominant
C. uvr ABC excinuclease is defective in this disease
D. It results in multiple skin cancers

Ans. B.

3595. Substitution of an adenine base by guanine in DNA is known as

A. Transposition
B. Transition
C. Transversion
D. Frameshift mutation

Ans. B.

3596. Substitution of a thymine base by adenine in DNA is known as

A. Transposition
B. Transition
C. Transversion
D. Frameshift mutation

Ans. C.

3597. A point mutation results from

A. Substitution of a base
B. Insertion of a base
C. Deletion of a base
D. All of these

Ans. A.

3598. Substitution of a base can result in a

A. Silent mutation
B. Mis-sense mutation
C. Nonsense mutation
D. All of these

Ans. D.

3599. A silent mutation is most likely to result from

A. Substitution of the first base of a codon
B. Substitution of the third base of a codon
C. Conversion of a nonsense codon into a sense codon
D. Conversion of a sense codon into a nonsense codon

Ans. B.

3600. The effect of a mis-sense mutation can be

A. Acceptable
B. Partially acceptable
C. Unacceptable
D. All of these

Ans. D.

3601. Amino acid sequence of the encoded protein is not changed in

A. Silent mutation
B. Acceptable mis-sense mutation
C. Both (A) and (B)
D. None of these

Ans. A.

3602. Haemoglobin S is an example of a/an

A. Silent mutation
B. Acceptable mis-sense mutation
C. Unacceptable mis-sense mutation
D. Partially acceptable mis-sense mutation

Ans. D.

3603. If the codon UAC on mRNA changes into UAG as a result of a base substitution in DNA, it will result in

A. Silent mutation
B. Acceptable mis-sense mutation
C. Nonsense mutation
D. Frameshift mutation

Ans. C.

3604. Insertion of a base in a gene can cause

A. Change in reading frame

B. Garbled amino acid sequence in the encoded protein

C. Premature termination of translation

D. All of these

Ans. D.

3605. A frameshift mutation changes the reading frame because the genetic code

A. Is degenerate
B. Is overlapping
C. Has no punctuations
D. Is universal

Ans. C.

3606. Suppressor mutations occur in

A. Structural genes
B. Promoter regions
C. Silencer elements
D. Anticodons of tRNA

Ans. D.

3607. Suppressor tRNAs can neutralize the effects of mutations in

A. Structural genes
B. Promoter regions
C. Enhancer elements
D. All of these

Ans. A.

3608. Mutations in promoter regions of genes can cause

A. Premature termination of translation

B. Change in reading frame of downstream structural gene

C. Decreased efficiency of transcription

D. All of these

Ans. C.

3609. Mitochondrial protein synthesis is inhibited by

A. Cycloheximide
B. Chloramphenicol
C. Diptheria toxin
D. None of these

Ans. B.

3610. All of the following statements about puromycin are true except

A. It is an alanyl tRNA analogue

B. It causes premature termination of protein synthesis

C. It inhibits protein synthesis in prokaryotes

D. It inhibits protein synthesis in eukaryotes

Ans. A.

3611. Leucine zipper motif is seen in some helical proteins when leucine residues appear at every

A. 3rd position B. 5th position

C. 7th position D. 9th position

Ans. C.

3612. Zinc finger motif is formed in some proteins by binding of zinc to

A. Two cysteine residues

B. Two histidine residues

C. Two arginine residues

D. Two cysteine and two histidine residues or two pairs of two cysteine residues each

Ans. D.

3613. Restriction endonucleases are present in

A. Viruses B. Bacteria

C. Eukaryotes D. All of these

Ans. B.

3614. Restriction endonucleases split

A. RNA B. Single stranded DNA

C. Double stranded DNA D. DNA-RNA hybrids

Ans. C.

3615. Restriction endonucleases can recognise

A. Palindromic sequences B. Chimeric DNA

C. DNA-RNA hybrids D. Homopolymer sequences

Ans. A.

3616. All of the following statements about restriction endonucleases are true except:

A. They are present in bacteria

B. They act on double stranded DNA

C. They recognize palindromic sequences

D. They always produce sticky ends

Ans. D.

3617. Which of the following is a palindromic sequence

A. 5 ATGCAG 3 B. 3 TACGTC 5

C. 5 CGAAGC 3 D. 3 GCTTCG 5

Ans. C.

3618. All of the following may be used as expression vectors except

A. Plasmid
B. Bacteriophage
C. Baculovirus
D. E.coli

Ans. D.

3619. A plasmid is a

A. Single stranded linear DNA
B. Single stranded circular DNA
C. Double stranded linear DNA
D. Double stranded circular DNA

Ans. D.

3620. Fragments of DNA can be identified by the technique of

A. Western blotting
B. Eastern blotting
C. Northern blotting
D. Southern blotting

Ans. D.

3621. A particular RNA in a mixture can be identified by

A. Western blotting
B. Eastern blotting
C. Northern blotting
D. Southern blotting

Ans. C.

3622. A radioactive isotope labeled cDNA probe is used in

A. Southern blotting
B. Northern blotting
C. Both (A) and (B)
D. None of these

Ans. C.

3623. An antibody probe is used in

A. Southern blotting
B. Northern blotting
C. Western blotting
D. None of these

Ans. C.

3624. A particular protein in a mixture can be detected by

A. Southern blotting
B. Northern blotting
C. Western blotting
D. None of these

Ans. C.

3625. The first protein synthesized by recombinant DNA technology was

A. Streptokinase
B. Human growth hormone
C. Tissue plasminogen activator
D. Human insulin

Ans. D.

3626. Monoclonal antibodies are prepared by cloning

A. Myeloma cells B. Hybridoma cells
C. T-Lymphocytes D. B-Lymphocytes

Ans. B.

3627. Myeloma cells are lacking in

A. TMP synthetase B. Formyl transferase
C. HGPRT D. All of these

Ans. C.

3628. Hybridoma cells are selected by culturing them in a medium containing

A. Adenine, guanine, cytosine and thymine
B. Adenine, guanine, cytosine and uracil
C. Hypoxanthine, aminopterin and thymine
D. Hypoxanthine, aminopterin and thymidine

Ans. D.

3629. Myeloma cells and lymphocytes can be fused by using

A. Calcium chloride B. Ethidium bromide
C. Polyethylene glycol D. DNA polymerase

Ans. C.

3630. Trials for gene therapy in human beings were first carried out, with considerable success, in a genetic disease called

A. Cystic fibrosis B. Thalassemia
C. Adenosine deaminase deficiency D. Lesch-Nyhan syndrome

Ans. C.

3631. Chimeric DNA

A. Is found in bacteriophages B. Contains unrelated genes
C. Has no restriction sites D. Is palindromic

Ans. B.

3632. Which of the following may be used as a cloning vector?

A. Prokaryotic plasmid B. Lambda phage
C. Cosmid D. All of these

Ans. D.

3633. The plasmid pBR322 has

A. Ampicillin resistance gene B. Tetracycline resistance gene
C. Both A and B D. None of these

Ans. C.

3634. Lambda phage can be used to clone DNA fragments of the size

A. Upto 3 kilobases
B. Upto 20 kilobases
C. Upto 45 kilobases
D. Upto 1,000 kilobases

Ans. B.

3635. DNA fragments upto 45 kilobases in size can be cloned in

A. Bacterial plasmids
B. Lambda phage
C. Cosmids
D. Yeast artificial chromosomes

Ans. C.

3636. A cosmid is a

A. Large bacterial plasmid
B. Viral plasmid
C. Hybrid of plasmid and phage
D. Yeast plasmid

Ans. C.

3637. Polymerase chain reaction can rapidly amplify DNA sequences of the size

A. Upto 10 kilobases
B. Upto 45 kilobases
C. Upto 100 kilobases
D. Upto 1,000 kilobases

Ans. A.

3638. The DNA polymerase commonly used in polymerase chain reaction is obtained from

A. E.coli
B. Yeast
C. T.aquaticus
D. Eukaryotes

Ans. C.

3639. Base sequence of DNA can be determined by

A. Maxam-Gilbert method
B. Sanger's dideoxy method
C. Both (A) and (B)
D. None of these

Ans. C.

3640. From a DNA-RNA hybrid, DNA can be obtained by addition of

A. DNA B protein and ATP
B. Helicase and ATP
C. DNA topoisomerase I
D. Alkali

Ans. D.

3641. Optimum temperature of DNA polymerase of T. aquaticus is

A. 30°C
B. 37°C
C. 54°C
D. 72°C

Ans. D.

3642. In addition to Taq polymerase, polymerase chain reaction requires all of the following except

A. A template DNA
B. Deoxyribonucleoside triphosphates
C. Primers
D. Primase

Ans. D.

3643. DNA polymerase of T. aquaticus is preferred to that of E. coli in PCR because

A. It replicates DNA more efficiently
B. It doesn't require primers
C. It is not denatured at the melting temperature of DNA
D. It doesn't cause errors in replication

Ans. C.

3644. Twenty cycles of PCR can amplify DNA:

A. 2^{20} fold
B. 20^2 fold
C. 20 x 2 fold
D. 20 fold

Ans. A.

3645. Transgenic animals may be prepared by introducing a foreign gene into

A. Somatic cells of young animals
B. Testes and ovaries of animals
C. A viral vector and infecting the animals with the viral vector
D. Fertilised egg and implanting the egg into a foster mother

Ans. D.

3646. Yeast artificial chromosome can be used to clone DNA sequences of the size

A. Upto 10 kb
B. Upto 45 kb
C. Upto 100 kb
D. Upto 1,000 kb

Ans. D.

3647. DNA finger printing is based on the presence in DNA of

A. Constant number of tandem repeats
B. Variable number of tandem repeats
C. Non-repititive sequences in each DNA
D. Introns in eukaryotic DNA

Ans. B.

3648. All the following statements about restriction fragment length polymorphism are true except

A. It results from mutations in restriction sites

B. Mutations in restriction sites can occur in coding or non-coding regions of DNA

C. It is inherited in Mendelian fashion

D. It can be used to diagnose any genetic disease

Ans. D.

3649. Inborn errors of urea cycle can cause all the following except

A. Vomiting B. Ataxia

C. Renal failure D. Mental retardation

Ans. D.

3650. A ketogenic amino acid among the following is

A. Leucine B. Serine

C. Threonine D. Proline

Ans. A.

3651. Carbon skeleton of the following amino acid can serve as a substance for gluconeogenesis

A. Cysteine B. Aspartate

C. Glutamate D. All of these

Ans. D.

3652. N-Formiminoglutamate is a metabolite of

A. Glutamate B. Histidine

C. Tryptophan D. Methionine

Ans. B.

3653. Homogentisic acid is formed from

A. Homoserine B. Homocysteine

C. Tyrosine D. Tryptophan

Ans. C.

3654. Which of the following is present as a marker in lysosomal enzymes to direct them to their destination?

A. Glucose-6-phosphate B. Mannose-6-phosphate

C. Galactose-6-phosphate D. N-Acetyl neuraminic acid

Ans. C.

3655. Marfan's syndrome results from a mutation in the gene coding:

A. Collagen B. Elastin

C. Fibrillin D. Keratin

Ans. B.

3656. Fibronectin is involved in

A. Cell adhension B. Cell movement

C. Both (A) and (B) D. None of these

Ans. B.

3657. Glycophorin is present in cell membranes of

A. Erythrocytes B. Platelets

C. Neutrophils D. Liver

Ans. A.

3658. Selectins are proteins that can recognize specific

A. Carbohydrates B. Lipids

C. Amino acids D. Nucleotides

Ans. A.

3659. Hunter's syndrome results from absence of

A. Hexosaminidase A B. Iduronate sulphatase

C. Neuraminidase D. Arylsulphatase B

Ans. B.

3660. A cancer cell is characterized by

A. Uncontrolled cell division B. Invasion of neighbouring cells

C. Spread to distant sites D. All of these

Ans. D.

3661. If DNA of a cancer cell is introduced into a normal cell, the recipient cell

A. Destroys the DNA B. Loses its ability to divide

C. Dies D. Changes into a cancer cell

Ans. D.

3662. A normal cell can be transformed into a cancer cell by all of the following except

A. Ionising radiation B. Mutagenic chemicals

C. Oncogenic bacteria D. Some viruses

Ans. C.

3663. Proto-oncogens are present in

A. Oncoviruses
B. Cancer cells
C. Healthy human cells
D. Prokaryotes

Ans. C.

3664. All the following statements about protooncogenes are true except

A. They are present in human beings
B. They are present in healthy cells
C. Proteins encoded by them are essential
D. They are expressed only when a healthy cell has been transformed into a cancer cell

Ans. D.

3665. Various oncogens may encode all of the following except:

A. Carcinogens
B. Growth factors
C. Receptors for growth factors
D. Signal transducers for growth factors

Ans. A.

3666. Ras proto-oncogene is converted into oncogene by

A. A point mutation
B. Chromosomal translocation
C. Insertion of a viral promoter upstream of the gene
D. Gene amplification

Ans. A.

3667. Ras proto-oncogene encodes

A. Epidermal growth factor (EGF)
B. Receptor for EGF
C. Signal transducer for EGF
D. Nuclear transcription factor

Ans. C.

3668. p53 gene:

A. A proto-oncogene
B. An oncogene
C. A tumour suppressor gene
D. None of these

Ans. C.

3669. Retinoblastoma can result from a mutation in

A. Ras proto-oncogene
B. erbB proto-oncogene
C. p 53 gene
D. RB 1 gene

Ans. D.

3670. Ames assay is a rapid method for detection of

A. Oncoviruses
B. Retroviuses
C. Chemical carcinogens
D. Typhoid

Ans. C.

3671. Amplification of dihydrofolate reductase gene in a cancer cell makes the cell

A. Susceptible to folic acid deficiency
B. Less malignant
C. Resistant to amethopterin therapy
D. Responsive to amethopterin therapy

Ans. C.

3672. The only correct statement about oncoviruses is

A. All the oncoviruses are RNA viruses
B. Reverse transcriptase is present in all oncoviruses
C. Viral oncogenes are identical to human protooncogens
D. Both DNA and RNA viruses can be oncoviruses

Ans. D.

3673. RB 1 gene is

A. A tumour suppressor gene
B. Oncogene
C. Proto-oncogene
D. Activated proto-oncogene

Ans. A.

3674. The major source of NH3 produced by the kidney is

A. Leucine
B. Glycine
C. Alanine
D. Glutamine

Ans. D.

3675. A prokaryotic ribosome is made up of ———- sub units.

A. 20 S and 50S
B. 30S and 50S
C. 30S and 60S
D. 20S and 50S

Ans. B.

3676. An Eukaryotic ribosome is made up of ——— sub unit.

A. 40S and 60S
B. 40S and 50S
C. 40S and 80S
D. 60S and 80S

Ans. A.

3677. The antibiotic which inhibits DNA dependent RNA polymerase is

A. Mitomycin C
B. Actinomycin D
C. Streptomycin
D. Puromycin

Ans. B.

3678. The antibiotic which cleaves DNA is

A. Actinomycin D
B. Streptomycin
C. Puromycin
D. Mitomycin C

Ans. D.

3679. The antibiotic which has a structure similar to the amino acyl end of tRNA tyrosine is

A. Actinomycin D
B. Streptomycin
C. Puromycin
D. Mitomycin C

Ans. C.

3680. An animal is in negative nitrogen balance when

A. Intake exceeds output
B. New tissue is being synthesized
C. Output exceeds intake
D. Intake is equal to output

Ans. C.

3681. When NH3 is perfused through a dog's liver ———— is formed, while ———— is formed in the birds liver.

A. Urea, Uric acid
B. Urea, allantoin
C. Uric acid, creatinine
D. Uric acid, Urea

Ans. A.

3682. Which among the following compounds is not a protein?

A. Insulin
B. Heparin
C. Mucin
D. Pepsin

Ans. B.

3683. Almost all the urea is formed in this tissue:

A. Kidney
B. Urethra
C. Uterus
D. Liver

Ans. D.

3684. A polyribosome will have about ———— individual ribosomes.

A. 20
B. 10
C. 5
D. 2

Ans. C.

3685. Genetic information originates from

A. Cistron of DNA
B. Codons of mRNA
C. Anticodons of tRNA
D. Histones of nucleoproteins

Ans. A.

3686. The genetic code operates through

A. The protein moiety of DNA
B. Cistrom of DNA
C. Nucleotide sequence of m RNA
D. The anticodons of tRNA

Ans. C.

3687. DNA synthesis in laboratory was first achieved by

A. Watson and crick
B. Khorana
C. A.Kornberg
D. Ochoa

Ans. C.

3688. Among the different types of RNA, which one has the highest M.W.?

A. mRNA
B. rRNA
C. yeast RNA
D. tRNA

Ans. B.

3689. From DNA the genetic message is transcribed into this compound:

A. Protein
B. mRNA
C. tRNA
D. rRNA

Ans. B.

3690. This compound has a double helical structure.

A. Deoxyribonucleic acid
B. RNA
C. Flavine-adevine dinucleotide
D. Nicotinamide adamine dinucleotide

Ans. A.

3691. The structural stability of the double helix of DNA is largely due to

A. Hydrogen bonding between adjacent purine bases
B. Hydrophobic bonding between staked purine and pyrinuidine nuclei
C. Hydrogen bonding between adjacent pyrimidine bases
D. Hydrogen bonding between purine and pyrimidine bases

Ans. D.

3692. Which of the following statements about nucleic acid is most correct?

A. Both pentose nucleic acid and deoxypentose nucleic acid contain the same pyrimidines

B. Both pentose nucleic acid and deoxypentose nucleic acid contain the same purines

C. RNA contains cytosine and thymine

D. DNA and RNA are hydrolysed by weak alkali

Ans. B.

3693. Acid hydrolysis of ribonucleic acid would yield the following major products:

A. D- deoxyribose, cytosine, adenine

B. D-ribose, thymine, guanine

C. D-ribose, cytosine, uracil, thymine

D. D-ribose, uracil, adenine, guanine, cytosine

Ans. D.

3694. RNA does not contain

A. Adenine
B. OH methyl cytosine
C. d-ribose
D. Uracil

Ans. B.

3695. Whcih of the following compound is present in RNA but absent from DNA?

A. Thymine
B. Cytosine
C. Uracil
D. Guanine

Ans. C.

3696. Nucleic acids can be detected by means of their absorption maxima near 260 nm. Their absorption in this range is due to

A. Proteins
B. Purines and pyrimidines
C. Ribose
D. Deoxyribose

Ans. B.

3697. Which of the following contains a deoxy sugar?

A. RNA
B. DNA
C. ATP
D. UTP

Ans. B.

3698. Transcription is the formation of

A. DNA from a parent DNA
B. mRNA from a parent mRNA
C. Pre mRNA from DNA
D. Protein through mRNA

Ans. C.

3699. Translation is the formation of

A. DNA from DNA
B. mRNA from DNA
C. Protein through mRNA
D. mRNA from pre mRNA

Ans. C.

3700. Sigma and Rho factors are required for

A. Replication
B. Transcription
C. Translation
D. Polymerisation

Ans. C.

3701. The genome of $\phi\times174$ bacteriophage is interesting in that if contains

A. No DNA
B. DNA with uracil
C. Single stranded DNA
D. Triple standard DNA

Ans. C.

3702. Okasaki fragments are small bits of

A. RNA
B. DNA
C. DNA with RNA heads
D. RNA with DNA heads

Ans. C.

3703. In addition to the DNA of nucleus there is DNA in

A. Mitochondrian
B. Endoplasmic reticulum
C. Golgi apparatus
D. Plasma membrane

Ans. A.

3704. The mitochondrial DNA is

A. Like the nuclear DNA in structure
B. Single stranded, linear
C. Double stranded, circular
D. Single stranded, circular

Ans. C.

3705. A synthetic RNA having the sequence of UUUUUU (Poly U) will give a protein having poly ———-.

A. Alanine
B. Phenylalanine
C. Glycine
D. Methionine

Ans. B.

3706. A mRNA of eukaryotes can code for

A. Only one polypeptide
B. Two polypeptides
C. Three polypeptides
D. Five polypeptides

Ans. A.

3707. mRNA of prokaryotes can code for

A. More than one polypeptide
B. Only one polypeptide
C. Many exons and introns
D. Introns only

Ans. A.

3708. DNA directed RNA polymerase is

A. Replicase
B. Transcriptase
C. Reverse transcriptase
D. Polymerase III

Ans. B.

3709. RNA directed DNA polymerase is

A. Replicase
B. Transcriptase
C. Reversetranscriptase
D. Polymerase–III

Ans. C.

3710. RNA synthesis requires

A. RNA primer
B. RNA template
C. DNA template
D. DNA primer

Ans. C.

3711. The mRNA ready for protein synthesis has the ——————- cap.

A. ATP
B. CTP
C. GTP
D. UTP

Ans. C.

3712. mRNA ready for protein synthesis has the poly —————— toil.

A. G
B. A
C. U
D. C

Ans. B.

3713. The codon for phenylalanine is

A. AAA
B. CCC
C. GGG
D. UUU

Ans. D.

3714. Blue print for genetic information resides in

A. mRNA
B. tRNA
C. rRNA
D. DNA

Ans. D.

3715. Genes are

A. RNA
B. DNA
C. lipoproteins
D. Chromoproteins

Ans. B.

3716. Codons are in

A. DNA
B. mRNA
C. tRNA
D. rRNA

Ans. B.

3717. The genetic code operates via

A. The protein moiety of DNA
B. The base sequences of DNA
C. The nucleotide sequence of mRNA
D. The base sequence of tRNA

Ans. C.

3718. Genetic information in human beings is stored in

A. DNA
B. RNA
C. Both (A) and (B)
D. None of these

Ans. A.

3719. If the amino group and a carboxylic group of the amino acid are attached to same carbon atom, the amino acid is called as

A. Alpha
B. Beta
C. Gamma
D. Epsilon

Ans. A.

3720. If in a nucleic acid there are more than 8000 nucleotides it is most likely

A. RNA
B. DNA
C. Both (A) and (B)
D. None of these

Ans. B.

3721. In RNA, apart from ribose and phosphate, all following are present except

A. Adenine
B. Guanine
C. Thymine
D. Cytosine

Ans. C.

3722. Which of the following gives a positive Ninhydrin test?

A. Reducing sugar
B. Triglycerides
C. α-amino acids
D. Phospholipids

Ans. C.

3723. A Gene is

A. A single protein molecule

B. A group of chromosomes

C. An instruction for making a protein molecule

D. A bit of DNA molecule

Ans. D.

3724. In DNA, genetic information is located in

A. Purine bases B. Pyrimidine bases

C. Purine and pyrimidine bases D. Sugar

Ans. C.

3725. Which one of the following is not a constituent of RNA?

A. Deoxyribose B. Uracil

C. Adenine D. Guanine

Ans. A.

3726. Which of the following are nucleo proteins?

A. Protamines B. Histones

C. Deoxy and Ribo nucleo proteins D. All of these

Ans. D.

3727. The tRNA constitutes ——— of total RNA in cell

A. 1–10% B. 10–20%

C. 30–50% D. 50–80%

Ans. B.

3728. Unit of genetic information:

A. DNA B. RNA

C. Cistron D. None of these

Ans. C.

3729. Anticodon sequence are seen in

A. tRNA and transcribed DNA strand

B. tRNA and complementary DNA strand

C. mRNA

D. mRNA and complementary DNA strand

Ans. A.

3730. Restriction enzymes have been found in

A. Humans B. Birds

C. Bacteria D. Bacteriophase

Ans. C.

3731. Sulphur is not present in

A. Thiamine B. Lipic acid

C. Thymine D. Biotin

Ans. C.

3732. Which one of the following binds to specific nucleotide sequences?

A. RNA polymerase B. Repressor

C. Inducer D. Restriction

Ans. A.

3733. Using written convertion which one of the following sequences is complimentary to TGGCAGCCT?

A. ACC GTC GGA B. ACC GUC GGA

C. AGG CTG CCA D. TGG CTC GGA

Ans. A.

3734. The mechanism of synthesis of DNA and RNA are similar in all the following ways except

A. They involve release of pyrophosphate from each nucleotide added

B. They require activated nucleotide precursor and Mg2+

C. The direction of synthesis is 5' '! 3'

D. They require a primer

Ans. A.

3735. Template-directed DNA synthesis occurs in all the following except

A. The replication fork B. Polymerase chain reaction

C. Growth of RNA tumor viruses D. Expression of oneogenes

Ans. C.

3736. Which one of the following causes frame shift mutation?

A. Transition B. Transversion

C. Deletion D. Substitution of purine to pyrimidine

Ans. C.

3737. Uric acid is the catabolic end product of

A. Porphyrine
B. Purines
C. Pyrimidines
D. Pyridoxine

Ans. A.

3738. Diphenylamine method is employed in the quantitation of

A. Nucleic acid
B. RNA
C. DNA
D. Proteins

Ans. C.

3739. Orcinol method is employed in the quantitation of

A. Nucleic acid
B. DNA
C. RNA
D. Proteins

Ans. C.

3740. Nucleic acid show strong absorption at one of the wavelength:

A. 280 nm
B. 220 nm
C. 360 nm
D. 260 nm

Ans. D.

3741. tRNA has

A. Clover leaf structure
B. Anticodon arm
C. Poly 'A' tay 3'
D. Cap at 5' end

Ans. A.

3742. Which one of the following contributes nitrogen atoms to both purine and pyrimidine rings?

A. Aspartate
B. Carbanoyl phosphate
C. Carbondioxide
D. Tetrahydrofolate

Ans. A.

3743. The four nitrogen atoms of purines are derived from

A. Urea and NH3
B. NH3, Glycine and Glutamate
C. NH3, Asparate and Glutamate
D. Aspartate, Glutamine and Glycine

Ans. D.

3744. A drug which prevents uric acid synthesis by inhibiting the enzyme Xanthine oxidase is

A. Aspirin
B. Allopurinal
C. Colchicine
D. Phenyl benzoate

Ans. B.

3745. In humans, the principal break down product of purines is

A. NH3 B. Allantin

C. Alanine D. Uric acid

Ans. D.

3746. In humans, the principal metabolic product of pyrimidines is

A. Uric acid B. Allantoin

C. Hypoxanthine D. β-alanine

Ans. D.

3747. In most mammals, except primates, uric acid is metabolized by

A. Oxidation to allantoin B. Reduction to NH3

C. Hydrolysis to allantoin D. Hydrolysis to NH3

Ans. A.

3748. All are true about Lesch-Nyhan syndrome except

A. Produces self-mutilation

B. Genetic deficiency of the enzyme (HGPRT)

C. Elevated levels of uric acid in blood

D. Inheritance is autosomal recessive

Ans. D.

3749. The formation of a peptide bond during the elongation step of protein synthesis results in the splitting of how many high energy bonds?

A. 1 B. 2

C. 3 D. 4

Ans. B.

3750. Translocase is an enzyme required in the process of

A. DNA replication B. RNA synthesis

C. Initiation of protein synthesis D. Elongation of peptides

Ans. D.

3751. Nonsense codons bring about

A. Amino acid activation B. Initiation of protein synthesis

C. Termination of protein synthesis D. Elongation of polypeptide chains

Ans. C.

3752. The anticodon region is an important part of the structure of

A. rRNA B. tRNA

C. mRNA D. hrRNA

Ans. B.

3753. Another name for reverse transcriptase is

A. DNA dependent DNA polymerase

B. DNA dependent RNA polymerase

C. RNA dependent DNA polymerase

D. RNA dependent RNA polymerase

Ans. C.

3754. In the 'lac operon' concept, which of the following is a protein?

A. Operator B. Repressor

C. Inducer D. Vector

Ans. B.

3755. The normal function of restriction endonucleases is to

A. Excise introns from hrRNA

B. Polymerize nucleotides to form RNA

C. Remove primer from okazaki fragments

D. Protect bacteria from foreign DNA

Ans. D.

3756. In contrast to Eukaryotic mRNA, prokaryotic mRNA is characterized by

A. Having 7-methyl guanosine triphosphate at the 5' end

B. Being polycystronic

C. Being only monocystronic

D. Being synthesized with introns

Ans. A.

3757. mRNA is complementary copy of

A. 5' - 3' strand of DNA+ B. 3' - 5' strand of DNA

C. Antisense strand of DNA D. tRNA

Ans. B.

3758. Synthesis of RNA molecule is terminated by a signal which is recognised by

A. α-factor B. β-factor

C. δ-factor D. Rho (ρ) factor

Ans. D.

3759. The binding of prokaryotic DNA dependent RNA polymerase to promoter sites of genes is inhibited by the antibiotic:

A. Streptomycin B. Rifampin

C. Aueromycin D. Puromycin

Ans. B.

3760. In E.coli the chain initiating amino acid in protein synthesis is

A. N-formyl methionine B. Methionine

C. Serine D. Cysteine

Ans. A.

3761. Amanitin the mushroom poison inhibits

A. Glycoprotein synthesis B. ATP synthesis

C. DNA synthesis D. mRNA synthesis

Ans. D.

3762. How many high-energy phosphate bond equivalents are required for amino acid activation in protein synthesis?

A. One B. Two

C. Three D. Four

Ans. B.

3763. Translation results in the formation of

A. mRNA B. tRNA

C. rRNA D. A protein molecule

Ans. D.

3764. The 'rho' (ρ) factor is involved

A. To increase the rate of RNA synthesis

B. In binding catabolite repressor to the promoter region

C. In proper termination of transcription

D. To allow proper initiation of transcriptide

Ans. C.

3765. Which one of the following binds to specific nucleotide sequences that are upstream and most distant from the start site?

A. RNA polymerase B. Repressor

C. Inducer D. Restriction

Ans. A.

3766. Ribosomes similar to those of bacteria found in

A. Plant nuclei B. Cardiac muscle cytoplasm

C. Liver endoplasmic reticulum D. Neuronal cytoplasm

Ans. A.

3767. The total body water in various subjects is relatively constant when expressed as percentage of the lean body mass and is about

A. 30% B. 40%

C. 50% D. 70%

Ans. D.

3768. The percentage of water contained in the body of an individual is less because of

A. High fat content B. Low fat content

C. High protein content D. Low protein content

Ans. A.

3769. In intracellular compartment the fluid present in ml/kg body weight is about

A. 100 B. 200

C. 250 D. 330

Ans. D.

3770. In extra cellular compartment, the fluid present in ml/kg of body weight is about

A. 120 B. 220

C. 270 D. 330

Ans. C.

3771. Fluid present in dense connective tissue and cartilage in ml/kg body weight is about

A. 10 B. 20

C. 45 D. 55

Ans. C.

3772. The total body water in ml/kg body weight in average normal young adult male is about

A. 200 B. 400

C. 600 D. 1000

Ans. C.

3773. The fluid present in bones which can not be exchanged readily because of relative avascularity is about

A. 20 ml/kg B. 25 ml/kg

C. 45 ml/kg D. 60 ml/kg

Ans. C.

3774. Water derived in gm from complete oxidation of each gm of carbohydrate is about

A. 0.15
B. 0.25
C. 0.35
D. 0.55

Ans. D.

3775. Each gm of protein on complete oxidation yields

A. 0.21 gm water
B. 0.31 gm water
C. 0.41 gm water
D. 0.51 gm water

Ans. C.

3776. The daily total body water derived from oxidation of food stuffs is about

A. 100 ml
B. 300 ml
C. 600 ml
D. 1000 ml

Ans. B.

3777. The daily water allowance for normal infant is about

A. 100–200 ml
B. 250–300 ml
C. 330–1000 ml
D. 1000–2000 ml

Ans. C.

3778. The daily water allowance for normal adult (60 kg) is about

A. 200–600 ml
B. 500–800 ml
C. 800–1500 ml
D. 1800–2500 ml

Ans. D.

3779. Insensible loss of body water of normal adult is about

A. 50–100 ml
B. 100–200 ml
C. 300–500 ml
D. 600–1000 ml

Ans. D.

3780. The predominant cation of plasma is

A. Na+
B. K+
C. Ca+
D. Mg++

Ans. A.

3781. The predominant anion of plasma is

A. HCO3–
B. Cl–
C. HPO4– –
D. SO4 – –

Ans. B.

3782. Vasopressin (ADH)

A. Enhance facultative reabsorption of water

B. Decreases reabsorption of water

C. Increases excretion of calcium

D. Decreases excretion of calcium

Ans. A.

3783. Action of kinins is to

A. Increase salt excretion
B. Decrease salt retention
C. Decrease water retention
D. Increase both salt and water excretion

Ans. D.

3784. The activity of kinins is modulated by

A. Prostaglandins
B. Ca++
C. Increased cAMP level
D. Increased cGMP level

Ans. A.

3785. An important cause of water intoxication is

A. Nephrogenic diabetes insipidus
B. Renal failure
C. Gastroenteritis
D. Fanconi syndrome

Ans. B.

3786. Minimum excretory urinary volume for waste products elimination during 24 hrs is

A. 200–300 ml
B. 200–400 ml
C. 500–600 ml
D. 800 ml

Ans. C.

3787. In primary dehydration

A. Intracellular fluid volume is reduced

B. Intracellular fluid volume remains normal

C. Extracellular fluid volume is much reduced

D. Extracellular fluid volume is much increased

Ans. A.

3788. An important cause of secondary dehydration is

A. Dysphagia
B. Oesophageal varices
C. Oesophageal varices
D. Gastroenteritis

Ans. D.

3789. Important finding of secondary dehydration is

A. Intracellular oedema B. Cellular dehydration
C. Thirst D. Muscle cramps

Ans. A.

3790. Urine examination in secondary dehydration shows

A. Ketonuria B. Low specific gravity
C. High specific gravity D. Albuminuria

Ans. B.

3791. The total calcium of the human body is about

A. 100–150 g B. 200–300 g
C. 1–1.5 kg D. 2–3 kg

Ans. C.

3792. Daily requirement of calcium for normal adult human is

A. 100 mg B. 800 mg
C. 2 g D. 4 g

Ans. B.

3793. Normal total serum calcium level varies between

A. 4–5 mg B. 9–11 mg
C. 15–20 mg D. 50–100 mg

Ans. B.

3794. The element needed in quantities greater than 100 mg for human beings is

A. Calcium B. Zinc
C. Selenium D. Cobalt

Ans. A.

3795. The mineral present in the human body in larger amounts than any other cation is

A. Sodium B. Calcium
C. Potassium D. Iron

Ans. B.

3796. The percentage of the total body calcium present in bones is

A. 1 B. 11
C. 55 D. 99

Ans. D.

3797. The percentage of calcium present in extracellular fluid is

A. 1
B. 5
C. 10
D. 50

Ans. A.

3798. The physiologically active form of calcium is

A. Protein bond
B. Ionised
C. Complexed with citrate
D. Complexed with carbonate

Ans. B.

3799. The normal concentration of calcium in C.S.F is

A. 1.5–2.5 mg/100 ml
B. 2.5–4 mg/100 ml
C. 4.5–5 mg/100 ml
D. 9–10 mg/100 ml

Ans. C.

3800. Absorption of calcium is increased on a

A. High protein diet
B. Low protein diet
C. High fat diet
D. Low fat diet

Ans. A.

3801. Calcium absorption is interfered by

A. Protein in diet
B. Phytic acid in cereals
C. Alkaline intestinal pH
D. Vitamin D

Ans. B.

3802. Calcium absorption is increased by

A. Vitamin D
B. Vitamin C
C. Vitamin K
D. Vitamin E

Ans. A.

3803. In serum product of Ca x P (in mg/100ml) in children is normally

A. 20
B. 30
C. 50
D. 60

Ans. C.

3804. In ricket, the product of Ca x P (in mg/ 100 ml) in serum is below

A. 30
B. 50
C. 70
D. 100

Ans. A.

3805. In man, the amount of calcium in gms filtered in 24 hrs period by the renal glomeruli is

A. 5 B. 10

C. 15 D. 20

Ans. B.

3806. The percentage of the calcium eliminated in feces is

A. 10–20 B. 30–40

C. 50–60 D. 70–90

Ans. D.

3807. Renal ricket is caused by renal tubular defect (usually inherited) which interferes with reabsorption of

A. Calcium B. Phosphorous

C. Sodium D. Chloride

Ans. B.

3808. After operative removal of the parathyroid glands resulting into hypoparathyroidism the concentration of the serum calcium may drop below

A. 11 mg B. 10 mg

C. 9 mg D. 7 mg

Ans. D.

3809. One of the principal cations of soft tissue and body fluids is

A. Mg B. S

C. Mn D. Co

Ans. A.

3810. The normal concentration of magnesium in whole blood is

A. 0–1 mg/100 ml B. 1–2 mg/100 ml

C. 2–4 mg/100 ml D. 4–8 mg/100 ml

Ans. C.

3811. The normal concentration of magnesium in C.S.F is about

A. 1 mg/100 ml B. 3 mg/100 ml

C. 5 mg/100 ml D. 8 mg/100 ml

Ans. B.

3812. The magnesium content of muscle is about

A. 5 mg/100 ml B. 10 mg/100 ml

C. 21 mg/100 ml D. 50 mg/100 ml

Ans. C.

3813. Intestinal absorption of magnesium is increased in

A. Calcium deficient diet
B. High calcium diet
C. High oxalate diet
D. High phytate diet

Ans. A.

3814. Deficiency of magnesium may occur with

A. Alcoholism
B. Diabetes mellitus
C. Hypothyroidism
D. Advanced renal failure

Ans. A.

3815. Hypermagnesemia may be observed in

A. Hyperparathyroidism
B. Diabetes mellitus
C. Kwashiorkar
D. Primary aldosteronism

Ans. B.

3816. The principal cation in extracellular fluid is

A. Sodium
B. Potassium
C. Calcium
D. Magnesium

Ans. A.

3817. The normal concentration of sodium (in mg/100 ml) of human plasma is

A. 100
B. 200
C. 250
D. 330

Ans. D.

3818. A decrease in serum sodium may occur in

A. Adrenocortical insufficiency
B. Hypoparathyroidism
C. Hyperparathyroidism
D. Thyrotoxicosis

Ans. A.

3819. Hypernatremia may occur in

A. Diabetes insipidus
B. Diuretic medication
C. Heavy sweating
D. Kidney disease

Ans. A.

3820. The metabolism of sodium is regulated by the hormone:

A. Insulin
B. Aldosterone
C. PTH
D. Somatostatin

Ans. B.

3821. The principal cation in intracellular fluid is

A. Sodium B. Potassium
C. Calcium D. Magnesium

Ans. B.

3822. The normal concentration of potassium in whole blood is

A. 50 mg/100 ml B. 100 mg/100 ml
C. 150 mg/100 ml D. 200 mg/100 ml

Ans. D.

3823. The normal concentration of potassium in cells in ng/100 ml is about

A. 100 B. 200
C. 350 D. 440

Ans. D.

3824. Potassium content of nerve tissue in mg/100 ml is about

A. 200 B. 330
C. 400 D. 530

Ans. D.

3825. One of the symptoms of low serum potassium concentration includes

A. Muscle weakness B. Confusion
C. Numbness D. Tingling of extremities

Ans. A.

3826. Potassium metabolism is regulated by the hormone:

A. Aldosterone B. PTH
C. Somatostatin D. Estrogen

Ans. A.

3827. A high serum potassium, accompanied by a high intracellular potassium occurs in

A. Adrenal insufficiency B. Any illness
C. Gastrointestinal losses D. Cushing's syndrome

Ans. A.

3828. Hypokalemia occurs in

A. Cushing's syndrome B. Addison's disease
C. Renal failure D. Advanced dehydration

Ans. A.

3829. Cardiac arrest may occur due to over doses of

A. Sodium
B. Potassium
C. Zinc
D. Magnesium

Ans. B.

3830. The normal concentration of chloride in mg/100 ml of whole blood is about

A. 200
B. 250
C. 400
D. 450

Ans. B.

3831. The normal concentration of chloride in mg/100 ml of plasma is about

A. 100
B. 200
C. 365
D. 450

Ans. C.

3832. The normal concentration of chlorine in mg/100 ml of C.S.F is about

A. 200
B. 250
C. 300
D. 440

Ans. D.

3833. Hypokalemia with an accompanying hypochloremic alkalosis may be observed in

A. Cushing's syndrome
B. Addison's disease
C. Hyptothyroidism
D. Malnutrition

Ans. A.

3834. Hypercholremia is associated with

A. Hyponatremia
B. Hypernatremia
C. Metabolic alkalosis
D. Respiratory acidosis

Ans. B.

3835. The exclusive function of iron in the body is confined to the process of

A. Muscular contraction
B. Nerve excitation
C. Cellular respiration
D. Blood coagulation

Ans. C.

3836. The normal pH of the blood is

A. 7.0
B. 7.1
C. 7.2
D. 7.4

Ans. D.

3837. At the pH of blood 7.4, the ratio between the carbonic acid and bicarbonate fractions is

A. 1 : 10 B. 1 : 20

C. 1 : 30 D. 1 : 40

Ans. B.

3838. Important buffer system of extracellular fluid is

A. Bicarbonate/carbonic acid

B. Disodium hydrogen phosphate/sodium dihydrogen phosphate

C. Plasma proteins

D. Organic Phosphate

Ans. A.

3839. The pH of body fluids is stabilized by buffer systems. The compound which will be the most effective buffer at physiologic pH is

A. Na2HPO4 pKa = 12.32 B. Na2HPO4 pKa=7.21

C. NH4OH pKa = 7.24 D. Citric acid pKa = 3.09

Ans. B.

3840. The percentage of CO2 carrying capacity of whole blood by hemoglobin and oxyhemoglobin is

A. 20 B. 40

C. 60 D. 80

Ans. C.

3841. The carbondioxide carrying power of the blood residing within the red cells is

A. 50% B. 60%

C. 85% D. 100%

Ans. C.

3842. Within the red blood cells the buffering capacity contributed by the phosphates is

A. 5% B. 10%

C. 20% D. 25%

Ans. D.

3843. The normal ratio between the alkaline phosphate and acid phosphate in plasma is

A. 2 : 1 B. 1 : 4

C. 20 : 1 D. 4 : 1

Ans. D.

3844. Of the total body water, intracellular compartment contains about

A. 50% B. 60%

C. 70% D. 80%

Ans. C.

3845. Osmotically active substances in plasma are

A. Sodium B. Chloride

C. Proteins D. All of these

Ans. D.

3846. Oncotic pressure of plasma is due to

A. Proteins B. Chloride

C. Sodium D. All of these

Ans. A.

3847. Oncotic pressure of plasma is about

A. 10 mm of Hg B. 15 mm of Hg

C. 25 mm of Hg D. 50 mm of Hg

Ans. C.

3848. Oedema can occur when

A. Plasma Na and Cl are decreased B. Plasma Na and Cl are increased

C. Plasma proteins are decreased D. Plasma proteins are increased

Ans. C.

3849. The water produced during metabolic reactions in an adult is about

A. 100 ml/day B. 300 ml/day

C. 500 ml/day D. 700 ml/day

Ans. B.

3850. The daily water loss through gastrointestinal tract in an adult is about

A. Less than 100 ml/day B. 200 ml/day

C. 300 ml/day D. 400 ml/day

Ans. A.

3851. Recurrent vomiting leads to loss of

A. Potassium B. Chloride

C. Bicarbonate D. All of these

Ans. B.

3852. Urinary water loss is increased in

A. Diabetes mellitus
B. Diabetes insipidus
C. Chronic glomerulonephritis
D. All of these

Ans. D.

3853. Diabetes insipidus results from

A. Decreased insulin secretion
B. Decreased ADH secretion
C. Decreased aldosterone secretion
D. Unresponsiveness of osmoreceptors

Ans. B.

3854. Thiazide diuretics inhibit

A. Carbonic anhydrase
B. Aldosterone secretion
C. ADH secretion
D. Sodium reabsorption in distal tubules

Ans. D.

3855. Furosemide inhibits reabsorption of sodium and chloride in

A. Proximal convoluted tubules
B. Loop of Henle
C. Distal convoluted tubules
D. Collecting ducts

Ans. B.

3856. A diuretic which is an aldosterone antagonist is

A. Spironolactone
B. Ethacrynic acid
C. Acetazolamide
D. Chlorothiazide

Ans. A.

3857. At pH 7.4, the ratio of bicarbonate : dissolved CO2 is

A. 1 : 1
B. 10 : 1
C. 20 : 1
D. 40 : 1

Ans. C.

3858. Quantitatively, the most significant buffer system in plasma is

A. Phosphate buffer system
B. Carbonic acid-bicarbonate buffer system
C. Lactic acid-lactate buffer system
D. Protein buffer system

Ans. B.

3859. In a solution containing phosphate buffer, the pH will be 7.4, if the ratio of monohydrogen phosphate : dihydrogen phosphate is

A. 4 : 1
B. 5 : 1
C. 10 : 1
D. 20 : 1

Ans. A.

3860. Buffering action of haemoglobin is mainly due to its

A. Glutamine residues
B. Arginine residues
C. Histidine residues
D. Lysine residues

Ans. C.

3861. Respiratory acidosis results from

A. Retention of carbon dioxide
B. Excessive elimination of carbon dioxide
C. Retention of bicarbonate
D. Excessive elimination of bicarbonate

Ans. A.

3862. Respiratory acidosis can occur in all of the following except

A. Pulmonary oedema
B. Hysterical hyperventilation
C. Pneumothorax
D. Emphysema

Ans. B.

3863. Respiratory alkalosis can occur in

A. Bronchial asthma
B. Collapse of lungs
C. Hysterical hyperventilation
D. Bronchial obstruction

Ans. C.

3864. Anion gap is the difference in the plasma concentrations of

A. (Chloride) – (Bicarbonate)
B. (Sodium) – (Chloride)
C. (Sodium + Potassium) – (Chloride + Bicarbonate)
D. (Sum of cations) – (Sum of anions)

Ans. C.

3865. All the following changes in blood chemistry can occur in severe diarrhea except

A. Decreased pH
B. Decreased bicarbonate
C. Increased pCO2
D. Increased chloride

Ans. C.

3866. Metabolic alkalosis can occur in

A. Severe diarrhoea
B. Renal failure
C. Recurrent vomiting
D. Excessive use of carbonic anhydrase inhibitors

Ans. C.

3867. One joule is the energy required to

A. Raise the temperature of 1 gm of water by 1°C

B. Raise the temperature of 1 kg of water by 1°C

C. Move a mass of 1 gm by 1 cm distance by a force of 1 Newton

D. Move a mass of 1 kg by 1 m distance by a force of 1 Newton

Ans. D.

3868. Organic compound of small molecular size is

A. Urea B. Uric acid

C. Creatinine D. Phosphates

Ans. A.

3869. Organic substance of large molecular size is

A. Starch B. Insulin

C. Lipids D. Proteins

Ans. D.

3870. Body water is regulated by the hormone:

A. Oxytocin B. ACTH

C. FSH D. Epinephrine

Ans. A.

3871. Calcium is required for the activation of the enzyme:

A. Isocitrate dehydrogenase B. Fumarase

C. Succinate thiokinase D. ATPase

Ans. D.

3872. Cobalt is a constituent of

A. Folic acid B. Vitamin B12

C. Niacin D. Biotin

Ans. B.

3873. Calcium absorption is inferred by

A. Fatty acids B. Amino acids

C. Vitamin D D. Vitamin B12

Ans. A.

3874. The average of pH of urine is

A. 5.6 B. 6.0

C. 6.4 D. 7.0

Ans. B.

3875. The macromolecules that require a template for their synthesis are

A. Carbohydrates
B. Lipids and carbohydrates
C. Proteins
D. Proteins and carbohydrates

Ans. D.

3876. The macromolecules whose monomers are bound by noncovalent forces are

A. Carbohydrates
B. Lipids
C. Carbohydrates and lipids
C. Lipids and nucleic acids

Ans. B.

3877. A nucleotide base not present in DNA is

A. Adenine
B. Guanine
C. Uracil
D. Thymine

Ans. C.

3878. The polarity of DNA chains is represented by

A. 3'-5'
B. 2'-5'
C. 1'-6'
D. 2'-3'

Ans. A.

3879. An amino acid that has a secondary amine and disrupts α helix formation is

A. Glycine
B. Phenylalanine
C. Serine
D. Proline

Ans. D.

3880. Adenosine is

A. A nitrogenous base
B. A ribonucleotide
C. A deoxyribonucleotide
D. None of these

Ans. A.

3881. The kind of nucleic acid that is represented by a cloverleaf model ?

A. Mitochondrial DNA
B. mRNA
C. tRNA
D. rRNA

Ans. C.

3882. Which of the following is not a characteristic of most DNA under physiological conditions ?

A. A pairs with T by hydrogen bonds
B. 20 A° diameter
C. 3.4 A° pitch
D. 10 base pairs per turn of helix

Ans. C.

3883. RNA molecules differ from DNA molecules in all but which of the following respects

A. Kinds of purines
B. Kinds of pyrimidines
C. Number of strands per molecules
D. Type of sugar

Ans. A.

3884. What type of function do protein porins perform ?

A. Cytoskeletons
B. Transport
C. Structural
D. None of the above

Ans. B.

3885. The degree of inhibition for non competitive inhibition of an enzyme catalyzed reaction ?

A. Increase with increase substrate concentration
B. Reaches with increase in substrate concentration
C. Reaches a maxima with increase in substrate concentration and then decreases
D. Dereases with increase in substrate concentration

Ans. C.

3886. Enzyme papain is used with success to

A. Increase meat production
B. Ripen papaya fruit
C. Leaven bread
D. Tenderize meat

Ans. D.

3887. Which of the following reactions used for the purpose of recycling enzymes in bioprocesses

A. Isomerization
B. Phosphorylation
C. Immobilization
D. Polymerization

Ans. C.

3888. Most industrial enzymes are obtained from

A. Plants
B. Microbes
C. Insects
D. Animal tissues

Ans. B.

3889. Ki indicates

A. Reaction velocity
B. Competition inhibition
C. Denaturation of enzyme
D. All of the above

Ans. B.

3890. The phenomenon by which the synthesis of a set of enzyme leading to a product from outside is known as

A. Repression
B. Suppression
C. Depression
D. None of these

Ans. A.

3891. De novo synthesis of an enzyme promoted by the substrate on which it acts is characterized by the term

A. Induction
B. Activation
C. Gratuity
D. Derepression

Ans. A.

3892. Out of total enzymes present in the cell mitochondria alone has

A. 4%
B. 70%
C. 90%
D. no enzymes

Ans. B.

3893. Enzymes, vitamins and hormones can be classified into a single category of biological chemicals because all of them

A. Aid in regulating metabolism
B. Are synthesized in organism
C. Are proteins
D. Enhance the oxidation metabolism

Ans. C.

3894. A nucleoside is

A. A nucleoside without sugar
B. A nucleoside without phosphate
C. A nucleoside without nitrogenous base
D. A nucleoside without sugar only

Ans. B.

3895. The adjacent nucleotides are joined by

A. Ionic bond
B. Hydrogen bond
C. Phosphodiester bond
D. All the above

Ans. C.

3896. According to Chargaff's rule, in a DNA molecule

A. The amount of adenine and thymine = the amount of guanine and cytosine
B. The amount of cytosine and guanine = the amount of adenine and cytosine
C. The amount of adenine and guanine = the amount of thymine and cytosine
D. All of these

Ans. C.

3897. Watson and Crick's double helical DNA is a

A. A DNA
B. B-DNA
C. Z –DNA
D. D-DNA

Ans. B.

3898. The two straínds in a DNA double helix are joined by

A. Hydrogen bonds between sugars
B. Phosphodiester bonds between sugars
C. Hydrogen bonds between bases
D. Phosphodisester bonds between sugars

Ans. C.

3899. Who all got the Nobel prize for discovering the structure of DNA double helix?

A. Watson and Crick
B. Watson, Crick and Wilkins
C. Watson, Crick and Franklin
D. Watson, Crick and Pauling

Ans. B.

3900. The diameter of DNA helix is

A. 10 A°
B. 21 A°
C. 1 nm
D. 2 nm

Ans. D.

3901. The distance between two adjacent nucleotide is

A. 6.8A°
B. 3.4 A°
C. 1.7 A°
D. 2A°

Ans. B.

3902. DNA is

A. Positively charged
B. Negatively charged
C. Neutral
D. None of the above

Ans. B.

3903. Which one of the following statement is correct ?

A. The two DNA strands are parallel and complementary
B. The two DNA strands are antiparallel and non-complementary
C. The two DNA strands are antiparallel and complementary
D. None of these

Ans. C.

3904. Enzymes are

A. Carbohydrate
B. RNA
C. Proteins
D. Fats

Ans. C.

3905. The term enzymes are coined by

A. Pasteur
B. Butchner
C. Urey Miller
D. Kuhne

Ans. D.

3906. The fastest enzymes is

A. Pepsin
B. Carbonic anhydrase
C. DNA gyrase
D. DNA polymerase

Ans. B.

3907. Fat is hydrolysed by the enzyme known as

A. Trypsin
B. Lipase
C. Pepsin
D. Amylase

Ans. B.

3908. The term apoenzyme is applicable to

A. Simple enzyme
B. Protein part of conjugate enzyme
C. Organic cofactor of a conjugate enzyme
D. Inorganic cofactor of a conjugate enzyme

Ans. B.

3909. Enzymes

A. Do not require activation energy
B. Do not change requirement of activation energy
C. Increase requirement of activation energy
D. Lowest requirement of activation energy

Ans. D.

3910. Zymogen is

A. Enzyme poison
B. Enzyme modulator
C. Enzyme precursor
D. Enzyme inhibitor

Ans. C.

3911. Allosteric enzyme possesses

A. Active site and an allosteric site

B. Active site and two types of allosteric sites

C. Active site and three types of allosteric sites

D. Three types of allosteric sites

Ans. B.

3912. Enzymes generally have

A. Same pH and temperature optima

B. Same pH but different temperature optima

C. Different pH but same temperature optima

D. Different pH and different temperature optima

Ans. A.

3913. The enzyme which forms the peptide bond is known as

A. Carbonic unhydrase B. Peptidase

C. Carbohydrase D. Peptidyl transferase

Ans. D.

3914. The tyrosinase is activated by

A. Iron B. Copper

C. Zinc D. Potassium

Ans. B.

3915. Lock and key theory of enzyme action was proposed by

A. Fisher B. Koshland

C. Kuhne D. Arrhenius

Ans. A.

3916. Trypsin is active in

A. Acidic B. Alkaline

C. Neutral D. None of these

Ans. B.

3917. Koshland's theory of enzyme action is known as

A. Reduced fit theory B. Lock and key theory

C. Induced fit theory D. Enzyme coenzyme theory

Ans. C.

3918. The enzymes involved in feedback inhibiton are called

A. Allosteric enzymes
B. Holoenzymes
C. Apoenzymes
D. Coenzymes

Ans. A.

3919. Which one of the following is a group of proteolytic enzymes ?

A. Bromelin and Papain
B. Cellulase and myrosinase
C. Maltase and diastase
D. Phosphatase and diastase

Ans. A.

3920. Enzymes having slightly different molecular structures but performing identical activity are

A. Holoenzymes
B. Apoenzymes
C. Isoenzymes
D. Coenzymes

Ans. C.

3921. Which factor is responsible for inhibition enzymatic process during feed back ?

A. Enzymes
B. End products
C. Temperature
D. Substrate

Ans. B.

3922. Which one of the following statements regarding enzyme inhibition is correct ?

A. Competitive inhibition is seen when a substrate competes with an enzyme for binding to an inhibitor protein
B. Noncompetitive inhibition of an enzyme can be overcome by adding large amount of substrate
C. Noncompetitive efficiency inhibitors often bind to the enzyme irreversibly
D. Competitive inhibiton is seen when the substrate and the inhibitor compete for the active site on the enzyme

Ans. D.

3923. The catalytic efficiency of two different enzymes can be compared by the

A. Formation of the product
B. Km value
C. Molecular size of the enzyme
D. pH of optimum value

Ans. B.

3924. The nuclease enzyme which begins its attack from free of a polynucleotide is

A. Polymerase
B. Kinase
C. Exonuclease
D. Endonuclease

Ans. C.

3925. The enzyme enterokinase helps in the conversion of

A. Caseinogens into casein
B. Trypsinogen into trypsin
C. Pepsigenogen in to pepsin
D. Proteins into polypeptides

Ans. B.

3926. Which of the following is a typical example of 'feedback inhibition ?

A. Cyanide and cytochrome reaction
B. Sulpha drugs and folic acid synthesizer bacteria
C. Allosteric inhibition of hexokinase by glucose 6 phosphate
D. Reaction between succinic dehydrogenase and succinic acid

Ans. C.

3927. Some of the enzymes which are associated in converting fats into carbohydrates are present in

A. Liposomes
B. Golgi bodies
C. Glyoxysomes
D. Microsomes

Ans. C.

3928. In which one of the following enzymes is copper necessarily associaged as an activator?

A. Tyrosinase
B. Lactic dehydrogenase
C. Carbonic unhydrase
D. Trypsinase

Ans. D.

3929. A peptide bond

A. Has a partial double bond character
B. Is ionized at physiological pH
C. Is stable to heating in strong acids
D. Occurs most commonly in the cos configuration

Ans. A.

3930. At neutral pH a mixture of amino acids in solution would be predominantly

A. Hydrophobic
B. Negative and monovalent
C. Hydrophobic
D. Dipolar ions

Ans. D.

3931. Which one of the following states of haemoglobin (Hb) binds oxygen with the greatest affinity ?

A. Hb
B. Hb(O)2
C. Hb(O2)2
D. Hb(O2)4

Ans. D.

3932. Which of the following amino acids is most compatible with an α helical structure?

A. Proline B. Tryptophan

C. Alanine D. Cysteine

Ans. C.

3933. Which of the following techniques is used to separate proteins based upon differences in their mass ?

A. Isoelectric focusing B. Western blotting

C. Ion exchange chromatography D. SDS gel electrophoresis

Ans. D.

3934. The greatest buffering capacity at physiological pH would be provided by a protein rich in which of the following amino acids ?

A. Lysine B. Aspartic acid

C. Valine D. Histidine

Ans. D.

3935. The site of enzyme modification by phosphorylation is the amino acid

A. Arginine B. Cysteine

C. Phenylalanine D. Serine

Ans. D.

3936. Which of the following reagents would be most useful in determining the N terminal amino acid of polypeptide ?

A. Trypsin B. Cyanogen bromide

C. 1 mol/L HCl D. Phenylisothiocyanate

Ans. D.

3937. Which of the following statement is correct ?

A. The helix can be composed of more than one polypeptide chain

B. β sheets exists only in the antiparallel form

C. Motifs are a type of secondary structure

D. β bends often contain proline

Ans. D.

3938. The highest concentration of cystine can be found in

A. Melanin B. Keratin

C. Myosin D. Collagen

Ans. B.

3939. if the percentage of adenine in a DNA sample is 20%, what would be the percentage of other bases ?

A. T=30%, G=20%, C=20%

B. T=40%, G=20%, C=20%

C. T=20%, G=30%, C=30%

D. T=20%, G=20%, C=40%

Ans. C.

3940. Which of the following statement is incorrect ?

A. DNA is the only biomolecule with self repair mechanism

B. DNA is autocatalytic

C. DNA is heterocatalytic

D. Increasing temeperature to 90-100°C breaks the phosphodiester bonds in DNA

Ans. D.

3941. In a DNA sample, the percentage on bases is G=30% and C=40%, the most probable explanation is

A. Mutation might have occurred

B. The DNA sample may be a bacterial genome

C. The DNA sample may be a viral genome

D. None of these

Ans. C.

3942. Which of the following statement is true ?

A. DNA bases varies from one species to another

B. DNA bases of a species does not change with age, nutritional state and environment

C. DNA base remains same in different tissues of the same individual

D. All of these

Ans. D.

3943. The negative charge of DNA is due to

A. Sugar, phosphate and amino acids

B. Deoxyribose sugar

C. Nitrogenous bases specifically adenine

D. Phosphate group

Ans. D.

3944. The amount of DNA in a cell can be altered by

A. Ecological factors

B. Environmental factors

C. Physiological factors

D. Can not be altered

Ans. D.

3945. The amount of DNA in a cell at the beginning of mitosis is

A. Half of the amount found in cells at G1 stage

B. Same as the amount found in cells at G1 stage

C. Twice the amount found in cells at G1 stage

D. Four times the amount found at G1 stage

Ans. C.

3946. The DNA found in all living organisms is

A. Left handed DNA
B. Right handed DNA
C. Both A and B
D. Z- DNA

Ans. B.

3947. The DNA strand is directly involved in the formation of all except

A. Protein
B. Another DNA strand
C. mRNA molecule
D. tRNA molecule

Ans. A.

3948. Which of the following statement is wrong

A. A-DNA is the dehydrated form of DNA

B. The naturally occurring DNA is B-DNA and is also called as wet DNA

C. Z DNA is also called zig zag DNA and is a right handed helix

D. Z DNA occurs in dehydrated high salt concentration

Ans. C.

3949. RNA is genetic material in

A. Viruses only

B. In some viruses and prokaryotes

C. In some viruses and some prokaryotes and rarely in eukaryotes

D. Only in some viruses

Ans. D.

3950. RNA is

A. Single stranded
B. Double stranded
C. Triple stranded
D. Both A and B

Ans. A.

3951. The sugar in RNA is

A. Deoxyribose
B. Ribose
C. Hexose
D. Fructose

Ans. B.

3952. Nucleotides in RNA are joined by

A. 3'5' phosphodiester bond
B. 3'4' phosphodiester bond
C. 3'2' phosphodiester bond
D. 3'6' phosphodiester bond

Ans. A.

3953. Thymine in DNA is replaced by

A. Guanine in RNA
B. Adenine in RNA
C. Cytosine in RNA
D. Uracil in RNA

Ans. D.

3954. The most abundant type of RNA in the cell is

A. rRNA
B. mRNA
C. tRNA
D. hnRNA

Ans. A.

3955. Which of the following RNA serves as adaptor molecule during protein synthesis?

A. rRNA
B. mRNA
C. tRNA
D. hnRNA

Ans. C.

3956. rRNA is synthesised in

A. Nucleus
B. Cytoplasm
C. RER
D. Nucleolus

Ans. D.

3957. cDNA is

A. Complementary to mRNA
B. Complementary to rRNA
C. Complementary to tRNA
D. Complementary to hnRNA

Ans. A.

3958. Amino acids are attached to the

A. Acceptor arm of tRNA
B. Anti-codon arm of tRNA
C. Codon arm of tRNA
D. None of these

Ans. A.

3959. Ribozymes are

A. Enzymes with catalytic activity
B. RNAs with catalytic activity
C. Proteins with catalytic activity
D. Nucleic acids with catalytic activity

Ans. B.

3960. RNA is primarily seen in

A. Nucleus
B. Cytoplasm
C. RER
D. SER

Ans. B.

3961. Ribose sugar in RNA is

A. D-ribose
B. L-ribose
C. Both L and D
D. None of these

Ans. A.

3962. Which of the virus has double stranded RNA as genetic material ?

A. Tobacco mosaic virus
B. Influenza virus
C. Rous Sarcoma virus
D. Reovirus

Ans. D.

3963. Ribosomes are composed of

A. DNA and RNA
B. RNA and proteins
C. DNA and proteins
D. RNA only

Ans. B.

3964. Fats are abundantly found in

A. Reproductive tissue
B. vegetative tissue
C. Both A and B
D. None of these

Ans. A.

3965. Natural lipids are readily soluble in

A. Oil
B. Mercury
C. Water
D. None of these

Ans. D.

3966. Which of the following is/are unsaturated fatty acids ?

A. Linoleic acid
B. Oleic acid
C. Palmitoleic acid
D. All of these

Ans. D.

3967. Fats can be stored in the cell without disturbing their

A. Hydroxyl bond
B. Aleurone layer
C. Osmotic relations
D. None of these

Ans. C.

3968. Liquid form of triglycerides at ordinary room temperature are called

A. Oils B. Solids

C. Fats D. None of these

Ans. A.

3969. The synthesis of glucose from fat is called

A. Glycolysis B. Kreb's cycle

C. Saponification D. Gluconeogenesis

Ans. D.

3970. Hydrolysis of fats by alkalies into fatty acids and glycerol is called

A. Coagulation B. saponification

C. Suspension D. Colloidal

Ans. B.

3971. The fats and oils are respectively rich in

A. Unsaturated fatty acids

B. Saturated fatty acids

C. Saturated and unsaturated fatty acids

D. None of these

Ans. C.

3972. β oxidation takes place in

A. Mitochondria B. Cytoplasm

C. Chloroplasts D. Nucleus

Ans. A.

3973. Which is a phospholipid

A. Lecithin B. Cholesterol

C. Sterol D. Steroid

Ans. A.

3974. The number of double bonds in Arachidonic acid

A. 1 B. 2

C. 3 D. 4

Ans. D.

3975. Essential fatty acids are

A. Linoleic acid B. Arachidonic acid

C. Linolenic acid D. All of these

Ans. D.

3976. The following is not a phospholipid

A. Sphingomyelin
B. Lecithin
C. Cephalin
D. Cerebroside

Ans. D.

3977. Examples of monounsaturated fatty acids are

A. Oleic acid
B. Arachidonic acid
C. Palmitic acid
D. Linolenic acid

Ans. A.

3978. High content of triglycerides are seen in

A. LDL
B. HDL
C. VLDL
D. Chylomicrons

Ans. D.

3979. The repeating units of proteins are

A. Glucose units
B. Amino acids
C. Fatty acids
D. Peptides

Ans. B.

3980. Amino acids are joined by

A. Peptide bond
B. Hydrogen bond
C. Ionic bond
D. Glycosidic bond

Ans. A.

3981. The primary structure of protein represents

A. Linear sequence of amino acids joined by peptide bond
B. 3 dimensional structure of protein
C. Helical structure of protein
D. Subunit structure of protein

Ans. A.

3982. Peptide bond is

A. Rigid with partial double bond character
B. Planer, covalent
C. Covalent
D. None of the above

Ans. D.

3983. Enzymes are

A. Proteins
B. Carbohydrates
C. Nucleic acids
D. DNA molecules

Ans. A.

3984. The first protein sequenced by Frederick Sanger is

A. Haemoglobin
B. Myoglobin
C. Insulin
D. Myosin

Ans. C.

3985. A dipeptide has

A. 2 amino acids and 1 peptide bond
B. 2 amino acids and 2 peptide bond
C. 2 amino acids and 3 peptide bond
D. 2 amino acids and 4 peptide bond

Ans. A.

3986. The most common secondary structure is

A. α helix
B. β pleated structure
C. β pleated structure parallel
D. β pleated structure non-parallel

Ans. A.

3987. Myoglobin is a

A. Protein with primary structure
B. Protein with secondary structure
C. Protein with tertiary structure
D. Protein with quaternary structure

Ans. C.

3988. Fibrous protein such as silk fibroin consists of polypeptide chains arranged in

A. α helix
B. β pleated structure
C. β helix
D. None of the above

Ans. B.

3989. α helix has

A. 3.4 amino acids residues per turn
B. 3.6 amino acids residues per turn
C. 3.8 amino acids residues per turn
D. 3.0 amino acids residues per turn

Ans. B.

3990. Tertiary structure is maintained by

A. Peptide bond
B. Hydrogen bond
C. Disulphide bond
D. All of the above

Ans. D.

3991. Haemoglobin has

A. Primary structure
B. Secondary structure
C. Tertiary structure
D. Quaternary structure

Ans. D.

3992. Disulphide bonds are formed between

A. Cysteine residues that are close together
B. Cystine residues that are close together
C. Proline residues that are close together
D. Histidine residues that are close together

Ans. A.

3993. The 3D structure of protein can be determined by

A. NMR
B. X ray crystallography
C. Both A and B
D. Spectroscopy

Ans. C.

3994. 4-hydroxy proline is present in

A. Collagen
B. Plant cell wall
C. Keratin
D. Both plant cell wall and collagen

Ans. D.

3995. Peptide bonds between amino acids are highly stable and have a half life of seven years in intracellular condition. This is due to

A. High activation energy required for hydrolysis
B. Low activation energy required for hydrolysis
C. Peptide bond is a covalent bond
D. Peptide bond is rigid and planar

Ans. A.

3996. Tripeptide consists

A. 3 amino acids and 3 peptide bonds
B. 2 amino acids and 3 peptide bonds
C. 3 amino acids and 2 peptide bonds
D. 3 amino acids and 4 peptide bonds

Ans. C.

3997. All the following statements are true except

A. Ornithine and citruline are uncommon amino acids

B. Ornithine is an intermediates in Urea cycle

C. Ornithine and citruline are uncommon amino acids present in many proteins

D. Both ornithine and citruline are intermediates in Urea cycle

Ans. C.

3998. The characteristic strong absorbance of 280 nm of protein is due to

A. All amino acids can absorb at 280 nm

B. Only tryptophan and tyrosine can absorb at 280 nm

C. Tryptophan is responsible for the absorbance

D. Tryptophan, tyrosine and phenylalanine can absorb at 280 nm

Ans. D.

3999. The formation of cystine occurs at

A. ER B. Golgi

C. Cytosol D. Mitochondria

Ans. A.

4000. Which of the following interaction contributes most in protein folding ?

A. Covalent bond B. Ionic bond

C. Hydrophobic interaction D. Vander walls interaction

Ans. C.

4001. Which of the following amino acid has pKa near neutrality ?

A. Tryptophan B. Arginine

C. Histidine D. Asparagine

Ans. C.

4002. Desmosine is an unusual amino acid found in

A. Myosin B. Elastin

C. Troponin D. Actin

Ans. B.

4003. How many small peptides are formed upon cleavage by trypsin if a protein has 5 lysine residues ?

A. 4 B. 5

C. 6 D. 7

Ans. C.

4004. EF-1α and EF-Tu are

A. Analogs
B. Homologs
C. Paralogs
D. Syllogs

Ans. B.

4005. All the statements regarding peptide bond are true except

A. Peptide bond is a covalent bond
B. Peptide bond is rigid and planar
C. Peptide bond has partial double bond character
D. Peptide bond is formed by non-condensation reaction

Ans. D.

4006. Which of the following amino acids are rarely present in alpha helix ?

A. Glycine and proline
B. Proline and tryptophan
C. Tryptophan and glycine
D. Proline only

Ans. A.

4007. PDI is an enzyme involve in

A. Protein synthesis
B. Protein degradation
C. Protein folding
D. Protein quaternary structure formation

Ans. C.

4008. A prosthetic group of a protein is a non protein structure that is

A. A ligand of the protein
B. A part of the secondary structure of the protein
C. A substrate of the protein
D. Permanently associated with the protein

Ans. D.

4009. In the binding of oxygen to myoglobin, the relationship between the concentration of oxygen and the fraction of binding sites occupied can best be described as

A. Hyperbolic
B. Linear with a negative slope
C. Linear with a positive slope
D. Sigmoidal

Ans. A.

4010. Myoglobin and the subunits of hemoglobin have

A. No obvious structural relationship
B. Very different primary and tertiary structures
C. Very similar primary and tertiary structures
D. Very similar tertiary structures but different primary structures

Ans. D.

4011. In hemoglobin, the transition from T state to R state (low to high affinity) is triggered by

A. Fe^{+2} binding
B. Heme binding
C. oxygen binding
D. Subunit association

Ans. C.

4012. Which of the following is not correct concerning cooperative bidning of a ligand to a protein ?

A. It is usually a form of allosteric interaction
B. It is usually associated with protein with multiple subunits
C. It rarely occurs in enzymes
D. It results in a nonlinear Hill Plot

Ans. C.

4013. The fundamental cause of sickle cell disease is a change in the structure of

A. Blood
B. Capillaries
C. Hemoglobin
D. Red cells

Ans. C.

4014. The proteins of the major histocompatibility complex bind and display

A. Antigen fragments
B. B cell fragments
C. Immunoglobin fragments
D. Macrophage fragments

Ans. A.

4015. A monoclonal antibody differs from a polyclonal antibody in that monoclonal antibodies

A. Are labeled with chemicals that can be visualized
B. Are produced by cells from the same organism that produced the antigen
C. Are synthesized by a population of identical or cloned cells
D. Are synthesized only in living organisms

Ans. C.

4016. The predominant structural feature in myosin molecules is

A. A β structure
B. An α structure
C. The Fab domain
D. The light chain

Ans. B.

4017. During muscle contraction, hydrolysis of ATP results in a change in the

A. Conformation of actin
B. Conformation of myosin
C. Structure of the myofibrils
D. Structure of the sarcoplasmic reticulum

Ans. B.

4018. The process of sorting and transporting newly synthesized proteins to correct destination in a cell is called

A. Protein sorting B. Protein targeting

C. Protein trafficking D. All of these

Ans. D.

4019. Protein required in the cytosol like the enzymes of glycolysis are synthesized on

A. Ribosomes on ER B. SER

C. Free ribosomes in the cytosol D. Ribosomes on nuclear membrane

Ans. C.

4020. Secretory proteins are synthesized by

A. Free ribosome B. Ribosomes on ER

C. Ribosomes on nuclear membrane D. All of the above

Ans. C.

4021. According to signal hypothesis, the signal peptide for a secretory protein is

A. Rich in hydrophobic amino acids at the centre of the signal peptide and is attached to the N terminus of the protein

B. Rich in hydrophilic amino acids at the centre of the signal peptide and is attached to the N terminus of the protein

C. Rich in hydrophobic amino acids at the centre of the signal peptide and is attached to the C terminus of the protein

D. Rich in sulphur containing amino acids at the centre of the signal peptide and is attached to the N terminus of the protein

Ans. A.

4022. Signal sequences are

A. Short peptide sequences that serves as an address for transporting newly synthesized proteins to the correct location

B. Glycoproteins that serves as an address for transporting newly synthesized protein to the correct location

C. Short peptide sequences to transport a protein to the nucleus

D. Short peptide sequences attached to a protein that initiates its degradation by digestive enzymes

Ans. A.

4023. The retention signal of proteins of endoplasmic reticulum consists of amino acids

A. Gly-Asp-Glu-Leu at the N terminus

B. Lys-Asp-Glu-Leu at the N terminus

C. Gly-Asp-Glu-Leu at the C terminus

D. Lys-Asp-Glu-Leu at the C terminus

Ans. D.

4024. Proteins tagged with mannose 6 phosphate are transported to

A. Nucleus
B. Lysosome
C. Mitochondrion
D. Golgi apparatus

Ans. B.

4025. Nuclear localization signal that ensures transport of a protein to nucleus is rich in

A. Lysine and arginine
B. Glutamine and asparagines
C. Serine and threonine
D. tryptophan and histidine

Ans. A.

4026. Proteins targeted to micochondrial matrix are tagged with matrix targeting sequence rich in

A. Serine and threonine
B. Serine, threonine, lysine and arginine
C. Serine,threonine, glutamine and asparagine
D. Serine, threonine, tryptophan and histidine

Ans. B.

4027. Protein purification refers to the

A. Purification of proteins
B. Separation of proteins from other biomolecules
C. Separation of a particular protein from other contaminating proteins
D. All of these

Ans. A.

4028. Protein separation techniques are often based on the following properties except

A. Solubility of the protein
B. Viscosity of the protein
C. Charge of protein
D. Specific binding affinity of the protein

Ans. B.

4029. Primary steps in protein purification includes

A. Homogenization
B. Differential centrifugation
C. Solubilization
D. All of these

Ans. D.

4030. Which of the following detergent is commonly used to release integral protein from its membranes ?

A. Urea
B. Dimethyl sulphoxide
C. Trition X100
D. Cyanogens bromide

Ans. C.

4031. Salting out process involves

A. Precipitation of proteins using ammonium sulphate

B. Precipitation of proteins using copper sulphate

C. Precipitation of proteins using sodium chloride

D. None of these

Ans. **A.**

4032. Which of the following separation method is suited from a protein sample with large differences in molecular mass ?

A. Dialysis B. Salting out process

C. Density gradient centrifugation D. Rate zonal centrifugation

Ans. **D.**

4033. In which of the following separation method where proteins are separated on the basis of their net charge

A. Affinity chromatography B. Ion exchange chromatography

C. Dialysis D. Gel filtration chromatography

Ans. **B.**

4034. In gel filtration chromatography, separation of proteins are based on their

A. Size and net charge B. Size and shape

C. Size and specific affinity D. Shape and net charge

Ans. **B.**

4035. The use of insulin hormone to purify its receptor is an example of

A. Ion exchange chromatography B. Affinity chromatography

C. Gel filtration chromatography D. Ligand mediated chromatography

Ans. **B.**

4036. In anion exchange chromatography

A. The column contains negatively charged beads where positively charged proteins bind

B. The column contains positively charged beads where negatively charged proteins bind

C. The column contains both positively and negatively charged beads where proteins bind depending on their net charge

D. All of these

Ans. **B.**

4037. For the study of a protein in detail, an effort is usually made to first

A. Conjugate the protein to a known molecule

B. Determine its amino acid composition

C. Determine its amino acid sequence

D. Determine its molecular weight

E. Purify the protein

Ans. E.

4038. In a mixture of the five proteins listed below, which should elute second in size exclusion (gel filtration) chromatography ?

A. Cytochrome C Mr =13000

B. Immunoglobulin G Mr = 145000

C. Ribonuclease A Mr = 13700

D. RNA polymerase Mr = 450000

E. Serum albumin Mr = 68500

Ans. B.

4039. By adding SDS (sodium dodecyl sulphate) during the electrophoresis of proteins, it is possible to

A. Determine a protein's isoelectric point

B. Determine an enzyme's specific activity

C. Determine the amino acid composition of the protein

D. Preserve a protein's native structure and biological activity

E. Separate proteins exclusively on the basis of molecular weight

Ans. E.

4040. To determine the isoelectric point of a protein first establish that a gel

A. Contains a denaturing detergent that can distribute uniform negative charges over the protein's surface

B. Exhibits a stable pH gradient when ampholytes become distributed in an electric field

C. Is washed with an antibody specific to the protein of interest

D. Neutralizes all ionic groups on a protein by titrating them with strong bases

E. Relates the unknown protein to a series of protein markers with known molecular weights

Ans. B.

4041. The first step in two dimensional gel electrophoresis generates a series of protein bands by isoelectric focusing. In a second step, a strip of this gel is turned 90 degrees, placed on another gel containing SDS, and electric current is again applied. In this second step

A. Proteins with similar isoelectric points become further separated according to their molecular weights

B. The individual bands become stained so that the isoelectric focus pattern can be visualized

C. The individual bands become visualized by interacting with protein specific antibodies in the second gel

D. The individual bands undergo a second, more intense isolectric focusing

E. The proteins in the bands separate more completely because the second electric current is in the opposite polarity to the first current

Ans. A.

4042. The term specific activity differs from the term activity in that specific activity

A. Is measured only under optimal conditions

B. Is the activity (enzyme units) in a milligram of protein

C. Is the activity (enzyme units) of a specific protein

D. Refers only to a purified protein

E. Refers to proteins other than enzymes

Ans. B.

4043. In isoelectric focusing, separation of proteins are based on

A. Relative content of positively charged groups

B. Relative content of negatively charged groups

C. Both a and b

D. pH

E. None of these

Ans. C.

4044. Which of the following statement is incorrect

A. In affinity chromatography lectins are used to purify a glycoprotein

B. The separation in gel filtration chromatography is based on size, shape and net charge of the protein

C. In ion exchange chromatography, the bound proteins are eluted using NaCl solution

D. In affinity chromatography, the binding of a protein to a ligand is by specific non-covalent interactions

E. All of these

Ans. B.

4045. Amino acids are

A. Building blocks of carbohydrates B. Building blocks of nucleic acids

C. Building blocks of proteins D. Building blocks of lipids

Ans. C.

4046. Amino acids has

A. Both amino group and carboxyl group

B. Both amino group and keto group

C. Amino group only

D. Carboxyl group only

Ans. A.

4047. The simplest amino acid is

A. Proline B. Methionine

C. Glycine D. Serine

Ans. C.

4048. Which of the amino acid is a α helix terminator ?

A. Tryptophan B. Phenylalanine

C. Tyrosine D. Proline

Ans. D.

4049. The first amino acid in a polypeptide chain is

A. Serine B. Valine

C. Alanine D. Methionine

Ans. D.

4050. Which of the following amino acid has the buffering capacity ?

A. Tryptophan B. Cysteine

C. Histidine D. Arginine

Ans. C.

4051. Which of the following is an α imino acid ?

A. Serine B. Threonine

C. Valine D. Proline

Ans. D.

4052. The naturally occurring form of amino acid in proteins

A. L- amino acids only B. D- amino acids only

C. Both L and D amino acids D. None of these

Ans. A.

4053. Sulphur containing amino acids are

A. Cysteine and methionine
B. Methionine and threonine
C. Cysteine and threonine
D. Cysteine and serine

Ans. A.

4054. Aromatic amino acids include

A. Phenylalanine, tyrosine and tryptophan
B. Phenylalanine, serine and tryptophan
C. Threonine, tyrosine and tryptophan
D. Asparagine, tyrosine and tryptophan

Ans. A.

4055. Positively charged basic amino acids are

A. Lysine and arginine
B. Lysine and asparagines
C. Glutamine and arginine
D. Lysine and glutamine

Ans. A.

4056. Acidic amino acids include

A. Arginine and glutamate
B. Aspartate and asparagines
C. Aspartate and lysine
D. Aspartate and glutamate

Ans. D.

4057. Amino acids with hydroxyl groups are

A. Serine and alanine
B. Alanine and valine
C. Serine and threonine
D. Valine and isoleucine

Ans. C.

4058. The 21st amino acid is

A. Hydroxy lysine
B. Hydroxy proline
C. Selenocysteine
D. Citrulline

Ans. C.

4059. Absorbance at 280 nm exhibited by protein is due to

A. Aliphatic amino acids
B. All amino acids
C. Nonpolar amino acids
D. Aromatic amino acids

Ans. D.

4060. Which one of the following statements is true when a cell is kept in a hypotonic solution ?

A. Water moves out of the cell

B. Size of the cell remains same

C. No movement of water takes place

D. Size of the cell increases

Ans. D.

4061. Which one of the following amino acids has a higher propensity for cis peptide bond formation ?

A. Histidine B. Cysteine

C. Glycine D. Proline

Ans. D.

4062. The length of an alpha helix composed of 36 amino acid residues is

A. 10 A^0 B. 54 A^0

C. 27 A^0 D. 360 A^0

Ans. B.

4063. Which one of the following amino acid residues is specifically recognized by chymotrypsin during peptide bond cleavage ?

A. Phe B. Leu

C. Val D. Asp

Ans. A.

4064. The terminal electron acceptor during mitochondrial respiration is

A. O2 B. FAD+

C. NAD+ D. ATP

Ans. A.

4065. During the biosynthesis of urea in the urea cycle, the two nitrogen atoms are derived from

A. Two free ammonium groups

B. Free ammonium group and aspartate

C. Both nitrogen atoms are derived from arginine

D. One nitrogen atom is derived from citulline and one from glutamate

Ans. B.

4066. In different types of tissue transplantations the rate of graft rejection in decreasing order is

A. Isograft >xenograft > allograft B. Allograft> Isograft >xenograft

C. xenograft > autograft > allograft D. xenograft > allograft > Isograft

Ans. D.

4067. Arrange the following in the decreasing order of their permeability coefficients across a lipid bilayer membrane

i. Urea
ii. Glucose
iii. H2O
iv. Na+
v. Tryptophan

A. i, iii, v, ii, iv
B. iii, v, ii, iv, i
C. iii, i, v, ii, iv
D. i, iii, iv, v, ii

Ans. C.

4068. A researcher wants to clone 3 DNA fragments of sizes 1.1 Mb, 0.097 Mb and 0.045 Mb. The choice of the vectors for cloning

A. Cosmid, Bacteriphage lambda, Bacteriphage P1
B. Yeast artificial chromosome, bacteriphage P1/ lambda, Cosmid
C. Bacterial artificial chromosome, Bacteriphage lambda, Yeast artificial chromosome
D. Only plasmids

Ans. B.

4069. Which of the following four enzymes given below cut the following DNA sequence?

5'-CCGATATCTCGAGGGC-3'

i. Bam HI (3'-CCTAG^G-5')
ii. Xho I (3'-GAGCT^C-5')
iii. Eco RI (3'-CTTAA^G-5')
iv. Eco RV (3'-CTA^TAG-5')

A. i & ii
B. i, iii & iv
C. ii & iv
D. I, ii &iii

Ans. C.

4070. An enzyme of 40 kDa is added to a substrate solution in a molar ratio of 1:3. The concentration of the enzyme in the mixture is 12 mg/ml. What would be the corresponding substrate concentration ?

A. 0.4 mM
B. 0.12 mM
C. 0.9 mM
D. 0.3 mM

Ans. C.

4071. A patient suffering from pneumonia and tuberculosis was found to have very low CD4+ T cells. In all probability the primary causative infectious agent belongs to

A. Klebsiella family
B. Mycobacterium family
C. Retrovirus family
D. Streptococcus family

Ans. C.

4072. Which of the following mineral element facilitates insulin binding to cell receptor site ?

A. Zinc
B. Selenium
C. Copper
D. Chromium

Ans. D.

4073. Which of the following is a folate analog ?

A. Carnosine
B. Aniserine
C. Azaserine
D. Methotrexate

Ans. D.

4074. ATP concentration is maintained relatively constant during muscle contraction by

A. Increasing the metabolic activity
B. The action of creatine phosphokinase
C. The action of adenylate kinase
D. All of the above

Ans. D.

4075. The cone of retina

A. Are responsible for colour vision
B. Are much more numerous than rods
C. Have red, blue and green light sensitive pigment that differ because of small difference in the retinal prosthetic group
D. Do not use transduction in signal transduction

Ans. A.

4076. The C21 steroid hormones include

A. Vitamin D3
B. Estradiol
C. Testosterone
D. Aldosterone

Ans. D.

4077. Which of the following oxidoreductases form hydrogen peroxide as one of its products?

A. Oxidases
B. Peroxidases
C. Dehydrogenases
D. Oxygenases

Ans. A.

4078. The mjor protein responsible for the storage of iron

A. Ferredoxin
B. Ferritin
C. Hemisiderine
D. Transferine

Ans. B.

4079. Which of the following is an excitatory neurotransmitter ?

A. Glutamate
B. GABA
C. Glycine
D. Taurine

Ans. A.

4080. Which of the following is not involved in enzyme regulation ?

A. Covalent modification
B. Competitive inhibition
C. Suicide inhibition
D. Allosteric activation

Ans. C.

4081. The preferred substrate for hexokinase is

A. Glucose
B. Fructose
C. Glucose and fructose are equally preferred
D. None of these

Ans. A.

4082. The general chemical formula of carbohydrate is

A. $(CH_2O)n$
B. $(CH_2O)2n$
C. (CHO)n
D. $CnH_{2n}O$

Ans. A.

4083. Which of the following is an aldotriose ?

A. Dihydroxyacetone
B. Glyceraldehyde
C. Ribulose
D. Erythrose

Ans. B.

4084. What is the molecular formula of sucrose ?

A. $C_{12}H_{22}O_{11}$
B. $C_{10}H_{20}O_{10}$
C. $C_6H_{12}O_6$
D. $C_{12}H_{20}O_{11}$

Ans. A.

4085. The glycosidic linkage between glucose molecule in maltose is

A. β_{1-4}
B. α_{1-2}
C. α_{1-4}
D. β_{1-4}

Ans. C.

4086. A keto pentose will have ———— sterioisomers.

A. 4
B. 6
C. 8
D. 10

Ans. A.

4087. The reserve food material of green algae is

A. Laminarin
B. Chrysolaminarin
C. Floridian starch
D. Starch

Ans. D.

4088. The only carbohydrate which is not having any chiral carbon atom is

A. Glyceraldehyde
B. Erythrose
C. Dihydroxyacetone
D. Erythrulose

Ans. C.

4089. Select the odd one from the following

A. Arabinose
B. Xylose
C. Lyxose
D. Erythrose

Ans. D.

4090. A pentose sugar reported to be present in heart cells

A. Xylose
B. Arabinose
C. Lyxose
D. Xylulose

Ans. C.

4091. Which of the following is an epimeric pair ?

A. D-glucose and D-mannose
B. D-glucose and D-galactose
C. D-glucose and L-glucose
D. Both A and B

Ans. D.

4092. Select the odd one from the following

A. Xylulose
B. Dihydroxyacetone
C. Glyceraldehyde
D. Ribulose

Ans. C.

4093. Which of the following sugar give a positive result with Seliwanoff test ?

A. Sucrose
B. Glucose
C. Galactose
D. Mannose

Ans. A.

4094. Which of the following is a keto tetrose ?

A. Erythrulose
B. Xylulose
C. Sorbose
D. Psicose

Ans. A.

4095. The glycosidic linkage between two glucose molecules in isomaltose is

A. α 1-4 B. β 1-4

C. α 1-6 D. β 1-6

Ans. C.

4096. Which of the following is an alpha lactone ?

A. Vit C B. Vit D

C. Vit A D. Vit K

Ans. A.

4097. A sweetner used in sugar less gums and candies

A. Ribitol B. Xylitol

C. Inositol D. mannitol

Ans. B.

4098. The glycosidic linkage in cellobiose is

A. α 1-4 B. β 1-4

C. α 1-6 D. β 1-6

Ans. B.

4099. Pick the odd one from the following

A. Deoxyribose B. Rhamnose

C. Fucose D. Altrose

Ans. D.

4100. Lectins are ————.

A. Sugars specific to proteins

B. Proteins specific to sugars

C. Enzymes specific to carbohydrates

D. Carbohydrates specific to enzymes

Ans. B.

4101. Which of the following is a keto triose ?

A. Dihydroxyacetone B. Glyceraldehyde

C. Ribulose D. Erythrose

Ans. A.

4102. Fructose is metabolized by

A. Fructose 1-phosphate pathway

B. Fructose 6-phosphate pathway

C. Glyceraldehyde 3-phosphate pathway

D. Both (a) and (b)

Ans. D.

4103. A common way that cells capture the energy released during the breakdown of large molecules is to add electrons to smaller, specialized molecules that can accept them. This process of electron acceptance is otherwise known as

A. Biosynthesis B. Metabolism

C. Reduction D. Catalysis

Ans. C.

4104. Humans are unable to digest

A. Starch B. Complex carbohydrates

C. Denatured proteins D. Cellulose

Ans. D.

4105. How many ATP equivalents per mole of glucose input are required for gluconeogenesis?

A. 2 B. 6

C. 8 D. 4

Ans. B.

4106. Which of the following compounds is responsible for coordinated regulation of glucose and glycogen metabolism?

A. NAD^+ B. Fructose 2,6 bisphosphate

C. Acetyl-CoA D. Fructose 1,6 bisphosphate

Ans. B.

4107. Gluconeogenesis requires a higher amount of ATP equivalents as compared to that produced by glycolysis because

A. Gluconeogenesis releases energy as heat

B. Glycolysis releases energy as heat

C. Glycolysis occurs in the mitochondria while gluconeogenesis occurs in the cytosol

D. All of the above

Ans. B.

4108. Which of the following is carried out when cAMP functions as a second messenger?

A. Acts second in importance to AMP

B. Activates all cytosolic protein kinases

C. Activates the cAMP-dependent protein kinase

D. Acts outside the cell to influence cellular processes

Ans. C.

4109. The production or break down of——— is often coupled with the metabolic reactions of biosynthesis and catabolism.

A. Aspirin B. DNA
C. ATP D. CO_2

Ans. C.

4110. The cells dependent solely on glucose as an energy source are

A. Muscle cells B. Brain cells
C. Kidney cells D. Liver cells

Ans. B.

4111. The main site for gluconeogenesis is

A. Kidney B. Liver
C. Brain D. Muscle

Ans. B.

4112. Which of the following statements about the energy needs of cells is false?

A. Without a continuous input of energy, cell disorder will increase
B. The laws of thermodynamics force cells to acquire energy
C. Many cellular reactions have an associated activation energy
D. The most usable energy for cells comes from the rapid combustion of glucose

Ans. D.

4113. In lysozyme catalysis, which of the following does not contribute?

A. The abnormally high pK_a of Glu35
B. The strained conformation of the D sugar
C. Formation of a covalent intermediate at Asp52
D. Formation of a covalent intermediate at Ser195

Ans. D.

4114. Cellulose fibers resemble with the protein structure in the form of

A. β-sheets B. α-helices
C. β-turns D. None of these

Ans. A.

4115. During vigorous exercise, pyruvate produced by glycolysis is converted to

A. Acetate B. Lactate
C. Monosodium phosphate D. Pyruvic acid

Ans. B.

4116. Glucagon and epinephrine

A. Inhibits gluconeogenesis and stimulates glycolysis

B. Stimulates gluconeogenesis and glycolysis

C. Stimulates gluconeogenesis and inhibits glycolysis

D. Inhibits gluconeogenesis and glycolysis

Ans. C.

4117. The NAG6 substrate is hydrolyzed by human lysozyme to form

A. 6 glucosamines + 6 acetic acids B. $NAG_4 + NAG_2$

C. $NAG_3 + NAG_3$ D. NAG_3

Ans. B.

4118. Gluconeogenesis uses

A. 3 ATPs and 2 GTPs per glucose B. 2 ATPs and 1 GTPs per glucose

C. 3 ATPs and 3 GTPs per glucose D. 4 ATPs and 2 GTPs per glucose

Ans. D.

4119. Saliva contains all of the following except

A. Hormones B. Amylase

C. Bacteria-killing enzymes D. Antibodies

Ans. A.

4120. The conversion of pyruvate to oxaloacetate

A. Requires biotin B. Involves the fixation of carbon dioxide

C. Occurs in the mitochondria D. All of the above

Ans. A.

4121. Gluconeogenesis is the

A. Formation of glycogen

B. Breakdown of glucose to pyruvate

C. Breakdown of glycogen to glucose

D. Synthesis of glucose from non-carbohydrate precursors

Ans. D.

4122. Hydrolysis of lactose yields

A. Galactose and fructose B. Galactose and glucose

C. Glucose and fructose D. Fructose and galactose

Ans. B.

4123. Two major products of pentose phosphate pathway are

A. Nicotinamide adenine dinucleotide and ribose 5-phosphate

B. Flavine adenine dinuclueotide and glucose 5-phosphate

C. FAD and CoA

D. NADPH and NAD

Ans. A.

4124. A catabolic intermediate which stimulates phosphofructokinase would stimulate

A. Gluconeogenesis
B. Glycolysis
C. Glycogen synthesis
D. None of these

Ans. B.

4125. Pyruvate is initially converted to which of the following in the gluconeogenesis?

A. Glycerol
B. Phosphoenol pyruvate
C. Oxaloacetate
D. Acetyl CoA

Ans. C.

4126. Boat and chair conformations are found

A. In pyranose sugars

B. In any sugar without axial -OH groups

C. In any sugar without equatorial -OH groups

D. Only in D-glucopyranose

Ans. A.

4127. The conversion of pyruvate to lactate is catalysed by

A. Pyruvate carboxylase
B. Lactate dehydrogenase
C. Pyruvate dismutase
D. Pyruvate decarboxylase

Ans. B.

4128. Which of the following can act as precursors for gluconeogenesis?

A. Lactate
B. Glycerol
C. Alanine
D. All of these

Ans. D.

4129. α -amylose is similar to

A. β-sheets
B. β-turned coils
C. α-helices
D. The hydrophobic core

Ans. C.

4130. Storage polysaccharide made by animals is

A. Amylopectin | B. Glycogen
C. Cellulose | D. Collagen

Ans. B.

4131. The glycosidic bond

A. In maltose is not hydrolyzed in lactose intolerant humans
B. In sucrose is hydrolyzed by bees
C. Joins glucose and fructose to form sucrose
D. Both B and C

Ans. D.

4132. The sugar which forms major component of nucleic acids is

A. Ribose | B. Galactose
C. Mannose | D. Maltose

Ans. A.

4133. Under aerobic condition pyruvate is converted by pyruvate dehydrogenase to

A. Phosphoenol pyruvate | B. Acetyl CoA
C. Lactate | D. Glyceraldehyde 3 phosphate

Ans. B.

4134. Which of the following is not a disaccharide?

A. Amylose | B. Cellobiose
C. Lactose | D. None of these

Ans. A.

4135. Hexokinase activity in glycolysis is inhibited by

A. Glucose 6- phosphate | B. Fructose 6-phosphate
C. Fructose 1,6 biphosphate | D. Phosphofructokinase

Ans. A.

4136. The ultimate source of energy that sustains living systems is

A. Glucose | B. Oxygen
C. Sunlight | D. Carbon dioxide

Ans. C.

4137. Citric acid accumulation would

A. Stimulate phosphofructokinase activity
B. Stimulate fructose 1,6 diphosphatase activity
C. Inhibit phosphofructokinase activity
D. Both (b) and (c)

Ans. D.

4138. Which of the following is not involved in the biosynthesis of DNA?

A. Energy from ATP
B. Mononucleotides
C. Carbonic anhydrase
D. Enzymes

Ans. C.

4139. Which of the following would be considered a part of metabolism?

A. Biosynthetic pathways that build DNA
B. Catabolic pathways that break down complex carbohydrates
C. The capture of light energy for use in making glucose
D. All of the above

Ans. D.

4140. Insulin

A. Stimulates gluconeogenesis and glycolysis
B. Stimulates gluconeogenesis and inhibits glycolysis
C. Inhibits gluconeogenesis and glycolysis
D. Inhibits gluconeogenesis and stimulates glycolysis

Ans. D.

4141. What is present in the stomach to prevent self-digestion?

A. Mucus
B. Acid
C. Enzymes
D. Hormones

Ans. A.

4142. The key enzyme in the regulation of fatty acid synthesis is

A. Acetyl CoA carboxylase
B. AMP activated proteinkinase
C. Protein phosphatase
D. None of these

Ans. A.

4143. Arachidonate has 20 carbon atoms with

A. 3 double bonds
B. 2 double bonds
C. 4 double bonds
D. 8 double bonds

Ans. C.

4144. In the intestine, the dietary fats are hydrolysed by

A. Triacylglycerol lipase
B. Adenylate cyclase
C. Pancreatic lipase
D. Protein kinase

Ans. C.

4145. HDLs are synthesized in

A. Blood
B. Liver
C. Intestine
D. Pancreas

Ans. B.

4146. Triacylglycerols are

A. Soluble in water
B. Insoluble in water
C. Soluble in water at elevated temperature
D. Partially soluble in water

Ans. B.

4147. Animals cannot convert fatty acids into glucose because

A. Acetyl CoA can not be converted to pyruvate
B. Absence of malate synthase
C. Absence of dehydrogenase
D. Absence of a-ketoglutarate dehydrogenase

Ans. A.

4148. In eukaryotes fatty acid breakdown occurs in

A. Mitochondrial matrix
B. Cytosol
C. Cell membrane
D. Endoplasmic reticulum

Ans. A.

4149. What is the major protein constituent of high-density lipoprotein (HDL)?

A. Apolipoprotein A-l
B. Apolipoprotein C-l
C. Apolipoprotein E
D. None of these

Ans. A.

4150. Phospholipid contains

A. Hydrophilic heads and hydrophobic tails
B. Long water-soluble carbon chains
C. Positively charged functional groups
D. Both (b) and (c)

Ans. A.

4151. Micelles of fatty acids in water are organized such that the ——— faces the solvent and the ———— are directed toward the interior

A. Carboxylic acid groups, hydrocarbon chains heads
B. Hydrophilic heads, hydrophobic tails
C. Hydrocarbon chains, carboxylic acid groups
D. Both (a) and (b)

Ans. D.

4152. Cholesterolemia means

A. Lack of functional LDL receptors

B. Lack of functional HDL receptor

C. High sensitivity to fatty food intake

D. None of the above

Ans. A.

4153. Fatty acids break down of eukaryotes occurs in

A. Mitochondrial matrix
B. Cell membrane
C. Cytosol
D. Endoplasmic reticulum

Ans. A.

4154. VLDLs are synthesized in

A. Blood
B. Liver
C. Intestine
D. Pancreas

Ans. B.

4155. Chylomicrons are synthesized in

A. Blood
B. Liver
C. Intestine
D. Pancreas

Ans. C.

4156. How many types of lipoproteins are there?

A. 2
B. 6
C. 8
D. 5

Ans. D.

4157. Fatty acid synthesis takes place in

A. Mitochondria
B. Cell membrane
C. Cytosol
D. Endoplasmic reticulum

Ans. C.

4158. Cholestrol is the precursor of

A. Steroid hormones
B. Vitamin A
C. Bile salts
D. Both (a) and (c)

Ans. D.

4159. Atherosclerosis can cause blood

A. Thinning
B. Clotting
C. Thickening
D. None of these

Ans. B.

4160. Palmitate has 16 carbon atoms with

A. 2 Double bonds
B. 3 Double bonds
C. One double bond
D. None of these

Ans. D.

4161. How many ATPs are formed during complete oxidation of palmitate?

A. 35
B. 96
C. 129
D. 131

Ans. C.

4162. The lowest energy value lipid for human nutrition is

A. Olive oil
B. Olestra
C. Margarine
D. Cardiolipih

Ans. B.

4163. How many classes of steroid hormones are there?

A. 3
B. 2
C. 4
D. 5

Ans. D.

4164. The number of water molecules consumed by the formation of phosphatidyl serine are

A. 0
B. 1
C. 2
D. 4

Ans. A.

4165. Synthesis of fatty acid takes place when

A. Fatty acid are plentiful
B. Carbohydrate is plentiful
C. Carbohydrate and energy are plentiful
D. None of these

Ans. C.

4166. Which of the following is called milk ejection hormone?

A. Prolactin
B. Vasopressin
C. Oxytocin
D. All of these

Ans. C.

4167. Which of the following two organelles look most alike structurally?

A. Nucleus and vesicle

B. Golgi apparatus and smooth endoplasmic reticulum ER

C. Vacuole and cytoskeleton

D. Lysosome and chloroplast

Ans. B.

4168. In terms of basic cell structure, what do an elephant and an oak tree have in common?

A. They both are eukaryotes

B. They both have a cell nucleus

C. They both have mitochondria

D. All of the above

Ans. D.

4169. Where in a eukaryotic cell, DNA can be found?

A. Nucleus

B. Mitochondrion

C. Vacuole

D. Both A and B

Ans. D.

4170. Which of the following structures is expected in a bacterium?

A. Nucleus

B. Plasma membrane

C. Golgi apparatus

D. Endoplasmic reticulum

Ans. B.

4171. Which of the following organelles is directly connected to the outer membrane of the nucleus in a eukaryotic cell?

A. Mitochondrion

B. Lysosome

C. Golgi apparatus

D. Endoplasmic reticulum

Ans. D.

4172. Microtubules, motor proteins, and actin filaments are all part of

A. The mechanism of photosynthesis that occurs in chloroplasts

B. The rough ER (endoplasmic reticulum) in prokaryotic cells

C. The cytoskeleton of eukaryotic cells

D. The process that moves small molecules across cell membranes

Ans. C.

4173. A certain cell organelle which is made of a double phospholipid bilayer that has many large pores in it, is most likely

A. The nuclear envelope

B. The plasma membrane

C. The mitochondrion

D. The cytoskeleton

Ans. A.

4174. Which of the following cell organelles are expected to be associated with motor proteins?

A. Smooth ER B. Vesicles

C. Plasma membrane D. Chloroplasts

Ans. B.

4175. According to the fluid mosaic model of cell membranes,

A. The most common type of molecules in the membrane are proteins

B. Basic membrane structure results from how the proteins interact with water

C. The membrane is a highly mobile mixture of phospholipids and proteins

D. The unique properties of cell types are determined by their phospholipids

Ans. C.

4176. The highly folded membranes found in such eukaryotic organelles as mitochondria and chloroplasts

A. Increase the surface area where key chemical processes can occur

B. Help the cell against physical damage

C. Make it possible to package large amounts of DNA within the cell

D. Assist with cell movement

Ans. A.

4177. In which of the following cell organelles, it is expected to find the biochemical reactions that harness energy from the breakdown of sugar molecules to synthesize large amounts of ATP?

A. Lysosome B. Vesicles

C. Mitochondria D. Plasma membrane

Ans. C.

4178. Which of the following macromolecules are found in the plasma membrane?

A. Lipids and proteins only B. Lipids, proteins, and carbohydrates

C. Proteins and carbohydrates only D. Proteins only

Ans. B.

4179. Thin layer chromatography is

A. Partition chromatography B. Electrical mobility of ionic species

C. Adsorption chromatography D. None of the above

Ans. C.

4180. In gas chromatography, the basis for separation of the components of the volatile material is the difference in

A. Partition coefficients
B. Conductivity
C. Molecular weight
D. Molarity

Ans. A.

4181. In reverse phase chromatography, the stationary phase is made

A. Non-polar
B. Polar
C. Either non-polar or polar
D. None of these

Ans. A.

4182. Ion exchange chromatography is based on the

A. Electrostatic attraction
B. Electrical mobility of ionic species
C. Adsorption chromatography
D. Partition chromatography

Ans. A.

4183. A combination of paper chromatography and electrophoresis involves

A. Partition chromatography
B. Electrical mobility of the ionic species
C. Both A and B
D. None of these

Ans. C.

4184. Additional mono saccharides are added in Golgi to produce

A. Either high mannose type oligosaccharide or a complex type
B. Either fructose type monosaccharide or a complex type
C. Either high sucrose type polysaccharide or a complex type
D. None of the above

Ans. A.

4185. Beta pleated sheets are examples of protein's

A. Primary structure
B. Secondary structure
C. Tertiary structure
D. Quaternary structure

Ans. B.

4186. Signal sequences are part of a protein that

A. Signal folding of the protein
B. Signal the protein synthesis on the ribosomes is ended
C. Transport proteins to other sites within the cell
D. Refold proteins in prion-associated diseases

Ans. C.

4187. Individuals with PKU disease are mentally retarded unless

A. Phenylalanine in the diet is restricted

B. Tyrosine in the diet is restricted

C. Homogentisic acid in the diet is restricted

D. None of the above

Ans. A.

4188. Marfan's syndrome is thought to be a mutation affecting

A. Hemoglobin synthesis

B. Collagen synthesis

C. Metabolism of homogentisic acid

D. Insufficient thyroid production

Ans. B.

4189. Cyclins are proteins that

A. Regulate ability of cells to invade tissue

B. Regulate passage from one stage of cell division to another

C. Regulate apoptosis of damaged cells

D. None of the above

Ans. B.

4190. Over 50% of common cancers are associated with damage to a protein, p53. This protein

A. Is a cyclin

B. Is a tumor supressor

C. Is an oncogene

D. Regulates apoptosis

Ans. B.

4191. Protein folding is

A. Automatic, mediated by the protein itself

B. Mediated by other proteins called chaperones

C. Mediated by the ribosomes

D. None of the above

Ans. B.

4192. Sickle cell disease is due to

A. A mutation in the beta chain of Hb

B. A mutation in the alpha chain of Hb

C. Infection with a parasite

D. None of the above

Ans. A.

4193. The four subunits of the hemoglobin (Hb) gene represent protein's

A. Primary structure
B. Secondary structure
C. Tertiary structure
D. Quaternary structure

Ans. D.

4194. Which of the following is a positively charged matrix for ion exchange chromatography?

A. CM cellulose
B. DEAE cellulose
C. Phosphocellulose
D. None of these

Ans. B.

4195. The complex of RNA polymerase, DNA template and new RNA transcript is called

A. Transcription bubble
B. Replication bubble
C. A translation bubble
D. None of these

Ans. A.

4196. RNA polymerase in prokaryotes has a removable

A. Alpha subunit
B. Beta subunit
C. Both (a) and (b)
D. Sigma subunit

Ans. D.

4197. Promoters for tRNAs are located

A. Upstream from the start codon
B. Downstream from the start codon
C. Both (a) and (b)
D. None of these

Ans. B.

4198. The binding of lac repressor to DNA could be considered to be analogous to

A. Competitive inhibition of an enzyme
B. Mixed-type inhibition of an enzyme
C. Uncompetitive inhibition of an enzyme
D. Allosteric effects in enzyme regulation

Ans. A.

4199. Rho-dependent termination of transcription in *E.coli*

A. Requires ATP
B. Requires about 50 nucleotides of uncomplexed mRNA
C. Both (a) and (b)
D. Removes mRNA and holoenzyme from the DNA

Ans. C.

4200. Enhancers are regions that

A. Bind RNA polymerase
B. Are adjacent to the TATA box
C. Are CAT box binding proteins
D. Modulate transcription

Ans. D.

4201. Transcription by *E.coli* polymerase occurs in

A. Four phases known as initiation, propagation, elongation and termination
B. Three phases known as initiation, elongation and termination
C. Two phases known as initiation and termination
D. None of the above

Ans. B.

4202. Which of the following is necessary for transcription to occur?

A. DNA molecule
B. RNA polymerase
C. DNA polymerase
D. Both DNA & RNA polymerase

Ans. D.

4203. Multiple copies of 5S genes, located at a chromosomal site distinct from the other rRNA genes

A. Are transcribed by rRNA polymerase III and the 5S rRNA
B. Are transcribed by rRNA polymerase II
C. Are transcribed by rRNA polymerase I and the 5S rRNA
D. Are transcribed by DNA polymerase I

Ans. A.

4204. Each tRNA molecule has a cloverleaf secondary structure consisting of

A. Three stem loops
B. Two stem loops
C. Four stem loops
D. Either (a) or (b)

Ans. A.

4205. What is a promoter?

A. A specific sequence of DNA to which a catabolic repressor binds
B. A specific sequence of DNA to which RNA polymerase binds
C. A specific DNA sequence to which a restriction endonuclease binds
D. None of the above

Ans. B.

4206. The function of the sigma factor of RNA polymerase is to
- A. Assure that transcription begins at the proper point
- B. Assure that transcription ends at the proper point
- C. Assure that translation begins at the proper point
- D. Assure that translation ends at the proper point

Ans. A.

4207. In both eukaryotes and prokaryotes, a promoter region that is rich in AT bases is called as
- A. CATT
- B. Shine Dalgarno region
- C. TATA box
- D. SV40 region

Ans. C.

4208. The RNA polymerases that transcribe bacterial DNA are
- A. Multisubunit enzymes
- B. Only active inside the cell
- C. Interchangable with DNA polymerases
- D. Highly glycosylated in their active forms

Ans. A.

4209. Immediately after transcription
- A. A methylated guanine cap is added to the 5' end of the transcript
- B. A methylated guanine cap is added to the 3' end of the transcript
- C. Both (a) and (b)
- D. A poly adenylation signal is added

Ans. A.

4210. Transcription factors are
- A. Promoters
- B. Proteins which bind to DNA and regulate transcription
- C. TATA boxes
- D. CATT boxes

Ans. B.

4211. The major function of RNA polymerase's sigma factor is
- A. Recognition of the translational stop sequence
- B. Recognition of the transcriptional start sequence
- C. Recognition of the transcriptional stop sequence
- D. Recognition of the translational start sequence

Ans. B.

4212. Most transcripts of protein coding genes are cleaved

A. At the 3' end just after a poly adenylation signal

B. At the 3' end just before a poly adenylation signal

C. At the 5' end immediately after a poly adenylation signal

D. At the 5' end immediately before a poly adenylation signal

Ans. A.

4213. RNA is synthesized on a DNA template in a process called ——— , which utilizes the enzyme —————.

A. Translation, RNA polymerase   B. Transcription, DNA polymerase

C. Transcription, RNA polymerase   D. Replication, DNA polymerase

Ans. C.

4214. The closed complex at bacterial promoters is

A. In equilibrium with free RNA polymerase and the promoter

B. Not affected by promoter mutations

C. Bound more tightly when repressors are present

D. Not affected by activator proteins

Ans. A.

4215. Transcription begins

A. At the start codon   B. Upstream from the start codon

C. Downstream from the start codon   D. None of these

Ans. B.

4216. Transcription results in

A. An amino acid chain   B. Messenger RNA

C. Complementary DNA   D. Okazaki fragments

Ans. B.

4217. RNA polymerase holoenzyme initiates transcription which involves

A. Recognition of the -10 sequence and -35 sequence

B. Recognition of the -10 sequence only

C. Recognition of the -35 sequence only

D. None of the above

Ans. A.

4218. The transcriptional regulatory proteins in eukaryotes which induce transcription usually have

A. At least two distinct domains of protein structure, a DNA binding domain and an activation domain

B. At least two distinct domains of protein structure and a DNA binding domain

C. At least one distinct domains of protein structure, a DNA binding domain and an activation domain

D. None of these

Ans. A.

4219. In prokaryotes, transcription is

A. Terminated by the stop codon B. Terminated by a protein called rho

C. Terminated by a poly A sequence D. Terminated by a start codon

Ans. B.

4220. In eukaryotes, there are three different RNA polymerases. The RNA polymerase responsible for transcription of mRNA is

A. RNA polymerase I B. RNA polymerase II

C. RNA polymerase III D. None of these

Ans. B.

4221. The nucleons of eukaryotic cell has

A. RNA polymerase I B. RNA polymerase II

C. RNA polymerase III D. All of these

Ans. D.

4222. Upstream regions which are essential for correct transcription are called

A. Enhancers B. Start codons

C. Promoters D. Transcription factors

Ans. C.

4223. Transcription of each set of rRNA genes by RNA polymerase l produces

A. A single 45S rRNA precursor molecule

B. A single 5S rRNA precursor molecule

C. A single 18S rRNA precursor molecule

D. A single 28S rRNA precursor molecule

Ans. A.

4224. The regions of a gene located at -10 and -35, with respect to the start of transcription, are termed

A. Start codons.
B. OriC regions.
C. Shine Dalgarno sequences.
D. Promoters.

Ans. D.

4225. Which of the following conditions would cause the release of the lac repressor protein from the lac operator site on DNA?

A. Presence of glucose in the growth media
B. Presence of lactose in the growth media
C. Presence of IPTG (isopropyl thiogalactoside) in the growth media
D. Both b and C

Ans. D.

4226. On the ribosome, mRNA binds

A. Between the subunits
B. To the large subunit
C. To the small subunit
D. None of these

Ans. C.

4227. Type I proteins (plasma membrane) have a

A. Cleavage N- terminal signal sequence and a hydrophobic stop transfer sequence
B. Cleavaged N- terminal signal sequence that doubles as the membrane anchoring sequence
C. Multiple signal sequence and a hydrophobic stop transfer sequence
D. Multiple signal sequence that doubles as the membrane anchoring sequence

Ans. A.

4228. Which of the following is not a necessary component of translation?

A. Anticodon
B. mRNA
C. Ligase
D. Amino acid

Ans. C.

4229. A polysome could be best described as

A. An active site of DNA synthesis.
B. An active site of protein synthesis.
C. An active site of lipid synthesis.
D. All of the above.

Ans. B.

4230. Eukaryotic mRNA binding to the ribosomes is facilitated by ———————.

A. The Shine Dalgarno sequence
B. The 7-methyl guanosine cap
C. tRNA
D. Poly A tail

Ans. B.

4231. Amino acids are joined together into a protein chain by which of the following?

A. Transfer RNA B. DNA polymerase
C. Hydrogen bonds D. Messenger RNA

Ans. A.

4232. Phosphorus is taken up by the cell during the process of

A. Carbohydrate synthesis. B. Protein synthesis,
C. Lipid synthesis. D. ATP synthesis.

Ans. D.

4233. Protein synthesis rates in prokaryotes are limited by the rate of mRNA synthesis. If RNA synthesis occurs at the rate of 50 nucleotides/sec, then rate of protein synthesis occurs at

A. 10 amino acids/sec B. 17 amino acids/sec
C. 25 amino acids/sec D. 50 amino acids/sec

Ans. B.

4234. The site of protein synthesis is

A. Ribosome B. Nucleus
C. Endoplasmic reticulum D. Chromosome

Ans. A.

4235. The structure in a bacterium that indicates an active site for protein synthesis is

A. A chromosome. B. A cell membrane,
C. A flagellum. D. A polysome.

Ans. D.

4236. The lac operon contains the z, y and a structural genes

A. Encoding p-galactosidase, galactose permeases and thio-galactosidase transacetylase respectively
B. Encoding P-galactosidase and galactose permeases
C. Encoding P-galactosidase only
D. None of the above

Ans. A.

4237. Proteins contain ——— different amino acids, whereas DNA and RNA are composed of——— different nucleotides

A. 20,64 B. 3,20
C. 4,20 D. 20,4

Ans. D.

4238. Which of the following is not necessary for protein synthesis to occur, once transcription is completed?

A. tRNA B. Ribosomes

C. mRNA D. DNA

Ans. D.

4239. Ribosomes select the correct tRNAs

A. Then bind to the appropriate mRNA

B. Solely on the basis of their anticodons

C. Depending on their abundance in the cytosol

D. With the least abundant anticodons

Ans. B.

4240. Signal peptide protein removal that is translocated across a membrane is accomplished by

A. fMet aminopeptidase B. Trypsin

C. Signal peptidase D. Chymotrypsin

Ans. C.

4241. The direction of amino acid transfer to the growing polypeptide chain is

A. From the A (aminoacyl tRNA site) site to the P (peptidyl tRNA site) site on the ribosome

B. From the P site to the A site on the ribosome

C. From the A site to the E (exit tRNA site) site on the ribosome

D. From the P site to the E site on the ribosome

Ans. B.

4242. The pathway of a tRNA during polypeptide elongation on the ribosome is

A. A site→P site→E site B. P site→entry site→exit site

C. A site→P site→entry site D. P site→A site→E site

Ans. A.

4243. Which of the following has unusual bases?

A. mRNA B. tRNA

C. rRNA D. hnRNA

Ans. B.

4244. The site on a bacterial chromosome that marks the termination point for chromosome replication is called

A. Ter B. A stop codon.

C. A stem-loop *D. Pau*

Ans. A.

4245. Degenerated codon differs mostly in

A. The identities of their second base B. The identities of their third base

C. The wobble position D. Both (b) and (c)

Ans. D.

4246. Translation in prokaryotes begins by the formation of a 30S initiation complex between the

A. 30S ribosomal subunit, mRNA, initiation factors and N-fMet tRNA

B. 30S ribosomal subunit, tRNA and initiation factors

C. 30S ribosomal subunit and mRNA only

D. 30S ribosomal subunit, mRNA and initiation factors

Ans. A.

4247. The anticodon of tRNA

A. Binds to rRNA

B. Binds to an amino acid

C. Binds to the Shine Dalgarno sequence

D. Binds to an mRNA codon

Ans. D.

4248. The peptidyl transferase reaction occurs

A. On the large subunit B. On the small subunit

C. Between the subunit D. None of these

Ans. A.

4249. Processive synthesis is a characteristic feature of

A. All DNA polymerases.

B. DNA Pol III at a replication fork.

C. Removal of RNA primers on Okasaki fragments.

D. DNA mismatch repair

Ans. B.

4250. Which site of the tRNA molecule binds to the mRNA molecule ?

A. Anticodon B. Codon

C. Amino acid D. 5 prime end

Ans. A.

4251. The first step in translation is

A. Binding of the two ribosomal subunits to each other

B. Binding of mRNA to the two ribosomal subunits

C. Binding of tRNA to the small ribosomal subunit

D. Binding of mRNA to the small ribosomal subunit

Ans. D.

4252. Which of the following amino acid starts all proteins synthesis ?

A. Glycine B. Proline

C. Thymine D. Methionine

Ans. D.

4253. The growing polypeptide chain is released from the ribosomes when

A. A chain terminating codon is reached

B. A chain terminating tRNA binds to the ribosome

C. The 7-methyl guanosine cap is reached

D. The poly A tail is reached

Ans. A.

4254. Which of the following RNAs bind to an amino acid?

A. mRNA B. tRNA

C. rRNA D. hnRNA

Ans. B.

4255. How many bases of nucleic acid determine a single amino acid?

A. Four B. One

C. Two D. Three

Ans. D.

4256. The ribosomes are composed of

A. Proteins B. RNA

C. Both A and B D. Lipids

Ans. C.

4257. Which is required for protein synthesis?

A. tRNA B. mRNA

C. rRNA D. All of these

Ans. D.

4258. Glycolytic pathway regulation involves

A. Allosteric stimulation by ADP

B. Allosteric inhibition by ATP

C. Feedback, or product, inhibition by ATP

D. All of the above

Ans. D.

4259. During catabolism, only about 40% of the energy available from oxidizing glucose is used to synthesize ATP. Remaining 60%

A. Is lost as heat

B. Is used to reduce NADP

C. Remains in the products of metabolism

D. Is stored as fat.

Ans. A.

4260. Why does the glycolytic pathway continue in the direction of glucose catabolism?

A. There are essentially three irreversible reactions that act as the driving force for the pathway

B. High levels of ATP keep the pathway going in a forward direction

C. The enzymes of glycolysis only function in one direction

D. Glycolysis occurs in either direction

Ans. A.

4261. The released energy obtained by oxidation of glucose is stored as

A. a concentration gradient across a membrane

B. ADP

C. ATP

D. NAD^+

Ans. C.

4262. A kinase is an enzyme that

A. Removes phosphate groups of substrates

B. Uses ATP to add a phosphate group to the substrate

C. Uses NADH to change the oxidation state of the substrate

D. Removes water from a double bond

Ans. B.

4263. For every one molecule of sugar glucose which is oxidized ———— molecule of pyruvic acid are produced.

A. 1
B. 2
C. 3
D. 4

Ans. B.

4264. In the glycogen synthase reaction, the precursor to glycogen is

A. Glucose-6-P
B. UTP-glucose
C. UDP-glucose
D. Glucose-1-P

Ans. C.

4265. The active form of glycogen phosphorylase is phosphorylated, while the dephosphorylation of which active form occurs?

A. Glycogen synthase
B. Glycogen semisynthase
C. Glycogen hydrolase
D. Glycogen dehydrogenase

Ans. A.

4266. The amount of energy received from one ATP is

A. 76 kcal
B. 7.3 kcal
C. 760 kcal
D. 1000 kcal

Ans. B.

4267. The enzymes of glycolysis in a eukaryotic cell are located in the

A. Intermembrane space
B. Plasma membrane
C. Cytosol
D. Mitochondrial matrix

Ans. C.

4268. When concentration of the reactants is higher than the equilibrium concentration then

A. The gibbs free energy will be positive
B. The gibbs free energy will be negative
C. More products will be formed
D. Both B and C

Ans. D.

4269. Which of the following is not true of glycolysis ?

A. ADP is phosphorylated to ATP via substrate level phosphorylation
B. The pathway does not require oxygen
C. The pathway oxidizes two moles of NADH to NAD^+ for each mole of glucose that enters
D. The pathway requires two moles of ATP to get started catabo-lizing each mole of glucose

Ans. C.

4270. In glycolysis, ATP is formed by the transfer of a high-energy phosphate from 1,3-bisphosphoglycerate to ADR . No such high-energy phosphate donor has ever been isolated in mitochondria because

A. The techniques for isolating the phosphate donor are not refined enough

B. No such phosphate donor exists

C. The high-energy phosphate donor is very short-lived and difficult to isolate

D. None of the above

Ans. B.

4271. ATP is from which general category of molecules ?

A. Polysaccharides B. Proteins

C. Nucleotides D. Amino acids

Ans. C.

4272. The glycolytic pathway (glucose $\rightarrow$2 pyruvate) is found

A. In all living organisms B. Primarily in animals excluding particles

C. Only in eukaryotes D. Only in yeast

Ans. A.

4273. Which of the following could act as an uncoupler of electron transport and ATP synthesis?

A. The Fo base-piece of ATP synthase (without the Fl subunit)

B. Dinitrophenol

C. Neither A nor B

D. Both A and B

Ans. D.

4274. Which of the following is not a mechanism for altering the flux of metabolites through the rate-determining step of a pathway?

A. Allosteric control of the enzyme activity

B. Diffusional coupling between adjacent active sites

C. Genetic control of the enzyme concentration

D. Covalent modification of the enzyme

Ans. B.

4275. Phosphofructokinase, the major flux-controlling enzyme of glycolysis is allosterically inhibited and activated respectively by

A. ATP and PEP B. AMP and Pi

C. ATP and ADP D. Citrate and ATP

Ans. C.

4276. Which of the following regulates glycolysis steps?

A. Phosphofructokinase B. Hexose kinase

C. Pyruvate kinase D. All of these

Ans. D.

4277. During glycolysis, the major energy generating step involves

A. Pyruvate kinase B. Phosphoglycerate kinase

C. Glyceraldehyde-3 -dehydrogenase D. Phosphofructokinase

Ans. C.

4278. Fructose-2,6-bisphosphate

A. Activates fructose-1,6-bisphosphatase

B. Activates phosphofructokinase

C. Inhibits fructose-1,6-bisphosphatase

D. Both B and C

Ans. D.

4279. Glucose from the breakdown of glycogen is obtained in

A. The liver by phosphorolysis B. The muscles by phosphorolysis

C. The muscles by hydrolysis D. Both (a) and (b)

Ans. D.

4280. Glycogen has

A. α-1,4 linkage B. α-1,6 linkages

C. α-1,4 and α-1,6 linkages D. α-1,4 and β-1,6 linkage

Ans. C.

4281. The symptoms of retinol excess are

A. Bone fragility B. Nausea

C. Weakness D. All of these

Ans. D.

4282. Main function of insulin hormone is to

A. Increase glycogen in liver B. Decrease glycogen in liver

C. Increase blood sugar D. Decrease blood sugar

Ans. D.

4283. Ascorbic acid acts as an

A. Reducing agent B. Oxidizing agent

C. Oxidizing and reducing agent both D. None of the above

Ans. A.

4284. A deficiency of thiamin produces the disease known as

A. Beri-beri
B. Scurvy
C. Cataract
D. Anemia

Ans. A.

4285. Acyl carrier protein (ACP) plays an important role in the biosynthesis of

A. Fatty acids
B. Amino acids
C. Sugars
D. Carbohydrates

Ans. A.

4286. Vitamin B_{12} (Cobalamin) is only synthesized by

A. Fishes
B. Micro-organisms
C. Plants
D. Animals

Ans. B.

4287. Which of the following are reduced coenzymes?

A. NADH and FADH2
B. NAD^+ and FAD
C. ATP and GTP
D. Coenzyme A and ubiquinone

Ans. A.

4288. The absence of ascorbic acid in the human diet gives rise to

A. Rickets
B. Pernicious anemia
C. Cataract
D. Beri-beri

Ans. B.

4289. Vitamins are essential because the organism

A. Can't synthesize these compounds at all
B. Can synthesize these compounds partially
C. Can't synthesize these compounds in the adequate amounts
D. None of the above

Ans. A.

4290. The prosthetic group biotin is a carrier of which type of molecule?

A. Activated carbon dioxide (CO_2)
B. Ammonia
C. Methyl group
D. Sulfhydryl group

Ans. A.

4291. Lipoic acid exists in

A. Oxidized form
B. Reduced form
C. Oxidized and reduced form both
D. None of these

Ans. C.

4292. Vitamin B_{12} is useful in the prevention and treatment of

A. Pernicious anemia B. Scurvy

C. Cataract D. Beri-beri

Ans. A.

4293. An example of a digestive hormone is

A. Lipase B. Pepsin

C. Amylase D. Gastrin

Ans. D.

4294. In the co-enzyme B_{12} the position occupied by a cyanide ion in vitamin B_{12} is bonded directly to the ———— of the ribose of adenosine.

A. Adenine B. 5-6 dimethylbenzimidazole

C. Hydroxycobalamin D. Cyanocobalamin

Ans. A.

4295. The reductant, NADH, transfers the electrons via a flavo-proteins to the specific disulfide (S-S) protein to form a dithiol (SH,SH) protein which converts vitamin

A. $B_{12}(Co^{2+})$to $B_{12}(Co)$ B. $B_{12}(Co)$ to $B_{12}(Co^{2+})$

C. $B_{12}(Co^{2+})$to $B_{12}(Co^{+})$ D. $B_{12}(Co^{+})$to $B_{12}(Co^{2+})$

Ans. C.

4296. An early sign of retinol deficiencies in man is

A. Night blindness B. Keratinization

C. Xeropthalmia D. None of these

Ans. A.

4297. An enzyme, L-folate reductase reduces folic acid to

A. Hydrofolic acid B. Dihydrofolic acid

C. Trihydrofolic acid D. Tetrahydrofolic acid

Ans. B.

4298. What compound of raw egg white causes a syndrome similar to vitamin B deficiency?

A. Avidin B. Betabindin

C. Ovalbumin D. Albumin

Ans. A.

4299. The disease Beriberi is due to a dietary deficiency in

A. Vitamin B_1 (thiamine) B. Vitamin B_2 (riboflavin)

C. Vitamin B_6 (pyridoxine) D. Vitamin B_{12}

Ans. A.

4300. Which of these is a symptom of vitamin A deficiency?

A. Osteoporosis
B. Impaired taste perception
C. Blindness
D. Impaired blood clotting

Ans. C.

4301. Vitamin-C is considered as a

A. Water soluble
B. Fat soluble
C. Fat and water soluble
D. None of these

Ans. A.

4302. The vitamin niacin is part of the ———— molecule.

A. Ferredoxin
B. Pyridoxal phosphate
C. Pyrophosphate
D. NAD^+

Ans. D.

4303. Which of these hormones is a catecholamine?

A. Follitropin
B. Norepinephrine
C. Tetraiodothyronine
D. Tetrahydrofolate

Ans. B.

4304. Dihydroorotate dehydrogenase contains

A. 4 flavins and 4 atoms of iron per molecule
B. 2 flavins and 4 atoms of iron per molecule
C. 2 flavins and 2 atoms of iron per molecule
D. 4 flavins and 2 atoms of iron per molecule

Ans. A.

4305. *E.coli* ACP has its molecular weight as around

A. 9000
B. 19000
C. 39000
D. 90,000

Ans. A.

4306. The vitamin riboflavin is part of the ———— molecule.

A. Ferredoxin
B. FAD
C. Pyridoxal phosphat
D. Pyrophosphate

Ans. B.

4307. The most prominent role that tocopherol has in *in-vitro* systems is as a strong

A. Antioxidants
B. Reducing agent
C. Oxidizing agent
D. All of these

Ans. A.

4308. Biotin occurs mainly in combined forms bound to protein through

A. ε-N-lysine moiety
B. ε-S-lysine moiety
C. ε-N-biotinyl-L-lysine
D. ε-N-lipoyl - L-lysine

Ans. A.

4309. Lipoic acid is a co-factor of the

A. Pyruvic dehydrogenase
B. α-ketoglutaric dehydrogenase
C. Both A and B
D. Di-hydroorotate dehydrogenase

Ans. C.

4310. β-carotene together with α-carotene, γ-carotene and cryptoxanthine are synthesized by

A. Plants
B. Animal
C. Plants and animals both
D. None of these

Ans. A.

4311. Vitamin-D deficiency can cause

A. Rickets
B. Pernicious anemia
C. Cataract
D. Beri-beri

Ans. A.

4312. A deficiency of Vitamin K results in a decreased level of

A. Prothrombin
B. Thrombin
C. Fibrin
D. Fibrinogen

Ans. A.

4313. The vitamin riboflavin, which occurs as a yellow pigment in egg yolk and milk become

A. Colorless on reduction with Zn in acid and regained its color on re-oxidation
B. Colorless on oxidation and regained its color on reduction with Zn in acid
C. More deep in color on reduction with Zn in acid and regained its color on re-oxidation
D. More deep in color on oxidation and regained its color on reduction with Zn in acid

Ans. A.

4314. Which of the following compounds/(s) belong/(s) to the vitamin B_6 group?

A. Pyridoxal
B. Pyridoxine
C. Pyridoxamine
D. All of these

Ans. D.

4315. What metal ion is specifically bound by vitamin B_{12}?

A. Cobalt
B. Copper
C. Zinc
D. Iron

Ans. A.

4316. A fat-soluble vitamin that regulates blood clotting is

A. Vitamin A
B. Vitamin K
C. Vitamin C
D. Niacin

Ans. B.

4317. Which of these is a vitamin A precursor?

A. Cobalamin
B. Pyridoxine
C. Beta-Carotene
D. Thiamine

Ans. C.

4318. In one iron-metalloflavoprotein, the iron is present as a

A. Heme-protein
B. Nonheme type
C. Both (a) and (b)
D. Flavin moiety

Ans. A.

4319. Vitamin K_1 was first isolated from alfalalfa and has the phytyl side chain consisting of

A. Four isoprene units
B. Six isoprene units
C. Nine isoprene units
D. Four isoprene units

Ans. A.

4320. Which of these molecules is vitamin H?

A. Biotin
B. Carnitine
C. Folic acid
D. None of these

Ans. A.

4321. The occurrence of metals such as iron or molybdenum in some flavoproteins can

A. Stabilize the semiquinone
B. De-stabilize the semiquinone
C. Form chelation
D. All of these

Ans. A.

4322. Models of end-linked Osaka VI Fibrinogen dimers, a bilayer dimer is linked at

A. Both ends by one disulfide bond
B. Either end via two disulfide bonds
C. Either end via a single disulfide bond
D. Both ends by two disulfide bonds

Ans. D.

4323. A deficiency of niacin causes

A. Pellagra B. Scurvy

C. Cataract D. Anemia

Ans. A.

4324. Selenium is an essential component of the enzyme glutathione peroxidase which

A. Scavenges toxic hydoperoxycompounds in tissues

B. Reduces toxic hydoperoxycompounds in tissues

C. Oxidizes toxic hydoperoxycompounds in tissues

D. None of the above

Ans. A.

4325. Who discovered vitamin C (ascorbic acid) ?

A. Paul Berg B. Linus Pauling

C. Albert Szent-Gyorgyi D. Kerry Mull is

Ans. C.

4326. Which of the following mineral is involved in protein metabolism and oxidation reactions ?

A. Molybdenum B. Manganese

C. Magnesium D. calcium

Ans. A.

4327. Which of the following mineral deficiency may result into impaired growth and development, skin lesions and loss of appetite ?

A. Zinc B. Cobalt

C. Iron D. Magnesium

Ans. A.

4328. Which of the following is not a function of iron ?

A. Oxygen transport B. Immune function

C. Brain function D. Gene regulation

Ans. D.

4329. Consumption of which nutrient leads to the multiplication of oral bacteria ?

A. Fat B. Carbohydrate

C. Protein D. Fluoride

Ans. B.

4330. Examples of goitrogenic foods are ———- and ————— .

A. Turnips and corn
B. Rutabagas and okra
C. Raw cabbage and turnips
D. Cassava and lettuce

Ans. **C.**

4331. Which of the following carbohydrate is effective in promoting the calcium absorption?

A. Lactose
B. Maltose
C. Sucrose
D. Xylose

Ans. **A.**

4332. What condition is caused by iodine deficiency during pregnancy and is characterized by stunted growth, deafness, and mental retardation?

A. Cretinism
B. Keshan disease
C. Multiple sclerosis
D. Crohn's disease

Ans. **A.**

4333. Iodine is a part of thyroid hormone and is essential for the prevention of

A. Goiter
B. Osteoporosis
C. Muscle weakness
D. Diarrhea

Ans. **A.**

4334. What transports copper from the intestinal cells to the liver?

A. Ceruloplasmin
B. Secretin
C. Acrolein
D. Albumin

Ans. **A.**

4335. Which group is most often affected with copper deficiency?

A. Elderly woman
B. Alcoholics
C. Active toddlers with limited
D. Preterm infants food variety

Ans. **A.**

4336. What is the main source of natural fluoride?

A. Mushrooms
B. Potatoes
C. Meat
D. Water

Ans. **D.**

4337. Which of the following mineral is involved in the enzyme -controlled energy yielding reactions of metabolism?

A. Calcium
B. Phosphorus
C. Iron
D. Copper

Ans. **B.**

4338. The mineral which aids in the utilization of iron and in hemoglobin synthesis is

A. Calcium
B. Phosphorus
C. Cobalt
D. Copper

Ans. D.

4339. The mineral which is considered important in maintaining electrical potential in nerves and membranes is

A. Magnesium
B. Manganese
C. Calcium
D. Iron

Ans. A.

4340. Wilson's disease is an example of——— and Menkes' syndrome is an example of———.

A. Zinc deficiency; zinc toxicity
B. Zinc toxicity; zinc deficiency
C. Copper deficiency; copper toxicity
D. Copper toxicity; copper deficiency

Ans. D.

4341. Which of the following is correct?

A. Cobalt is part of vitamin B_{12}.
B. Cobalt will not replace the need for vitamin B_{12} in humans
C. Both (a) and (b)
D. Cobalt will replace the need for vitamin B_{12} in humans

Ans. C.

4342. Which of the following is required as a component of blood hemoglobin?

A. Iron
B. Magnesium
C. Calcium
D. Copper

Ans. A.

4343. Adding ———————— to a breakfast of cereal will help your body absorb iron.

A. Milk
B. Orange juice
C. Coffee
D. Water

Ans. B.

4344. Which of the following ion is required for the development of sound teeth with resistance to tooth decay?

A. Fluoride ion
B. Sodium ion
C. Chloride ion
D. Magnesium ion

Ans. A.

4345. Which of the following two beverages contribute 20 to 30 percent of our daily manganese intake?

A. Milk or tea B. Cola or coffee

C. Tea or orange juice D. Milk or orange juice

Ans. A.

4346. An endemic disease of cardiomyopathy in children is attributed to

A. Low Se in the environment B. Low intake of iron

C. High Se in the environment D. High intake of iron

Ans. A.

4347. Which of the following statement is correct?

A. Sodium and chloride are the chief extracellular ions of the body

B. Sodium and chloride are primarily involved in maintaining osmotic equilibrium and body fluid volume.

C. Chloride ion is necessary for the production of hydrochloric acid of gastric juice.

D. All of these

Ans. D.

4348. Which of the following is necessary for the clotting of blood, functions of certain enzymes and control of fluids through cell membranes?

A. Calcium B. Magnesium

C. Copper D. Cobalt

Ans. A.

4349. Selenium deficiency leads to

A. Liver necrosis B. Diarrhea

C. Multiple sclerosis D. Crohn's disease

Ans. A.

4350. Manganese is a key component of all of the following enzymes except

A. Arginase B. Pyruvate carboxylase

C. Ceruloplasmin D. Mn-superoxide dismutase

Ans. C.

4351. Which of the following vitamin is essential for the absorption of calcium from the intestinal tract?

A. Vitamin D B. Vitamin E

C. Vitamin B_{12} D. Vitamin B_6

Ans. A.

4352. Which trace mineral is a component of the enzyme that activates vitamin A in the eye?

A. Zinc
B. Iron
C. Iodine
D. Chromium

Ans. A.

4353. Chronic consumption of excess selenium can lead to

A. Brittle hair and nails.
B. Muscle weakness,
C. TPN
D. Diarrhea.

Ans. B.

4354. Normal glucose metabolism requires

A. Chromium
B. Manganese
C. Magnesium
D. Calcium

Ans. A.

4355. Manganese is needed for

A. Normal bone structure
B. Reproduction and functioning of central nervous system
C. Both A and B
D. Muscle strengthening

Ans. C.

4356. What is the specificity of the Clostripain protease?

A. It cleave after Arg residues
B. It cleave after His residues
C. It cleave after Lys residues
D. None of the above

Ans. A.

4357. The proteolysis rate enhancement by chymotrypsin ($\sim 10^{10}$ folds) corresponds to a reduction in activation energy of about

A. 40 kJ/mol
B. 49 kJ/mol
C. 58 kJ/mol
D. 88 kJ/mol

Ans. C.

4358. Which of the following is false statement with regard to comparison between Serine and HIV proteases?

A. Both use nucleophilic attack to hydrolyze the peptide bond
B. Both require water to complete the catalytic cycle
C. Both forms an acyl-enzyme intermediate
D. Both show specificity for certain amino acid sequences

Ans. C.

4359. The nucleophile in serine proteases is

A. Serine
B. Water
C. Both A and B
D. Asparagine

Ans. C.

4360. The role of Asp 102 and His 57 during trypsin catalysis is to

A. Neutralize the charge on the other's side chain
B. Keep the specificity pocket open
C. Function as a proton shuttle
D. Clamp the substrate into the active site

Ans. C.

4361. The cleavage specificity of trypsin and chymotrypsin depend in part on the

A. Proximity of ser 195 to the active site or specificity pocket
B. Size, shape, and charge of the active site or specificity pocket
C. Presence of a low-barrier hydrogen bond in the active site or specificity pocket
D. Absence of water in the active site

Ans. B.

4362. The *E.coli* pyruvic acid dehydrogenase complex is reported to

A. Decatalyze the oxidation of pyruvic acid to acetyl Co A and CO_2
B. Catalyze the oxidation of pyruvic acid to acetyl Co A and CO_2
C. Retard the reduction of pyruvic acid to acetyl Co A and CO_2
D. Catalyze the reduction of pyruvic acid to acetyl Co A and CO_2

Ans. B.

4363. Which of the common features are shared between serine and aspartate proteases?

A. Both require water to complete the catalytic cycle
B. Both use a base to activate the nucleophile
C. Both show specificity for certain amino acid sequences
D. All of the above

Ans. D.

4364. Before they can react, many molecules need to be destabilized. This state is typically achieved through

A. Changing the three-dimensional shape of the molecule
B. Oxidizing the molecules by removing electrons
C. Changing the reaction from a biosynthetic to a catabolic pathway
D. The input of a small amount of activation energy

Ans. D.

4365. Common feature in all serine proteases is a

A. Hydrophobic specificity pocket B. Hydrophilic specificity pocket

C. Cluster of reactive serine residues D. Single reactive serine residue

Ans. D.

4366. How is the enzyme COX-1 important in human health?

A. It helps to transport carbon dioxide in the blood

B. It is critical for the biosynthesis of DNA

C. It is a chemical derivative of aspirin

D. It catalyzes the production of hormones that maintain the stomach lining

Ans. D.

4367. A nicked RNA molecule can be ligated by

A. T4 RNA ligase B. DNA polymerase

C. T4 DNA ligase D. all of these

Ans. C.

4368. The tertiary structure of yeast tRNA

A. Involves extensive base stacking interactions

B. Resembles the 3-dimensional structure of other tRNAs

C. Is maintained mostly by non-Watson-Crick base pairing

D. All of the above

Ans. D.

4369. Which of following RNA characteristically contains unusual purines and pyrimidmes?

A. rRNA B. nRNA

C. mRNA D. tRNA

Ans. D.

4370. The anticodon is a structure on

A. mRNA B. tRNA

C. Aribosome D. rRNA

Ans. B.

4371. The genetic material of retroviruses such as HIV is

A. DNA B. RNA

C. Protein D. All of these

Ans. B.

4372. Retroviruses replicate via ———— intermediate

A. RNA
B. DNA
C. mRNA
D. rDNA

Ans. B.

4373. During RNA synthesis, the DNA template sequence 5'Tp Ap Gp Cp 3' Would be transcribed to produce which of the following RNA sequence?

A. 5'-Ap Tp Cp Gp-3'
B. 5'-Gp Cp Up Ap-3'
C. 5'-Gp Cp Tp Ap-3'
D. 5'-Ap Up Cp Gp-3'

Ans. B.

4374. RNA instability in alkaline solutions is due to

A. Adenine
B. Ribose
C. Uracil
D. Single strand nature

Ans. B.

4375. In RNA, uracil pairs with

A. Adenine
B. Cytosine
C. Thymine
D. Guanine

Ans. A.

4376. Two features of the tRNA molecule associated, in converting the triplet codon to an amino acid, are

A. In the T Loop and D stem and loop
B. In the anticodon loop and D stem loop
C. In the anticodon loop and the 3' CCA end
D. None of the above

Ans. C.

4377. Which of the following is the smallest of the RNAs ?

A. Messenger RNA
B. Transfer RNAs
C. Ribosomal RNAs
D. All of these

Ans. B.

4378. The mRNA from which of the following would contain a poly-A tail?

A. A restriction endonuclease from *E.coli*
B. Bacterial alpha-amylase
C. Human insulin
D. Bacteriophage DNA ligase

Ans. C.

4379. What is the average size (in bp) of a mature t-RNA?

A. 80 bp
B. 100 bp
C. 120 bp
D. 140 bp

Ans. A.

4380. What modified base is at the 5' extremity of a capped eukaryotic m-RNA?

A. 1-methyl-adenosine
B. 2'-O-methyl-guanosine
C. 7-methyl-guanosine
D. 1-methyl-guanosine

Ans. C.

4381. What is the function of messenger RNA?

A. It carries amino acids
B. It is a component of the ribosomes
C. It is a direct copy of a gene
D. It is the genetic material of some organisms

Ans. C.

4382. Hydrogen bonds in α-helices are

A. More numerous than Vander Waals interactions
B. Not present at Phe residues
C. Analogous to the steps in a spiral staircase
D. Roughly parallel to the helix axis

Ans. D.

4383. The peptide bond in proteins is

A. Only found between proline residues
B. Usually cis unless proline is the next amino acid
C. Usually trans unless proline is the next amino acid
D. Is planar because of steric hinderance

Ans. C.

4384. The molecular formula for glycine is $C_2H_5O_2N$. What would be the molecular formula for a linear oligomer made by linking ten glycine molecules together by condensation synthesis?

A. $C_{20}H_{50}O_{20}N_{10}$
B. $C_{20}H_{32}O_{11}N_{10}$
C. $C_{20}H_{40}O_{10}N_{10}$
D. $C_{20}H_{68}O_{29}N_{10}$

Ans. B.

4385. Which of the following is an example of tertiary structure in a protein?

A. A multimeric protein

B. An α-helix

C. A β -pleated sheet

D. A globular domain

Ans. D.

4386. The peptide, Val-Lys-Glu-Met-Ser-Trp-Arg-Ala, was digested with cyanogen bromide (CNBr) to produce:

A. Val-Lys + Glu-Met-Ser + Trp-Arg-Ala

B. Val-Lys-Glu-Met-Ser-Trp + Arg-Ala

C. Val-Lys-Glu-Met + Ser-Trp-Arg-Ala

D. Val-Lys-Glu + Met-Ser-Trp-Arg-Ala

Ans. C.

4387. In deoxy hemoglobin (Hb), the Fe (II) is coordinated to

A. Four nitrogens of heme, the proximal His, and a water molecule

B. Four nitrogens of heme and to a water molecule

C. Two nitrogens of heme and to three His residues in Hb

D. Two nitrogens of heme and to three water molecules

Ans. A.

4388. In the β-pleated sheet

A. Hydrogen bonds are formed between the peptide bonds

B. Adjacent polypeptide chains can either be parallel or antiparallel

C. The polypeptide chain is fully extended

D. All of the above

Ans. D.

4389. The Ramachandran Plot illustrates the fact that

A. The peptide bond is planar

B. The F & Y angles can assume any value in a peptide

C. The F & Y angles can assume only a single value in a protein

D. The F & Y angles can assume approximately three different values

Ans. D.

4390. The resonance structures that can be drawn for the peptide bond indicate that the peptide bond

A. Is stronger than an ordinary single bond

B. Has partial double bond character

C. Both A and B

D. Is still not completely understood

Ans. C.

4391. The major element of secondary structure in myoglobin and hemoglobin is

A. The β-strand
B. The α-helix
C. The reverse turn
D. All of these

Ans. B.

4392. An oil drop with a polar coat is a metaphor referring to the three dimensional structure of

A. Fibrous proteins
B. Collagen
C. Globular proteins
D. Silk protein

Ans. C.

4393. What was the first protein whose complete tertiary structure was determined ?

A. Lysozyme
B. Myoglobin
C. Pancreatic ribonuclease
D. Pancreatic DNase

Ans. B.

4394. The peptide bond in proteins is

A. Planar, but rotates to three preferred dihedral angles
B. Nonpolar, but rotates to three preferred dihedral angles
C. Nonpolar, and fixed in a trans conformation
D. Planar, and usually found in a trans conformation

Ans. D.

4395. In β-pleated sheet structures neighbouring

A. Chains lie in a flat plane
B. Neighboring residues are hydrogen bonded
C. Neighboring chains are connected by a-helices
D. Neighboring chains are hydrogen bonded

Ans. D.

4396. The same peptide, Val-Lys-Glu-Met-Ser-Trp-Arg-Ala. was digested with chymotrypsin to produce

A. Val-Lys + Glu-Met-Ser + Trp-Arg-Ala.
B. Val-Lys-Glu-Met-Ser-Trp + Arg-Ala.
C. Val-Lys-Glu-Met-Ser + Trp-Arg-Ala.
D. Val-Lys-Glu-Met + Ser-Trp-Arg-Ala.

Ans. B.

4397. Disulfide bonds most often stabilize the native structure of

A. Extracellular proteins
B. Dimeric proteins
C. Hydrophobic proteins
D. Intracellular proteins

Ans. A.

4398. Secondary structure in protein refers to

A. Linear sequence of amino acids joined together by peptide bond
B. Three dimensional arrangement of all amino acids in polypeptide chain
C. Regular folding of regions of the polypeptide chain
D. Protein made up of more than one polypeptide chain

Ans. C.

4399. Heme is the binding pocket of myoglobin and hemoglobin and is composed of

A. Negatively charged residues
B. Polar residues
C. Hydrophobic residues
D. Positively charged residues

Ans. C.

4400. What is the effect of a decrease in pH on hemoglobin oxygen affinity?

A. Decrease in oxygen affinity
B. Increase in oxygen affinity
C. No effect on oxygen affinity
D. Increase affinity in muscle cell otherwise decrease

Ans. A.

4401. What is the proportion of glycine residues in collagenous regions?

A. One-fourth
B. One-third
C. Half
D. One-tenth

Ans. B.

4402. Which of the following statements is incorrect?

A. Protein G contains both α-helix and β-sheet
B. Protein G contains only α-helix
C. Fatty acid binding protein contains largely β-sheet
D. Hemoglobin contains four sub-units

Ans. B.

4403. The oxygen binding curves of hemoglobin and myoglobin

A. Allow maximum transfer of oxygen to the tissues

B. Are a consequence of the quaternary structure of hemoglobin

C. Both A and B

D. Are identical

Ans. C.

4404. The nature of peptide bond can be best explained as

A. Partial double bond B. Truly double bond

C. Hydrogen bond D. Van der waals force

Ans. A.

4405. Which of the following statement is incorrect?

A. Hemoglobin and myoglobin are the two oxygen binding proteins

B. Hemoglobin transports O_2 in the blood

C. Myoglobin stores O_2 in muscles

D. None of the above

Ans. D.

4406. Which hemoglobin chain replaces the beta chain in embryonic hemoglobulin?

A. Delta B. Epsilon

C. Gamma D. Alfa

Ans. B.

4407. Hemoglobin has quaternary structure and is made up of

A. Six polypeptide chains, two α-chains and four β-chains

B. Two polypeptide chains, one α-chains and one β-chains

C. Four polypeptide chains, two α-chains and two β-chains

D. Five polypeptide chains, two α-chains and three β-chains

Ans. C.

4408. The oxygen in hemoglobin and myoglobin is bound to

A. The iron atom in the heme group B. The nitrogen atoms on the heme

C. Histidine residues in the protein D. Lysine residues in the protein

Ans. A.

4409. Which of the three subunits of the G proteins binds GDP and GTP?

A. Alpha B. Beta

C. Gamma D. Delta

Ans. A.

4410. If the F and Y angles of each peptide unit in a protein are known, which of the following may also be determined?

A. Complete secondary structure B. Complete tertiary structure

C. Complete quaternary structure D. Thermodynamic stability

Ans. A.

4411. The different orders of protein structure are determined by all of the following bond types except

A. Peptide bonds B. Phospho-diester bonds

C. Disulfide bridges D. Hydrogen bonds

Ans. B.

4412. The heme is held in place by a bond between

A. The Fe^{2+} and cysteine B. The Fe^{3+} and histidine

C. The Fe^{3+} and cysteine D. The Fe^{2+} and histidine

Ans. D.

4413. When the amino acid alanine (R-group is CH_3) is added to a solution with a pH of 7.3, alanine becomes

A. A cation B. Nonpolar

C. A zwitterions D. An isotope

Ans. C.

4414. What is the end product of leucine metabolism?

A. Acetyl-CoA B. Pyruvic acid

C. Oxaloacetic acid D. Acetyl carnitine

Ans. A.

4415. What is the heaviest of the twenty amino acids?

A. Phenylalanine B. Tryptophan

C. Tyrosine D. Histidine

Ans. B.

4416. Which of the following amino acids can form hydrogen bonds with their side (R) groups?

A. Asparagine B. Aspartic acid

C. Glutamine D. All of these

Ans. D.

4417. The isoelectric point of an amino acid is defined as the pH

A. Where the molecule carries no electric charge

B. Where the carboxyl group is uncharged

C. Where the amino group is uncharged

D. Of maximum electrolytic mobility

Ans. A.

4418. Molecules that bear charged groups of opposite polarity are known as

A. Zwitterions B. Ambions

C. Ion conversion D. Amphions

Ans. A.

4419. What is the product of the catabolic breakdown of Arginine?

A. Alpha-ketoglutarate B. Fumarate

C. Oxaloacetate D. Succinate

Ans. A.

4420. Which amino acids would most likely reside in the membrane-anchoring domain of a membrane embedded protein?

A. Isoleucine, valine and phenylalanine

B. Phenylalanine, valine, and aspartate

C. Leucine, threonine, and lysine

D. Lysine, arginine and histidine

Ans. A.

4421. An essential amino acid is one that

A. Is essentially easy to synthesize

B. Is essential to flagella motion

C. The body cannot synthesize

D. The body can synthesize under essential conditions

Ans. C.

4422. D-Alanine and L-Alanine are technically known as

A. Anomers B. Enantiomers

C. Epimers D. Polymer

Ans. B.

4423. Which of the following pairs of amino acids would carry a negative charge on their side chain at pH 8.0?

A. Asparagine & Glutamine
B. Leucine & Glycine
C. Histidine & Lysine
D. Aspartate & Glutamate

Ans. D.

4424. In a polypeptide average mass of an amino acid residue is

A. 110 daltons
B. 118 daltons
C. 80 daltons
D. 150 daltons

Ans. A.

4425. Which pair of amino acids absorbs the most UV light at 280 nm?

A. Threonine and Histidine
B. Trptophan and Tyrosine
C. Cystein and Asparagine
D. Phenylalnine and Proline

Ans. B.

4426. Which of the following is a nonstandard amino acid?

A. Cysteine
B. Isoleucine
C. Hydroxyproline
D. Histidine

Ans. C.

4427. Which of the following is an essential amino acid ?

A. Tryptophan
B. Methionine
C. Lysine
D. All of these

Ans. D.

4428. Protein fluorescence arises primarily from which residue ?

A. Arginine
B. Tryptophan
C. Tyrosine
D. Phenylalanine

Ans. B.

4429. Which of the following amino acid is known as half-cystine residue ?

A. Cysteine
B. Isoleucine
C. Valine
D. Histidine

Ans. A.

4430. Which of the following is not an essential amino acid ?

A. Aspartic acid
B. Glutamic acid
C. Glycine|
D. All of these

Ans. D.

4431. Which of the following is not a sensible grouping of amino acids based on their polarity properties?

A. Ala, Leu, and Val
B. Arg, His, and Lys
C. Phe, Trp, and Tyr
D. Asp, Ile, and Pro

Ans. D.

4432. Proteins and macromolecular structures take on their higher order structures

A. By self-assembly
B. With the help of molecular chaperons
C. With the help of precursor sequences that are removed from the final structures
D. All of the above

Ans. D.

4433. What is the product of the catabolic breakdown of Alanine?

A. Fumarate
B. Oxaloacetate
C. Pyruvate
D. Malate

Ans. C.

4434. How many different amino acids are there?

A. 3
B. 20
C. 100
D. An infinite number

Ans. B.

4435. Amino acids required in the human diet and not synthesized by the body are called

A. Specialized
B. Trace
C. Essential
D. Accessory

Ans. C.

4436. Which of the following amino acid contain an imidazolium moiety?

A. Alanine
B. Valine
C. Cysteine
D. Histidine

Ans. D.

4437. The sequence of letters 'WYQN' will represent

A. Tryptophan, tyrosine, glutamic acid, asparagine
B. Tryptophan, tyrosine, glutamine, asparagine
C. Tryptophan, glutamine, tryptophan, asparagine
D. Glutamine, tyrosine, tryptophan, aspartic acid

Ans. B.

4438. The sulphur containing side chain of cysteine is

A. Ampiphillic, highly reactive and capable of reacting with another cysteine

B. Hydrophillc, highly reactive and capable of reacting with another cysteine

C. Hydrophobic, highly reactive and capable of reacting with another cysteine

D. None of the above

Ans. C.

4439. Which of the following is a nonprotein amino acid?

A. Dopamine B. Hydroxylysine

C. Cystine D. None of these

Ans. A.

4440. Serine and threonine are polar amino acids due to

A. Reactive hydroxyl group in the side chain

B. Reactive alcoholic group in the side chain

C. Reactive keto group in the side chain

D. Reactive aldehyde group in the side chain

Ans. A.

4441. Which of the following is not the hydrophobic and aromatic amino acid?

A. Phenylalanine B. Tyrosine

C. Tryptophan D. None of these

Ans. D.

4442. Stereo chemical configuration of all α-amino acids derived from proteins is

A. L B. D

C. L and D D. None of these

Ans. A.

4443. The α-amino acids have a carboxyl group with a pK around ————, and an amino group with a pK near ————.

A. 1.1, and 12.1 B. 6.5, and 8.0

C. 3.3, and 10.5 D. 2.2, and 9.4

Ans. D.

4444. Coomassie Blue stains the proteins by reacting with

A. Arginine residues B. Free c-termini

C. Peptide bonds D. Aromatic ring

Ans. A.

4445. Which amino acid when exposed to ninhydrin produces a brown color?

A. Asparagine B. Proline

C. Alanine D. Valine

Ans. A.

4446. How many molecules of ATPs are synthesized per NADH oxidation?

A. 2 B. 1

C. 3 D. 4

Ans. C.

4447. Why is the TCA cycle the central pathway of metabolism of the cell ?

A. It occurs in the center of the cell

B. Its intermediates are commonly used by other metabolic reactions

C. All other metabolic pathways depend upon it

D. None of the above

Ans. B.

4448. In what form does the product of glycolysis enter the TCA cycle ?

A. AcetylCoA B. Pyruvate

C. NADH D. Glucose

Ans. A.

4449. Malate-asparatate shuttle operates in

A. Lungs and liver B. Heart and liver

C. Pancreas and liver D. None of these

Ans. B.

4450. Oxidation of a molecule involves

A. Gain of electron B. Loss of electron

C. Gain of proton D. Loss of proton

Ans. B.

4451. During cellular respiration, most of the ATP made, is generated by

A. Oxidative phosphorylation B. Photophosphorylation

C. Glycolysis D. Substrate-level phosphorylation

Ans. A.

4452. Important function of cholesterol is to

A. Modulate fluidity B. Enhance blood circulation

C. Prevent bile salts formation D. None of these

Ans. A.

4453. To stop ATP synthesis which chemical is generally used?

A. DNSA

B. 2,4 dinitrophenol

C. DDT

D. None of the chemical can stop ATP synthesis

Ans. B.

4454. The enzymes of the TCA cycle in a eukaryotic cell are located in the

A. Nucleus
B. Mitochondria
C. Plasma membrane
D. Lysosomal bodies

Ans. B.

4455. Citric acid cycle occurs in

A. Cytoplasm
B. Mitochondria
C. Endoplasmic reticulum
D. Golgi bodies

Ans. B.

4456. Most multi-cellular organisms obtain energy for the synthesis of ATP during oxidative phosphorylation from

A. High energy phosphate compounds

B. A proton gradient across the inner mitochondrial membrane

C. A proton gradient across the cell membrane

D. A proton gradient across the outer mitochondrial membrane

Ans. B.

4457. Standard redox potential for a substance is measured under standard condition and is expressed as

A. Mili-Ampere
B. Volt
C. Without unit
D. Ohm

Ans. B.

4458. Most of the enzymes of the citric acid cycle in a eukaryotic cell are located in the

A. Inner mitochondrial membrane
B. Cytosol
C. Mitochondrial matrix
D. Intermembrane space

Ans. C.

4459. A positive redox potential means substance has

A. Lower affinity for electron
B. Higher affinity for electron
C. Lower affinity for proton
D. Higher affinity for proton

Ans. B.

4460. The end product of glycolysis is pyruvate, which enters the citric acid cycle after being converted to

A. Acetic acid
B. Acetyl-CoA
C. Acetaldehyde
D. None of these

Ans. B.

4461. Energy that is released from glucose during respiration but not transferred to ATP bonds can be detected as

A. CO_2
B. AMP
C. ADP
D. Heat

Ans. D.

4462. Which of the following is involved in energy production?

A. Generation of proton gradients across membranes
B. Transport of electrons on organic molecules
C. Conversion of compounds with high energy to those of low energy
D. All of the above

Ans. D.

4463. Which of the following enzyme does not take part in the TCA cycle?

A. Citrate synthase
B. Iso-citrate dehydrogenase
C. Pyruvate dehydrogenase
D. Malate dehydrogenase

Ans. C.

4464. The first intermediate in TCA cycle is

A. Succinate
B. Fumerate
C. Citrate
D. Malate

Ans. C.

4465. Cholesterol can be synthesized *de novo* in

A. Pancreas
B. Intestine
C. Liver
D. Cell membrane

Ans. C.

4466. Which one of the following is not the intermediate of Kreb's cycle?

A. Isocitrate
B. Succinate
C. Fumarate
D. Stearate

Ans. D.

4467. Which one is not the main protein in electron transport chain?

A. NADH dehydrogenase
B. Cytochrome bc1 complex
C. Cytochrome oxidase
D. Citrate synthease

Ans. D.

4468. How many ATPs are produced during citric acid cycle?

A. 10
B. 13
C. 12
D. 8

Ans. C.

4469. The $FADH_2$ and NADH produced by the oxidation of one acetyl-CoA results in the synthesis of about

A. 3 ATPs
B. 6 ATPs
C. 11 ATPs
D. 15 ATPs

Ans. C.

4470. In eukaryotes, electron transport occurs in

A. Membranes and mitochondria
B. Endoplasmic reticulum
C. Cytoplasm
D. All of the above

Ans. A.

4471. The catabolism of sugars and fatty acids is similar because

A. both of these compounds are funnelled through the TCA/citric acid cycle
B. both of these compounds generate redox energy during catabolism
C. both of these compounds generate chemical energy during catabolism
D. all of the above

Ans. A.

4472. Number of asymmetric carbon atoms in glucose is

A. One
B. Two
C. Three
D. Four

Ans. D.

4473. The specific gravity of urine normally ranges from

A. 0.900–0.999
B. 1.003–1.030
C. 1.000–1.001
D. 1.101–1.120

Ans. B.

4474. Specific gravity of urine increases in

A. Diabetes mellitus
B. Chronic glomerulonephritis
C. Compulsive polydypsia
D. Hypercalcemia

Ans. A.

4475. The sugar which forms major component of nucleic acids is

A. Ribose
B. Galactose
C. Mannose
D. Maltose

Ans. A.

4

Famous Scientists

1. Father of microbiology is

   A. Louis Pasteur B. Lister

   C. A.V. Leeuwenhock D. Robert Koch

Ans. C.

2. The antiseptic method was first demonstrated by

   A. Lwanowski B. Lord Lister

   C. Edward Jenner D. Beijerinck

Ans. B.

3. Small pox vaccine was first discovered by

   A. Robert Koch B. Louis Pasteur

   C. Lister D. Edward Jenner

Ans. D.

4. The term mutation was coined by

   A. Pasteur B. Darwin

   C. Hugo devries D. Lamarck

Ans. C.

5. Compound microscope was discovered by

   A. Antony von B. Pasteur

   C. Hans Janssen D. None of these

Ans. C.

6. Father of Medical Microbiology is

   A. Pasteur B. Jenner

   C. Koch D. A.L.Hock

Ans. C.

7. Phagocytic phenomenon was discovered by

A. Louis Pasteur B. Alexander Fleming

C. Metchnikoff D. Robert Koch

Ans. C.

8. Hybridoma technique was first discovered by

A. Kohler and Milstein B. Robert Koch

C. 'D' Herelle D. Land Steiner

Ans. A.

9. Griffith (1928) reported the phenomenon of transformation first in

A. H. influenzae B. Bacillus species

C. Pneumococci D. E.coli

Ans. C.

10. Monoclonal antibodies are associated with the name of

A. Burnet B. Medwar

C. Milstein & Kohler D. Owen

Ans. A.

11. Hanging drop method for motility study was first introduced by

A. Robert Koch B. Louis Pasteur

C. Jenner D. Leeuwenhoek

Ans. D.

12. Term vaccine was coined by

A. Robert Koch B. Pasteur

C. Needham D. None of these

Ans. B.

13. The inventor of Microscope is

A. Galileo B. Antony von Leeuwenhoek

C. Pasteur D. Koch

Ans. B.

14. Modern concepts of chemotherapy was proposed by

A. Paul Ehrlich B. Joseph Lister

C. Elie Metchnikoff D. None of these

Ans. A.

15. L – forms are discovered by

A. Klein Berger B. Louis Pasteur

C. Robert Koch D. Antony von Leeuwenhock

Ans. A.

16. The causative organism of rocky mountain spotted fever was first described by

A. Howard Ricketts B. da Rocha-lima

C. Both a and b D. Robert Koch

Ans. C.

17. The term bacteriophage was coined by

A. De'Herelle B. F.W. Twort

C. Beijernick D. Jwanosky

Ans. A.

18. Viral infection of bacteria was discovered by

A. De'Herelle B. F.W. Twort

C. Beijernick D. Jwanoksy

Ans. B.

19. Electron Microscope was discovered by

A. Prof. Fritz B. Janssen and Hans

C. Knoll and Ruska D. None of these

Ans. C.

20. Who perfected a magnetic lens in 1927

A. Gabor B. Broglie

C. Busch D. None of these

Ans. A.

21. Mycorrhiza was first observed by

A. Funk B. Frank

C. Fisher D. Crick

Ans. B.

22. The transfer of genetic material during transformation is proved basing on Griffith's experiment by

A. Avery, Macleod & Mc.Carthy B. Lederberg & Taulum

C. Zinder & Lederberg D. Watson & Crick

Ans. A.

23. Anaphylaxia was first observed by

A. Parter & Richet
B. Coombs
C. Gell
D. None of these

Ans. A.

24. Vibrio Cholerae was discovered by

A. Koch
B. Metchnikoff
C. John Snow
D. Virchow

Ans. B.

25. E. coli was first isolated by

A. Louis Pasteur
B. Escherich
C. Shiga
D. Robert Koch

Ans. B.

26. Mycobacterium tuberculosis was first discovered by

A. Robert Koch
B. Edward Jenner
C. Louis Pasteur
D. None of these

Ans. A.

27. Mycobacterium leprae was discovered by

A. Robert Koch
B. Hansen
C. Edward Jenner
D. Louis Pasteur

Ans. B.

28. Streptococcus pneumoniae was isolated by

A. Robert Koch
B. Edward Jenner
C. Antony von Leewenhock
D. Louis Pasteur

Ans. D.

29. B. anthracis was isolated by

A. Louis Pasteur
B. Robert Koch
C. Antonyvon Leewenhok
D. None of these

Ans. B.

30. Staphylococcus aureus was identified by

A. Rosenberg
B. Louis Pasteur
C. Passet
D. Sir Alexander Ogston

Ans. D.

31. Pseudomonas aeruginosa was first named by

A. Schroeter and Gessard B. Robert Koch

C. Louis Pasteur D. Edward Jenner

Ans. A.

32. T. pallidum was discovered by

A. Robert Koch B. Schaudinn and Hoffman

C. Louis Pasteur D. Edward Jenner

Ans. B.

33. Neisseria gonorrhoeae was first described by

A. Neisser in 1879 B. Pasteur in 1878

C. Robert Koch D. None of these

Ans. B.

34. Rh factor of the blood was discovered by scientist

A. Louis Pasteur B. Landsteiner and Wiener

C. Janskey D. Moss

E. None of these

Ans. B.

35. Who isolated Streptococcus pneumonia for the first time ?

A. Robert Koch B. Edward Jenner

C. Antony von Leewenhock D. Louis Pasteur

Ans. D.

36. Who discovered M. tuberculosis ?

A. Koch B. Jenner

C. Pasteur D. Virchow

Ans. A.

37. M. leprae was discovered by ——

A. Pasteur B. Jenner

C. Koch D. Hansen

Ans. D.

38. Antibodies were discovered by —

A. Edelman B. Porter

C. Edelman &Porter D. Edelman & Hess

Ans. C.

39. Who discovered B.anthracis ?

A. Koch B. Pasteur

C. Jenner D. Hansen

Ans. A.

40. Scientist who disproved theory of spontaneous generation

A. Koch B. Pasteur

C. Jenner D. Hansen

Ans. B.

41. Germ theory was proposed by —

A. Koch B. Pasteur

C. Jenner D. Hansen

Ans. A.

42. Who discovered the importance of Agar in culture media ?

A. Ehrlich B. Petri

C. Finley D. Hess

Ans. D.

43. Diphtheria toxin was identified by :

A. Von Behring B. Finley

C. Hess D. Pasteur

Ans. A.

44. The theory of immunity was proposed by

A. Koch B. Ehrlich

C. Hess D. Hansen

Ans. B.

45. Who isolated E. coli for the first time ?

A. Escherich B. Robert Koch

C. Jenner D. Pasteur

Ans. A.

46. What is Caduceus ?

A. A parasitic nematode B. Symbol of medicine

C. A method of surgery D. A method of anaesthesia

Ans. B.

47. Who discovered archaebacteria ?

A. Carl Woese B. Edelman

C. Ehrlich D. Pasteur

Ans. A.

48. Scientist who demonstrated that open tubes of broth remained free of microbes when air was free of dust

A. Tyndal B. Pasteur

C. Petri D. Francesco Redi

Ans. A.

49. Who discovered bacterial transformation ?

A. Jenner B. B.Griffith

C. C.Messelson D. D.Tautum

Ans. B.

50. Who is known as the father of microbiology ?

A. Pasteur B. Koch

C. Leewenhoek D. Robert Hook

Ans. C.

51. Who is known as father of medical microbiology ?

A. Koch B. Pasteur

C. Jenner D. Tautum

Ans. A.

52. Antiseptic properties were first described by

A. Jenner B. Pasteur

C. Lister D. Beijernic

Ans. C.

53. Who developed smallpox vaccine for the first time ?

A. Koch B. Jenner

C. Pasteur D. Lister

Ans. B.

54. Who discovered the process of phagocytosis ?

A. Mechnikov B. Koch

C. Pasteur D. A.Fleming

Ans. A.

55. Scientist(s) who proved DNA and not protein as genetic material.

A. Hershey B. Beadle and Tatum

C. Pasteur D. Jenner

Ans. A.

56. Who developed hybridoma technology for the first time ?

A. Landsteiner B. Fire and Mello

C. Kohler and Milstein D. D'Herelle

Ans. C.

57. Who developed the concept of specific toxicity?

A. Pasteur B. B. Fleming

C. C. Watson D. D. Ehrlich

Ans. D.

58. Which were the investigators lived at the same time?

A. Koch and Pasteur B. Darwin and Woese

C. Van Leeuwenhoek and Ricketts D. Berg and Hooke

Ans. A.

59. The word cell was first used by

A. Robert Hooke B. Theodor Schwann

C. Louis Pasteur D. Ronald Ross

Ans. A.

60. Carl Woese and his colleague are best known for establishing

A. The five kingdom system B. The three domain system

C. The prokaryote-eukaryote system D. The plant-animal system

Ans. B.

61. Who was awarded with Nobel prize for contribution towards of 3D structure of DNA along with Watson and Crick

A. Rosalind Franklin B. Maurice Wilkins

C. Linus Pauling D. Temin

Ans. B.

62. Andrew Z Fire and Graig C Mello got Nobel prize in medicine for the discovery of

A. Split gene B. Transposons

C. Ribozymes D. RNA interference mechanisms

Ans. D.

63. Stanley Prusiner, Nobel winner of 1997 discovered bizarre infectious protein particle called as

A. Prions B. Viroids

C. Virusoids D. Proteosomes

Ans. A.

64. The key enzyme that helped K. Mullis in the invention of PCR was

A. Ligase B. Taq polymerase

C. Restriction endonuclease D. Vent polymerase

Ans. B.

65. All enzymes are proteins that was the concept before the discovery of ribozymes or catalytic RNAs by

A. Roberts and Sharp B. Cech and Altman

C. Alwin and Towbin D. Sanger

Ans. B.

66. Bacterial conjugation was discovered by

A. Beadle and Tatum B. Meselson and Stahl

C. Lederberg and Tatum D. Griffith

Ans. C.

67. The first confirmation regarding the status of DNA as genetic material was given by the work of Avery, Macleod and McCarty on

A. E. coli B. Diplococcus pneumonia

C. Klebsiella D. T 2 phage

Ans. B.

68. DNA fingerprinting using BKM-probe was developed by

A. Alec Jeffrey B. K. Mullis

C. Watson D. Lalji Singh

Ans. D.

69. Central Dogma of biology was put forward by

A. Watson B. Crick

C. Temin D. Khorana

Ans. B.

70. The discovery of restriction enzyme paved way towards the development of modern biotechnology or rDNA technology. The discoverers are

A. K. Mullis and Mc Clintock B. Arber, Nathans and Smith

C. Milstein and Saiki D. Sanger, Maxam and Gilbert

Ans. B.

71. Father of bacteriological techniques

A. Robert Koch B. Gram

C. Buchner D. Pasteur

Ans. A.

72. In 2006, the Nobel prize for RNA interference phenomenon was won for the work carried out on

A. D. Melanogaster B. A. Thaliana

C. C. elegans D. S. Pombe

Ans. C.

73. Who developed the concept of specific toxicity?

A. Fleming B. Pasteur

C. Ehrlich D. Watson

Ans. C.

74. Insulin was prepared by scientists in

A. 1968 B. 1970

C. 1978 D. 1975

Ans. C.

75. Scientist Louis Pasteur proposed that microbial activity is cause of all fermentations in

A. 1869 B. 1857

C. 1862 D. 1867

Ans. B.

76. Scientist who proposed that microbial activity is cause of all fermentations is

A. Ibn al Haithem B. Gregor Mendel

C. Louis Pasteur D. Ian Wilmot

Ans. C.

77. Answer the followings :

1. Father of Biology
2. Father of Modern biology
3. Father of Antibiotics
4. Father of Taxonomy
5. Father of Immunology
6. Father of Microbiology

7. Father of Modern Microbiology
8. Father of Medical Microbiology
9. Father of Pathology
10. Father of Bacteriology
11. Father of Virology
12. Father of Embryology
13. Father of Modern Embryology
14. Father of Physiology
15. Father of Modern Experimental Physiology
16. Father of Genetics
17. Father of Modern Genetics
18. Father of Human / biochemical Genetics
19. Father of Experimental Genetics
20. Father of Haploid /Neurospora Genetics
21. Father of Ecology
22. Father of Cloning
23. Father of Plant Anatomy
24. Father of Histology
25. Father of Cytology
26. Father of Modern Cytology
27. Father of Paleontology
28. Father of Modern Paleontology
29. Father of Concept of Evolution
30. Father of Botany
31. Father of Modern Botany
32. Father of Zoology
33. Father of Biochemistry
34. Father of Epidemiology
35. Father of Plant Pathology
36. Father of Modern Pathology
37. Father of Genetic Engineering
38. Father of Gene therapy
39. Father of Ethology
40. Father of Endocrinology
41. Father of Eugenics
42. Father of Gerantology

43. Father of Palynology
44. Father of Stress Physiology
45. Father of Electrocardiography
46. Father of DNA fingerprinting
47. Father of Mycology
48. Father of Bryology
49. Father of ATP cycle
50. Father of Anatomy
51. Father of Modern Anatomy
52. Father of Radiation Biology
53. Father of Homeopathy
54. Father of Ayurveda
55. Father of Surgery/ Plastic Surgery
56. Father of blood circulation
57. Father of Medicine
58. Father of blood groups
59. Father of Polio Vaccine
60. Father of Green Revolution

Ans.

1.	Father of Biology	Aristotle
2.	Father of Modern biology	Linnaeus
3.	Father of Antibiotics	Alexander Fleming
4.	Father of Taxonomy	Carolus Linnaeus
5.	Father of Immunology	Edward Jenner
6.	Father of Microbiology	A.V. Leeuwenhoek
7.	Father of Modern Microbiology	Louis Pasteur
8.	Father of Medical Microbiology	Robert Koch
9.	Father of Pathology	Rudolph Virchow
10.	Father of Bacteriology	Robert Koch
11.	Father of Virology	W. M. Stanley
12.	Father of Embryology	Aristotle
13.	Father of Modern Embryology	Ernst Von Baer
14.	Father of Physiology	Stephan Hales
15.	Father of Modern Experimental Physiology	Calude Bernard
16.	Father of Genetics	Gregor Mendel
17.	Father of Modern Genetics	Bateson
18.	Father of Human / biochemical Genetics	Arachibald Garrod

19. Father of Experimental Genetics	T.H. Morgan
20. Father of Haploid /Neurospora Genetics	Dodge
21. Father of Ecology	Theophrastus
22. Father of Cloning	Ian Wilmut
23. Father of Plant Anatomy	Grew
24. Father of Histology	Malpighi
25. Father of Cytology	Robert Hooke
26. Father of Modern Cytology	Swanson
27. Father of Paleontology	Leonard da Vinci
28. Father of Modern Paleontology	Cuvier
29. Father of Concept of Evolution	Empedocles
30. Father of Botany	Theophrastus
31. Father of Modern Botany	Bauhin
32. Father of Zoology	Aristotle
33. Father of Biochemistry	Liebig
34. Father of Epidemiology	John Snow
35. Father of Plant Pathology	De Bary
36. Father of Modern Pathology	Rudolf Virchow
37. Father of Genetic Engineering	Paul Berg
38. Father of Gene therapy	Anderson
39. Father of Ethology	Konard Lorentz
40. Father of Endocrinology	Thomas Addison
41. Father of Eugenics	Galton
42. Father of Gerantology	Korenchevsk
43. Father of Palynology	Erdtman
44. Father of Stress Physiology	Hans Selye
45. Father of Electrocardiography	Einthoven
46. Father of DNA fingerprinting	Alec Jeffery
47. Father of Mycology	Micheli
48. Father of Bryology	Hedwig
49. Father of ATP cycle	Lipmann
50. Father of Anatomy	Herophilus
51. Father of Modern Anatomy	Andreas Vesalius
52. Father of Radiation Biology	HJVS Muller
53. Father of Homeopathy	Hahnemann
54. Father of Ayurveda	Charaka

55. Father of Surgery/ Plastic Surgery — Susruta
56. Father of blood circulation — William Harvey
57. Father of Medicine — Hippocrates
58. Father of blood groups — Landsteiner
59. Father of Polio Vaccine — Jonas Salk
60. Father of Green Revolution — Norman Borlaug

5

Genetic Engineering

1. One of the standard cloning vector widely used in gene cloning is

   A. Ti pasmid B. EMBL 3

   C. pBR 322 D. EMBL 4

Ans. C.

2. Transgenic animals are for improvement of the quality of

   A. Milk B. Meat

   C. Eggs D. All of the above

Ans. D.

3. Different methods of strain improvement are

   A. Protoplast fusion B. Recombinant DNA technique

   C. Genetic recombination D. All of these

Ans. D.

4. Protoplasts can be prepared from

   A. Gram positive bacteria B. Gram negative bacteria

   C. Both a & b D. None of these

Ans. B.

5. Tumour inducing plasmids are extensively used in production of

   A. Avirulent phases B. Single cell proteins

   C. Transgenic plants D. Nitrogen fixing bacteria

Ans. C.

6. A population of cells derived from a single cell are called

   A. Monoclonal cells B. Clones

   C. Protoplasts D. Sub culture

Ans. B.

7. In which of the following microorganism, conjunction tube was not produced during conjunction process?

A. Thiobaillus thiooxidence
B. T. Ferroxidance
C. Tetrahymena thermophila
D. Cryptaporiclium

Ans. A.

8. During mitosis, synapsis occurs in the phase called

A. Telophase
B. Anaphase
C. Prophase
D. None of the above

Ans. C.

9. Centromere is that part of chromosome where

A. Nucleoli are formed
B. Crossing over takes places
C. Chromatids are attached
D. Naking occurs

Ans. C.

10. Somatic cell of the adult body are haploid in many except

A. Vertebrates
B. Invertebrates
C. Fungi
D. Vascular plants

Ans. C.

11. Maximum application of animal cell culture technology today is in the production of

A. Insulin
B. Interferons
C. Vaccines
D. Edible proteins

Ans. C.

12. The cells having F plasmid in the chromosomes were termed as

A. Hfr
B. F–
C. Hbr
D. C+

Ans. A.

13. The enzyme required for DNA from RNA template:

A. RNA polymerase
B. Reverse transcriptase
C. DNA polymerase
D. Terminal transferase

Ans. B.

14. The most important function of a gene is to synthesize

A. Enzymes
B. Hormones
C. RNA
D. DNA

Ans. A.

15. One of the genes present exclusively on the X-chromosome in humans is concerned with

A. Baldness B. Red-green colour blindness

C. Facial hair/moustache in males D. Night blindness

Ans. B.

16. Peptide linkages are formed in between

A. Nucleotides B. Amino acids

C. Glucose molecules D. Sucrose

Ans. B.

17. In genetic engineering breaks in DNA are joined by enzymes known as

A. Restriction enzymes B. Ligases

C. Nucleases D. Hydrolase

Ans. B.

18. DNA transfer from one bacterium to another through phages is termed as

A. Transduction B. Induction

C. Transfection D. Infection

Ans. A.

19. Which one of the following mutagens act only on replicating DNA?

A. Ethidium bromide B. Nitrosogeranidine

C. Acridine orange D. None of above

Ans. C.

20. The technique involved in comparing the DNA components of two samples is known as

A. Monoclonal antibody techniques B. Genetic finger printing

C. Recombinant DNA technology D. Polymerase chain reaction

Ans. B.

21. Plasmids are ideal vectors for gene cloning as

A. They can be multiplied by culturing

B. They can be multiplied in the laboratory using enzymes

C. They can replicate freely outside the bacterial cell

D. They are self replicating within the bacterial cell

Ans. D.

22. Humans normally have 46 chromosomes in skin cells. How many autosomes would be expected in a kidney cell?

A. 46 B. 23

C. 47 D. 44

Ans. D.

23. The widely used yeast for the production of single cell protein is

A. Saccharomyces cerevisiae B. Rhizopus

C. Candida utilis D. All of the above

Ans. C.

24. Analysis of protein antigen is by

A. Southern blot B. Northern blot

C. Western blot D. None of these

Ans. C.

25. A mutation that produces termination codon is

A. Mis-sense mutation B. Neutral mutation

C. Non-sense mutation D. Reverse mutation

Ans. C.

26. During conjunction the genetic material will be transferred through

A. Cell wall B. Medium

C. Pili D. Capsule

Ans. C.

27. Lederberg and Tatum (1946) described the phenomena of

A. Conjunction B. Transformation

C. Mutation D. Plasmids

Ans. A.

28. First crop plant whose genome was sequenced ————————.

Ans. Rice. Oryza glaberrima (African rice) in 2010.

29. First whole genome sequenced organism ————————.

Ans. Bacteriophage ϕx174 in 1977.

30. First bacteria whose genome was sequenced ————————.

Ans. H. influenza in 1995 using short gun method.

31. First multicellular organism (also 1st animal, 1st invertebrate) whose genome was sequenced ————————.

Ans. Caenor habditis elegans in 1998.

32. First Eukaryote (1st unicellular eukaryote) whose genome was sequenced —.

Ans. S. cerevisiae in 1996.

33. First insect whose genome was sequenced ——————.

Ans. Drosophila melanogaster.

34. First plant whose genome was sequenced ——————.

Ans. Arabidopsis thaliana.

35. Which year was human genome sequencing completed ?

Ans. 2003.

36. Proof reading is done by ———— subunits of E. coli DNA polymerase III.

A. α subunit
B. ε subunit
C. Chi subunit
D. Tau subunit

Ans. B.

37. ———— type of sigma factor is involved in the expression of housekeeping gene in E. coli.

A. Sigma 70
B. Sigma 54
C. Sigma 48
D. Sigma 32

Ans. A.

38. The phenomenon of transformation was first described in

A. E. coli
B. B. subtilis
C. Pneumococci
D. Vibrio

Ans. C.

39. The phenomenon of transformation was first described in

A. E. coli
B. B. subtilis
C. Pneumococci
D. Vibrio

Ans. C.

40. The efficiency of amplification in PCR in later cycles is reduced due to

A. Reduction in substrate concentration
B. Insufficient enzyme and time to synthesize mass quantity of DNA
C. Build up of PCR product which competes with primers for hybrid formation
D. All of these

Ans. D.

41. The original enzyme(s) used in PCR reaction is/are known as

A. E. coli DNA polymerase B. E. coli RNA polymerase

C. Taq polymerase D. all of these

Ans. A.

42. RNA populations can also be used as PCR templates after reverse transcription into

A. c DNA B. t RNA

C. m DNA D. r RNA

Ans. A.

43. The cloning step in PCR/sequencing analysis of microbial communities is necessary for

A. The amplification process

B. Preventing contamination by outside DNA

C. Separating the different rRNA gene sequences in the mixture

D. None of these

Ans. C.

44. The template for PCR is

A. RNA B. single stranded DNA

C. Double stranded DNA D. None of these

Ans. C.

45. The human genome project was initiated by

A. NIH and DOE B. NIH and EBI

C. NIH and DDBJ D. DOE and DDBJ

Ans. A.

46. The prime objective of HGP was

A. To find out the exact functions of proteins in humans

B. To sequence the entire base pairs that makes up the 23 chromosomes

C. To sequence the entire base pairs that makes up the 24 chromosomes

D. To find out the active genes in human genome

Ans. C.

47. HGP was also focused on identifying

A. SNPs B. VNTRs

C. Minisatellites D. Junk DNA

Ans. A.

48. At the initial stage of HGP, the estimated time and budget was

A. 30 years & $100 billion B. 15 years & $15 billion

C. 10years & $ 6 billions D. 15 years & $ 3 billion

Ans. D.

49. The private company involved in the human genome sequencing in parallel with HGP is

A. Roche B. Gilead

C. Celera D. Genentech

Ans C.

50. According to HGP, human genome consists of approximately

A. 100000 genes B. 50000 genes

C. 30000 genes D. 20000 genes

Ans. D.

51. The first draft of HGP was published in 2001 in the journal

A. Science B. Cell

C. Nature D. Molecular biology

Ans. C.

52. DNA base pairs in the Human Genome are about

A. $2X10^7$ B. $3X10^9$

C. $4X10^8$ D. $7X10^7$

Ans. B.

53. The Cre-Lox system uses one of the following

A. DNA kinase B. Creatine phosphatise

C. DNA recombinase D. S1 nuclease

Ans. C.

54. Which of the following is a dual resistance vector ?

A. M13 B. pUC18

C. pUC19 D. pBR 322

Ans. D.

55. Alec Jeffery's name is associated with

A. DNA sequencing B. RNA sequencing

C. DNA fingerprinting D. Site directed mutagenesis

Ans. C.

56. Yeast Two Hybrid system involves the use of
A. Domains of transcription factors B. Histone proteins
C. Two point crossovers D. Homologous recombination

Ans. A.

57. The method of plasmid isolation by alkaline lysis was published by
A. Mandel and Higa B. Temin and Baltimore
C. Tatum and Lederberg D. Birnboim and Doly

Ans. D.

58. The antisense gene involved in the production of Flavr Savr is
A. Polygalacturonase B. Lactamase
C. Adenosine deaminase D. Glutathione transferase

Ans. A.

59. The genetically engineered 'Golden rice' synthesize large amount of
A. Vitamin K B. Betacarotene
C. Vitamin C D. Beta galactosidase

Ans. B.

60. His-tagged proteins can be eluted from Ni columns using
A. Imidazole B. Ammonium hydroxide
C. 6X SSC D. 0.25 N HCL

Ans. A.

61. Which of the following DNA repair mechanism is known as the 'cut and patch mechanism'?
A. Photoreactivation B. Nucleotide excision repair
C. Base excision repair D. Mismatch repair

Ans. B.

62. DNA helicase enzyme involved in base excision repair mechanism is ———
A. DNA replicase I B. DNA replicase II
C. DNA replicase III D. DNA replicase IV

Ans. C.

63. In mismatch repair mechanism, which of the following protein recognize DNA mismatches in the genomic DNA ?
A. MutH B. MutS
C. MutL D. UvrD

Ans. B.

64. The main difference between nucleotide excision repair (NER) and base excision repair (BER) is

A. In NER double strand breaks are repaired whereas in BER single strand breaks repaired

B. NER is a light dependent reaction whereas BER is light independent process

C. In NER phosphodiester backbone is first cleaved whereas in BER phosphodiester backbone is cleaved later

D. All of these

Ans. C.

65. Which enzyme is responsible for photoreactivation of DNA ?

A. photoligase B. Photoreductase

C. Photooxidase D. Photolyase

Ans. D.

66. Which of the following enzyme(s) is involved in base excision repair ?

A. DNA glycosylase B. AP endonuclease

C. AP exonuclease D. A, B & C

E. A & B.

Ans. E.

67. Xeroderma pigmentosum in human is associated with mutation in

A. Photoreactivation B. Nucleotide excision repair

C. Base excision repair D. Mismatch repair

Ans. B.

68. In eukaryotes, the mismatch repair mechanism is initiated and directed by

A. Methylated DNA strand B. Acetylated DNA strand

C. Strand specific nicks D. Double strand breaks

Ans. C.

69. In DNA excision repair mechanism which of the following proteins first recognize DNA lesions ?

A. UvrA B. UvrB

C. UvrC D. UvrD

Ans. A.

70. Which of the following statement is true regarding the nucleotide excision repair (NER) mechanism ?

A. NER mechanism is present only in eukaryotes

B. NER present only in prokaryotes

C. NER present in both prokaryotes and eukaryotes but the exact mechanisms varies

D. NER present in both prokaryotes and eukaryotes with similar molecular mechanism in both

Ans. C.

71. Photolyase enzyme involved in the photoreactivation can remove ——

A. UV induced double strand breaks B. UV induced thymine dimers

C. Mismatch in DNA D. Single strand breaks in DNA

Ans. B.

72. DNA polymerase enzyme involved in base excision repair mechanism is —

A. Pol α B. Pol β

C. Pol γ D. Polδ

Ans. B.

73. DNA polymerase enzyme involved in mismatch repair system of E. coli is ——

A. DNA Pol-I B. DNA Pol-II

C. DNA Pol-III D. DNA Pol- β

Ans. C.

74. A critical enzyme used directly in the synthesis of dTMP (thymidine) is

A. Carbamoyl phosphate B. Aspartate Transcarbamoylase

C. Dihydrooratase D. Thymidylate synthetase

Ans. D.

75. In which phase of the cell cycle does DNA replication occur ?

A. G0 B. G1

C. S D. G2

Ans. C.

76. The enzyme responsible for initiating DNA replication in prokaryotes is

A. DNA polymerase I B. DNA polymerase III

C. Polymerase beta D. Primase

Ans. D.

77. In pyrimidine synthesis, eukaryotes can use uracil to feedback inhibit which of the following enzymes ?

A. Carbamoyl phosphate synthase B. Aspartate transcarbamoylase

C. Dihydrooratase D. Thymidylate synthase

Ans. A.

78. All of the following are required for purine de novo synthesis except

A. CO2 B. Glycine

C. Glutamine D. Isoleucine

Ans. D.

79. The enzyme responsible for continuing DNA replication in prokaryotes, once it is initiated is

A. DNA polymerase I B. DNA polymerase III

C. Polymerase beta D. Polymerase delta

Ans. B.

80. Antibiotics such as Ciprofloxacin and Fluoroquinolines work by inhibiting a specific enzyme. This enzyme is necessary to relieve torsional strain that is caused by the unwinding of the helix. What is the name of the enzyme ?

A. DNA ligase B. DNA gyrase

C. Single stranded binding protein D. Primase

Ans. B.

81. Which of the following technique is primarily undertaken to amplify DNA ?

A. PCR B. Microarray

C. Southern blotting D. Northern blotting

Ans. A.

82. Which of the following, in high concentrations, can overcome purine de novo inhibition ?

A. Ribose-5-phosphate B. PRPP

C. 5-Phosphoribosyl 1 amine D. GDP

Ans. B.

83. All of the following are used in PCR except

A. Taq polymerase B. Restriction enzyme

C. Oligonucleotide primers D. Deoxynucleotide triphosphates

Ans. B.

84. The following are features of DNA replication except

A. Semi-conservative
B. Semi-discontinuous
C. Unidirectional
D. Chain growth in the 5'-3' direction

Ans. C.

85. Which out of the following mechanisms is involved in the production of variety of immunoglobulins each specific for a specific antigen?

A. Class switching
B. Gene amplification
C. Gene arrangement
D. RNA editing

Ans. C.

86. Which of the following is a common enzyme for de novo as well as salvage pathway of purine biosynthesis ?

A. Amidotransferase
B. PRPP synthetase
C. HGPRTase
D. Adenylosuccinate synthetase

Ans. B.

87. Which of the following does not have introns ?

A. DNA
B. Nonprocessed pseudogenes
C. Processed mRNA
D. Primary RNA transcript

Ans. C.

88. Which of the following is not true of RNA synthesis ?

A. The key enzyme is RNA enzyme
B. The energy is supplied by ring cleavage
C. The RNA sequence is complementary to the template strand of DNA
D. The RNA sequence is of opposite polarity to the template strand of DNA

Ans. B.

89. If the molar amount of G in a DNA sample is 20%, what is the molar amount of T in the sample?

A. 20%
B. 30%
C. 40%
D. 60%

Ans. B.

90. Which of the following subunits of the bacterial RNA polymerase is responsible for promoter recognition ?

A. Alpha
B. Beta
C. Gamma
D. Sigma

Ans. D.

91. What is true of the melting temperature of G-C pairs compared to A-T pairs in DNA?

A. The Tm are equal

B. Tm of G-C is less than the Tm of A-T

C. Tm of G-C is greater than the Tm of A-T

D. None of the above

Ans. C.

92. A boy came to the hospital after eating wild mushroom. The poison associated with mushroom most likely directly inhibit—

A. hn RNA
B. tRNA
C. DNA
D. mRNA

Ans. A.

93. DNA methylation is associated with

A. CpG islands
B. CAT box
C. TATA box
D. Increasing gene transcription

Ans. A.

94. Alternative splicing

A. Creates protein from multiple segments of DNA on different chromosomes

B. Is the reason why the human genome is much more complex than other species

C. Creates different proteins from a single gene

D. Is not tissue specific

Ans. C.

95. All of the following are involved in translating information into proteins except

A. rRNA
B. siRNA
C. tRNA
D. snRNA

Ans. B.

96. Which histone is not part of the nucleosome ?

A. H1
B. H2A
C. H2B
D. H3

Ans. A.

97. Which of the following is an inhibitor of prokaryotic transcription ?

A. Ciprofloxacin
B. Etoposide
C. Erythromycin
D. Rifampicin

Ans. D.

98. Choose the nucleoside analogue used as an anticancer drug out of the following

A. Methotrexate B. 6-Mercaptopurine

C. Vinblastin D. Cytosine Arabinoside

Ans. D.

99. Which amino acid reside is in abundance in histones?

A. Arginine B. Aspartic acid

C. Tryptophan D. Phenylalanine

Ans. A.

100. Which out of the following techniques is used for the detection of gene of interest

A. Southern blotting B. Northern blotting

C. PCR D. DNA foot printing

Ans. A.

101. Triple repeat sequence disease occurs in

A. Alzheimer's disease B. Cystic fibrosis

C. Ataxia telangectasia D. Huntington's chorea

Ans. D.

102. Northern blotting is used for separation of

A. DNA B. mRNA

C. protein D. protein DNA interaction

Ans. B.

103. How does puromycin inhibit protein synthesis?

A. It binds to A site and stop the elongation

B. It affect the peptidyl transferase activity.

C. It degrades the t-RNA

D. It is responsible for loading termination codon

Ans. A.

104. The shape of a DNA molecule is

A. Double helix B. Triple helix

C. No helix D. Linear

Ans. A.

105. Cytochrome C releases to cytoplasm during

A. Apoptosis B. Mitosis

C. Meiosis D. Cytosis

Ans. A.

106. What is the main reason for cyanide poisoning?

A. Inhibition of electron transport chain

B. Inhibition of Fatty acid transport chain

C. Inhibition of Nucleic acid transport chain

D. Inhibition of Nucleic acid transport chain

Ans. A.

107. DNA replication takes place during

A. G1 phase B. G2 phase

C. M phase D. S phase

Ans. D.

108. The term "Molecular biology" was first used by

A. Warren Weaver in 1938 B. Warren Buffet

C. Watson and Crick D. Watson and Crick

Ans. A.

109. RNAPII can exist in two forms

A. Protein and vitamin

B. RNAPII0, with a highly phosphorylated CTD, and RNAPIIA, with a nonphosphorylated CTD

C. RNAP 1 and RNAP 2

D. Protein and RNA

Ans. B.

110. Single letter code for Alanine is

A. A B. B

C. C D. D

Ans. A.

111. Single letter code for phenylalanine is

A. P B. B

C. C D. F

Ans. D.

112. Single letter code for Tryptophan is

A. T B. B

C. C D. W

Ans. D.

113. In DNA Adenine coupled with

A. T B. G

C. C D. W

Ans. A.

114. DNA is a long polymer made from repeating units of

A. Nucleotides B. Nucleosides

C. Nucleorides D. Nucleophyte

Ans. A.

115. Topoisomerases are enzymes with

A. Both nuclease and ligase activity

B. Both polymerase and cutting activity

C. Both transcription and ligase activity

D. Both unwinding and polymerase activity

Ans. A.

116. Who could not win the Nobel Prize in Physiology or Medicine for discovery of DNA structure

A. Franklin B. Watson

C. Crick D. Wilkins

Ans. A.

117. Who is not associated with discovery of DNA structure ?

A. Linus Pauling B. Watson

C. Crick D. Wilkins

Ans. A.

118. Single letter code for Selenocysteine is

A. P B. B

C. C D. U

Ans. D.

119. Where will you keep collagen triple helix in Ramchandran plot

A. Top right B. Bottom right

C. Bottom left D. Top left

Ans. D.

120. t-RNA gene is synthesized by

A. RNA polymerase I B. RNA polymerase II

C. RNA polymerase III D. DNA polymerase III

Ans. C.

121. Micro RNA was first discovered in

A. Yeast B. Bacteria

C. C. elegans D. Mouse

Ans. C.

122. Micro RNA generally contain

A. 22 hundred nucleotide B. 22 thousand nucleotide

C. 22 nucleotide D. 22 million nucleotide

Ans. C.

123. How does puromycin inhibit protein synthesis?

A. It binds to a site and stop the elongation.

B. It affect the peptidyl transferase activity

C. It degrades the t-RNA

D. It is responsible for loading termination codon

Ans. A.

124. The shape of a DNA molecule is

A. Double helix B. Triple helix

C. No helix D. Linear

Ans. A.

125. Cytochrome C releases to cytoplasm during

A. Apoptosis B. Mitosis

C. Meiosis D. Cytosis

Ans. A.

126. What is the main reason for cyanide poisoning

A. Inhibition of electron transport chain

B. Inhibition of fatty acid transport chain

C. Inhibition of nucleic acid transport chain

D. Inhibition of fatty acid metabolism

Ans. A.

127. The technique of obtaining large number of plantlet by tissue culture method is called

A. Plantlet culture B. Micropropagation

C. Organ culture D. Macropropagation

Ans. B.

128. Maximum application of animal cell culture technology is in the production of

A. Insulin B. Interferons

C. Edible proteins D. Vaccines

Ans. D.

129. What is true for monoclonal antibodies ?

A. These antibodies obtained from one parent and for one antigen

B. These antibodies obtained from many parents and for many antigens

C. These antibodies obtained from different parents and for one antigen

D. These antibodies obtained from one parent and for many antigens

Ans. C.

130. Two bacteria found to be very useful in genetic engineering experiments are

A. Nitrobacter and Azotobacter B. Rhizobium and Diplococcus

C. Nitrosomonas and Klebsiella D. E. coli and Agrobacterium

Ans. D.

131. A genetically engineered microorganism used successfully in bioremediation of oil spills is a species of

A. Trichoderma B. Bacillus

C. Xanthomonas D. Pseudomonas

Ans. D.

132. Probiotics are

A. Cancer inducing microbes B. Safe antibiotics

C. New kind of food allergens D. Live microbial food supplement

Ans. D.

133. The process involved in the RNA formation on the DNA template is

A. Transcription B. Translation

C. Replication D. Transformation

Ans. A.

134. The enzyme required for transcription is

A. Restriction enzymes B. DNA polymerase

C. RNA polymerase D. RNAase

Ans. C.

135. Transcription is the transfer of genetic information from

A. DNA to RNA B. tRNA to mRNA

C. DNA to mRNA D. mRNA to tRNA

Ans. C.

136. RNA required for the protein synthesis

A. mRNA B. tRNA

C. rRNA D. All of these

Ans. D.

137. A promoter site on DNA

A. Initiates transcription B. Regulates termination

C. Codes for RNA D. Transcribes repressor

Ans. A.

138. Sigma factor is component of

A. DNA ligase B. DNA polymerase

C. RNA polymerase D. Endonuclease

Ans. C.

139. What is the function of tRNA in relation to protein synthesis ?

A. Inhibits protein synthesis

B. Proof reading

C. Identifies amino acids and transport them to ribosomes

D. All of these

Ans. C.

140. RNA polymerase has polymerase chains

A. 2 B. 3

C. 4 D. 5

Ans. D.

141. Which site of tRNA molecule hydrogen bonds to a mRNA molecule ?

A. Codon B. Anticodon

C. 5' end of the tRNA molecule D. 3' end of the tRNA molecule

Ans. B.

142. The DNA chain acting as template for RNA synthesis has the following order of bases, AGCTTCGA. What will be the order of

A. TCGAAGCT B. UGCUAGCT

C. TCGAUCGU D. UCGAAGCU

Ans. D.

143. A human cell containing 22 autosomes and a Y chromosome is

A. A sperm
B. An egg
C. A somatic cell of a female
D. A somatic cell of a male

Ans. A.

144. If the DNA content of a diploid cell in the G1 phase of the cell cycle is X, then the DNA content of the same cell at metaphase of meiosis I would be

A. X
B. 2X
C. 0.5 X
D. 0.25 X

Ans. B.

145. How many different combination of maternal and paternal chromosomes can be packaged in gametes made by an organism with a diploid number of 8 (2n=8) ?

A. 2
B. 4
C. 8
D. 16

Ans. D.

146. Homologous chromosomes move toward opposite poles of a dividing cell during

A. Mitosis
B. Meiosis I
C. Meiosis II
D. Fertilization

Ans. B.

147. Meiosis II is similar to mitosis in that

A. Sister chromatids separate during anaphase
B. The daughter cells are diploid
C. Homologous chromosomes synapse
D. DNA replication before the division

Ans. A.

148. Mitochondrial DNA is advantageous for evolutionary studies because

A. It is inherited only through the female parent and thus evolves in a way that allows trees of relationship to be easily constructed
B. It is inserted into the X chromosomes
C. It evolves more slowly than the gene in the nucleus
D. It first appeared in humans and is not found in other animals

Ans. A.

149. Which of the following amino acids interact with the DNA or RNA backbone (i.e. phosphate)?

A. Ile and Val
B. Lys and Arg
C. Leu and Ala
D. Cys and Met

Ans. B.

150. Which of the following are similar between transcription in prokaryotes and eukaryotes?

A. RNA polymerase produces mRNA which grow in the 5'-3' direction

B. RNA polymerase bind to ribosomes to allow transcription

C. A polytail is added to the 3' end of messenger RNAs

D. Introns are present in genes which are spliced out after transcription

Ans. A.

151. Translation involves

A. Mapping genes in bacteria using a viral carrier

B. Reading a DNA strand and making an mRNA copy

C. Taking up DNA into a cell and changing its genetic make up

D. Reading an mRNA to yield an amino acid sequence in a protein

Ans. D.

152. The normal function of a promoter is to

A. Bind the small subunit of the ribosome

B. Serve as an origin of DNA replication

C. Serve as an acceptor for transfer RNA

D. Serve as the a binding site for RNA polymerase

Ans. D.

153. The process of DNA replication involves

A. Multiple origins of replication per chromosome in eukaryotes

B. Binding of ribosomes to origins of replication

C. Continuous synthesis on both strand of the double helix

D. Conservative replication with one original double helix and one totally new double helix as products

Ans. A.

154. Which of the following biomolecule has self repair mechanisms ?

A. DNA, RNA and protein
B. DNA and RNA
C. DNA only
D. DNA and protein

Ans. C.

155. Which of the following chemicals induce depuration

A. Methyl ethane sulphonate
B. Nitrosoguanidine
C. Ethyl ethane sulphonate
D. All of these

Ans. D.

156. Which of the following mechanism of DNA polymerase helps in preventing error during DNA replication ?

A. Rechecking B. Proof checking

C. Proof reading D. All of these

Ans. C.

157. The protein(s) involved in mismatch repair are

A. Mut S B. Mut H

C. Mut L D. All of these

Ans. D.

158. Which of the following dimer formation is most common

A. Thymidine dimer B. Cytidine dimer

C. Both A & B D. None of these

Ans. A.

159. Dimer repair mechanism include

A. Excision repair B. Photoreactivation

C. Recombination repair D. All of these

Ans. D.

160. Thymidine dimmers are often corrected by light induced repair mechanism. The enzyme involved in the process is

A. photolyase B. photoligase

C. DNA glycosylase D. All of these

Ans. A.

161. Which of the following is dark repair ?

A. Nucleotide excision repair (NER) B. Base excision repair

C. Both A and B D. None of these

Ans. C.

162. DNA glycosylase is an enzyme involved in base excision repair. The function is

A. Addition of correct base B. Addition of correct nucleotide

C. Removal of incorrect base D. Removal of phosphodiester bond

Ans. C.

163. Recombinational repair is often due to

A. Incorporation of many incorrect nucleotides by DNA polymerase

B. Many cytidine dimer and associated large gaps in a strand

C. Many thymidine dimer formation and associated large gaps in a strand

D. All of these

Ans. B.

164. Which is the DNA polymerase involved in BER

A. DNA polymerase α
B. DNA polymerase β
C. DNA polymerase δ
D. DNA polymerase £

Ans. B.

165. Which of the following is a bypass repair system

A. BER
B. NER
C. SOS
D. Recombinational repair

Ans. C.

166. DNA repair mechanism is absent in

A. Nuclear genome
B. Mitochondrial genome
C. Chloroplast genome
D. Both B and C

Ans. D.

167. umuC, umuD gene family and RecA proteins are involved in

A. BER
B. NER
C. SOS repair
D. Recombinational repair

Ans. C.

168. The distortion in DNA helix due to pyrimidine dimer formation is called as

A. Nick
B. Single stranded breaks
C. Kink
D. None of the above

Ans. C.

169. Organic farming is the technique of raising crops through uses of

A. Manures
B. Biofertilizers
C. Resistant varieties
D. All of these

Ans. D.

170. Pyrethrin is got from

A. Azardirachta indica
B. Urtica dioca
C. Tagetus erecta
D. Chrsamthemum cinerarifolium

Ans. D.

171. Which one is green manure/biofertilizer

A. Sesbania
B. Rice
C. Oat
D. Maize

Ans. A.

172. Azolla is used as biofertilizer as it has

A. Rhizobium | B. Cyanobacteria
C. Mycorrhiza | D. Large quantity of humus

Ans. B.

173. The most quickly available source of nitrogen to plants are

A. Amide fertilizers | B. Ammonia fertilizers
C. Nitrate fertilizers | D. Ammonia nitrate fertilizer

Ans. C.

174. Most effective pesticide is

A. Carbamates | B. Organophosphates
C. Organochlorines | D. All of these

Ans. B.

175. Which is true for DDT ? It is

A. Not a pollutant | B. An antibiotic
C. An antiseptic agent | D. A non degradable pollutant

Ans. D.

176. Which is major component of Bordeaux mixture ?

A. Copper sulphate | B. Sodium chloride
C. Calcium chloride | D. Magnesium sulphate

Ans. A.

177. Which one is correctly matched ?

A. Carbamates-malathion | B. Organophosphates-carbofuran
C. Carbamates-malathion | D. Organochloride-endosulphan

Ans. D.

178. IPM stands for

A. Integrated pest manufacture | B. Integrated plant management
C. Integrated plant manufacture | D. Integrated pest management

Ans. D.

179. Green manuring increases the crop yield by

A. 5-10% | B. 15-25%
C. 30-50% | D. 80-90%

Ans. C.

180. Insecticides generally attack

A. Respiratory system
B. Nervous system
C. Muscular system
D. Circulatory system

Ans. A.

181. Organisms associated with sorghum and cotton, which provide nuturion to them are

A. Azospirillium, Azotobacter
B. Anabaena, Rhizobium
C. Rhizobium, Azotobacter
D. Anabaena, Azotobacter

Ans. A.

182. Azolla as biofertilizer, increases the yield of rice fields by

A. 10%
B. 20%
C. 30%
D. 50%

Ans. D.

183. DNA sequencing is done by

A. Maxam and Gilbert method
B. Sanger dideoxy method
C. Both A and B
D. Watson and Crick

Ans. C.

184. A vector should have which of the following properties

i. MCS
ii. Small size
iii. Multiple ori
iv. Low replication speed

A. i, ii, iii
B. ii, iii, iv
C. i, ii, iv
D. i, iii, iv

Ans. C.

185. DNA staining is done by

A. Crystal violet
B. Giemsa staining
C. Methylene blue
D. Feulgen staining

Ans. D.

186. Which of the following is not a restriction enzyme ?

A. Eco RI
B. Bam HI
C. DNA ligase
D. Pst I

Ans. C.

187. Use of alkaline phosphatase is to

A. Remove terminal phosphates from 3' end
B. Remove terminal phosphates from 5' end
C. Remove terminal phosphate from both end
D. All of these

Ans. D.

188. The uptake of plasmid DNA into bacterial cells is facilitated in the presence of

A. Calcium chloride
B. Magnesium chloride
C. Potassium chloride
D. All of these

Ans. D.

189. Taq polymerase is used in PCR because of its

A. Low thermal stability
B. High fidelity
C. High speed
D. High thermal stability

Ans. D.

190. Introduction of recombinant DNA into bacterial cell by using current is called

A. Transformation
B. Transfection
C. Electroporation
D. Transduction

Ans. C.

191. Nick translation is done by

A. DNA polymerase I
B. DNA polymerase II
C. DNA ligase
D. Kinase

Ans. A.

192. Telomeric sequences are found in

A. HAC
B. BAC
C. YAC
D. PAC

Ans. C.

193. DNA fingerprinting was developed by

A. Francis Crick
B. Khorana
C. Alec Jeffrey
D. James Watson

Ans. C.

194. The technique to distinguish the individuals based on their DNA print patterns is called

A. DNA fingerprinting
B. DNA profiling
C. Molecular fingerprinting
D. All of these

Ans. D.

195. DNA fingerprinting relies on

A. Difference in patterns of genes between individuals
B. Difference in order of genes between individuals
C. Difference in junk DNA patterns between individuals
D. All of these

Ans. C.

196. Minisatellites are

A. 10-40 bp sized short sequences within the genes

B. Short coding repetitive regions on the eukaryotic genome

C. Short non-coding repetitive sequences present throughout the chromosome

D. Are regions of chromosomes after secondary constriction

Ans. C.

197. Each individual has a unique DNA fingerprint as individuals differ in

A. Number of minisatellites on chromosome

B. Location of minisatellites on chromosome

C. Size of minisatellites on chromosome

D. All of these

Ans. D.

198. The correct order of procedures in DNA profiling is

A. DNA isolation → PCR amplification → electrophoresis → southern blotting → autoradiography → analysis of DNA print pattern

B. DNA isolation → restriction digestion → PCR amplification → electrophoresis → southern blotting → autoradiography → analysis of DNA print pattern

C. DNA isolation → PCR amplification → restriction digestion → electrophoresis → southern blotting → autoradiography → analysis of DNA print pattern

D. DNA isolation → restriction digestion → PCR amplification → southern blotting → electrophoresis → autoradiography → analysis of DNA print pattern

Ans. B.

199. DNA profiling to demonstrate the similarity between different animal species with reference to some specific protein coding DNA sequence is called

A. Zoo blot B. Phylogenetic blot

C. Animal profiling D. Animal blot

Ans. A.

200. DNA profiling is used

A. In forensic studies and in cases of disputed parentage

B. In pedigree analysis and to study migration pattern

C. To confirm cell line identity

D. All of these

Ans. D.

201. The DNA fingerprint pattern of a child is

A. Exactly similar to that of both of the parents

B. 100% similar to the father's DNA print

C. 100% similar to mother's DNA print

D. 50% bands similar to father and rest similar to mother

Ans. D.

202. DNA profiling technique to demonstrate the similarity between different plant species with reference to some specific protein coding DNA sequences is called

A. Phytoblot B. Garden blot

C. Plant profiling D. All of these

Ans. B.

203. The procedure of aligning two sequences by searching for patterns that is in the same order in the sequences

A. Sequence alignment B. Pair wise alignment

C. Multiple sequence alignment D. All of these

Ans. B.

204. Alignment method suitable for aligning closely related sequence is

A. Multiple sequence alignment B. Pair wise alignment

C. Global alignment D. Local alignment

Ans. C.

205. The alignment procedure that tries to align the entire sequence is

A. Multiple sequence alignment B. Pair wise alignment

C. Global alignment D. Local alignment

Ans. C.

206. The alignment method suitable for finding out conserved patterns in DNA or protein sequences is

A. Multiple sequence alignment B. Pair wise alignment

C. Global alignment D. Local alignment

Ans. D.

207. The procedure of aligning many sequences simultaneously is called

A. Multiple sequence alignment B. Pair wise alignment

C. Global alignment D. Local alignment

Ans. A.

208. Sequence alignment helps scientists

A. To trace out evolutionary relationships

B. To infer the functions of newly synthesized genes

C. To predict new members of gene families

D. All of these

Ans. D.

209. The alignment procedure that tries to align regions with high level of matches without considering the alignment of rest of the sequences is

A. Multiple sequence alignment B. Pair wise alignment

C. Global alignment D. Local alignment

Ans. D.

210. All are sequence alignment tools except

A. Rasmol B. BLAST

C. FASTA D. Clustal W

Ans. A.

211. Which of the following is sequence alignment tool provided by NCBI

A. Chime B. BLAST

C. FASTA D. Clustal W

Ans. B.

212. Which of the following is a multiple sequence alignment tool

A. Clustral W B. Chime

C. Dismol D. PDP

Ans. A.

213. Which of the following enzyme is used to synthesize DNA using a mRNA template

A. Taq polymerase B. Alkaline phosphatise

C. Reverse transcriptase D. Nuclease

Ans. C.

214. Which of the following enzyme is used to cut DNA molecule internally

A. Restriction enzymes B. Restriction endonuclease

C. Restriction exonuclease D. Ribonuclease H

Ans. B.

215. Which type of restriction enzymes are commonly used in rDNA technology ?

A. Type I B. Type II

C. Type III D. Type IV

Ans. C.

216. Which of the following enzyme is used to join two DNA molecule

A. Nuclease B. Restriction enzymes

C. Lyases D. Ligases

Ans. D.

217. Which is the enzyme used to remove phosphate group from the 5' end of the DNA ?

A. Restriction enzymes B. Alkaline phosphatase

C. Polynucleotide kinase D. Ribonuclease H

Ans. B.

218. The enzyme that adds mononucleotide triphosphates to the 3' OH group of a DNA fragment is

A. Polynucleotide kinase B. Terminal nucleotidyl transferase

C. Terminal phosphoryl transferase D. All of these

Ans. B.

219. The RNA strand in RNA-DNA hybrid is removed by

A. RNase B. RNase H

C. Nuclease D. None of these

Ans. B.

220. Klenow enzyme is the product of enzymatic breakdown of

A. DNA polymerse I B. DNA polymerse II

C. DNA polymerse III D. RNA polymerase

Ans. A.

221. Selective degradation of single stranded DNA is carried out by the enzyme

A. Nuclease B. Ribonuclease

C. S1 Nuclease D. Deoxyribonulcease

Ans. C.

222. Which of the following is an RNA dependent DNA synthetase ?

A. DNA polymerase I B. DNA polymerase II

C. Reverse transcriptase D. All of these

Ans. C.

223. Which of the following is a thermostable DNA polymerase ?

A. Taq polymerase B. Vent polymerase

C. Pfu polymerase D. All of these

Ans. D.

224. Eco R I is a

A. Endonuclease
B. Polymerase enzyme
C. Ligase
D. Exonuclease

Ans. A.

225. Deoxy position of Deoxyribose in DNA is

A. 1st carbon
B. 2nd carbon
C. 3rd carbon
D. 5th carbon

Ans. B.

226. Which of the following transgenic crop occupies the largest area in the world ?

A. Herbicide tolerant soybean
B. Herbicide tolerant maize
C. Insect resistant cotton
D. Insect resistant potato

Ans. A.

227. The gene responsible for dwarfing character in rice is

A. Tift 23A
B. Norin 10
C. Dee-gee-woo-gen
D. Opaque 2

Ans. C.

228. Aroma in rice is due to

A. Acetyl choline
B. 4-benzyl pyrroline
C. 2-ethyl -1-pyrroline
D. 2-acetyl-1-pyrroline

Ans. D.

229. Rifampicin is a specific inhibitor of

A. Bacterial RNA polymerase
B. RNA polymerase II
C. RNA polymerase I
D. RNA polymerase III

Ans. A.

230. The Philadelphia chromosome is

A. An example of gene amplification
B. A product of a reciprocal translocation
C. A characteristic of Burkitt's lymphoma
D. An example of duplication

Ans. B.

231. Independently folded functional unit of a protein is called a

A. Motif
B. Fold
C. Domain
D. Module

Ans. C.

232. Most predominant antibody in serum is

A. IgG B. IgA

C. IgE D. IgD

Ans. A.

233. Which of the following organisms is used in Ames test ?

A. E. coli B. Streptococcus aureus

C. Pseudomonas aeruginosa D. Salmonella typhimurium

Ans. D.

234. Which of the following antibiotic attaches to 50S ribosome and inhibits peptidyl-transferase activity ?

A. Penicillin B. Chloramphenicol

C. Trimethoprim D. Amphotericin

Ans. B.

235. In a population of 200 individuals which is at equilibrium, the frequency of one of the alleles under study is 0.11. What is the expected frequency of heterozygous individual ?

A. 0.89 B. 0.0979

C. 0.1958 D. 0.842

Ans. C.

236. Antibodies which can cross placenta and are involved in allergic reactions, respectively are

A. IgG and IgA B. IgM and IgE

C. IgG and IgE D. IgD and IgM

Ans. C.

237. cis-trans isomerisation of the peptide bond preceding an amino acid X is known to be critical in the folding of

A. Isoleucine B. Tryptophan

C. Proline D. Histidine

Ans. C.

238. Which one of the following repetitive motifs is responsible for the formation of triple helix in collagen ?

A. Ala-X-Y B. Gly-X-Y

C. Cys-X-Y D. Pro-X-Y

Ans. B. Collagen consists of 3 polypeptide chains. It contains a repeating tripeptide sequence of Gly-X-Y where X is always proline and Y is always hydroxyl proline.

239. Pyrosequencing derives its name from the fact that

A. The bases are detected by pyrolysis

B. It uses enzyme apyrase to detect the bases

C. It detects pyrophosphate released during base incorporation

D. It generates programs as output

Ans. C.

240. In the course of cell cycle, the level of the protein cyclin abruptly falls during

A. G1 B. G2

C. S D. M

Ans. D.

241. Si RNA interfere at

A. Transcriptional level B. Post transcriptional level

C. DNA replication level D. Translational level

Ans. B.

242. Mobile genetic elements present in human genome are

i) LINES ii) SINES

iii) P elements iv) IS elements

A. ii, iii B. i, ii

C. i, iii D. ii, iv

Ans. B.

243. The enzyme(s) that can be used in 5' end labelling of DNA are

A. Alkaline phosphatase B. DNA ligase

C. Terminal transferase D. Polynucleotide kinase

Ans. A, D.

244. The number of replicons in a typical mammalian cell is

A. 40-200 B. 400

C. 1000-2000 D. 50000-100000

Ans. A.

245. What product will result from complete hydrolysis of soluble dextran?

A. Sucrose B. Fructose

C. Glucose and Fructose D. Glucose

Ans. D.

246. The mobility of DNA in agarose gel electrophoresis is solely based on its

A. Charge B. Conformation

C. Size D. None of the above

Ans. C.

247. Which of the following fluorescent probes is used to monitor the progress of amplification of real time PCR ?

A. SYBR Green B. FITC

C. Cyan Blue D. Rhodamine

Ans. A.

248. Expression of which of the following reporter genes does not require addition of specific substrate for detection

A. Luciferase B. Glucuronidase

C. Beta Glucosidase D. Green fluorescent protein

Ans. A.

249. Zinc fingers are characteristic of

A. Blood clotting proteins B. RNA chaperons

C. DNA binding protein D. Lysosomal hydrolyses

Ans. C.

250. The technique used to identify specific DNA sequence in bacterial colonies is

A. Colony hybridization B. In situ hybridization

C. Dot blot technique D. Western blotting

Ans. A.

251. Southern hybridization is

A. Used to identify a specific protein B. Used to identify a specific DNA

C. Used to identify a specific RNA D. Used to identify both DNA and RNA

Ans. B.

252. Which of the following statements are true regarding Southern blotting

A. Developed by E.M. Southern

B. DNA-DNA hybridization is the basis

C. The transfer of DNA from gel to nitrocellulose paper is called blotting

D. All of these

Ans. D.

253. Application of Southern blotting includes

A. DNA fingerprinting B. Preparation of RFLP map

C. Identification of transferred genes D. All of these

Ans. D.

254. The technique used to detect the presence of DNA or RNA in a nonfractionated DNA sample is

A. Colony hybridization B. In situ hybridization

C. Dot blot technique D. Western blotting

Ans. C.

255. Northern hybridization is

A. Used to identify a specific protein B. Used to identify a specific DNA

C. Used to identify a specific RNA D. Used to identify both DNA and RNA

Ans. C.

256. In Northern hybridization probe hybridization forms

A. DNA-DNA hybrid B. RNA-DNA hybrid

C. Both A and B D. None of these

Ans. C.

257. All are differences in procedure between Northern and Southern hybridization except

A. DBM membrane is used in Northern hybridization

B. RNA:DNA hybrids are formed in Northern hybridization

C. Initially fragments are separated by electrophoresis in Northern hybridization

D. DNA denaturation is required before blotting in Southern hybridization

Ans. C.

258. In Western blotting

A. Agrose gel is commonly used B. Polyacrylamide gel is commonly used

C. Both A and B D. High resolution gel

Ans. B.

259. For glycoproteins, most commonly used probe is

A. Antibody B. Lectin

C. Antigen D. Interferon

Ans. B.

260. For protein detection, most commonly used probe is

A. Antibody B. Lectin

C. Antigen D. Interferon

Ans. A.

261. ELISA is based on

A. Antibody –antibody interaction B. Antigen-protein interaction

C. Lectin-antibody interaction D. All of these

Ans. A.

262. The technique used to locate specific genes in chromosomes

A. Colony hybridization B. In situ hybridization

C. Dot blot technique D. Western blotting

Ans. B.

263. The separation technique of charged molecules under the influence of electric current is called

A. Colony hybridization B. Electrophoresis

C. Dot blot technique D. Western blotting

Ans. B.

264. The linking of antibiotic resistance gene with plasmid vector became possible with

A. DNA ligase B. Exonucleases

C. Endonucleases D. DNA polymerases

Ans. A.

265. Human insulin is commercially produced from a transgenic species of

A. Rhizobium B. Escherichia

C. Mycobacterium D. Saccharomyces

Ans. B.

266. A transgenic food crop which may help in solving the problem of night blindness in developing countries is

A. Bt soybean B. Flav Savr tomatoes

C. Golden rice D. Starlink maize

Ans. C.

267. What is antisense technology ?

A. When a piece of RNA that is complementary in sequence is used to stop expression of a specific gene

B. RNA polymerase producing DNA

C. Production of somaclonal variants in tissue cultures

D. A cell displaying a foreign antigen used for synthesis of antigens

Ans. A.

268. Which of the following plant species you would select for the production of bioethanol ?

A. Zea mays B. Jatropa

C. Brassica D. Pongamia

Ans. A.

269. Cry I endotoxins obtained from B.thuringiensis are effective against

A. Nematodes B. Flies

C. Bolt worms D. Mosquitoes

Ans. C.

270. Which of the following is commonly used in transfer of foreign DNA into crop plants ?

A. Trichoderma harzianum B. Penicillium texpansum

C. Agrobacterium tumefaciens D. Meloidogyne incognita

Ans. C.

271. Which of the following are used in gene cloning ?

A. Iomasomes B. Mesosomes

C. Nucleoids D. Plasmids

Ans. D.

272. Which one of the following is used as vector for cloning genes into higher organisms?

A. Retrovirus B. Baculovirus

C. Salmonella typhimurium D. Rhizopus nigricans

Ans. A.

273. Gel electrophoresis is used for

A. Construction of recombinant DNA by joining with cloning vectors

B. Cutting of DNA into fragments

C. Separation of DNA fragments according to their size

D. Isolation of DNA molecules

Ans. C.

274. Who discovered rDNA technology ?

A. Har Gobind Khorana B. J.D.Watson

C. Sutton and Boveri D. Stanley Cohen and Herbert Boyer

Ans. D.

275. Match the name of the scientist with their contributions and choose the correct answer

A. Walter Sutton — 1. Discovered penicillin

B. Stanley Cohen — 2. Discovered double helical structure of DNA

C. Alexander Fleming — 3. Discovered the chromosomal basis of heredity

D. James D.Watson — 4. Discovered rDNA

A. a2, b1, c4, d3 B. a3, b4, c1, d2

C. a1, b3, c2, d4 D. a4, b3, c2, d1

Ans. B.

276. Which of the following is a plasmid ?

A. Sal I B. Bam HI

C. Eco RI D. pBR322

Ans. D.

277. Restriction enzymes are

A. DNA unwinding enzymes B. DNA joining enzymes

C. DNA cleaving enzymes D. None of these

Ans. C.

278. The enzyme used to join the DNA fragments

A. Topoisomerase B. DNA ligase

C. DNA polymerase D. Reverse transcriptase

Ans. B.

279. Which of the following is used as vector in gene therapy for SCID ?

A. Arbovirus B. Rotavirus

C. Parovovirus D. Retrovirus

Ans. D.

280. Ti plasmid used in genetic engineering is obtained from

A. Bacillus thuringiensis B. Agrobacterium rhizogenes

C. Agrobacterium tumefaciens D. Bacillus subtilis

Ans. C.

281. The vector for T-DNA is

A. Thermus aquaticus B. Bacillus tumefaciens

C. Agrobacterium tumefaciens D. E. coli

Ans. C.

282. cry II Ab and cry I Ab produce toxins that control

A. Corn borer and tobacco budworms respectively

B. Nematodes and tobacco budworms respectively

C. Cotton bollworms and corn borer respectively

D. Corn borer and cotton bollworms respectively

Ans. C.

283. In genetic engineering, a DNA segment of interest, is transferred to the host cell through a vector. Tick the right answer

i. bacterium ii. Plasmid iii. Plasmodium iv. Bacteriophage

A. i, ii, iv
B. ii, iv
C. i, iv
D. i only

Ans. B.

284. Genetic engineering is possible because

A. We can cut DNA at specific sites by endonucleases like DNase I

B. Restriction endonucleases purified from bacteria can be used in vitro

C. The phenomenon of transduction in bacteria is well understood

D. we can see DNA by electron microscope

Ans. B.

285. Restriction endonucleases are

A. Used to in vitro DNA synthesis

B. Used in genetic engineering

C. Synthesized by bacteria

D. Present in mammalian cells for degradation of DNA

Ans. B.

286. Transgenic animals are those which are

A. Foreign RNA in all its cells
B. Foreign DNA in some of its cells
C. Foreign DNA in all its cells
D. Both A & B.

Ans. C.

287. The first transgenic plant was

A. Tobacco
B. Pea
C. Flax
D. cotton

Ans. A.

288. Which of the following is related to genetic engineering ?

A. Plastid B. Plasmid

C. Heterosis D. Mutation

Ans. B.

289. First cloned animal

A. Dolly sheep B. Dog

C. Mule D. Cat

Ans. A.

290. Which of the following bases in plasmids discovered so far

A. 50 Kb B. 500 Kb

C. 5 Kb D. 5 bases

Ans. B.

291. Plasmid has been used as vector because

A. It has antibiotic resistance gene

B. It is circular DNA which have capacity to join to eukaryotic DNA

C. Both ends show replication

D. It can move between prokaryotic and eukaryotic cells

Ans. B.

292. The bacteria generally used for genetic engineering is

A. Bacillus B. Pseudomonas

C. Clostridium D. Agrobacterium

Ans. D.

293. Which of the following cut the DNA from specific places

A. E. coli restriction endonuclease II B. Ligase

C. Exonuclease D. Alkaline phosphatise

Ans. A.

294. For mitochondrial structure and function mt-DNA species

A. 10% B. 20%

C. 30% D. 40%

Ans. A.

295. Which of the following reagent is useful for visualizing DNA ?

A. Uracil B. DNA polymerase

C. Diphenylamine D. Ethidium bromide

Ans. D.

296. Most plant cells are surrounded by a rigid cell wall made primarily of

A. Monosaccharide B. Pectin

C. Chitins D. Polysaccharides

Ans. D.

297. The organelle that functions in the breakdown of cells and tissues is the

A. Episome B. Mitochondrion

C. Centrosomes D. Lysosomes

Ans. D.

298. Endoplasmic reticulum

A. Is found only in animals

B. Is a system of membrane bound channels

C. Is called rough if mitochondria is attached to it

D. Is a site of ATP production

Ans. B.

299. The function of nucleus includes

A. Cellular respiration

B. Synthesis of proteins

C. Housing the hereditary information

D. Synthesis of carbohydrates

Ans. C.

300. Baculoviruses

A. RNA viruses B. DNA viruses

C. Both A & B D. None of the above

Ans. B.

301. Secondary metabolites like antibiotics are not essential for

A. Log phase growth B. Exponential growth

C. Both A & B D. None of these

Ans. C.

302. Which of the following vector is suitable for DNA sequencing

A. EMBL B. PBR 322

C. M13 D. Lamda

Ans. C.

303. During which process the free end of the chromosome move from Hfr donor in to the F cell across an intracellular bridge called piles

A. Transformation
B. Transduction
C. Conjugation
D. All the above

Ans. C.

304. Francis Jacob and Monod proposed

A. Lock and key hypothesis
B. Gene for protein synthesis
C. Operon synthesis
D. None of the above

Ans. C.

305. Which of the following is not a desired characteristic of a vector

A. Unique restriction site
B. Large size
C. Gene that confer antibiotic resistance
D. Autonomous replication

Ans. B.

306. Which of the following chemical is used for preparation of competent cell ?

A. HCl
B. NaCl
C. CaCl2
D. Glycine

Ans. C.

307. Endochitinase can be used as an

A. Antibacterial
B. Antiviral
C. Antifungal
D. Antinematodal

Ans. C.

308. The direct DNA uptake by the protoplast is stimulated by

A. Cellulose
B. Sucrose
C. PEG
D. Mannose

Ans. C.

309. Which of the following is an herbicide resistant gene ?

A. Bar
B. Hpt
C. Chitinase
D. Oxidase

Ans. A.

310. Restriction enzymes that cut straight across the DNA produce

A. Nick
B. Sticky end
C. Blunt end
D. None of these

Ans. C.

311. Lambda has short single stranded 5' projection of

A. 8 nucleotide length
B. 10 nucleotide length
C. 12 nucleotide length
D. 14 nucleotide length

Ans. C.

312. In Agrobacterium mediated plant transformation which one of the following is used to check the Agrobacterium growth

A. PPT
B. Kanamycin
C. Timentin
D. Penicillin

Ans. C.

313. The T-DNA region of all the Ti and Ri plasmid are flanked by direct repeat sequence

A. 15 bp
B. 20 bp
C. 25 bp
D. 35 bp

Ans. C.

314. Most commonly used strategy to develop transgenic plant against any viral disease is to engineer a

A. Antisense RNA for viral genome
B. Coat or capsid protein gene
C. Direct DNA transfer to viral gene
D. Liposome mediated transfer of viral RNA

Ans. B.

315. Replication of DNA by rolling cycle mechanism give rise to a

A. Blunt end DNA
B. Theta structure
C. Concatamer
D. Single strand DNA with nick

Ans. C.

316. The gene transferred from E. coli to tobacco to increase the level of manitol is

A. Manitol dehydrogenase
B. Manitol carboxylase
C. Manitol oxygenase
D. Manitol hydrolase

Ans. A.

317. Relaxed plasmid

A. Have oly single copy per cell
B. Can not be purified
C. Does not exist in bacteria
D. Have multiple copies per cell

Ans. D.

318. In vitro packaging is required for which one of the following vector

A. BAC B. YAC

C. PAC D. None of these

Ans. C.

319. Cosmids have the Cos site of

A. Lambda B. Plasmid

C. ML3 D. YAC

Ans. A.

320. Thiobacillus thioxidans grows on

A. Iron B. Sulphur

C. Aluminium D. Pyrites

Ans. D.

321. Which of the following characteristic differentiate lysosome from other cell organelles ?

A. Lysosome is a micro organelle

B. Lysosome is a single membrane bounded organelle

C. Lysosomes present only in plants

D. All of the above

Ans. B.

322. The main function of carotenoid in photosynthesis is

A. Light absorption

B. prevention of photooxidation of chlorophyll

C. Act as light absorbing centre

D. Act as source of electron

Ans. B.

323. Most essential features required to maintain a plasmid in a host cell is

A. Ability to transfect cells

B. Antibiotic resistance

C. Origin of replication and marker for selection

D. Capacity to insert into the host genome

Ans. C.

324. Abzymes are

A. Zymogens B. inactive proteinases

C. antibody with catalytic activity D. RNA with catalytic activity

Ans. C.

325. Which of the following organelle is absent in plants ?

A. Mitochondria
B. Peroxisomes
C. Glyoxysomes
D. Lysosomes

Ans. D.

326. Cytoplast is

A. Enucleated protoplast
B. A cytoplasmic hybrid
C. A cell without cell wall
D. A cell without vacuole

Ans. A.

327. Individuals of a species inhabiting the same geographic area is called

A. Allopatric
B. Sympatric
C. Parapatric
D. Metapatric

Ans. B.

328. Microtubules are the main components of

A. Spindle apparatus
B. Muscle network
C. Nuclear membrane complex
D. Actin network

Ans. A.

329. In an ant colony, the male individuals will be

A. Haploid
B. Diploid
C. Triploid
D. Polyploid

Ans. A.

330. An important characteristic of a house keeping gene

A. They are all inducible gene
B. They are permanently kept inactive in somatic cells
C. All expressed in all cells
D. They are positively regulated gene

Ans. C.

331. Which of the following cancer can be prevented by vaccination ?

A. Oral cancer
B. Cervical cancer
C. Breast cancer
D. Colon cancer

Ans. B.

332. Individuals having X chromosome and short arm of Y chromosome are males, while individuals having X chromosome and long arm of Y chromosome are female. This shows that –

A. Genes for maleness are located on short arm of Y chromosome

B. Genes for maleness are located on long arm of Y chromosome

C. Genes for maleness are located on the X chromosome

D. Male determining genes are located on Y chromosome

Ans. A.

333. Xeroderma pigmentosum is a genetic disorder caused by error in ——.

A. Base excision repair mechanism B. Nucleotide excision repair mechanism

C. Direct repair mechanism D. DNA replication mechanism

Ans. B.

334. Which of the following antibiotic inhibit 80S ribosomes

A. Tetracycline B. Streptomycin

C. Cyclohexamide D. Chloramphenicol

Ans. C.

335. The toxic mechanism of diphtheria toxin is by ——.

A. ADP ribosylation of EF-2

B. ADP ribosylation of EF-1α

C. blocking the activity of RNA polymerase

D. blocking DNA replication process

Ans. A.

336. A major functional difference between the succinyl CoA-synthetase of plant and animal cell mitochondria is that

A. Does not produce ATP in plant cells

B. Produce UTP in plant cells

C. Produce ATP in plant and GTP in animals

D. Produce GTP in plant and ATP in animals

Ans. C.

337. Which one of the following is not considered as a potential pollutant?

A. CO B. CO2

C. SO2 D. NOx

Ans. B.

338. As per the IUCN red data list, which taxa contains maximum number of endangered and critically endangered species ?

A. Amphibians B. Reptiles

C. Mammals D. Birds

Ans. A.

339. In molecular systematic of animals, which of the following candidate gene have been extensively used ?

A. DNA polymerase
B. Cytochrome C
C. RNA polymerase
D. Collagen

Ans. B.

340. As we move from one geographical region to next neighbouring region, species diversity tends to change. It is termed as

A. α diversity
B. β diversity
C. γ diversity
D. δ diversity

Ans. B.

341. In stomach, the mucus which protect the epithelial lining of stomach, is secreted by

A. Goblet cells
B. Parietal cells
C. Microvilli
D. Aciner cells

Ans. A.

342. Chitin is a major cell wall component of————.

A. Bacteria
B. Arthropods
C. Fungus
D. Mollusks

Ans. C.

343. The anti-cancer drug obtained from Catharanthus roseus is ———.

A. Taxol
B. Vincristine
C. Colchicine
D. Serpentine

Ans. B.

344. An oligonucletide DNA sequence tagged with fluorescent tag used to identify unknown gene by hybridization is termed as

A. Probe
B. Reporter gene
C. Ligand
D. cDNA

Ans. A.

345. Bacteria undergo multiplication by

A. Binary fission
B. Mitosis
C. Fission and mitosis
D. Fragmentation

Ans. A.

346. Bacterial DNA polymerase I lack which of the following activity ?

A. 5'-3' polymerase activity
B. 3'-5' polymerase activity
C. 5'-3' exonuclease activity
D. 3'-5' exonuclease activity

Ans. B.

347. When releasing factor binds to stop codon on m-RNA during translation the synthesized peptide chain is transferred to

A. tRNA
B. Water
C. H+
D. Amino acid

Ans. B.

348. The radio isotope which is usually incorporated into thymine to study DNA replication process is

A. ^{32}P
B. ^{35}S
C. ^{3}H
D. ^{14}C

Ans. C.

349. Globular proteins when treated with organic solvents get denatured. The main interaction which is affected on treatment with organic solvent is

A. Hydrogen bonds
B. Covalent bonds
C. Ionic interactions
D. Hydrophobic interactions

Ans. D.

350. Which region of visible light is most useful for phtotosynthesis ?

A. Blue and red
B. Green and red
C. Violet and blue
D. Green and blue

Ans. A.

351. Fog, which is commonly observed during winter is mainly seen at

A. Low altitude with pollution
B. High altitude without pollution
C. High altitude with pollution
D. Low altitude without pollution

Ans. D.

352. Natural killer cells can be detected in human peripheral blood using

A. Anti-cd3 antibody
B. Anti-cd25 antibody
C. Anti-cd69 antibody
D. Anti-cd16 antibody

Ans. D.

353. Deoxy position of deoxyribose in DNA is at

A. 1st carbon
B. 3rd carbon
C. 2nd carbon
D. 5th carbon

Ans. C.

354. Which of the following non-coding RNAs is involved in RNA editing ?

A. Sn RNA B. Si RNA

C. gRNA D. Mi RNA

Ans. C.

355. Which of the following techniques is used for the evaluation of phylogenetic trees?

A. Null hypothesis B. Bootstrapping

C. Chi-square D. Probability

Ans. B.

356. One Pam means one accepted point mutation per

A. 10^2 residues B. 10 residues

C. 10^3 residues D. 10^4 residues

Ans. A.

357. Intestinal flora can not digest

A. Cellulose B. Lignin

C. Pectin D. Starch

Ans. D.

358. All the following are malignant neoplasms except

A. Papilloma B. Liposarcoma

C. Squamous cell carcinoma D. Neuroblastoma

Ans. A.

359. Replication of papillomavirus is restricted to

A. Epithelial cells B. Nerve cells

C. Fibroblasts D. Reticuloendothelial cells

Ans. A.

360. A mammalian cell has an outstretched double stranded DNA of 1.2 meters which duplicates in 4 h. If it duplicates @ 20 μm/min, how many origins of replication are there in the DNA?

A. 2500 B. 250

C. 25 D. 1

Ans. B.

361. Sperm DNA is covered by

A. Lipids B. Protamines

C. Carbohydrates D. Histones

Ans. B.

362. Testosterone hormone necessary for spermatogenesis is secreted by

A. Sertoli cell
B. Leydig cell
C. Spermatozoa
D. Cowpers gland

Ans. B.

363. Cholesterol contributes to which of the following properties of biological membranes?

A. Membrane rigidity
B. Membrane fluidity
C. Membrane permeability
D. Membrane osmolarity

Ans. B.

364. Penicillin resistant bacteria produce beta lactamase which inactivates penicillin by

A. Esterifying the carboxyl group
B. Oxidizing S atom
C. Hydrolysing the side chain
D. Hydrolyzing the C-N bond

Ans. D.

365. Pseudomurein present in cell wall of

A. Streptococci
B. Staphylococci
C. Methanococci
D. Micrococci

Ans. C.

366. Bacteria that can penetrate the intact corneal epithelium is

A. P. aeruginosa
B. Staphylococcus aureus
C. L. monocytogenes
D. Yersinia pestis

Ans. B.

367. Which of the following bacterial toxins does not have ADP-ribosyl transferase activity ?

A. Cholera toxin
B. Diphtheria toxin
C. Exotoxin A
D. S. aureus alpha toxin

Ans. D.

368. The oxygen carrying protein of invertebrate is

A. Hemoglobin
B. Hemocyanin
C. Myoglobin
D. Ceruloplasmin

Ans. B.

369. The bond length of hydrogen bond in water is approximately

A. 0.177 nm
B. 0.177A°
C. 1.77 nm
D. 0.77 um

Ans. A.

370. Which is the most preferred carbon source for E. coli

A. Glucose B. Glycerol

C. Galactose D. Sucrose

Ans. A.

371. Interferons

A. Activate B cells to make virus specific antibodies

B. Are Th2 cytokines

C. Are virus proteins that interfere with activation of cytotoxic cells

D. Inhibit virus replication by infected cells

Ans. D.

372. Activated form of insulin contains

A. 2 inter chain disulphide bonds

B. 2 intra chain and 1 inter chain disulphide bonds

C. 1 intra chain and 2 inter chain disulphide bonds

D. Two intra chain disulphide bonds

Ans. C.

373. Which of the following is not considered as prion disease ?

A. Kuru B. CJD

C. BSE D. Alzeimer

Ans. D.

374. It was found that normal stem cells isolated from brain have a doubling time of 24hours whereas tumor derived cells have a doubling time of 12 hours. Both these cells types were grown in the presence of radioactive thymidine for 24 hours, following which they were grown in normal media. After the end of a week, radioactivity per cell will be

A. Double in stem cells as compared to cancer cells

B. Half in stem cells as compared to cancer cells

C. Same in both stem and cancer cells

D. None in stem cells and high level in cancer cells

Ans. B.

375. The average size of 70S ribosomes of prokaryotes are

A. 200 A° B. 250 A°

C. 290 A° D. 303 A°

Ans. A.

376. Which of the following is an example for chemolithotroph ?

A. Acidithiobacillus ferrooxidans B. B.nitrosomonas

C. C.nitrobacter D. All of the above

Ans. D.

377. Which of the following is an example for denitrifying bacteria ?

A. Nitrosomonas B. Nitrobacter

C. Pseudomonas D. All of the above

Ans. C.

378. Who introduced the group Archaea for a group of prokaryotes on the basis of phylogenetic analysis of 16S rRNA ?

A. Roger Stainer B. Carl Woese

C. C.B.van Niel D. Theodor Escherich

Ans. B.

379. Who discovered endoplasmic reticulum ?

A. Keith Porter B. K. Mereschkowsky

C. C.Golgi D. G.E. Palade

Ans. A.

380. Acrosome in sperm cell is a modified

A. Lysosome B. Peroxisome

C. Golgi D. None of these

Ans. C.

381. Calmodulin is a calcium binding messenger protein of eukaryotic cells. A single calmodulin protein at a time can bind ——— Ca+2 ions.

A. 1 B. 2

C. 3 D. 4

Ans. D.

382. The H-O-H bond angle of water molecule is ——

A. 103.5° B. 104.5°

C. 105.5° D. 109.5°

Ans. B.

383. At a time a single water molecule can form — hydrogen bonds with other water molecules

A. 1 B. 2

C. 3 D. 4

Ans. D.

384. pH below pI amino acid will be————.

A. Cationic
B. Anionic
C. No charge
D. Net charge zero

Ans. A.

385. Which of the following is an example for a ribozyme ?

A. Transpeptidase
B. Glutamyl transpeptidase
C. Peptidyl transferase
D. All of the above

Ans. C.

386. An auto immune disease that affects the thyroid gland

A. Tay-Sach disease
B. Addition's disease
C. Graves' disease
D. Behcet's disease

Ans. C.

387. Weil-Felix test is used for the diagnosis of

A. Rickettsial infection
B. Pertussis
C. Cholera
D. African sleeping sickness

Ans. A.

388. The 20 different amino acids in the protein are normally coded by

A. 60 codons
B. 61 codons
C. 62 codons
D. 64 codons

Ans. B.

389. Cleavage of DNA by EcoRI endonuclease results in the formation of

A. Two 3'-OH ends and two 5'-phosphate ends
B. One 3'-OH end and one 5'-phosphate end
C. Two 3'-phosphate ends and two 3'-OH ends
D. One 3'-OH end and two 5'-phosphate end

Ans. A.

390. Which of the following amino acids is coded by maximum number of codons ?

A. Leucine
B. Tryptophan
C. Valine
D. Alanine

Ans. A.

391. Which of the following amino acids in a protein forms a 'salt bridge'?

A. Tyr-Phe
B. Cys-Cys
C. Lys-Glu
D. Ala-Val

Ans. C.

392. The reason for the melting of DNA double helix at specific temperature is
   A. Loss of base stacking energy
   B. The double helix is intrinsically unstable
   C. The single helix is more stable than double helix
   D. The double helix is a co-operative structure stabilized by hydrogen bonds and base pairing

Ans. D.

393. Which of the following RNA is involved in gene expression regulation ?
   A. rRNA B. 5.5 S RNA
   C. tRNA D. miRNA

Ans. D.

394. If the ratio of (A+G)/(T+C) in one strand of DNA is 0.70, what is the same ratio in the complementary strand ?
   A. 0.70 B. 1.43
   C. 0.35 D. 0.30

Ans. B.

395. How many different transfer RNA molecules are possible in a hypothetical organism where the ribosome detect a quadruplet instead of a triplet codon including the start and stop codon ?
   A. 64 B. 128
   C. 20 D. 256

Ans. D.

396. If a species contain 23% adenine in its DNA, then the percentage of guanine in its DNA would be
   A. 23 B. 46
   C. 54 D. 27

Ans. D.

397. During photosynthesis the source of O2 is
   A. Water B. CO2
   C. Glucose D. Chlorophyll

Ans. A.

398. Which of the following bacteria is not naturally competent ?
   A. B.subtilis B. E. coli
   C. Streptococcus pneumoniae D. Haemophilus influenza

Ans. B.

399. The enzyme used in SoLiD sequencing technology is

A. Sequenase B. DNA polymerase

C. DNA ligase D. Taq polymerase

Ans. C.

400. Which of the following chemotherapeutic drugs has neurotoxicity

A. Vincristine B. Cyclophosphamide

C. Anthracyclines D. Adriamycin

Ans. A.

401. Which of the following does not contribute to protein diversity ?

A. RNA editing B. RNA splicing

C. RNA interference D. Alternative initiation of translation

Ans. C.

402. A mRNA is 336 bases long including the initiation and termination codon. The number of amino acids in the polypeptide translated from this is

A. 110 B. 333

C. 111 D. 600

Ans. A.

403. Specific biomolecules which show easily detectable differences among different strains of a species or among different species is termed as

A. DNA fingerprinting B. Molecular markers

C. Molecular scissors D. RFLP

Ans. B.

404. Molecular markers include

A. RFLP B. RAPD

C. AFLP D. All of these

Ans. D.

405. Molecular markers are used to construct

A. Chromosome maps B. Cytogenetic maps

C. Physical maps D. All of these

Ans. D.

406. The variation in the restriction DNA fragment lengths between individuals of a species is called

A. Restriction fragment length polymorphism (RFLP)

B. Random amplified polymorphic DNA

C. Amplified fragment length polymorphism

D. Simple sequence repeats

Ans. A.

407. RFLP is used to

A. Construct high resolution linkage maps

B. Identify single gene disease

C. Construct QTL maps

D. All of these

Ans. D.

408. Locations of quantitative genes on chromosomes are called

A. Qualitative trait loci

B. Quantitative trait loci

C. Both A & B

D. None of these

Ans. B.

409. RAPD is a

A. DNA sequencing based method

B. Restriction digestion based method

C. PCR based method

D. All of these

Ans. C.

410. The set of DNAs generated by using random primers in a PCR reaction is called

A. RAPD

B. RFLP

C. AFLP

D. in situ hybridization

Ans. A.

411. All the statements are true regarding RFLP and RAPD except

A. RAPD is a quick method compared to RFLP

B. RFLP is more reliable than RAPD

C. Species specific primers are required for RAPD

D. Radioactive probes are not required in RAPD

Ans. C.

412. DNA of eukaryotic organisms has several repeating units of short sequences called

A. Random repeats

B. Tandem repeats

C. Mini satellites

D. All of these

Ans. B.

413. The variation in number of tandem repeats between 2 or more individuals is called

A. Variable number of tandem repeats (VNTRs)

B. Restrict fragment length polymorphisms (RFLPs)

C. Simple sequence repeats (SSRs)

D. Amplified fragment length polymorphism (AFLP)

Ans. A.

414. Simple sequence repeats are

A. 1-6 bp long sequences distributed along the chromosome

B. Also called micro satellites

C. Individual specific in number and position

D. All of these

Ans. D.

415. AFLP is a

A. PCR based method

B. Method to detect polymorphism in the DNA throughout the genome

C. Method that detects the presence or absence of a fragment

D. All of these

Ans. D.

416. The variant fragment that distinguish one individual from another one is called

A. Variant length B. Marking fragment

C. Differing fragment D. All of these

Ans. B.

417. Any DNA molecule that has the ability to replicate in an appropriate host cell to which the desired gene are integrated for cloning is called as

A. Plasmid B. Linker

C. Vector D. Adaptor

Ans. C.

418. Which of the following statement is true

A. A vector should have an origin of replication

B. A vector should have selectable markers

C. A vector should have unique restriction sites

D. All of these

Ans. D.

419. Expression vectors differ from a cloning vector in having

A. An origin of replication B. Suitable marker genes

C. Unique restriction sites D. Control elements

Ans. D.

420. Extra chromosomal double stranded circular DNA molecules present in bacteria which is widely used as a vector is called

A. Phagemid B. Cosmid

C. Plasmid D. Bacterial vectors

Ans. C.

421. The first engineered plasmid vector is

A. pBR322 B. pUC vectors

C. pSC 101 D. pUC19

Ans. C.

422. The most popular and widely used engineered plasmid vector is

A. pBR322 B. pUC vectors

C. pSC 101 D. pUC19

Ans. A.

423. In pBR 322, pBR stands for

A. Plasmid bacterial recombination B. Plasmid bacterial replication

C. Plasmid Boliver and Rodriguez D. Plasmid Baltimore and Rodriguez

Ans. C.

424. Phase M13 vectors are widely used for

A. Obtaining single stranded copies of cloned DNA suitable for DNA sequencing

B. Obtaining double stranded copies of cloned DNA suitable for DNA sequencing

C. Obtaining fragments of cloned DNA suitable for DNA sequencing

D. Obtaining double stranded copies of cloned DNA suitable for electrophoresis

Ans. A.

425. Cosmid is plasmid with

A. A minimum of 250 bp of lambda DNA that includes cos site

B. A minimum of 250 bp of M13 DNA that includes cos site

C. A minimum of 100 bp of lambda that includes cos site

D. A minimum of 250 bp of T4 phage DNA that includes cos site

Ans. A.

426. Vectors designed to replicate in cells of two different species are called

A. Plasmids B. Transfer vectors

C. Shuttle vectors D. Phagemids

Ans. C.

427. Autonomously replicating sequences (ARS) is a characteristic feature of

A. Plasmid vectors
B. Phage vectors
C. E. coli vectors
D. Yeast vectors

Ans. D.

428. Which of the following are vectors for animals

A. SV40 vectors and bovine papillomavirus vectors
B. CMV vectors and Gemini vectors
C. Lambda phage and M13 vectors
D. All of these

Ans. A.

429. The vectors commonly used for sequencing human genome

A. Yeast artificial chromosome
B. Plasmid
C. CMV vectors
D. M13 vectors

Ans. A.

430. Ti plasmid that is used as a plant vector is obtained from

A. Agrobacterium tumefaciens
B. Agrobacterium rhizhogenes
C. Agrobacterium radiobacter
D. Thermus aquaticus

Ans. A.

431. The most common vectors for plants are

A. SV40 vectors and bovine papillomavirus vectors
B. Cauliflower mosaic virus (CMV vectors) and Gemini vectors
C. Lambda phage and M13 phage vectors
D. T4 phage vectors

Ans. B.

432. The process involved in the RNA formation on the DNA template is

A. Transcription
B. Translation
C. Replication
D. Transformation

Ans. A.

433. The enzyme required for transcription is

A. Restriction enzymes
B. DNA polymerase
C. RNA polymerase
D. RNase

Ans. C.

434. Transcription is the transfer of genetic information from

A. DNA to RNA
B. tRNA to mRNA
C. DNA to mRNA
D. mRNA to tRNA

Ans. C.

435. RNA required for the protein synthesis

A. mRNA
B. rRNA
C. tRNA
D. All of these

Ans. D.

436. A promoter site on DNA

A. Initiates transcription
B. Regulates termination
C. Codes for RNA
D. Transcribes repressor

Ans. A.

437. Sigma factor is component of

A. DNA ligase
B. DNA polymerase
C. RNA polymerase
D. Endonuclease

Ans. C.

438. What is the main function of tRNA in relation to protein synthesis ?

A. Inhibits protein synthesis
B. Proof reading
C. Identifies amino acids and transport them to ribosomes
D. All of these

Ans. C.

439. RNA polymerase has polypeptide chains

A. 2
B. 3
C. 4
D. 5

Ans. D.

440. Which site of tRNA molecule hydrogen bonds to a mRNA molecule ?

A. Codon
B. Anticodon
C. 5’ ends of the tRNA molecule
D. 3’ ends of the tRNA molecule

Ans. B.

441. The DNA chain acting as template for RNA synthesis has the following order of bases, AGCTTCGA.What will be the order of bases in mRNA

A. TCGAAGCT
B. UGCUAGCT
C. TCGAUCGU
D. UCGAAGCU

Ans. D.

442. Protein synthesis refers to the
   A. Process of formation of amino acids directly from a DNA template
   B. Process of formation of mRNA from DNA template
   C. Process of formation of amino acids from mRNA
   D. Process of duplicating DNA required for protein synthesis

Ans. C.

443. Which of the following is not a requirement for protein synthesis ?
   A. Ribosomes B. Peptidyl transferase
   C. Spliceosome D. Seryl-tRNS synthetase

Ans. C.

444. The enzyme involved in activation of serine is
   A. Peptidyl transferase B. Amino acyl-tRNA synthetase
   C. Peptide polymerase D. Seryl-tRNA synthetase

Ans. D.

445. Which is the source of energy for amino acid activation ?
   A. ATP B. GTP
   C. CTP D. TTP

Ans. A.

446. Which of the following statement is correct ?
   A. Termination codon has no tRNA
   B. Activated amino acid binds to the 5' end of respective tRNA molecule
   C. CTP is required for amino acid activation
   D. There is only one amino acyl-tRNA synthetase in a cell

Ans. A.

447. The preinitiation complex in prokaryotes include
   A. Initiation factors, mRNA, 30S subunit, 50S subunit, ATP
   B. Initiation factors, mRNA, 30S subunit, GTP
   C. Initiation factors, 30S subunit, 50S subunit, ATP
   D. Initiation factors, mRNA, 50S subunit, GTP

Ans. B.

448. Peptide bond formation between amino acids of growing polypeptide chain is catalysed by
   A. Peptidyl transferase B. Amino acyl-tRNA synthetase
   C. Peptide polymerase D. Peptidyl synthetase

Ans. A.

449. Translocation in protein synthesis begins with the
   A. Movement of tRNA from A site to P site
   B. Movement of dipeptidyl tRNA from A site to P site
   C. Movement of tRNA from P site to A site
   D. Movement of tRNA from P site to E site

Ans. B.

450. Peptidyl transferase involved in peptide bond formation is located in the
   A. 3' region
   B. Smaller subunit of ribosome
   C. Larger subunit of ribosome
   D. Near Shine Dalgarno sequence

Ans. C.

451. The amino acids are assembled into polypeptide chains on
   A. mRNA
   B. Nucleus
   C. Ribosome
   D. DNA template

Ans. C.

452. Which of the following release factor recognizes stop codons UGA and UAA ?
   A. Sigma factor
   B. RF1
   C. RF2
   D. RF3

Ans. C.

453. Protein binding regions of DNA are identified by one of the following techniques?
   A. Finger printing
   B. Foot printing
   C. Southern blotting
   D. Western blotting

Ans. B.

454. Transposon is known as
   A. IS element
   B. Jumping gene
   C. Conservative gene
   D. Co-integrate gene

Ans. B.

455. The uptake of plasmid DNA into the bacterial cell is facilitated by the presence of—— in the medium
   A. Calcium Chloride
   B. Potassium Chloride
   C. Magnesium Chloride
   D. None of these

Ans. A.

456. The travel of gene expression and gene activation can be measured using which of the following ?
   A. Reporter gene
   B. Marker gene
   C. Gene sequences
   D. Promoter element

Ans. B.

457. The enzyme required to obtain wall free/naked protoplasts are

A. Cellulase and proteinase
B. Cellulase and Pectinase
C. Cellulase and Amylase
D. Amylase and Pectinase

Ans. B.

458. A synchronous culture is one in which the majority of cells proceed through

A. Lag phase
B. Log phase
C. Exponential phase
D. Each cell cycle phase (G1, S, G2 and M)

Ans. D.

459. DNA molecules, identical except for different numbers of superhelical turns are called

A. Chain isolers
B. Topoisomers
C. Helical isomers
D. Geometrical isomers

Ans. B.

460. Application of embryo culture is in

A. Clonal propagation
B. Production of alkaloids
C. Production of soma clonal variation
D. Overcoming hybridization barrier

Ans. D.

461. Haploid culture are got from

A. Leaves
B. Root tips
C. Pollen grain
D. Bud

Ans. C.

462. Differentiation of shoot in plant culture is controlled by

A. High auxin-cytokinin ratio
B. High cytokinin - auxin ratio
C. High gibberellins-cytokinin ratio
D. High gibberellins- auxin ratio

Ans. B.

463. Which of the following is an amine hormone ?

A. Progesterone
B. Thyroxine
C. Oxypurin
D. Insulin

Ans. B.

464. T.O. Diener discovered a

A. Free infectious DNA
B. Infectious protein
C. Bacteriophage
D. Free infectious RNA

Ans. D.

465. Montreal Protocol aim at

A. Biodiversity conservation
B. Bontrol of water pollution
C. Bontrol of carbon dioxide emission
D. Reduction of ozone depleting substances

Ans. D.

466. Which one of the following is not used in organic farming ?

A. Glomus
B. Oscillatoria
C. Snail
D. Earth worm

Ans. C.

467. Which of the following is the most important discovery that leads to the development of rDNA technology ?

A. Discovery of double helix model by Watson and Crick
B. Discovery of DNA as genetic material
C. Discovery of restriction enzymes
D. All of the above

Ans. C.

468. Who discovered restriction enzymes

A. Watson and Crick
B. Jacob and Monad
C. Nathan, Arber and Smith
D. Boyer and Cohen

Ans. C.

469. Restriction enzymes are enzymes

A. Capable of cutting DNA molecule
B. Capable of adding nucleotides to the 3'OH end
C. Capable of restricting protein synthesis
D. Capable of joining DNA molecules

Ans. A.

470. Restriction enzymes capable of making internal cuts in a DNA molecule is called

A. Restriction exonuclease B. Restriction endonuclease

C. Both A & B D. S1 nuclease

Ans. B.

471. Restriction enzymes are also called

A. Molecular knives B. Molecular scissors

C. Molecular scalpels D. All of these

Ans. D.

472. The sequence recognized by the restriction enzymes to cut the DNA is called

A. Recognition site B. Restriction site

C. Both A & B D. Cleavage site

Ans. C.

473. Which of the following are true regarding restriction enzyme

A. Restriction enzyme are used to cut DNA molecule

B. Restriction enzyme are used to construct restriction maps

C. Restriction enzyme are used in RFLP

D. All of these

Ans. D.

474. The type of restriction enzymes used in rDNA technology is

A. Type I B. Type II

C. Type III D. All of these

Ans. B.

475. Which of the following statements are true regarding restriction enzymes

A. Type I and II enzymes cut far away from the restriction sites

B. Type II cuts DNA within restriction sites

C. Eco R I is a Type II restriction enzyme

D. All of these

Ans. D.

476. Restriction sites of type II enzymes

A. Generally are palindromic sequences

B. Consists of 4-6 bp

C. Mostly are palindromes with rotational symmetry

D. All of these

Ans. D.

477. Single stranded unpaired extensions formed by restriction enzyme upon cleavage is called as

A. Blunt ends
B. Flush ends
C. Sticky ends
D. None of these

Ans. C.

478. Which of the following ions are required for the activity of Type II restriction enzymes ?

A. Ca^{++}
B. Mg^{++}
C. Cl^{-2}
D. Mn^{++}

Ans. B.

479. Restriction enzymes

A. Are present in bacteria and are involved in host restriction system
B. Cleave viral DNA inside bacterium
C. Are enzymes involved in defence against bacteriophages
D. All of these

Ans. D.

480. Nathen, Arber and Smith were awarded with Nobel prize for physiology and medicine in the year

A. 1970
B. 1974
C. 1978
D. 1980

Ans. C.

481. The first Type II enzyme isolated was

A. Eco RI
B. Hind III
C. Bam HI
D. Sal I

Ans. B.

482. If the percentage of adenine in a DNA sample is 20%, what would be the percentage of other bases ?

A. T=30%, G=20%, C=30%
B. T=40%, G=20%, C=20%
C. T=20%, G=30%, C=30%
D. T=20%, G=20%, C=40%

Ans. C.

483. Which of the following statement is incorrect ?

A. DNA is the only biomolecule with self repair mechanism
B. DNA is autocatalytic
C. DNA is heterocatalytic
D. increasing temperature to 90-100oC breaks phosphodiester bonds in DNA

Ans. D.

484. In a DNA sample, the percentage on bases is G=30% and C=40%. The most probable explanation is

A. Mutation might have occurred

B. The DNA sample may be a bacterial genome

C. The DNA sample may be a viral genome

D. None of these

Ans. C.

485. Which of these following statement is true ?

A. DNA bases varies from one species to another

B. DNA bases of a species does not change with age nutritional state and environment

C. DNA base remains same in different tissues of the same individual

D. All of these

Ans. D.

486. The negative change of DNA is due to

A. Sugar phosphage and amino acids

B. Deoxyribose sugar

C. Nitrogenous bases specifically adenine

D. Phosphate group

Ans. D.

487. The amount of DNA in a cell can be altered by

A. Ecological factors

B. Environmental factors

C. Physiological factors

D. Can not be altered

Ans. D.

488. The amount of DNA of a cell at the beginning of mitosis is

A. Half of the amount found in cells at G1 stage

B. Same as the amount found in cells at G1 stage

C. Twice the amount found in cells at G1 stage

D. 4 Times the amount found in cells at G1 stage

Ans. C.

489. The DNA found in all living organisms is

A. Left handed DNA

B. Right handed DNA

C. Both A & B

D. Z- DNA

Ans. B.

490. The DNA strand is directly involved in the formation of all except

A. Protein B. Another DNA strand

C. mRNA molecule D. tRNA molecule

Ans. A.

491. Which of the following statement is wrong ?

A. A –DNA is the dehydrated form of DNA

B. The naturally occurring DNA is B-DNA and is also called as wet DNA

C. Z- DNA is also called zig-zag DNA and is a right handed helix

D. Z-DNA occurs in dehydrated high salt concentration

Ans. C.

492. In animal cell cultures, the addition of serum to media is essential for providing

A. Growth factors B. Amino acid for protein synthesis

C. Nucleotide for DNA synthesis D. All of these

Ans. A.

493. Recombinant DNA human health care product developed for treating haemophiliacs is

A. Interferon B. Lymphokines

C. Coagulation factor IX D. Phytohaemagglutinin

Ans. C.

494. Which of the following has been produced commercially from mammalian culture?

A. Insulin B. Rennin

C. Plasminogen activator D. Antibacterial antibody

Ans. C.

495. A heterogenous protein for its expression in the milk of a transgenic animal should be under the control of the promoter of the gene for

A. Preproinsulin B. Lac Z

C. Beta globin D. Beta lactoglobulin

Ans. D.

496. Aminopterine is used during the production of hybridoma cells because it

A. Blocks the salvage pathway

B. Prevents the growth of B cells

C. Prevents the growth of myeloma cells

D. Blocks the synthesis of Ig by B cells

Ans. A.

497. Antibody diversity is generated by

A. Allelic exclusion
B. Protein splicing
C. Somatic mutation
D. Interchromosomal recombination

Ans. A.

498. Reverse vaccinology indicates

A. From antibody to vaccine development
B. From genome sequence to vaccine development
C. From antigenic polysaccharide to vaccine development
D. From antigenic protein to vaccine development

Ans. D.

499. The culture fluid of 1000 to 5000 clones of hybridoma are screened for monoclonal antibody by P. antigen capture analysis Q. Western blot analysis R. Northern blot analysis S. Antibody capture analysis

A. P, Q
B. Q, R
C. R, S
D. P, S

Ans. D.

500. All of the following are produced by animal cells in culture and help the cells adhere to the culture dish except

A. Collagen
B. Glycoprotein
C. Phospholipase A
D. Hyaluronic acid

Ans. C.

501. Which of the following technique is used in DNA fingerprinting ?

A. Western blotting
B. Southern blotting
C. Northern blotting
D. Eastern blotting

Ans. B.

502. Arrange the following in correct order

1. Southern blotting (a) Alwine
2. Western blotting (b) E.M. Southern
3. Northern blotting (c) A.Jeffrey
4. DNA fingerprinting (d) Towbin

A. 1a2c3d4b
B. 1b2d3a4c
C. 1b2a3d4c
D. 1b2c3a4d

Ans. B.

503. Labelled antibodies are used to detect

A. Detect the presence of a particular DNA molecule in Southern blotting

B. Detect the presence of a particular RNA molecule in Southern blotting

C. Detect the presence f a particular protein molecule in Southern blotting

D. Detect the presence of a particular protein molecule in Western blotting

Ans. D.

504. Which of the following technique is suitable for identifying mRNA molecule in a sample

A. Western blotting B. Southern blotting

C. Northern blotting D. Eastern blotting

Ans. C.

505. Which of the following technique does not involve electrophoresis for the separation of biomolecules

A. Dot blotting B. Southern blotting

C. Northern blotting D. Western blotting

Ans. A.

506. Probe is a

A. Protein for detecting a specific DNA molecule

B. Short piece of labelled DNA which are complementary to the nucleic acid strand to be detected

C. Short piece of labelled DNA or RNA which are complementary to the nucleic acid strand to be detected

D. None of these

Ans. C.

507. Which of the following technique is most suitable for detecting the presence of a gene product

A. Dot blotting B. Southern blotting

C. Plaque blotting D. Western blotting

Ans. D.

508. Aminobenzyloxymethyl filter paper is commonly used for transfer in

A. Dot blotting B. Southern blotting

C. Northern blotting D. Western blotting

Ans. C.

509. Arrange the following in correct order

1. Southern blotting (a) RNA-DNA hybrid
2. Western blotting (b) DNA-DNA hybrid
3. Northern blotting (c) Southern blotting
4. DNA fingerprinting (d) Antigen-antibody reaction

A. 1 a 2c 3d 4b B. 1 b 2d 3a 4c
C. 1 b 2a 3d 4c D. 1 b 2c 3a 4d

Ans. B.

510. The sugar in RNA is

A. Deoxyribose B. Fructose
C. Glucose D. Ribose

Ans. D.

511. The building blocks of RNA is called

A. Amino acids B. Monomers
C. Nucleosides D. Nucleotides

Ans. D.

512. RNA is found in

A. Nucleolus B. Cytoplasm
C. Mitochondria D. All of these

Ans. D.

513. A ribonucleotide consists of

A. Ribose sugar, phosphate and amino acids
B. Glucose, phosphate and amino acids
C. Ribose sugar, phosphate and nitrogenous base
D. Sugar, phosphate and lipid

Ans. C.

514. Which of the following statement is incorrect

A. RNA is single stranded
B. RNA is the only genetic material in viruses
C. RNA is the only genetic material in some viruses
D. All of these

Ans. C.

515. The bonds involve in RNA.

A. Hydrogen bonds
B. Phosphodiester bond
C. Both A & B
D. None of these

Ans. B.

516. The nitrogenous bases in RNA include

A. Adenine, Guanine, Cytosine and thymine
B. Adenine, Guanine, Cytosine and Uracil
C. Adenine, Cytosine and thymine
D. Depends on the environment

Ans. B.

517. In RNA pyramidines are

A. Adenine and Guanine,
B. Thymine and Uracil
C. Adenine and Uracil
D. Cytosine and Uracil

Ans. D.

518. Which of the following statement is incorrect

A. Cytosine and thymine are the only pyrimidines
B. Pyrimidines are one ringed structures
C. Purines are two ringed structures
D. Cytosine, thymine and uracil are pyramidines

Ans. A.

519. Which of the following DNA repair mechanism is known as the 'cut and patch' mechanism?

A. Photoreactivation
B. Nucleotide excision repair
C. Base excision repair
D. Mismatch repair

Ans. B.

520. DNA helicase enzyme involved in base excision repair mechanism is —

A. DNA helicase I
B. DNA helicase II
C. DNA helicase III
D. DNA helicase IV

Ans. C.

521. The main difference between nucleotide excision repair (NER) and base excision repair (BER) is

A. In NER double strand breaks are repaired whereas in BER single strand breaks repaired

B. NER is a light dependent reaction whereas BER is light independent process

C. In NER phosphodiester backbone is first cleaved whereas in BER phosphodiester backbone is cleaved later

D. All of these

Ans. C.

522. Which enzyme is responsible for photoreactivation of DNA ?

A. Photoligase B. Photoreductase

C. Photooxidase D. Photolyase

Ans. D.

523. Which of the following enzyme(s) is involved base excision repair ?

A. DNA glycosylase B. AP endonuclease

C. A, B, & C D. A & B

Ans. D.

524. Xeroderma pigmentosum in human is associated with a mutation in

A. Photoreactivation B. Nucleotide excision repair

C. Base excision repair D. Mismatch repair

Ans. B.

525. Which of the following enzymes are used to join bits of DNA ?

A. DNA ligase B. DNA polymerase

C. Primase D. Endonuclease

Ans. A.

526. Semi conservative replication of DNA was first demonstrated in

A. E. coli B. Streptococcus pneumonia

C. Salmonella typhimurium D. Drosophila melanogaster

Ans. A.

527. Mode of DNA replication in E. coli is

A. Conservative and unidirectional B. Semiconservative and unidirectional

C. Conservative and bidirectional D. Semiconservative and bidirectional

Ans. D.

528. When DNA replication starts

A. The phosphodiester bonds between the adjacent nucleotides break

B. The bonds between the nitrogen base and deoxyribose sugar break

C. The leading strand produces Okazaki fragments

D. The hydrogen bonds between the nucleotides of two strand break

Ans. D.

529. During the replication of DNA, the synthesis of DNA on lagging strand takes place in segment, these segments are called

A. Satellite segments
B. Double helix segments
C. Kornberg segments
D. Okazaki segments

Ans. D.

530. The elongation of the leading strand during DNA synthesis

A. Progresses away from the replication fork
B. Occur in 3'-5' direction
C. Produces Okazaki fragment
D. Depend on the action of DNA polymerase

Ans. D.

531. Eukaryotes differ from prokaryotes in mechanism of DNA replication due to

A. Different enzyme for synthesis of lagging and leading strand
B. Use of DNA primer rather than RNA primer
C. Unidirectional rather than bidirectional replication
D. Discontinuous rather than semidiscontinuous replication

Ans. D.

532. True replication of DNA is possible due to

A. Hydrogen bonding
B. Phosphate backbone
C. Complementary base pairing rule
D. None of the above

Ans. C.

533. Unwinding of DNA is done by

A. Helicase
B. Ligase
C. Hexonuclease
D. Topoisomerase

Ans. A.

534. DNA synthesis can be specifically measured by estimating the incorporation of radio labelled

A. Uracil
B. Thymine
C. Adenine
D. Deoxyribose sugar

Ans. B.

535. Genetic code is

A. The sequence of nitrogenous bases in mRNA molecule that codes for protein
B. A triplet code
C. Non-overlapping
D. All of these

Ans. B.

536. The enzyme involved in the amino acid activation is

A. ATP synthetase
B. Aminoacyl tRNA synthetase
C. Aminoacyl mRNA synthetase
D. Aminoacyl rRNA synthetase

Ans. B.

537. Which of the following molecule acts as adaptor molecule during protein synthesis?

A. rRNA
B. mRNA
C. tRNA
D. tRNA 7 mRNA

Ans. C.

538. The unpaired nucleotides produced by the action of restriction enzymes are referred to have

A. Sticky ends
B. Single strands
C. Restriction fragments
D. Ligases

Ans. A.

539. Which of the following is not true of small inbreeding populations?

A. They tend to loose genetic diversity
B. There is an increased incidence of recessive diseases
C. Alleles may become fixed
D. Mutation is increased

Ans. D.

540. Which of these genes codes for a protein that plays a role in growth?

A. DCP1
B. SCLC6A4
C. KRTHA1
D. GH1

Ans. D.

541. Which of the following pair will produce complementary sticky ends?

A. Eco RI & MspI
B. Msp I & HPA II
C. Sau 3A & Bam HI
D. Mbo I & Sau 3A

Ans. C.

542. A human cDNA library

A. Contains DNA for specific human proteins
B. Contains DNA for virtually all of the human proteins in vectors
C. Cannot be used to obtain human genes because it would be radioactive
D. None of the above

Ans. B.

543. What enzyme forms covalent bonds between restriction fragments?

A. DNA primase B. DNA helicase

C. DNA polymerase D. DNA ligase

Ans. D.

544. Which of the following can be diagnosed by amniocentesis?

A. Down's syndrome B. Cystic Fibrosis

C. Sickle cell anemia D. All of these

Ans. D.

545. Reverse transcripase from HIV does not

A. Uses RNA as a template B. Has a 5' to 3' polymerase activity

C. Has a 3'- 5' exonuclease activity D. Requires a primer

Ans. C.

546. Which of the following amino acids can interact with the DNA or RNA nucleotide bases via hydrogen bonding?

A. Asn and Gln B. Cys and Met

C. Lys and Leu D. Ile and Val

Ans. A.

547. Different DNA polymerases play distinct roles in DNA replication and repair in both prokaryotic and eukaryotic cells. All known DNA polymerases synthesize DNA only in the —————— by the addition of dNTPs to a performed primer strand of DNA.

A. Positive direction B. 3' to 5' direction

C. 5' to 3' direction D. Negative direction

Ans. C.

548. In prokaryotes the first amino acid in the polypeptide chain is

A. Methionine B. N-methyl methionine

C. N-formyl methionine D. None of these

Ans. C.

549. In prokaryoties, the ribosomal binding site on mRNA is called

A. Hognes sequence B. Shine-Dalgarno sequence

C. Pribnow sequence D. TATA box

Ans. B.

550. During translation, the role of enzyme peptidyl transferase is
   A. Transfer of phosphate group
   B. Amino acid activation
   C. Peptide bond formation between adjacent amino acids
   D. Binding of ribosome subunits to mRNA

Ans. C.

551. Polysomes are
   A. Aggregation of ribosmes
   B. Aggregation of lysosomes
   C. mRNA molecules to which many ribosomes are attached simultaneously
   D. All of these

Ans. C.

552. Which is the energy rich molecule required for initiation of translation
   A. ATP   B. GTP
   C. CTP   D. AMP

Ans. B.

553. In eukaryotes, translation is initiated by binding of ribosome to the
   A. Pribnow box   B. Hognes box
   C. 5'cap   D. Poly A tail

Ans. C.

554. hsp 60 and hsp70 are proteins involved in
   A. Initiation of translation   B. Elongation of translation
   C. Termination of translation   D. Protein folding

Ans. D.

555. Tetracycline blocks protein synthesis by
   A. Inhibiting binding of aminoacyl tRNA to ribosome
   B. Inhibiting initiation of translation
   C. Inhibiting peptidyl transferase
   D. Inhibiting translocase enzyme

Ans. A.

556. In which phase of the cell cycle does DNA replication occur ?
   A. G0   B. G1
   C. S   D. G2

Ans. C.

557. The enzyme responsible for initiating DNA replication in prokaryotes is

A. DNA polymerase I
B. DNA polymerase III
C. Polymerase beta
D. Primase

Ans. D.

558. The enzyme responsible for continuing DNA replication in prokaryotes once it is initiated

A. DNA polymerase I
B. DNA polymerase III
C. Polymerase beta
D. Polymerase delta

Ans. B.

559. Antibiotics such as Ciprofloxacin and Fluoroquilones act by inhibiting — enzyme

A. DNA ligase
B. Topoisomerase (DNA gyrase)
C. Single stranded binding protein
D. Primase

Ans. B.

560. All of the following are required for purine de novo synthesis except

A. CO2
B. Glycine
C. Glutamine
D. Isoleucine

Ans. D.

561. Which of the following is a common enzyme for de novo as well as salvage pathway of purine biosynthesis ?

A. Amidotransferase
B. PRPP synthetase
C. HGPRTase
D. Adenylosuccinate synthetase

Ans. B.

562. Which of the following does not have introns ?

A. DNA
B. Nonprocessed pseudogenes
C. Processed mRNA
D. primary RNA transcript

Ans. C.

563. Which of the following is not true of RNA synthesis ?

A. The key enzyme is RNA polymerase
B. The energy is supplied by the ring cleavage
C. The RNA sequence is complementary to the template strand of DNA
D. The RNA sequence is of opposite polarity to the template strand of DNA

Ans. B.

564. If the molar amount of G in a DNA sample is 20%, what is the molar amount of T in the sample ?

A. 20% B. 30%

C. 40% D. 60%

Ans. B.

565. Which is true of the melting temperature of G-C pairs compared to A-T pairs in DNA ?

A. The Tm is equal

B. Tm of G-C is less than the Tm of A-T

C. Tm of G-C is more than the Tm of A-T

D. None of these

Ans. C.

566. The poison associated with toxic mushrooms usually inhibits

A. hn RNA B. tRNA

C. DNA D. mRNA

Ans. A.

567. DNA methylation is associated with

A. CpG islands B. CAT box

C. TATA box D. increasing gene transcription

Ans. A.

568. All of the following are involved in translating information into proteins except

A. rRNA B. siRNA

C. tRNA D. snRNA

Ans. B.

569. Which histone is not part of the nucleosome ?

A. H1 B. H2A

C. H2B D. H3

Ans. A.

570. Which of the following is an inhibitor of prokaryotic transcription ?

A. Ciprofloxacin B. Etoposide

C. Erythromycin D. Rifampicin

Ans. D.

571. The nucleoside analogue used as an anticancer drug

A. Methotrexate B. 6-Mercaptopurine

C. Vinblastin D. Cytosine Arabinoside

Ans. D.

572. Which amino acid is in abundance in histone ?

A. Arginine B. Aspartic acid

C. Tryptophan D. Phenylalanine

Ans. A.

573. Which of the following technique is used for the detection of gene of interest

A. Southern blotting B. PCR

C. Northern blotting D. DNA foot printing

Ans. A.

574. Which of the following is an example of post translational modification ?

A. Splicing B. Class switching

C. Subunit aggregation D. Base modification

Ans. C.

575. Triple repeat sequence disease occurs in

A. Alzheimer's disease B. Cystic fibrosis

C. Ataxia telangectasia D. Huntington's chorea

Ans. D.

576. Northern blot is used for separation of

A. DNA B. mRNA

C. Protein D. Protein DNA interaction

Ans. B.

577. First use of pure microbiological process in an industrial procedure was made by Chaim Weizmann in

A. 1921 B. 1925

C. 1917 D. 1907

Ans. C.

578. Application of biotechnology procedures in medical processes is classified as

A. White biotechnology B. Red biotechnology

C. Blue biotechnology D. Green biotechnology

Ans. B.

579. Field of biotechnology which is applied to industrial processes is known as

A. White biotechnology
B. Red biotechnology
C. Blue biotechnology
D. Green biotechnology

Ans. A.

580. Example of green biotechnology

A. Industrial antibiotics
B. Industrial chemicals
C. Industrial catalysts
D. BT corn and pesticides

Ans. D.

581. Process of using natural bacteria in mining industry is known as

A. Biodegradation
B. Biogenomics
C. Bioremediation
D. Bioleaching

Ans. D.

582. First use of pure microbiological process in an industrial procedure was made by

A. Alexander Fleming
B. Louis Pasteur
C. Charles Darwin
D. Chaim Weizmann

Ans. D.

583. Mold Penicillin was discovered by Alexander Fleming in

A. 1931
B. 1928
C. 1935
D. 1939

Ans. B.

584. Example of red biotechnology is

A. Antibiotics
B. Pesticides
C. Industrial catalysts
D. Bt cotton

Ans. A.

585. Example of white biotechnology is

A. Bt cotton
B. Use of enzymes in industry
C. Use of pesticides
D. Use of antibiotics

Ans. B.

586. Fungi has

A. Large central vacuole
B. Many small vacuole
C. No active vacuole is found
D. Contractile vacuole

Ans. A.

587. Process of manipulating genes usually outside normal reproductive process is known as

A. Genetic modification B. Gene targeting

C. Genome recombination D. Gene linking

Ans. A.

588. First genetically modified organism generated was

A. Fish B. Bacteria

C. Mice D. Virus

Ans. B.

589. Transfer of genes from one species to another can be studied through

A. Bacteria B. Vectors

C. Fungi D. All of these

Ans. B.

590. Casein is converted to yoghurt because of

A. Lactic acid B. Salicylic acid

C. Benzoic acid D. Picric acid

Ans. A.

591. Enzymes found in fungi are

A. Protease B. Amylase

C. Maltase D. All of these

Ans. D.

592. During milk fermentation lactose is converted to lactic acid through

A. Lactobacillus B. Streptococcus

C. Lactococcus D. Streptobacillus

Ans. A.

593. Transformation method of plants and animals in which plants and animals are given shocks is known as

A. Microinjection B. Genome breeding

C. Electroporation D. Genome engineering

Ans. C.

594. To produce penicillin the main fermentable source in culture is

A. Glucose B. Lactose

C. Sulphate D. Sugars

Ans. B.

595. Vibrio bacteria are a variation of

A. Cocci
B. Bacilli
C. Spirilla
D. Vibrious

Ans. B.

596. Link between composers and decomposers is called as

A. Nitrogen cycle
B. Water cycle
C. Carbon cycle
D. Fertility restoration process

Ans. C.

597. Viruses are not considered cells because

A. They can not divide
B. They do not have nucleus
C. They do not have a protoplasm
D. They are non living things

Ans. C.

598. Pruteen is made by mixing bacteria in

A. Ethanol
B. Methanol
C. Vaseline
D. Petroleum

Ans. B.

599. Techniques of inserting DNA into plants is known as

A. Bioinjection
B. Biofission
C. Biogenetic
D. Biodiffusion

Ans. B.

600. Function of streptococcus during milk fermentation is to

A. Produce aerobic environment
B. Produce anaerobic environment
C. Form lactic acid
D. All of these

Ans. B.

601. Examples of rod shaped viruses include

A. Influenza virus
B. Bacteriophages
C. TMV
D. Norwalk virus

Ans. C.

602. First genetically modified mice is generated in

A. 1964
B. 1968
C. 1974
D. 1978

Ans. C.

603. Antibodies are produced commercially by mixing a lymphocyte with

A. A bacteria B. A fungus

C. A tumour cell D. A non living tissue

Ans. C.

604. Yeasts are

A. Unicellular fungi B. Multicellular fungi

C. Bicellular fungi D. Tricellular fungi

Ans. A.

605. Fusarium is made through a culture medium of

A. Lactose B. Glucose

C. Galactose D. Maltose

Ans. B.

606. First genetically modified pet was sold in USA in

A. 2003 B. 2004

C. 2006 D. 2008

Ans. A.

607. In penicillin production pH of the culture medium is maintained between

A. 5 & 6 B. 4 & 6

C. 6 & 7 D. 4 & 5

Ans. A.

608. Chitin is a form of

A. Complex peptone B. Complex DNA

C. Complex plasmids D. Complex carbohydrate

Ans. D.

609. In anaerobic environment, sugar in dough is converted into

A. Glucose B. Water

C. Alcohol D. CO

Ans. C.

610. The restriction enzymes consist of the following enzymatic elements

A. Nuclease and protease B. Nuclease and kinase

C. Nuclease and methylase D. Nuclease and polymerase

Ans. C.

611. A mRNA that includes coding regions of more than one gene

A. Poysomes B. Polycistronic

C. Polylinker D. Polyadenylated

Ans. B.

612. RNA molecule that can catalyze chemical reactions, often cutting other RNAs

A. Ribonuclease B. Ribozyme

C. R-Zyme D. Ribofactor

Ans. B.

613. A gene from one genome that has been incorporated into the genome of another organism

A. Tra gene B. Cis gene

C. Mob gene D. Transgene

Ans. D.

614. Eukaryotic promoter region analogous to the Pribnow box

A. Shine-Delgarno sequence B. Pribnow box

C. TATA box D. CAAT box

Ans. C.

615. The bar gene generally used as a selectable marker gene during the transgenic development imparts

A. Antibiotic resistance B. Drug resistance

C. Herbicide resistance D. High amino acid tolerance

Ans. C.

616. The deletion of genes governing auxin and cytokinin production from T-DNA of a Ti plasmid is known as

A. Disharming B. Disarming

C. Dearming D. Deharming

Ans. B.

617. The DNA of an elephant and the DNA of a mango tree will probably differ in all of the following

A. Sequence of DNA nucleotides

B. Length of DNA molecules

C. Number of DNA molecules

D. Kinds of nucleotides utilized in forming DNA

Ans. D.

618. The lac operon in E. coli is involved in
   A. Regulating the expression of a gene
   B. Controlling DNA replication
   C. Regulating the translation of mRNA
   D. Controlling the formation of ribosomes

Ans. A.

619. Genetic variation can be introduced into bacteria by all of the following methods except:
   A. Transduction
   B. Mutation
   C. Transformation
   D. DNA amplification

Ans. D.

620. Which of the following would most likely cause a mutation with the greatest deleterious effect?
   A. An insertion of a nucleotide triplet into a DNA strand that codes for an mRNA
   B. A single addition of a nucleotide in a DNA strand that codes for an mRNA
   C. A deletion of a nucleotide triplet from a DNA strand that codes for an mRNA
   D. All of these

Ans. B.

621. All of the following enzymes are involved in DNA replication except:
   A. Helicase
   B. Primase
   C. DNA polymerase
   D. RNA polymerase

Ans. D.

622. Which of the following is true?
   A. A messenger RNA molecule has the form of a double helix
   B. Ribosomes contain RNA nucleotides and amino acids
   C. The uracil nucleotide consists of the uracil nitrogen base, a deoxyribose sugar and a phosphate group.
   D. In eukaryotes, DNA is manufactured in the nucleus and RNA is manufactured in the cytoplasm.

Ans. B.

623. A recombinant DNA molecule is produced by Recombinant DNA Technology by
   A. Joining of two DNA fragments
   B. Joining of two or more DNA fragments
   C. Both a and b
   D. Joining of two or more DNA fragments originating from different organisms

Ans. D.

624. The gene formed by the joining of DNA segments from two different sources are called as

A. Recombinant gene
B. Joined gene
C. Both a and b
D. Chimaeric gene

Ans. D.

625. Which of the following enzyme is used to cut DNA molecule in rDNA technology

A. Ligase
B. Phosphatase
C. Ribonuclease
D. Restriction enzymes

Ans. D.

626. Who created the first rDNA molecule

A. Nathan, Arber and Smith
B. Watson, Crick and Wilkins
C. Boyer and Cohen
D. Paul Berg

Ans. D.

627. The DNA molecule to which the gene of insert is integrated for cloning is called

A. Carrier
B. Transformer
C. Vector
D. None of these

Ans. C.

628. The DNA segment to be cloned is called

A. Gene segment
B. DNA fragment
C. DNA insert
D. All of these

Ans. C.

629. Which of the following statements are true regarding rDNA technology

A. rDNA technology is used to obtain large number of copies of specific DNA fragments
B. rDNA technology is used to obtain large quantities of the protein produced by the concerned gene
C. rDNA technology is used to integrate gene of interest into chromosomes where it expresses itself
D. All of these

Ans. D.

630. The first successful transformation of rDNA molecule into a bacterium was carried out by

A. Nathan, Arber and Smith
B. Watson, Crick and Wilkins
C. Boyer and Cohen
D. Paul Berg

Ans. C.

631. The plasmid used by Cohen and Boyer for their transformation experiment was

A. pSC 101 B. PUC 17

C. pBR 322 D. E. coli plasmids

Ans. A.

632. The mechanism of intake of DNA fragments from the surrounding medium by a cell is called

A. Transformation B. Transduction

C. Both A and B D. Conjugation

Ans. A.

633. Gene cloning refers to the

A. Production of large number of copies of the gene being cloned

B. Production of asexual progeny from a single individual or a cell

C. Both a and b

D. None of these

Ans. A.

634. Paul Berg's gene splicing experiment created the first rDNA molecule which was

A. A T4 phage fragment incorporated into SV40 vector

B. A lambda phage fragment incorporated into SV40 vector

C. A T4 phage fragment incorporated into pSC 101 vector

D. A lambda phage fragment incorporated into pSC 101 vector

Ans. B.

635. Which of the following enzyme is used to synthesize DNA using an mRNA template

A. Taq polymerase B. Alkaline phosphatase

C. Reverse transcriptase D. Nuclease

Ans. C.

636. Which of the following enzyme is used to cut DNA molecule internally

A. Restriction enzymes B. Restriction endonuclease

C. Restriction exonuclease D. Ribonuclease H

Ans. B.

637. The enzyme that adds mononucleotide triphosphates to the 3' OH group of a DNA fragment is

A. Polynucleotide kinase B. Terminal nucleotidyl transferase

C. Terminal phosphoryl transferase D. All of these

Ans. B.

638. The RNA strand in the RNA-DNA hybrid is removed by

A. RNAse B. RNase-H

C. Nuclease D. None of these

Ans. B.

639. Klenow enzyme is the product of enzymatic breakdown of

A. DNA polymerase I B. DNA polymerase II

C. DNA polymerase III D. RNA polymerase

Ans. A.

640. Selective degradation of single stranded DNA is carried out by the enzyme

A. Nuclease B. Ribonuclease

C. SI nuclease D. Deoxyribonuclease

Ans. C.

641. Which of the following is an RNA dependent DNA synthetase ?

A. DNA polymerase I B. DNA polymerase II

C. Reverse transcriptase D. All of these

Ans. C.

642. Which of the following is a thermo stable DNA polymerase

A. Taq polymerase B. Vent polymerase

C. Pfu polymerase D. All of these

Ans. D.

643. Eco RI is a

A. Restriction endonuclease B. Polymerase enzyme

C. Ligase D. Exonuclease

Ans. A.

644. Two bacteria most useful in genetic engineering are

A. Rhizobium and Azobacter B. Nitrosomonas and Klebsiella

C. Escherichia and Agrobacterium D. Rhizobium and Diplococcus

Ans. C.

645. What is the source of Eco RI

A. E. coli RI B. E. coli RI 13

C. E. coli RI Y 13 D. E. coli RI X 13

Ans. C.

646. First clinical gene therapy was given in 1992 to a 4 years girl for

A. Adenine deficiency
B. Growth deficiency
C. Adenosine deaminase deficiency
D. adenosine deficiency

Ans. C.

647. The most common monomer of carbohydrate is a molecule of

A. Glucose
B. Maltose
C. Amylase
D. Amylopectin

Ans. A.

648. The six most common atoms in organic molecules are

A. C, H, O, He, Ca and S
B. C,H,O,N, P and S
C. C,H,O, Mg, Mn and S
D. C,H,O,N, P and K

Ans. B.

649. Cholesterol is a

A. Saturated fat
B. Unsaturated fat
C. Steroid
D. Essential oil

Ans. C.

650. The part of a DNA molecule that varies among DNA molecules is its

A. Sugar
B. Phosphates
C. Glycerol
D. Nitrogenous bases

Ans. A.

651. Which is a linear polysaccharide ?

A. Glycogen
B. Cellulose
C. Starch
D. Amylase

Ans. B.

652. Ribose is a pentose sugar found in

A. NAD
B. FAD
C. RNA
D. All of these

Ans. D.

653. The most abundant monosaccharide in nature is

A. Lactose
B. Glucose
C. Maltose
D. Sucrose

Ans. B.

654. DNA is unique among molecules is that it can

A. Form multiplepolymer complexes B. Stay apart and reform

C. Replicate itself D. Withstand very high temperature

Ans. C.

655. Which of the following is a polysaccharide ?

A. Glucose B. Glycogen

C. Amylose D. Lactose

Ans. B.

656. Pomato is a grafted plant of

A. Poppy and Potato B. Potato and tomato

C. Poppy and tamarind D. Poppy and tomato

Ans. B.

657. Preserving germplasm in frozen state is

A. Cryopreservation B. Cold storage

C. In situ preservation D. Vernalisation

Ans. A.

658. Protein helping in opening of DNA double helix in front of replication fork

A. DNA gyrase B. DNA polymerase I

C. DNA ligase D. DNA topoisomerase

Ans. A.

659. Pyrimidine base present in RNA in place of thymine of DNA is

A. Uracil B. Adenine

C. Cytosine D. Guanine

Ans. A.

660. Restriction endonuclease is employed for cutting

A. A single stranded DNA B. Double stranded DNA

C. RNA segment D. mRNA

Ans. B.

661. Restriction endonuclease are

A. Used in genetic engineering for uniting two DNA molecules

B. Used for in vitro DNA synthesis

C. Present in mammalian cells for degeneration of DNA of dead cells

D. Synthesized by bacteria for their defence

Ans. D.

662. Restriction endonuclease are used in genetic engineering because they

A. Can join DNA fragment

B. Cut DNA at specific base sequence

C. Cut DNA at variable sites

D. Are proteolytic enzymes which degrade harmful proteins

Ans. B.

663. Reverse transcriptase is

A. RNA dependent RNA polymerase B. DNA dependent DNA polymerase

C. DNA dependent RNA polymerase D. RNA dependent DNA polymerase

Ans. D.

664. RNA contains

A. Hexose B. Ribose

C. Fructose D. Glucose

Ans. B.

665. RNA does not possess

A. Uracil B. Thymine

C. Adenine D. Cytosine

Ans. B.

666. RNA that picks up specific amino acid from amino acid pool of cytoplasm to carry it to ribosome during protein synthesis is

A. tRNA B. mRNA

C. rRNA D. gRNA

Ans. A.

667. Semiconservative DNA/chromosome replication using ^{14}N was demonstrated by

A. Messelson B. Tylor

C. Messelson and Stahl D. Hershey and Chase

Ans. C.

668. Similarity between DNA and RNA is that both have

A. Similar sugars B. Similar mode of replication

C. Similar pyrimidines D. Polymers of nucleotides

Ans. D.

669. Structure of DNA was given by

A. Kornberg B. Nirenberg

C. Watson and Crick D. Holley and Nirenberg

Ans. C.

670. Successive nucleotides are covalently linked through

A. Glycosidic bonds
B. Phosphodiester bonds
C. Hydrogen bonds
D. Nitrogen bonds

Ans. B.

671. Termination of polypeptide chain is brought about by

A. UUG, UAG and UCG
B. UAA, UAG and UGA
C. UUG, UGC and UCA
D. UCG, GCG and ACC

Ans. B.

672. The basic unit of a nucleic acid is

A. Pentose sugar
B. Nucleoid
C. Nucleoside
D. Nucleotide

Ans. D.

673. The codon for anticodon 3' UUUA5' is

A. 5' AAAU 3'
B. 5' UUUA3'
C. 3' UAAD5'
D. 3' AUUU5'

Ans. A.

674. The common feature amongst nucleus, chloroplast and mitochondria is

A. Lamellae
B. DNA
C. Cristae
D. All the above

Ans. B.

675. The enzyme taking part in joining two ends of DNA is

A. Ligase
B. Polymerase
C. Gyrase
D. Helicase

Ans. A.

676. In a DNA molecule cytosine is 18% . Percentage of adenine would be

A. 32%
B. 64%
C. 36%
D. 18%

Ans. A.

677. In AGCT of DNA hydrogen bonds and base pairings occur between

A. A-U, C-G
B. A-C, G-T
C. A-G, C-T
D. A-T, C-G

Ans. D.

678. In callus culture, roots can be induced by the supply of

A. Auxin and no cytokinin

B. Higher concentration of auxin and lower concentration of cytokinin

C. Higher concentration of cytokinin and lower concentration of auxin

D. Both auxin and cytokinin in equal proportions

Ans. B.

679. In DNA, adenine pairs with

A. Guanine B. Thymine

C. Cytosine D. Uracil

Ans. B.

680. In DNA, guanine lies opposite

A. Guanine B. Thymine

C. Cytosine D. Uracil

Ans. C.

681. In double helix of DNA, the two DNA strands are

A. Coiled around a common axis B. Coiled around each other

C. Coiled differently D. Coiled over protein sheath

Ans. A.

682. In RNA thymine is replaced by

A. Adenine B. Guanine

C. Cytosine D. Uracil

Ans. D.

683. In tissue/bacterial culture glassware and nutrients are sterilized through

A. Water bath at 200°C B. Dry air over at 200°C

C. Water bath at 100°C D. Autoclave

Ans. D.

684. In tissue culture, callus can be induced to form shoot or root by altering the ratio of

A. Auxin to cytokinin B. Cytokinin to ethylene

C. Auxin to gibberellins D. Gibberellins to cytokinin

Ans. A.

685. Initiation codon of protein synthesis (in eukaryotes) is

A. GUA B. GCA

C. CCA D. AUG

Ans. D.

686. Introduction of foreign genes for improving genotype is

A. Tissue culture B. Immunization

C. Biotechnology D. Genetic engineering

Ans. D.

687. It is now possible to breed plants and animals with desired characters through

A. Genetic engineering B. Chromosome engineering

C. Ikebana technique D. Bonsai technique

Ans. A.

688. Most abundant RNA of the cell is

A. tRNA B. rRNA

C. mRNA D. tRNA

Ans. B.

689. Nitrogen bases of DNA are

A. ATUC B. UTGC

C. ATGC D. AUGC

Ans. C.

690. Nonsense codon takes part in

A. Terminating message of gene controlled protein synthesis

B. Formulation of unspecified amino acids

C. Conversion of sense DNA into nonsense one

D. Releasing tRNA from polypeptide chain

Ans. A.

691. Nucleosides are

A. Sugar + phosphoric acid

B. Purine/pyrimidine +sugar +phosphate

C. Purine/pyrimidine +phosphoric acid

D. Purine/pyrimidine + sugar

Ans. D.

692. Nucleotides present in one turn of DNA helix are

A. 4 B. 8

C. 10 D. 9

Ans. C.

693. Okazaki segments are formed during

A. Transduction B. Transcription

C. Replication D. Translation

Ans. C.

694. Plants developed in vitro culture from pollen grains are

A. Androgenic plants B. Pollen plants

C. Male plants D. Sterile plants

Ans. A.

695. Plants are vectors for gene cloning because they

A. Self replicate in bacterial cells

B. Replicated freely outside bacterial cells

C. Can be multiplied in culture

D. Can be multiplied in laboratories using enzymes

Ans. A.

696. Distance between two successive nitrogenous bases or base pairs of DNA is

A. 34A° B. 3.4A°

C. 10A° D. 5A°

Ans. B.

697. DNA and RNA are similar in having

A. Similar nucleotides B. Similar pyrimidines

C. Similar purines D. Similar sugars

Ans. C.

698. DNA and RNA show similarity in having

A. Polymers of nucleotides B. Similar pyrimidines

C. Double strands D. Similar sugars

Ans. A.

699. DNA does not occur in

A. Nucleus B. Ribosomes

C. Mitochondria D. Plastids

Ans. B.

700. DNA duplex shows

A. Right handed coiling and parallel B. Right handed coiling and antiparallel

C. Left handed coiling and antiparallel D. Left handed coiling and parallel

Ans. B.

701. DNA is composed of repeating units of

A. Ribonucleosides
B. Deoxyribonucleosides
C. Ribonucleotides
D. Deoxyribonucleotides

Ans. D.

702. DNA replication in eukaryotes commences

A. From both ends of a chromosome simultaneously
B. Several sites along DNA of a chromosome simultaneously
C. From centromere to either end
D. From one end of chromosome to the other

Ans. B.

703. DNA replication is

A. Conservative and discontinuous
B. Semiconservative and semidiscontinuous
C. Semiconservative and discontinuous
D. Conservative

Ans. C.

704. DNA resembles RNA as both have

A. Polymers of nucleotides
B. Similar sugars
C. Similar pyrimidine bases
D. Ability to replicate

Ans. A.

705. DNA sequence is ATG. What would be the sequence of bases in anticodon of tRNA

A. ATG
B. AUG
C. UAC
D. TAC

Ans. B.

706. DNA sequence is TAG. What shall be the sequence in anticodon of tRNA

A. UAG
B. ATC
C. ATG
D. UAC

Ans. A.

707. DNA sequence of ATTCGATG is transcribed as

A. AUUCGAUG
B. UAAGCUAC
C. CAUCGAAU
D. GUAGCUUA

Ans. B.

708. DNA strand with nitrogen base sequence ATTGCC will be transcribed as ___

A. UAACGG
B. ATCGCC
C. ATTGCA
D. AGGACC

Ans. A.

709. Double chained DNA strand is made radioactive in both its chains. It is allowed to replicate twice in non-radioactive medium. The result

A. All strands have radioactivity
B. Half the strands have radioactivity
C. Three strands have radioactivity
D. Radioactivity is absent in all the strands

Ans. B.

710. Double helical structure of DNA was proposed by

A. Kornberg
B. Nirenberg
C. Watson and Crick
D. Wilkins and Franklin

Ans. C.

711. Functional unit of gene that specifies synthesis of one polypeptide is

A. Codon
B. Cistron
C. Recon
D. Muton

Ans. B.

712. Gene is segment of

A. RNA
B. DNA
C. RNA or DNA
D. Both RNA and DNA

Ans. B.

713. Genetically engineered bacteria are being used in commercial production of

A. Melatonin
B. Testosterone
C. Human insulin
D. Thyroxin

Ans. C.

714. Haploid plant cultures are got from

A. Leaves
B. Root tip
C. Pollen grain
D. Buds

Ans. C.

715. Hydrogen bonds present between cytosine and guanosine are

A. 2
B. 3
C. 1
D. 4

Ans. B.

716. The sequence of other strand of DNA will be when one strand has sequence of AGCTTCGA

A. TCGAAGCT B. GCTAAGCT
C. TAGCATAT D. GATCCTAG

Ans. A.

717. A nucleoside is formed by

A. Pentose sugar, phosphate and nitrogen base
B. Phosphate and nitrogen base
C. Pentose sugar and phosphate
D. Pentose sugar and nitrogen base

Ans. D.

718. A nucleotide is formed of

A. Purine, Pyrimidine and phosphate
B. Purine, sugar and phosphate
C. Nitrogen base, sugar and phosphate
D. Pyrimidine, sugar and phosphate

Ans. C.

719. A Riboside is

A. Base + phosphate B. Ribose + phosphate
C. Ribose + phosphate + base D. Ribose + base

Ans. D.

720. A segment of DNA has 120 adenine and 120 cytosine bases. The total number of nucleotides present in the segment is

A. 120 B. 240
C. 60 D. 480

Ans. D.

721. A strand of DNA has base sequence CATGACTAG. The base sequence on the other strand would be

A. CATTAGGAC B. GTACTGATC
C. GATGTCATC D. TACACTGCT

Ans. B.

722. A totipotent cell means

A. An undifferentiated cell capable of developing into a system or entire plant
B. An undifferentiated cell capable of developing into an organ
C. An undifferentiated cell capable of developing into complete embryo
D. Cell which lacks the capability to differentiate into an organ or system

Ans. A.

723. Adenine is

A. Purine
B. Pyrimidine
C. Nucleoside
D. Nucleotide

Ans. A.

724. Amino acid binding site of tRNA is

A. 5' end
B. Anticodon loop
C. DHU loop
D. –CCA 3' end

Ans. D.

725. Anticodon occurs in

A. tRNA
B. mRNA
C. mtRNA
D. rRNA

Ans. A.

726. Bacterial plasmid contains

A. RNA
B. RNA + protein
C. DNA
D. photosynthetic structure

Ans. C.

727. Base pairs present in one turn of DNA are

A. 12
B. 11
C. 10
D. 9

Ans. C.

728. Best method to determine paternity is

A. Protein analysis
B. Chromosome counting
C. Gene counting
D. DNA fingerprinting

Ans. D.

729. Callus is

A. Tissue that forms embryo
B. An insoluble carbohydrate
C. Tissue that grows to form embryoid
D. Unorganized actively dividing mass of cells maintained in culture

Ans. D.

730. Chemical knives/ molecular scissors of DNA are

A. Restriction endonucleases
B. Polymerases
C. Ligases
D. Transcriptases

Ans. A.

731. Chemofusion and electrofusion are employed in

A. Eugenics
B. Protoplast fusion
C. Cloning
D. Mutations

Ans. B.

732. Choose the correct statement

A. DNA is hereditary material
B. RNA is hereditary material
C. DNA is hereditary material but where it is absent RNA can function as hereditary material
D. Both DNA and RNA are hereditary materials

Ans. C.

733. Development of shoot and root in tissue culture is determined by

A. Cytokinin and auxin ratio
B. Enzymes
C. Temperature
D. Plant nutrients

Ans. A.

734. Distance between two base pairs of DNA is

A. 34 nm
B. 3.4 nm
C. 0.68 nm
D. 0.34 nm

Ans. D.

735. Distance between two strands of DNA is

A. 34A°
B. 20A°
C. 3.4A°
D. 340A°

Ans. B.

736. Hirudin is obtained from the transgenic plant

A. Brassica napus
B. Hibiscus rosasinesis
C. Raphanus sativus
D. Vinca rosea

Ans. A.

737. Bt cotton is

A. Cloned plant
B. Transgenic plant
C. Hybrid plant
D. Mutated plant

Ans. B.

738. Dolly sheep was genetically similar to

A. The mother from which nucleated fertilized egg was taken
B. The mother from which nuclear DNA of udder cell was taken
C. The surrogate mother
D. Both surrogate mother and nuclear donor mother

Ans. B.

739. Genome is

A. Genes on nuclear DNA

B. Nuclear DNA +Mitochondrial DNA

C. Nuclear DNA + Chloroplast DNA

D. Nuclear DNA + Mitochondrial DNA + Chloroplast DNA

Ans. D.

740. A technique of using very small metal particles coated with desired gene in the gene transfer is called

A. Electroporation B. Microinjection

C. Liposome D. Biolistics

Ans. D.

741. The complete set of chromosomal and extrachromosomal genes of an organisms is called

A. Genome B. Gene pool

C. Gene bank D. Gene library

Ans. A.

742. The study of all the proteins coded by the genome is called

A. Proteome B. Proteomics

C. Genome D. Protein formation

Ans. B.

743. Sequencing of genomic DNA is included under

A. Structural genomics B. Functional genomics

C. Proteomics D. Transgenesis

Ans. A.

744. Genome expression, regulation and phenotype production are studied in second phase of genome analysis called

A. Structural genomics B. Functional genomics

C. proteomics D. Transmeiosis

Ans. B.

745. A flowering plant lily have —— more DNA than humans

A. 10 times B. 15 times

C. 18 times D. 13 times

Ans. C.

746. In forensic science which of the following is used

A. Bacterial cloning B. DNA foot printing

C. DNA fingerprinting D. DNA cloning

Ans. C.

747. DNA fingerprinting is based on

A. Occurrence of VNTRs B. Knowledge of human karyotype

C. Cloned DNA D. Recombinant DNA

Ans. A.

748. VNTRs represents

A. New terminal regions in DNA

B. Functional genes in the DNA

C. Split genes in the sample DNA

D. Specific non-coding sequences with unique tandem repeats

Ans. D.

749. Which ones produce androgenic haploids in anther cultures ?

A. Anther wall B. Tapetal layer of anther wall

C. Connective tissue D. Young pollen grains

Ans. D.

750. Variations observed during tissue culture of some plants are known as

A. Clonal variations B. Somatic variations

C. Somaclonal variations D. Tissue culture variations

Ans. C.

751. Virus free plants can be obtained through

A. Antibiotic treatment B. Bordeaux mixture

C. Root tip culture D. Shoot tip culture

Ans. D.

752. Raisin of plants from a small tissue in culture is known as

A. Macroproduction B. Micropropagation

C. Tissue culture D. Mass production

Ans. B.

753. Biopatents are

A. Right to use invention B. Right to use biological entities

C. Right to use products D. Right to use process

Ans. B.

754. African plant Pentadiplandra is used as —

A. Low calories sweetener B. 2000 times sweeter agent

C. Sweetener for diabetic patients D. All the above

Ans. D.

755. Which organism was used as bioweapon derived from—

A. Clostridium B. Yersinia pestis

C. Fusarium species D. Green algae

Ans. C.

756. A set standards used to regulate own or community activity in relation to biological world is

A. Biopotency B. Biopiracy

C. Biowar D. Bioethics

Ans. D.

757. Biopiracy means

A. Use of biopatents

B. Thefts of plants and animals

C. Stealing of bioresources

D. Exploitation of bioresources without authentic permission

Ans. D.

758. Bioethics is related to

A. Preventing biopiracy

B. Regulation of unethical activities like gene cloning in animals

C. Preventing theft of living materials

D. Moral guidance to the problems in biology

Ans. B.

759. Three dimensional shape of tRNA is

A. L shaped B. Clove leaf like

C. X shaped D. Y shaped

Ans. B.

760. The term cistern, muton and recon were introduced by

A. Watson and Crick B. S. Benzer

C. Meselson D. Morgan

Ans. B.

761. Extranuclear genetic material is found in

A. Plastid and nucleus
B. Mitochondria and plastids
C. Nucleus and cytoplasm
D. Mitochondria and nucleus

Ans. B.

762. The molecular formulae of deoxyribose sugar and ribose sugar respectively are

A. $C_5 H_{10} O_4$ and $C_5H_{10}O_6$
B. $C_5 H_{10} O_4$ and $C_5H_{10}O_5$
C. $C_5 H_{10} O_5$ and $C_5H_{10}O_4$
D. $C_5 H_{10} O_5$ and $C_5H_{10}O_4$

Ans. B.

763. The nitrogen bases which pair with two hydrogen bonds are

A. Adenine and thymine
B. Adenine and Cytosine
C. Cytosine and Guanine
D. Cytosine and Adenine

Ans. A.

764. DNA differs from RNA in

A. Presence of deoxyribose sugar
B. Presence of thymine base
C. Property of replication
D. All the above

Ans. D.

765. The distance between two successive nitrogenous base pairs is

A. 34A°
B. 36 A°
C. 20A°
D. 3.4 A°

Ans. D.

766. In nucleoside, nitrogen base is attached to pentose sugar at

A. Carbon 1 of pentose sugar
B. Carbon 2 of pentose sugar
C. Carbon 4 of pentose sugar
D. Carbon 5 of pentose sugar

Ans. A.

767. If the strand of DNA has 35 nucleotide how many phosphodiester bonds would exist

A. 34
B. 35
C. 24
D. 70

Ans. A.

768. In eukaryotic DNA replication, lagging strand is formed by

A. RNA fragments
B. Okazaki fragments
C. DNA fragments
D. Nucleotide fragments

Ans. B.

769. The enzyme DNA polymerase can work only in

A. 3' - 5' direction
B. 5' - 3' direction
C. Both the direction
D. 5' - 5' direction

Ans. B.

770. Enzyme required for removing RNA primer during DNA replication is

A. DNA primase
B. DNA ligase
C. DNA polymerase I
D. DNA polymerase III

Ans. C.

771. During DNA replication, the reunion or recoiling of separated DNA strand is prevented by

A. Helix destabilizing protein
B. Single strand binding protein
C. ep protein
D. Both A and B

Ans. D.

772. The enzyme that cuts the bonds of DNA molecule at the origin of replication is

A. Endonuclease
B. DNA polymerase
C. DNA gyrase
D. DNA ligase

Ans. A.

773. Which of the following enzyme is required to release the tension imposed by uncoiling of strands ?

A. Endonuclease
B. DNA ligase
C. DNA gyrase
D. DNA helicase

Ans. C.

774. The cellular composition of mRNA is

A. 5-10%
B. 3-5%
C. 10-20%
D. 70-80%

Ans. B.

775. Formation of mRNA from DNA is called

A. Transformation
B. Transduction
C. Translation
D. Transcription

Ans. D.

776. The ratio of purines and pyrimidines in mRNA is not 1:1 because the nitrogenous bases are

A. Unpaired
B. Paired
C. Paired only in loops
D. Paired in stems

Ans. A.

777. The codons which may present at 3' end of mRNA is
A. UAA
B. UAG
C. UGA
D. Any one of these

Ans. D.

778. Which of the following is not tool of genetic engineering ?
A. Vectors
B. Enzymes
C. Foreign DNA
D. GMO

Ans. D.

779. The recombinant DNA technology a plasmid vector is cleaved by
A. Modified DNA ligase
B. A heated alkaline solution
C. The same enzyme that cleave the donor DNA
D. The different enzyme other than that cleave the donor DNA

Ans. C.

780. The most common plasmid vector used in genetic engineering is
A. PBR 328
B. PBR 322
C. PBR 325
D. PBR 330

Ans. B.

781. Nif gene for nitrogen fixation in cereal crops like wheat, jowar etc is introduced by cloning
A. Rhizobium meliloti
B. Bacillus thuringiensis
C. Rhizopus
D. Rhizophora

Ans. A.

782. Eco RI is an
A. Ligase
B. Polymerase
C. Restriction enzyme
D. Gyrase

Ans. C.

783. The transgenic plant flavr savr tomato carries an artificial gene for
A. Delay ripening process
B. Longer shelf life
C. Added flavours
D. All of these

Ans. D.

784. The work on GFP widely used as a reporter gene won the Nobel Prize in
A. Medicine/Physiology -2000
B. Chemistry-2008
C. Physics-2008
D. Biochemistry-2007

Ans. B.

785. The method of plasmid isolation by alkali lysis was published by

A. Mandel and Higa B. Sharp and Lederberg

C. Temin and Baltimore D. Birboim and Doly

Ans. D.

786. The group associated with first man made recombinant molecules :

A. Daniel Nathans, Arber and Kary Mullis

B. Paul Berg, Annie Chang, Boyer, Stanley Cohen

C. Temin, Brenner and Sharp

D. Hunt, Nurse, Hartwell

Ans. B.

787. In 2006, the Nobel prize for RNA interference was won for the work carried out on

A. D. melanogaster B. A. thaliana

C. C. elegans D. S. pombe

Ans. C.

788. The first crop plant genome sequenced

A. Maize B. Wheat

C. Rice D. Barley

Ans. C.

789. The first transgenic plant produced

A. Rice B. Maize

C. Cotton D. Tobacco

Ans. D.

790. The number of human genome project and completion of rough draft of sequence was in

A. 1992-2000 B. 1990-2000

C. 1990-2001 D. 1991-2001

Ans. B.

791. Who discovered recombinant DNA (rDNA) technology ?

A. Har Gobind Khorana B. J.D.Watson

C. Sulton and Boveri D. Stanley Cohen and Herbert Boyer

Ans. D.

792. Match the name of the scientist with their contributions and choose the correct answer

A. Walter Sutton — 1. Discovered penicillin

B. Stanley Cohen — 2. Discovered double helical structure of DNA

C. Alexander Flemming — 3. Discovered the chromosomal basis of heredity

D. James D.Watson — 4. Discovered rDNA

A. a2, b1, c4, d3 B. a3, b4, c1, d2

C. a1, b3, c2, d4 D. a4, b3, c2, d1

Ans. B.

793. Which of the following is a plasmid ?

A. Sal I B. Bam HI

C. Eco RI D. pBR322

Ans. D.

794. Restriction enzymes are

A. DNA unwinding enzymes B. DNA joining enzymes

C. DNA cleaving enzymes D. None of these

Ans. C.

795. The enzyme used to join the DNA fragments

A. Topoisomerase B. DNA ligase

C. DNA polymerase D. Reverse transcriptase

Ans. B.

796. Which of the following is used as vector in gene therapy for SCID ?

A. Arbovirus B. Rotavirus

C. Parvovirus D. Retrovirus

Ans. D.

797. Ti plasmid used in genetic engineering is obtained from

A. Bacillus thurigiensis B. Agrobacterium rhizogenes

C. Agrobacterium tumefaciens D. Bacillus subtilis

Ans. C.

798. The vector for T DNA is

A. Thermus aquaticus B. Bacillus rhizogenes

C. Agrobacterium tumefaciens D. E. coli

Ans. C.

799. Cry II Ab and cry I Ab produce toxins that control

A. Corn borer and tobacco budworms respectively

B. Nematodes and tobacco budworms respectively

C. Cotton bullworms and Corn borer respectively

D. Corn borer and Cotton bullworms respectively

Ans. C.

800. In genetic engineering, a DNA segment of interest is transferred to the host cell through a vector. Consider the following four agents (i-iv) in this regard and select the correct option about which one or more these can be used as a vector/ vectors

i) Bacterium
ii) Plasmid
iii) Plasmodium
iv) Bacteriophages

A. i, ii, iv
B. ii and iv
C. i and iv
D. i only

Ans. B.

801. Highest capacity vector is

A. Cosmid
B. YAC
C. Yeast integrative vector
D. Bacteriophage vector

Ans. B. Cosmid A plasmid with a cos site of lambda phage insert size 30-45 kb.

YAC yeast artificial chromosome insert size 1 Mb.

Bacteriopahge vectors refers to lambda and M13 phage vectors.

M13 vectors used to obtain single stranded copies of cloned DNA that are suited for DNA sequencing.

BAC Bacterial artificial chromosome insert size 300 kb.

802. The C value denotes the total number of DNA in a

A. Diploid
B. Haploid
C. Aneuploid
D. Polyploid

Ans. B.

803. Cdc mutants are useful for the study of

A. Chromosome breakpoint
B. B.Apoptosis
C. Various stages of cell cycle
D. Homeodomain

Ans. C. Cdc means cell division cycle.

804. RNA is very much susceptible to hydrolysis in alkali because

A. It contains Uracil residues in its structure

B. Its 2'OH groove participate in intramolecular cleavage of phosphodiester backbone

C. Cleavage occurs in the glycosidic bonds of purine bases

D. Cleavage occurs in the glycosidic bonds of pyrimidine bases

Ans. B. DNA is more stable than RNA because of H in the 2' position in DNA rather than OH in RNA.

805. Which one of the following is not a requirement of a PCR ?

A. DNA template   B. dNTPs

C. MgCl2   D. Taq polymerase

Ans. C. Although it is required for DNA polymerase but it can be avoided.

806. The heterozygosity of any locus can be ascertained by

A. SNPs   B. RFLPs

C. FISH analysis   D. Either RFLP analysis or SNP

Ans. D.

SNP single nucleotide polymorphism refers to the variation in the lengths of some DNA between the individuals due to single base changes. Application DNA fingerprinting.

RFLP refers to the variation in the restriction fragment length between individuals of a species.

FISH (Fluorescence in situ hybridization) : Hybridizing fluorescence labelled DNA probes onto human chromosome preparations allows genes to be mapped directly to their chromosomal locations.

807. Antibody diversity is generated by

A. Protein spicing   B. Somatic mutations

C. Allelic exclusion   D. Interchromosomal recombination

Ans. B.

808. The precursor for penicillin G biosynthesis during fermentation process is

A. Phenylacetic acid   B. Acetic acid

C. Phenoxy acetic acid   D. None of the above

Ans. C.

809. Which of the following process require energy ?

A. Ligation   B. Restriction digestion

C. Hybridization   D. Transformation

Ans. A.

810. Viral replication within cells is inhibited by

A. IL-4 B. IL-1

C. IFN-alpha D. TNF-alpha

Ans. C.

811. In the course of cell cycle, the level of the protein cyclin abruptly falls during

A. G1 phase B. G2 phase

C. S phase D. M phase

Ans. D.

812. The basic functional unit of human kidney is

A. Nephridia B. Nephron

C. Henle's loop D. None of the above

Ans. B.

813. Proximal and distal convoluted tubules are parts of

A. Oviduct B. Vas deferens

C. Nephron D. Seminiferous tubules

Ans. C.

814. Brush border is characteristic of

A. Neck of nephron B. Collecting tube

C. Proximal convoluted tubule D. All of the above

Ans. C.

815. A red blood cell was kept in a solution for a few minutes where it got burst. The solution was

A. Hypotonic B. Isotonic

C. Hypertonic D. Concentrated sugar solution

Ans. A.

816. Concentration of urine depends upon which organ ?

A. Bowman's capsule

B. Length of Henle's loop

C. P.C.T.

D. Network of capillaries arising from glomerulus

Ans. B.

817. A person is undergoing prolonged fasting. His urine will be found to contain abnormal quantities of

A. Fat B. Amino acid

C. Glucose D. Ketone

Ans. D.

818. Reabsorption of useful substances from glomerular filtrate occur in

A. Collecting tube
B. Loop of Henle
C. Proximal convoluted tubule
D. Distal convoluted tubule

Ans. C.

819. Conversion of ammonia to urea is done by

A. Arginine cycle
B. Fumaric cycle
C. Citrulline cycle
D. Ornithine cycle

Ans. D.

820. Angiotensinogen is a protein produced and secreted by

A. Liver cells
B. Macula densa cells
C. Endothelial cells
D. Juxtaglomerular cells

Ans. A.

821. A person who is on a longer hunger strike and surviving only on water will have

A. Less amino acids in his urine
B. More glucose in his blood
C. Less urea in his urine
D. More sodium in his urine

Ans. C.

822. A micro array is an ordered array of microscopic elements on a planer substrate that allows the specific binding of

A. Gene or gene products
B. Whole genome
C. Both A & B
D. None of these

Ans. A.

823. Biochips are made up of

A. Semi-conducting molecules inserted into the protein frame work
B. Conducting molecules inserted into the protein frame work
C. Non-conducting molecules inserted into the protein frame work
D. Any of the above

Ans. A.

824. Hypoxanthine can be measured by

A. Hypoxanthine sensor
B. Amorphous silicon ISFET
C. Urea sensor
D. Alcohol sensor

Ans. A.

825. Which of the following technology is used for micro array manufacturing?

A. Photolithography
B. Inkjetting
C. Contact printing
D. All of these

Ans. D.

826. Which of the following adaptations would be desirable for a farmer to breed into a crop of wheat?

A. Early ripening
B. Resistance to disease
C. Resistance to pests
D. All of these

Ans. D.

827. Microbiosensors are based on

A. Ions effect
B. Ion sensitive field effect transistor
C. Piezoelectric effect
D. Magnetic effect

Ans. B.

828. To qualify as a micro array the analytical device must be

A. Ordered
B. Microscopic
C. Planer and specific
D. All of these

Ans. D.

829. Microarrays are also known as

A. Biochips
B. DNA chips
C. Gene chips
D. All of these

Ans. D.

830. Single stranded circular RNA encapsidated with a larger RNA in a plant virus is

A. A virion
B. A viroid
C. A virusoid
D. None of these

Ans. C.

831. Microarray analysis involves biological assays based on

A. Gels
B. Filters
C. Purification columns
D. Small glass chips

Ans. D.

832. Which of the following is correct about micro biosensors?

A. Implantation in human body and are suitable for in-vivo measurements
B. Can be integrated on one chip and are useful for measuring various substrates in a small amount of sample solution simultaneously
C. It is possible to develop disposable transducers for biosensors through mass production
D. All of these

Ans. D.

833. Human insulin formed by recombinant DNA technology is known as

A. H insulin
B. R insulin
C. Humulin
D. Huinsulin

Ans. C.

834. How many nucleotides are there in ss RNA molecule of picorna virus causing FMD?

A. 1000
B. 5000
C. 8000
D. 10000

Ans. C.

835. Recombinant vaccine for Hepatitis B virus has been synthesized against which of the following antigen?

A. Viral core antigen (HBcAg)
B. Viral surface antigen (HBsAg)
C. E antigen (HBeAg)
D. All the above

Ans. B.

836. Chemically synthesized DNA sequences for the two chains are separately inserted into the plasmid pBR 322 by the side of

A. β-Galactosidase
B. Galactokinase
C. Acid phosphatise
D. Glucokinase

Ans. A.

837. Human growth hormone (hGH) is secreted by

A. Pituitary gland
B. Hypothalamus
C. Pancreas
D. None of these

Ans. A.

838. The promoter used for cloning HBV surface antigen is

A. Galactokinase
B. Alcohol dehydrogenase 1
C. β-galactosidase
D. Polyhedron

Ans. B.

839. Recombinant vaccine for HBV was produced by cloning viral genes in

A. Plasmids
B. Cosmids
C. Autonomously replicating plasmid of yeast
D. Phagemids

Ans. C.

840. The first therapeutic product formed by means of recombinant DNA technology is

A. Human growth hormone
B. Insulin
C. Hepatitis B vaccine
D. Vaccine for foot and mouth disease

Ans. B.

841. Which one of the following capsid protein of picorna virus is immunogenic in nature?

A. VP1
B. VP2
C. VP3
D. VP4

Ans. A.

842. The two chains are joined together to constitute native insulin using

A. Sodium dissulphonate and sodium sulphite
B. Sodium dissulphonate and sodium sulphate
C. Sodium sulphate and sodium sulphite
D. Sodium sulphate only

Ans. A.

843. In India first genetically engineered vaccine against HBV was developed by

A. Ranbaxy Pvt Ltd
B. Shantha Biotechnics Pvt. Ltd
C. Dabur Pvt Ltd
D. Glaxo Pvt. Ltd

Ans. B.

844. The recombinant hGH lacks

A. Terminal glutamine
B. Terminal lysine
C. Terminal methionine
D. Terminal arginine

Ans. C.

845. How is human insulin synthesized using recombinant DNA technology?

A. By using chemically synthesized DNA sequences for the two chains separately
B. By isolating DNA from the islets of Langerhans of pancreas
C. By using cDNA for insulin
D. By using chemically synthesized DNA sequences for the complete insulin protein

Ans. A.

846. The two chains of insulin can be separated by detaching it from b-galactosidase using

A. Hydrogen chloride
B. Cyanogens bromide
C. Peptidase
D. Protease

Ans. B.

847. Technique which uses homologous recombination to delete, add or change a gene is known as

A. Gene bundling B. Gene linking

C. Gene targeting D. Gene replication

Ans. C.

848. Name of first genetically modified organism was

A. Glow virus B. Globacteria

C. Glomice D. Glofish

Ans. D.

849. Microorganisms used in biotechnology

A. Shall not grow rapidly in cheap culture medium

B. Shall be readily manipulated

C. Shall not be pathogenic

D. All of these

Ans. C.

850. If genetic material from same species is used or species that can naturally breed with host then organism generated is

A. Clone genes B. Transgenic

C. Cisgenic D. Cross genes

Ans. C.

851. To transfer genes from one species to another, especially useful are

A. Vectors B. Plasmids

C. Double stranded DNA molecules D. Both A and B

Ans. D.

852. If genetic material of another species is added into host then organism resulting from this is classified as

A. Clone genes B. Transgenic

C. Cisgenic D. Cross genes

Ans. B.

853. First genetically modified organism is generated in

A. 1973 B. 1990

C. 1983 D. 1989

Ans. A.

854. Organism that is generated through processes of genetic engineering is classified as

A. Genetically replicated organism B. Clones organism
C. Mutation organism D. Genetically modified organism

Ans. D.

855. Process of replacing defective genes with effective genes is known as

A. Transgenic fusion B. Transgenic budding
C. Transgenic injection D. Gene therapy

Ans. D.

856. Element which allows easy visualization of genetic modification products is known as

A. Green fluorescent protein B. Blue fluorescent protein
C. White fluorescent protein D. Red fluorescent protein

Ans. A.

857. Enzyme which is used to remove or knockout genes is known as

A. Nucleolus B. Nuclease
C. Nucleotide D. Clones

Ans. B.

858. Technique of inserting DNA (Deoxyribonucleic Acid) into animal cells is known as

A. Microinjection B. Macro injection
C. Fusion injection D. Genome injection

Ans. A.

859. In penicillin production, pH of culture medium is maintained between

A. 5 and 6 B. 4 and 6
C. 6 and 7 D. 4 and 5

Ans. A.

860. First genetically modified pet was sold in United States in

A. 2003 B. 2008
C. 2006 D. 2004

Ans. A.

861. Antibodies are produced commercially by mixing a lymphocyte with

A. A bacteria B. A fungus
C. A tumor cell D. A non-living tissue

Ans. C.

862. First genetically modified mice is generated in

A. 1968 B. 1964

C. 1974 D. 1978

Ans. C.

863. Technique of inserting Deoxyribonucleic Acid (DNA) into plants is known as

A. Bio injection B. Bio-fission

C. Bio genetic D. Bio diffusion

Ans. B.

864. Function of streptococcus during milk fermentation is to

A. Produce aerobic environment B. Produce anaerobic environment

C. Form lactic acid D. All of these

Ans. B.

865. To produce penicillin, main fermentable source in culture is

A. Glucose B. Lactose

C. Sulphate D. Sugars

Ans. B.

866. Pruteen is made by mixing bacteria in

A. Ethanol B. Methanol

C. Vaseline D. Petroleum

Ans. B.

867. Transformation method of plants and animals in which plants and animals are given shocks is known as

A. Microinjection B. Genome breeding

C. Electroporation D. Genome engineering

Ans. C.

868. Transfer of genes from one species to another can be studied through

A. Bacteria B. Vectors

C. Fungi D. All of these

Ans. B.

869. Before discharging decomposed sewage into rivers and seas,

A. Water is filtered B. Pathogens are removed

C. pH of sewage is neutralized D. Both A and B

Ans. D.

870. Casein is converted to yoghurt because of

A. Lactic acid
B. Salicylic acid
C. Benzoic acid
D. Picric acid

Ans. A.

871. The enzyme needed in biological systems for joining two molecules is called

A. Ligase
B. Diastases
C. Polymerases
D. Hydrolase

Ans. A.

872. RNA does not contain

A. Uracil
B. Adenine
C. Hydroxy methyl cytosine
D. Phosphate

Ans. C.

873. In mammalian cells, ribosomal RNA is produced mainly in the

A. Nucleus
B. Nucleolus
C. Ribosome
D. Golgi apparatus

Ans. B.

874. A major advance in the detection of food borne pathogens is the use of standardized pathogen DNA patterns, or "food borne pathogen ————".

A. Fingerprinting
B. Plasmid patterns
C. Chromosomal patterns
D. Polymerase chain reaction
E. All of the above

Ans. A.

875. First discovered, Type II restriction endonuclease was

A. Hinf I
B. Eco K
C. Hind II
D. EcoRI

Ans. C.

876. Which of the following techniques can be used to determine the defective gene responsible for developing cancer?

A. Western blot
B. Southern blot
C. Northern blot
D. Eastern blot

Ans. B.

877. Some genetic diseases cannot be diagnosed by changes in restriction sites. Some of these can be detected by allele-specific oligonucleotide probes. These are

A. Copies of the gene with an altered sequence so that a restriction site is inserted

B. Mutagenized copies of a gene

C. Short sequences that will hybridize only to a specific base sequence

D. PCR-amplified variable numbers of tandem repeats (VNTRs)

Ans. C.

878. In order to insert a foreign gene into a plasmid, both must ———.

A. Have identical DNA sequences

B. Originate from the same type of cell

C. Be cut by the same restriction enzyme

D. Be of the same length

Ans. C.

879. Which of the following genetic diseases would be amenable to genetic engineering?

A. Down's syndrome B. Muscular dystrophy

C. Cystic fibrosis D. Cri du Chat

Ans. C.

880. X-rays cause

A. The formation of thymine dimers B. Ionization of water in the cell

C. Heat D. None of the above

Ans. B.

881. The order for the construction of a cDNA fragment from mRNA is to

A. Bind oligo-dT, treat with reverse transcriptase, digest with RNase, add G residues to the 3' end, bind oligo-dC, treat with DNA polymerase

B. Treat with reverse transcriptase, digest with RNase, add G residues to the 3' end, bind oligo-dC, treat with DNA polymerase and bind oligo-dT

C. Digest with RNase, add G residues to the 3' end, treat with reverse transcriptase, add G residues to the 3' end and treat with DNA polymerase

D. Bind oligo-dC, treat with reverse transcriptase, digest with RNase, add G residues to the 3' end, bind oligo-dT and treat with DNA polymerase

Ans. A.

882. Why is golden rice pale yellow in color?

A. It is rich in chlorophyll a. B. It is rich in beta-carotene.

C. It is rich in chlorophyll b. D. It is rich in phycobilins.

Ans. B.

883. Which type of restriction enzymes do not usually require ATP?

A. Type I
B. Type II
C. Type III
D. Type IV

Ans. B.

884. An example of a restriction fragment length polymorphism is

A. An Eco RI cuts DNA at a different sequence than Hind III
B. Different length fragments of DNA resulting from loss or gain of a restriction site
C. Cystic fibrosis results from a three base deletion in most cases but in other cases, other mutations are involved
D. All of the above

Ans. B.

885. Knockout mice are created by

A. Mutagenizing a mouse and selecting for mutant offspring
B. Creating a chimera by fusing cells from two different cell lines
C. Infecting the mouse with a retrovirus
D. Transfecting embryonic stem cells with an altered gene sequence

Ans. D.

886. A plasmid

A. Is a circular DNA molecule
B. Always contains an origin of replication
C. Usually contains one or more restriction sites
D. All of the above

Ans. D.

887. Under which of the following conditions would population gene frequencies remain the same?

A. Selection for homozygotes
B. Small population size
C. Active migration between groups
D. Random mating

Ans. D.

888. Plant transformation can be obtained by

A. Combining plant and animal cells in culture
B. Shooting DNA into plant cells with a gun
C. Using the E. coli bacterium to infect plant roots
D. Infecting plants with a tobacco mosaic virus

Ans. B.

889. An expression vector

A. Always contains an origin of replication

B. Usually contains a gene that confers antibiotic resistance to the bacterial host

C. Always contains DNA segments for the regulation of mRNA production

D. All of the above

Ans. D.

890. The unpaired nucleotides produced by the action of restriction enzymes are referred to have

A. Sticky ends B. Single strands

C. Restriction fragments D. Ligases

Ans. A.

891. Which of the following is not true of small inbreeding populations?

A. They tend to loose genetic diversity

B. There is an increased incidence of recessive diseases

C. Alleles may become fixed

D. Mutation is increased

Ans. D.

892. Which of these genes codes for a protein that plays a role in growth?

A. DCP1 B. SCLC6A4

C. KRTHA1 D. GH1

Ans. D.

893. Which of the following pair will produce complementary sticky ends?

A. Eco RI & MspI B. Msp I & HPA II

C. Sau 3A & Bam HI D. Mbo I & Sau 3A

Ans. C.

894. A human cDNA library

A. Contains DNA for specific human proteins

B. Contains DNA for virtually all of the human proteins in vectors

C. Cannot be used to obtain human genes because it would be radioactive

D. None of the above

Ans. B.

895. What enzyme forms covalent bonds between restriction fragments?

A. DNA primase B. DNA helicase

C. DNA polymerase D. DNA ligase

Ans. D.

896. Which of the following can be diagnosed by amniocentesis?

A. Down's syndrome
B. Cystic Fibrosis
C. Sickle cell anemia
D. All of these

Ans. D.

897. The type II restriction endonucleases, bind to DNA sites

A. Using H-bonds for specificity
B. That are usually palindromic
C. Using non-sequence-dependent backbone interactions
D. All of the above

Ans. D.

898. The enzyme that joins DNA cuts is called

A. Joinase
B. Ligase
C. DNA phosphorylase
D. Reverse transcriptase

Ans. B.

899. Cleavage of DNA by EcoRI endonuclease results in the formation of

A. Two 3'-OH ends and two 5'-phosphate ends
B. One 3'-OH end and one 5'-phosphate end
C. Two 3'-phosphate ends and two 3'-OH ends
D. One 3'-OH end and two 5'-phosphate end

Ans. A.

900. For gene transfer to be effective, transforming DNA must be

A. Incorporated into the bacterial chromosome
B. Incorporated into a viral genome
C. Free in the bacterial cytoplasm
D. None of the above

Ans. A.

901. Double stranded DNA denaturation with specified limit of temperature is

A. Reversible reaction
B. Irreversible reaction
C. Either A or B
D. None of these

Ans. A.

902. From a single molecule of DNA, PCR can make

A. One additional copy
B. Hundreds of copies
C. Thousands of copies
D. Millions of copies

Ans. D.

903. Genomic libraries are made from

A. Genomic DNA of an organism B. Genomic RNA of an organism

C. Genomic cDNA of an organism D. Genomic mRNA of an organism

Ans. A.

904. Bacteriophages are

A. Cells in the blood that eat bacteria B. A class of bacteria

C. Bacterial viruses D. None of the above

Ans. C.

905. Specialized transduction occurs when

A. The bacteriophage incorporates randomly in the bacterial chromosome

B. The bacteriophage never incorporates into the bacterial chromosome

C. The bacteriophage always incorporates at the same position in the bacterial chromosome

D. None of the above

Ans. C.

906. PCR is used

A. To diagnose genetic diseases B. To solve crimes

C. To study gene function D. All of these

Ans. D.

907. To clone into a plasmid vector, both the plasmid and the foreign DNA are cut

A. With the same restriction enzyme and mixed together

B. With different restriction enzyme and mixed together

C. With the combination of enzymes and then seperated

D. With the combination of enzymes and mixed together

Ans. A.

908. PCR can be used to amplify a specific fragment of DNA from which of the following?

A. A drop of blood B. A hair follicle

C. A fragment of skin D. All of these

Ans. D.

909. Transformation means

A. Formation of a pilus

B. Acquiring DNA from the bacterial cell environment

C. Plasmid containing a F factor

D. F+ and F- strains of bacteria

Ans. B.

910. Restriction maps

A. Allows comparison between DNA molecules without the need to determine nucleotide sequence

B. Allows comparison between DNA molecules but requires to determine nucleotide sequence

C. Does not allow comparison between DNA molecules

D. None of the above

Ans. A.

911. A PCR cycle consists of

A. Three steps, denaturation, primer annealing and elongation

B. Three steps, denaturation, initiation and elongation

C. Three steps, primer annealing, elongation and termination

D. Three steps, initiation, elongation and termination

Ans. A.

912. How many ds DNA molecule can be produced, which comprise precisely the target region in double strand form during 4th cycle of PCR?

A. Two ds DNA molecule B. Three ds DNA molecule

C. Eight ds DNA molecule D. Four ds DNA molecule

Ans. D.

913. PCR can be used in

A. Cloning

B. Sequencing

C. Medical diagnosis and forensic medicine

D. All of the above

Ans. D.

914. PCR (Polymerase Chain Reaction) can make multiple copies of

A. DNA B. RNA

C. Protein D. Carbohydrate

Ans. A.

915. PCR is an abbreviation for

A. Protein Change Reaction B. Polymerase Chain Reaction

C. Positive Charge Reaction D. Preliminary Change Rate

Ans. B.

916. PCR amplifies millions of copies of

A. A short fragment of DNA

B. The entire genome (all the DNA in a sample)

C. Both (a) and (b)

D. Short chain RNA

Ans. A.

917. Southern blotting involves

A. Electrophoresis of DNA molecules and then blotting the separated DNA bands followed by incubation

B. Electrophoresis of DNA molecules and then blotting the separated RNA bands followed by incubation

C. Electrophoresis of DNA molecules followed by incubation

D. Electrophoresis of RNA molecules and then blotting the separated RNA bands followed by incubation

Ans. A.

918. Bactriophages absorb to a bacterial surface and inject the phage DNA through the

A. Cell wall into cytosol

B. Cell wall into plasmamembrane

C. Both (a) and (b)

D. Cell wall into endoplasmic reticulum

Ans. A.

919. In a PCR reaction after four cycles, each molecule of a duplex DNA will give rise to

A. 16 single strands of DNA

B. 16 double stranded DNA

C. 18 single strands of DNA

D. 18 double stranded DNA

Ans. A.

920. The PCR, polymerase chain reaction is becoming the method of choice for

A. Alteration of gene

B. Screening gene

C. Sterilization of gene

D. All of these

Ans. B.

921. Northern blotting is

A. Widely different than southern blotting

B. Another name for southern blotting

C. Analogous to southern blotting

D. None of the above

Ans. C.

922. What technique can be used to determine the murderer who left blood with the victim?

A. DNA sequencing
B. PCR amplification
C. Western blot
D. RFLP mapping

Ans. B.

923. DNA fragments in a restriction digest can be separated by electrophoresis in

A. Poly acrylamide
B. Agarose gel
C. Both A and B
D. None of these

Ans. C.

924. Which of the following techniques was carried out by Nirenberg and Matthaei in 1961 to determine the first codon?

A. In vitro synthesis of a polypeptide using UUUUU
B. Labeled peptide binding to a ribosome
C. Mixed co-polymer mRNA synthesis
D. None of the above

Ans. A.

925. Bacterial protein called catabolic activator protein (CAP) is an example of

A. Negative control of gene expression
B. Positive control of gene expression
C. Second type of positive control of gene expression
D. None of the above

Ans. C.

926. How many different codons are possible?

A. 3
B. 20
C. 64
D. An infinite number

Ans. C.

927. The genetic code is

A. Universal
B. Universal except for rare exceptions in mitochondria and some protozoa
C. Species-specific
D. Kingdom-specific

Ans. B.

928. Which of the following has been used as an evidence that primitive life forms lacked both DNA and enzymes?

A. RNA can both code genetic information and act as a catalyst

B. DNA and enzymes are only present in the most advanced cells

C. Advanced cells lack RNA

D. All of the above

Ans. A.

929. Crick demonstrated that the genetic code involved three bases and suggested that the code was degenerated. What experimental technique Crick conducted to suggest genetic code degeneration?

A. Gel electrophoresis
B. Density gradient centrifugation
C. Frameshift mutagenesis
D. Restriction digests of the rII gene

Ans. C.

930. Codon that specify the amino acids often differs in the

A. First base
B. Second base
C. Third base
D. None of these

Ans. C.

931. In some organelles in eukaryotes, the genetic code for some codons

A. Differs from that used in prokaryotes

B. Are same

C. Are partially same

D. None of the above

Ans. A.

932. The codons which do not specify an amino acid are called

A. Initiation code
B. Termination code
C. Propagation code
D. None of these

Ans. B.

933. The genetic code is degenerated. Which of the following codons represents the principle of degeneracy?

A. UAA and UAC
B. AUG and AUA
C. CAU and CAC
D. UUA and UUC

Ans. C.

934. The sequence of one strand of DNA is: 5' ATTGCCA 3', what is the sequence of the other strand?

A. 5' TAACGGT 3'
B. 5' TGGCAAT 3'
C. 5' ATTGCCA 3'
D. 5' UAAGCCU3'

Ans. B.

935. In prokaryotes, AUG encodes

A. Methionine
B. N-formyl methionine
C. A stop codon
D. Alanine

Ans. B.

936. How many amino acids will be encoded by 5' GAU GGU UGA UGU 3' sequence?

A. One
B. Two
C. Three
D. Four

Ans. B.

937. In protein synthesis in prokaryotes

A. The initiating amino acid is N- formyl methionine
B. The initiating amino acid is methionine
C. The initiating amino acid is phenyl alanine
D. None of the above

Ans. A.

938. AUG codes for methionine act as a

A. Initiation code
B. Elongation code
C. Termination code
D. Propagation code

Ans. A.

939. Translation begins

A. At the replication fork
B. On the lagging strand
C. At the start codon
D. In nucleus

Ans. C.

940. Sex lethal (sxl) in Drosophila is transcribed when

A. The X autosome balance is less than 0.5
B. The X autosome balance is 1 or greater
C. The X autosome balance equals 0.5
D. None of the above

Ans. B.

941. A mutation in the tip binding site of the repressor would result in

A. Constitutive trp operon expression

B. Inducible trp operon expression

C. No operon expression

D. None of the above

Ans. A.

942. The first protein complex to bind to the TATA box is

A. Transcription factor IIA B. Transcription factor IIB

C. Transcription factor IID D. All of these

Ans. C.

943. Which of the following is not part of the lac operon?

A. I B. O

C. P D. none of these

Ans. A.

944. The lac operon is transcribed in which segments?

A. 1 B. 2

C. 3 D. 4

Ans. A.

945. A frameshift mutation occurs in the sigma subunit gene transcribed as part of SPOl early genes. What will be the immediate result?

A. Early genes will not be translated

B. Middle genes will not be transcribed

C. The bacterial host will lyse immediately

D. Infection will proceed as usual

Ans. C.

946. In the presence of high levels of tryptophan

A. Attenuator allows transcription of trp structural genes

B. Attenuator propogates transcription

C. Attenuator terminates transcription

D. None of the above

Ans. C.

947. Tubulin is regulated by

A. Binding of tubulin to tubulin mRNA

B. Splicing of the tubulin transcript

C. Binding of tubulin to the tubulin translational product

D. Binding of tubulin to DNA

Ans. C.

948. Transcription factors are

A. Regions of DNA in the promoter area

B. Regions of DNA in the enhancer area

C. Any protein which binds to DNA

D. Proteins which bind DNAand initiate transcription

Ans. D.

949. Genes which need to be coordinately regulated but are not in operons may be regulated by

A. Common transcription factor binding domains

B. TATA boxes

C. CAAT regions

D. GC regions

Ans. A.

950. What are genes?

A. The functional unit of inheritance B. A fragment of DNA

C. A portion of a chromosome D. All of the above

Ans. D.

951. Which of the following is not a transcription factor?

A. Helix-turn-helix proteins B. Zinc finger proteins

C. Leucine zipper proteins D. Steroid hormones

Ans. D.

952. Sex determination in Drosophila involves

A. Alternate splicing B. Methylation

C. Gene amplification D. None of these

Ans. A.

953. Enhancers differ from promoters in that

A. They initiate transcription

B. They are adjacent to the start codon

C. Their orientation can be inverted without effect

D. They are restricted to a specific gene

Ans. C.

954. Methylated gene are

A. Active B. Silent

C. Dynamic D. Either A or B

Ans. B.

955. Which of the following occur in the presence of glucose?

A. Lac Z gene expression is increased

B. cAMP increases

C. Binding of CAP-cAMP complex to the promoter area decreases

D. None of the above

Ans. C.

956. Sex hormones activate transcription of specific genes by

A. Binding to a transcription factor B. Binding to RNA polymerase

C. Binding to DNA enhancer region D. Binding to DNA promoter region

Ans. A.

957. The lac operon is translated into ———— proteins.

A. 1 B. 2

C. 3 D. 4

Ans. C.

958. In the presence of tryptophan in the cell, the repressor is ————

A. Bound to tryptophan

B. Bound to DNA

C. Bound to both DNA and tryptophan

D. Bound to neither tryptophan nor DNA

Ans. C.

959. Catabolite activating protein exerts —— control on transcription of the lac operon genes.

A. Positive B. Negative

C. May be positive or negative D. None of these

Ans. A.

960. DNA is methylated at

A. AC sequences
B. TATA sequences
C. CAAT sequences
D. CG sequences

Ans. D.

961. Why are several structural genes regulated as a unit in bacteria?

A. An accident of evolution
B. It allows coordinating regulation of genes with a common function
C. The bacteria chromosome is so small; many different genes must be controlled by the same promoter
D. None of the above

Ans. B.

962. Alternate splicing of RNA transcripts is a mechanism to regulate

A. Tubulin
B. Tachykinins
C. DNA methylation
D. Leucine zippers

Ans. B.

963. Agarose gel electrophoresis and pulsed field gel electrophoresis may be used to resolve respectively

A. 2000 kb and 20kb DNA
B. 1000 kb and 10kb DNA
C. 20 kb and 2000 kb DNA
D. 10 kb and 1000 kb DNA

Ans. C.

964. The IPTG is a gratuitous inducers of b-galactosidase, and x-gal is a chromogenic substrate. When a-complementation occurs which colour is produced?

A. Blue
B. White
C. Brown
D. No colour is produced

Ans. A.

965. Different form of a plasmid, on an agarose gel, after electrophoresis may be in which of the following sequence in decreasing molecular weight?

A. Open circular, super coiled, linear plasmid DNA
B. Linear plasmid, open circular, super coiled plasmid
C. Open circular, super coiled, linear plasmid DNA
D. Open circular, linear plasmid, super coiled plasmid

Ans. B.

966. What radioactive molecule is used to end-label an oligonucleotide?

A. (alpha)-^{32}P-ATP B. (alpha)-^{32}P-dUTP

C. (gamma)-^{32}P-ATP D. Any of these

Ans. C.

967. Which of the following radioactive element is generally involved in RIA?

A. Tritium B. Carbon-14

C. Iodine-125 D. All of these

Ans. D.

968. What is approximately the half life of 32-Phosphorus?

A. 14 days B. 28 days

C. 42 days D. 30 days

Ans. A.

969. DNA- footprinting is a suitable technique for identifying which of the following?

A. Particular mRNA in mixture B. Particular t-RNA in mixture

C. Introns within DNA D. Protein binding site within DNA

Ans. D.

970. Which of these restriction enzymes produce blunt ends?

A. SalI B. EcoRV

C. XhoI D. HindIII

Ans. B.

971. The RP13 gene of chromosome 17 codes for a protein ————.

A. Involved in glucose transport

B. That is a component of hair and nails

C. Involved in eye development

D. Involved in the determination of personality

Ans. C.

972. Isoschizomers recognize

A. Same recognition sequence but different recognition site

B. Same recognition site and recognition sequence

C. Same recognition site and different recognition sequence

D. Different recognition site and different recognition sequence

Ans. B.

973. Restriction enzymes are named for

A. The person who discovered
B. The bacterium they are derived from
C. The viral DNA that they attack
D. None of the above

Ans. B.

974. Which of these genes codes for a protein that plays a role in white blood cell function?

A. DCP1
B. MPO
C. GLUT4
D. RP13

Ans. B.

975. When populations are small, gene frequencies can change from generation to generation and some alleles may become fixed in a population. This is called—.

A. Assortative mating
B. Inbreeding
C. Heterosis
D. Genetic drift

Ans. D.

976. Which of the following is correct in terms of determination of location of genetic traits?

A. Known protein coding sequences are too far apart to allow linkage determination for most new genes
B. Restriction sites allow DNAs to be digested
C. Protein-coding genes are always associated with a restriction pattern
D. None of the above

Ans. A.

977. In gel electrophoresis, DNA molecules migrate from ——— to ——— ends of the gel.

A. Negative ... positive
B. Basic ... acidic
C. Long ... short
D. Positive to negative

Ans. A.

978. Restriction enzymes

A. Protect bacteria from viral infection
B. Cut DNA in a staggered fashion
C. Cut DNAs producing a blunt end
D. All of the above

Ans. D.

979. First discovered, Type II restriction endonuclease was

A. Hinf I
B. Eco K
C. Hind II
D. EcoRI

Ans. C.

980. Which of the following techniques can be used to determine the defective gene for developing cancer?

A. Western blot
B. Southern blot
C. Northern blot
D. Eastern blot

Ans. B.

981. The transfer of antibiotic-resistant genes from genetically engineered bacteria to disease causing bacteria ————.

A. Would be of no concern if it occurred.
B. Has occurred
C. Can never occur
D. Seems unlikely

Ans. D.

982. Both DNA gel electrophoresis and SDS-PAGE of proteins are similar because

A. In both cases molecules migrate to the anode
B. Both techniques rely on a constant charge to mass ratio
C. Both techniques utilize the sieving properties of gels
D. All of the above

Ans. D.

983. Some genetic diseases cannot be diagnosed by changes in restriction sites. Some of these can be detected by allele-specific oligonucleotide probes. These are

A. Copies of the gene with an altered sequence so that a restriction site is inserted
B. Mutagenized copies of a gene
C. Short sequences that will hybridize only to a specific base sequence
D. PCR-amplified variable numbers of tandem repeats (VNTRs)

Ans. C.

984. In order to insert a foreign gene into a plasmid, both must ————.

A. Have identical DNA sequences
B. Originate from the same type of cell
C. Be cut by the same restriction enzyme
D. Be of the same length

Ans. C.

985. Which of the following genetic diseases would be amenable to genetic engineering?

A. Down's syndrome
B. Muscular dystrophy
C. Cystic fibrosis
D. Cri du Chat

Ans. C.

986. X-rays cause

A. The formation of thymine dimers
B. Ionization of water in the cell
C. Heat
D. None of the above

Ans. B.

987. The order for the construction of a cDNA fragment from mRNA is to

A. Bind oligo-dT, treat with reverse transcriptase, digest with RNase, add G residues to the 3' end, bind oligo-dC, treat with DNA polymerase
B. Treat with reverse transcriptase, digest with RNase, add G residues to the 3' end, bind oligo-dC, treat with DNA polymerase and bind oligo-dT
C. Digest with RNase, add G residues to the 3' end, treat with reverse transcriptase, add G residues to the 3' end and treat with DNA polymerase
D. Bind oligo-dC, treat with reverse transcriptase, digest with RNase, add G residues to the 3' end, bind oligo-dT and treat with DNA polymerase

Ans. A.

988. The TP53 gene of chromosome 17 codes for a protein ——————.

A. That plays a role in the digestive process
B. Involved in glucose transport
C. Involved in the regulation of the cell cycle
D. That is like a white blood cell protein

Ans. C.

989. Which type of restriction enzymes do not usually require ATP ?

A. Type I
B. Type II
C. Type III
D. Type IV

Ans. B.

990. An example of a restriction fragment length polymorphism is

A. An Eco RI cuts DNA at a different sequence than Hind III
B. Different length fragments of DNA resulting from loss or gain of a restriction site
C. Cystic fibrosis results from a three base deletion in most cases but in other cases, other mutations are involved
D. All of the above

Ans. B.

991. Knockout mice are created by

A. Mutagenizing a mouse and selecting for mutant offspring

B. Creating a chimera by fusing cells from two different cell lines

C. Infecting the mouse with a retrovirus

D. Transfecting embryonic stem cells with an altered gene sequence

Ans. D.

992. A plasmid

A. Is a circular DNA molecule

B. Always contains an origin of replication

C. Usually contains one or more restriction sites

D. All of the above

Ans. D.

993. Under which of the following conditions would population gene frequencies remain the same?

A. Selection for homozygotes

B. Small population size

C. Active migration between groups

D. Random mating

Ans. D.

994. Plant transformation can be obtained by

A. Combining plant and animal cells in culture

B. Shooting DNA into plant cells with a gun

C. Using the E. coli bacterium to infect plant roots

D. Infecting plants with a tobacco mosaic virus

Ans. B.

995. An expression vector

A. Always contains an origin of replication

B. Usually contains a gene that confers antibiotic resistance to the bacterial host

C. Always contains DNA segments for the regulation of mRNA production

D. All of the above

Ans. D.

996. The type II restriction endonucleases, bind to DNA sites

A. Using H-bonds for specificity

B. That are usually palindromic

C. Using non-sequence-dependent backbone interactions

D. All of the above

Ans. D.

997. The enzyme that joins DNA cuts is called

A. Joinase
B. Ligase
C. DNA phosphorylase
D. reverse transcriptase

Ans. B.

998. The original enzyme(s) used in PCR reaction is/are known as

A. E. coli RNA polymerase
B. E. coli DNA polymerase
C. All of these
D. Taq polymerase

Ans. B.

999. How is human insulin synthesized using recombinant DNA technology?

A. By isolating DNA from the islets of Langerhans of pancreas
B. By using chemically synthesized DNA sequences for the two chains separately
C. By using chemically synthesized DNA sequences for the complete insulin protein
D. By using cDNA for insulin

Ans. A.

1000. The two chains are joined together to constitute native insulin using

A. Sodium dissulphonate and sodium sulphate
B. Sodium dissulphonate and sodium sulphite
C. Sodium sulphate only
D. Sodium sulphate and sodium sulphite

Ans. B.

1001. Which of the following repairs nicked DNA by forming a phosphodiester bond between adjacent nucleotides?

A. DNA gyrase
B. Helicase
C. DNA ligase
D. Topoisomerases

Ans. C.

1002. DNA replication rates in prokaryotes are approximately of the order of

A. 1000 bases per second
B. 10 bases per second
C. 10,000 bases per second
D. 1,000 bases per second

Ans. B.

1003. During which of the following process a new copy of a DNA molecule is precisely synthesized?

A. Transcription
B. Transformation
C. Replication
D. Translation

Ans. C.

1004. The replication of chromosomes by eukaryotes occurs in a relatively short period of time because

A. The eukaryotic replication machinery is 1000 times faster than the prokaryotes

B. The eukaryotes have more amount of DNA for replication

C. Eukaryotic DNA is always single stranded

D. Each chromosome contains multiple replicons

Ans. D.

1005. Both strands of DNA serve as templates concurrently in

A. Excision repair B. Replication

C. None of these D. Mismatch repair

Ans. B.

1006. Proofreading activity to maintain the fidelity of DNA synthesis

A. Is a function of the 3'-5' exonuclease activity of the DNA polymerases

B. Occurs after the synthesis has been completed

C. Occurs in prokaryotes but not eukaryotes

D. Requires the presence of an enzyme separate from the DNA polymerases

Ans. A.

1007. Electroporation is

A. The process of combining foreign DNA to an electrically charged vector molecule

B. The process of separating charged molecules through a gel maintained in an electric field

C. The process of multiplication of the cells

D. The application of high voltage pulses

Ans. D.

1008. The deliberate modifications of an organism's genetic information by directly changing its nucleic acid content is a subject matter of

A. Population genetics B. Genetic engineering

C. Protein engineering D. Microbiology

Ans. B.

1009. Which of the following is obtained using processed mRNA molecules as a template?

A. mDNA B. rDNA

C. tDNA D. cDNA

Ans. D.

1010. In genetic engineering, a chimera is

A. A plasmid that contains foreign DNA

B. An enzyme that links DNA molecules

C. A fungi

D. A virus that infects bacteria

Ans. A.

1011. The piece of equipment, that introduces DNA into cells via DNA-coated microprojectiles is known as

A. DNA probe
B. Laser
C. Inoculating needle
D. Gene gun

Ans. D.

1012. A molecular technique in which DNA sequences between two oligonucleotide primers can be amplified is known as

A. Northern blotting
B. Southern blotting
C. DNA replication
D. Polymerase chain reaction

Ans. D.

1013. Problems in obtaining large amounts of proteins encoded by recombinant genes can often be overcome by using

A. Expression vectors
B. BACS
C. All of these
D. YACS

Ans. A.

1014. Nucleotide bases and aromatic amino acids absorb light respectively at

A. 260 and 280 nm
B. 280 and 260 nm
C. 260 and 270 nm
D. 270 and 280 nm

Ans. A.

1015. Processive synthesis is a characteristic feature of

A. DNA Pol III at a replication fork

B. All DNA polymerases

C. DNA mismatch repair

D. Removal of RNA primers on Okazaki fragments

Ans. A.

1016. Which of the following is not a transcription factor?

A. Zinc finger proteins
B. Helix turn helix proteins
C. Steroid hormones
D. Leucine zipper proteins

Ans. C.

1017. First step of genetic engineering is

A. Isolation of gene of interest
B. Insertion of gene into vector
C. Growth of GMO
D. Expression of gene

Ans. A.

1018. In first step of genetic engineering, special enzymes that are used to separate identified gene are called

A. Expressed nucleases
B. Inserted nucleases
C. Restriction endonuclease
D. Isolated nucleases

Ans. C.

1019. Particular enzyme produced by genetic engineering which is used to dissolve clots of blood is called

A. Interferon
B. Urokinase
C. Thymosin
D. Beta-endorphin

Ans. B.

1020. 2nd step of genetic engineering is

A. Growth of GMO
B. Expression of gene
C. Isolation of gene interest
D. Insertion of gene into vector

Ans. D.

1021. Fourth step of genetic engineering is

A. Growth of GMO
B. Expression of gene
C. Isolation of gene interest
D. Insertion of gene into vector

Ans. B.

1022. Last step of genetic engineering is

A. Isolation of gene interest
B. Insertion of gene into vector
C. Transfer of recombinant DNA
D. Expression of gene

Ans. D.

1023. Third step of genetic engineering is

A. Isolation of gene interest
B. Insertion of gene into vector
C. Transfer of recombinant DNA
D. Expression of gene

Ans. C.

6

Immunology

1. Interferon is formed by

   A. Lymphocytes B. Lymphoblasts

   C. Fibroblasts D. All of these

Ans. D.

2. Histones are found in

   A. Prokaryotes B. Eukaryotes

   C. Viruses D. None of these

Ans. B.

3. Phagocytes are

   A. Monocytes B. Macrophages

   C. Basophils D. All of these

Ans. D.

4. The microorganism engulfed by phagocyte resides in a vacuole is known as

   A. Phagosome B. Lysosome

   C. both a and b D. None of these

Ans. A.

5. Toxic products in phagolysosome are

   A. H2SO4 B. Singlet O2

   C. Superoxide radicals D. All of these

Ans. D.

6. During destruction of antigen particle in phagolysosome the product formed in phagolysosome

   A. Acetic acid B. Lactic acid

   C. Citric acid D. None of these

Ans. B.

7. The coating of a bacterium with antibody or complement that leads to enhanced phagocytosis of the bacterium by phagocytes is called

A. Opsonisation B. Aggulation

C. CFT D. None of these

Ans. A.

8. Infection that results in pus formation are called

A. Focal infection B. Acute infection

C. Pyogenic infection D. Chronic infection

Ans. C.

9. Presence of viable bacteria in the blood stream is called

A. Viraemia B. Septicaemia

C. Bacteraemia D. Bactericidal

Ans. C.

10. Presence of viruses in the blood stream is known as

A. Viraemia B. Bacteraemia

C. Septicaemia D. Pyemia

Ans. A.

11. Opsonin is the

A. Cell wall component B. Plasma component

C. Serum component D. Cytoplasm component

Ans. C.

12. β-haemolytic bacteria is

A. Streptococcus pyogenes B. Str. pneumoniae

C. Str. viridans D. Str. Faecalis

Ans. A.

13. Influenza virus is identified by using

A. Haemaggulutinin inhibition test B. Tissue culture method

C. Embryonated eggs D. Plaque formation

Ans. A.

14. "Prozone phenomenon" is encountered in

A. A typical mycobacteria B. Brucella

C. Streptococcus D. Bordetella pertusis

Ans. B.

15. Coagulase test is used for

A. Salmonella B. Staphylococcus

C. Bordetella D. Pneumococcus

Ans. B.

16. Lab diagnosis of Leishmaniasis is done by

A. CFT B. Peripheral smear

C. Blood culture D. All of these

Ans. D.

17. Freeze-etch particles (used in preparing cell for electron microscopy) can be located in the

A. Cytoplasm B. Cell wall

C. Cell membrane D. Nucleus

Ans. C.

18. Which of the following can provide naturally acquired passive immunity for the new born.

A. IgA B. IgG

C. IgE D. IgM

Ans. B.

19. Complement based agglutination reaction is known as

A. Haemagglutination B. Complement fixation

C. Conglutination D. Schultz Dale Phenomenon

Ans. B.

20. Reverse transcriptase is an enzyme involved in the synthesis of

A. cDNA B. Soluble RNA

C. mRNA from DNA D. Nucleotides

Ans. A.

21. The major immunoglobulin present in the human serum is

A. IgG B. IgA

C. IgE D. IgG

Ans. A.

22. Reaginic type antibody is

A. IgG B. IgA

C. IgM D. IgE

Ans. D.

23. Blood group antigens are
   A. Species specific B. Isospecific
   C. Autospecific D. Organ specific

Ans. B.

24. The reaction of soluble antigen with antibody is known by
   A. Precipitation B. Flocculation
   C. Agglutination D. Complement fixation

Ans. A.

25. Agglutination reaction is strongest with the immunoglobulin:
   A. IgM B. IgG
   C. IgA D. IgD

Ans. A.

26. The use of monoclonal antibodies is
   A. Immunotherapy B. Gene therapy
   C. Blood transfusion D. Organ transfusion

Ans. A.

27. Hybridoma technique is used for
   A. Monoclonal antibodies B. Polyclonal antibodies
   C. Both a and b D. None of these

Ans. A.

28. Test used for AIDS is
   A. Widal test B. ELISA
   C. Aggluatination D. CFT

Ans. B.

29. In Counter immunoelectrophoresis
   A. Electrophoresis will drive the antibody and antigen parallel to each other
   B. Electrophoresis will drive the antibody and antigen toward each other
   C. The antibody will migrate towards anode
   D. The antibody will migrate towards cathode

Ans. B.

30. What is the ELISA test intended to measure?
   A. Antibody to HIV only
   B. Antigen to HIV only
   C. Presence of free, circulating virus in the patient
   D. Antibodies directed against HLA molecules

Ans. A.

31. Immunoaffinity chromatography can be used in biochemical applications to

A. Break down antibody structure

B. Purify protein antigen

C. Break down antigen and analyze quantitatively

D. None of the above

Ans. B.

32. Antibody having high valency is

A. IgG
B. IgA
C. IgD
D. IgM

Ans. D.

33. Antigenic specificity is due to

A. Chemical complexity
B. Solubility
C. Steric configuration
D. All of these

Ans. C.

34. Antibodies are

A. Proteins
B. Glycoproteins
C. Phospholipids
D. None of these

Ans. B.

35. General purpose antibody is

A. IgA
B. IgG
C. IgM
D. IgD

Ans. B.

36. Antibody present in colostrums is

A. IgG
B. IgA
C. IgM
D. IgE

Ans. B.

37. Which antibody is called millionaire molecule?

A. IgA
B. IgM
C. IgG
D. IgD

Ans. B.

38. IgE is discovered by

A. Ishizaka
B. Porter
C. Richet
D. None of these

Ans. A.

39. Serological reactions are useful for

A. Detection of antigens B. Detection of antibodies

C. Both a and b D. None of these

Ans. C.

40. When a particular antigen is mixed with antibody in the presence of an electrolyte at suitable temperature and pH the particles are clumped, this is called:

A. Precipitation B. Agglutination

C. Electrophoresis D. CIE

Ans. B.

41. Toxins and viruses can be detected by

A. Precipitation B. Agglutination

C. Neutralisation D. None of these

Ans. C.

42. Which is most antigenic?

A. Exotoxins B. Endotoxins

C. Viruses D. All of these

Ans. A.

43. Shick test is used for the detection of

A. Diphtheria B. T.B.

C. Cholera D. Typhoid

Ans. A.

44. Very effective, less time consuming and at a time so many samples can be detected by

A. ELISA B. CFT

C. Neutralization D. Agglutination

Ans. A.

45. B-cells are involved in

A. Humoral immunity B. Cell-mediated immunity

C. Active immunity D. Passive immunity

Ans. A.

46. Example for cell-mediated immunity are

A. Tuberculin type B. Contact dermatitis

C. Granulomatous D. All of these

Ans. A.

47. Mountax reaction is used for detection of

A. T.B. B. Diphtheria

C. Cholera D. None of these

Ans. A.

48. Anthrax vaccine is prepared by

A. Attenuated bacilli B. Killing the bacilli

C. Live bacilli D. None of these

Ans. A.

49. Attenuated, oral poliomyelitis vaccine is

A. BCG B. Measles vaccine

C. Sabin vaccine D. TAB vaccine

Ans. C.

50. Killed polio vaccine is

A. Sabin vaccine B. Salk

C. BCG D. TAB

Ans. B.

51. Measles vaccine is given to children at the age of

A. 1 year B. 7 months

C. between 9 months and 10 years D. None of these

Ans. C.

52. Pertussis vaccine is

A. Heat killed B. Formalin killed

C. Attenuated D. live

Ans. B.

53. DPT is

A. Triple vaccine B. Double vaccine

C. Tetanus toxoid D. All of these

Ans. A.

54. DPT, is used as vaccine for

A. Diphtheria B. Pertussis vaccine

C. Tetanus toxoid D. All of these

Ans. D.

55. DPT is given to children at the age of 16-24 months, a the dose is

A. 0.5 ml at intervals of 4 weeks B. A booster dose of 0.5 ml

C. Both a and b D. None of these

Ans. B.

56. If more than one kind of immunizing agent is included in the vaccine, it is

A. Cellular vaccine B. Recombinant vaccine

C. Mixed vaccine D. Toxoid vaccine

Ans. C.

57. Which one of the following fungi is the most serious threat in a bone marrow transplant unit?

A. Candida albicans B. Aspergillus

C. Blastomyces D. Cryptococus

Ans. B.

58. Direct microscopic count can be done with the aid of

A. Neubauer chamber B. Anaerobic chamber

C. Mineral oil D. Olive oil

Ans. A.

59. The image obtained in a compound microscope is

A. Real B. Virtual

C. Real inverted D. Virtual inverted

Ans. B.

60. Enzymes responsible for alcoholic fermentation

A. Ketolase B. Zymase

C. Peroxidase D. Oxidase

Ans. B.

61. Which type of spores are produced sexually?

A. Conidia B. Sporangiospores

C. Ascospores D. None of these

Ans. C.

62. Bacterial transformation was discovered by

A. Lederberg and Tatum B. Beadle and Tatum

C. Griffith D. None of these

Ans. A.

63. Primary mediators in anaphylaxis

A. Histamine B. Serotonin

C. Heparin D. All of these

Ans. D.

64. Arthus reaction was discovered by

A. Maurice Arthus B. Von Perquit

C. Richet D. Porter

Ans. A.

65. Serum sickness reaction was discovered by

A. Maurice Arthus B. Von Perquit

C. Richet D. Porter

Ans. B.

66. Hybridoma technique was developed by

A. Kohler & Milstein B. Niels Jerne

C. Both a and b D. None of these

Ans. A.

67. If the vectors transmit the infection mechanically they are called

A. Biological vectors B. Mechanical vectors

C. Biological reservoir D. Both a and c

Ans. B.

68. Reduction of virulence is known as

A. Exaltation B. Attenuation

C. Both a and b D. None of these

Ans. B.

69. Enhancement of virulence is known as

A. Exaltation B. Attenuation

C. Both a and b D. None of these

Ans. A.

70. The virulence of a pathogen is usually measured by

A. LD B. MLD

C. ID D. All of the above

Ans. D.

71. The lethal dose required to kill 50% of the lab animals tested under standard called

A. ID B. LD50

C. ID50 D. MLD

Ans. B.

72. The most important virulence factors are

A. Adhesions B. Invasiveness

C. Toxigenicity D. Enzymes

E. All of the above

Ans. E.

73. The ability of a pathogen to spread in the host tissues after establishing the infection is known as

A. Adhesion B. Invasiveness

C. Toxigenicity D. None of these

Ans. B.

74. Which is the following enzyme acts as a spreading factor?

A. Hyaluronidase B. Coagulase

C. Catalase D. DNase

Ans. A.

75. The phenomenon of transformation was first described in

A. E. coli B. B.subtilis

C. Pneumococci D. Vibrio

Ans. C.

76. Which type of interferon is produced by T lymphocytes?

A. α B. β

C. γ D. γ and β

Ans. C.

77. The major Ig family to which a particular Ig belongs can be determined by sequential analysis of the 110 amino acids beginning from the

A. amino terminus of the heavy chain

B. amino terminus of the light chain

C. C terminal of the heavy chain

D. C terminal of the light chain

E. None of these

Ans. C.

78. A(n) ——— is a multisubunit protein produced by B cells that binds to foreign substances and alters components of the immune system.

A. Antibody
B. Cytokine
C. Antigen
D. None of the above

Ans. A.

79. T cells provides the — response

A. Humoral response
B. Cellular response
C. Inherited response
D. Progressive response

Ans. B.

80. A transplant that occurs between species, such as human and a pig, is called a(n)

A. Autograft
B. Isograft
C. Allograft
D. Xenograft

Ans. D.

81. Which blood type can be transfused to an individual whose blood type is unknown?

A. AB+
B. AB-
C. O+
D. O-

Ans. D.

82. A couple expecting their second child is worried about Rh incompatibility. Their first child was Rh +. They have their blood typed. Which result would be cause for alarm?

A. Both parents Rh-
B. Both parents Rh-
C. Man Rh- and woman Rh+
D. Man Rh+ and woman Rh-

Ans. D.

83. Allergens stimulate the production of ____ antibodies that bind to mast cells, causing them to release allergy mediators.

A. IgA
B. IgD
C. IgE
D. IgG

Ans. C.

84. Which antibody type protects against bacteria, viruses, and toxins, especially in secondary immune responses?

A. IgA
B. IgD
C. IgE
D. IgG

Ans. D.

85. Severe combined immune deficiencies affect which branch of the immune system?

A. Humoral response B. Cellular response

C. Both A & B D. None of the above

Ans. C.

86. Which of the following statements about crowd diseases is true?

A. Crowd diseases are very difficult to bring under control and may linger for many months

B. The diseases that killed early Native Americans cannot be classified as crowd diseases

C. Crowd diseases tend to pass from those who live in large societies to those who live in smaller, more isolated societies.

D. We don't expect new crowd diseases to emerge in the future

Ans. C.

87. Humoral immunity can be boosted using

A. Monoclonal antibody technology B. Treatment with interferon.

C. Treatment with interleukin-2 D. Treatment with cytokines

Ans. A.

88. Which of the following is not an HLA-linked disease?

A. Narcolepsy B. Ankylosing spondylitis

C. Reiter's disease D. All of the above

Ans. D.

89. Which of the following is not part of the nonspecific, innate defence?

A. Phagocytosis B. Unbroken skin

C. Inflammatory response D. Fever

Ans. B.

90. ———— are cytokines that cause fever, temporarily maintaining a higher body temperature that directly kills some infecting bacteria and viruses.

A. Interferons B. Interleukins

C. TNF D. Collectins

Ans. B.

91. The specific parts of the antibody molecule that bind the antigen are called

A. Interleukins B. Heavy chains

C. Antigen binding sites D. Idiotypes

Ans. C.

92. Helper T cells secrete ——— which stimulate white blood cells to mature in bone marrow

A. Interferons
B. Interleukins
C. TNF
D. Colony stimulating factor

Ans. D.

93. ——— cells coordinate innate and acquired immune responses

A. Th cells
B. Tc cells
C. $\gamma\ \delta$ cells
D. B cells

Ans. C.

94. Mutations encoding ——— cause inherited immune deficiencies

A. Cytokine genes
B. T cell receptors
C. Antibody genes
D. All of the above

Ans. D.

95. People who cannot produce a complete ——— protein resist HIV infection.

A. CD4
B. CCR5
C. Cytotoxin
D. AIDS

Ans. B.

96. A transplant that occurs between identical twins is called a(n)

A. Autograft
B. Isograft
C. Allograft
D. Xenograft

Ans. B.

97. Bioweapons

A. Have been used for centuries
B. Employ pathogens to harm innocent people
C. Are inexpensive and fairly easy to produce
D. All of the above are true regarding bioweapons

Ans. D.

98. Which of the below provide evidence suggesting that allergies may be a holdover of an immune function that was important in the past?

A. People with allergies have higher levels of eosinophils
B. People with allergies have higher levels of t cells
C. People with allergies have lower levels of eosinophils
D. People with allergies have lower levels of T cells

Ans. A.

99. The polio vaccine uses

A. An attenuated pathogen
B. An inactivated toxin
C. Part of the pathogen surface
D. Naked DNA from pathogen

Ans. A.

100. Monoclonal antibodies are produced by a fused cell consisting of

A. A B cell and a T cell
B. A B cell and a cancer cell
C. A mast cell and a macrophage
D. None of the above

Ans. B.

101. B cells secrete

A. Antibodies
b. Cytokines
C. Antigens
d. Helper T cells

Ans. A.

102. A major advancement in transplantation technology occurred in 1984 when—— —— was transplanted into "Baby Fae."

A. A baboon liver
B. Baboon bone marrow
C. A baboon heart
D. A pig liver

Ans. C.

103. Specific immunity can be acquired either naturally or artificially and involves

A. All of the below.
B. Antibodies.
C. Antigens.
D. The classical complement pathway.

Ans. A.

104. Which does not provide long term immunity?

A. Artificially acquired active immunity
B. Artificially acquired passive immunity
C. Naturally acquired active immunity
D. None of the above

Ans. B.

105. An epitope is

A. A B-cell
B. A hapten
C. An antibody
D. The antigen determinant site

Ans. D.

106. An immunoglobulin is a

A. Carbohydrate
B. Fatty acid
C. Glycoprotein
D. Protein

Ans. C.

107. Isotypes refer to variations in the:

A. Heavy chain constant region. B. Heavy chain variable region.

C. Light chain constant region. D. Light chain variable region.

Ans. A.

108. The Fc region mediates all of the below except binding to

A. Antigen. B. Lysosomes.

C. Some phagocytic cells. D. Various cells of the immune system.

Ans. A.

109. Which of the following is the major immunoglobulin in human serum, accounting for 80% of the immunoglobulin pool?

A. IgA B. IgD

C. IgG D. IgM

Ans. C.

110. Which immunoglobulin is the least prevalent?

A. IgA B. IgD

C. IgE D. IgM

Ans. C.

111. Which of the following is useful to stimulate antibody production?

A. An adjuvant B. A hapten

C. Antiserum D. Purified antigen

E. Crude antigen

Ans. A.

112. Compared to the secondary antibody response, the primary response

A. attains a higher IgG titer.

B. has a longer lag phase.

C. persists for a longer plateau period.

D. produces antibodies with a higher affinity for the antigen.

Ans. B.

113. Viral replication within cells is inhibited by

A. IL-4 B. IL-1

C. IFN-alpha D. TNF-alpha

Ans. C.

114. For brucellosis, 2 ME agglutination test is used to identify

A. IgG
B. IgM
C. IgA
D. IgE

Ans. A.

115. Agglutination test for Brucella mainly identifies which class of antibodies?

A. IgG
B. IgM
C. IgA
D. IgE

Ans. B.

116. ——— protects foetus.

A. IgA
B. IgD
C. IgE
D. IgG
E. IgM

Ans. A.

117. ——— found in tears.

A. IgA
B. IgD
C. IgE
D. IgG
E. IgM

Ans. A.

118. The plasma cells and memory cells are associated with

A. Inflammation
B. CMI
C. HI
D. Complement cascade

Ans. C.

119. Which is true for antibodies ?

A. Inflammation
B. Cell mediated response
C. Humoral response
D. Complement cascade

Ans. C.

120. Epitopes are

A. Specific partof antigen that is reactive
B. Part of the antigen to which antibody binds
C. Small molecules that couple to carrier protein
D. The protein of antigen that is displayed on MHC

Ans. B.

121. Which of these cytokines is also known under the name cachectin?

A. Interferon gamma
B. Interleukin 2
C. Tumor necrosis factor (TNF)
D. None of the above

Ans. C.

122. ——— is found to mast cells and B cells ?

A. IgA
B. IgG
C. IgD
D. IgM
E. IgE

Ans. C.

123. The portion of the antigen molecule which is recognized by antibody is known as

A. Hapten
B. Epitope
C. Complement
D. Variable region

Ans. B.

124. All the following statements about haptens are true except

A. They have high molecular weights
B. They cannot elicit an immune response by themselves
C. When combined with some other large molecule, they can elicit an immune response
D. Once an immune response develops, the free hapten can be recognized by the antibody

Ans. A.

125. Antigens and haptens have the following similarity:

A. They have high molecular weights
B. They can elicit immune response by themselves
C. They can elicit an immune response only in association with some other large molecule
D. Once an immune response develops, free antigen and free hapten can be recognized by the antibody

Ans. D.

126. The minimum number of polypeptide chains in an immunoglobulin is

A. Two
B. Four
C. Five
D. Six

Ans. B.

127. Light chains of immunoglobulins are of following types:

A. Alpha and kappa B. Alpha and gamma

C. Lambda and delta D. Kappa and lambda

Ans. D.

128. Immunoglobulins are classified on the basis of

A. Type of light chains B. Type of heavy chains

C. Types of light and heavy chains D. Molecular weight

Ans. B.

129. The molecular weight of light chains is

A. 10,000–15,000 B. 20,000–25,000

C. 25,000–50,000 D. 50,000–75,000

Ans. B.

130. The molecular weight of heavy chains is

A. 20,000–25,000 B. 25,000–50,000

C. 50,000–70,000 D. 70,000–1,00,000

Ans. C.

131. The variable region of light chains is the

A. N-terminal quarter B. N-terminal half

C. C-terminal quarter D. C-terminal half

Ans. B.

132. The variable region of light chains has

A. One hypervariable region B. Two hypervariable regions

C. Three hypervariable regions D. Four hypervariable regions

Ans. C.

133. The variable region of heavy chains has

A. One hypervariable region B. Two hypervariable regions

C. Three hypervariable regions D. Four hypervariable regions

Ans. D.

134. The most abundant immunoglobulin in plasma is

A. IgA B. IgG

C. IgM D. IgD

Ans. B.

135. The largest immunoglobulin is

A. IgA B. IgG
C. IgM D. IgD

Ans. C.

136. The plasma concentration of IgA is

A. 1–5 mg/dl B. 40–200 mg/dl
C. 60–500 mg/dl D. 700–1,500 mg/dl

Ans. C.

137. An immunoglobulin found in exocrine secretions is

A. IgA B. IgG
C. IgM D. IgE

Ans. A.

138. Allergic reactions are mediated by

A. IgA B. IgG
C. IgD D. IgE

Ans. D.

139. An immunoglobulin which can cross the placental barrier is

A. IgA B. IgM
C. IgD D. None of these

Ans. D.

140. IgM possesses

A. Two light chains and two heavy chains
B. Four light chains and four heavy chains
C. Six light chains and six heavy chains
D. Ten light chains and ten heavy chains

Ans. D.

141. The immunoglobulin having the longest half-life is

A. IgA B. IgG
C. IgM D. IgE

Ans. B.

142. The half-life of IgG is

A. 2–3 days B. 5–6 days
C. 8–10 days D. 20–25 days

Ans. D.

143. Recognition of antigen is the function of

A. Variable region of light chains

B. Variable regions of light and heavy chains

C. Constant region of heavy chains

D. Constant regions of light and heavy chains

Ans. B.

144. The effector function of antibody is performed by

A. Variable region of light chains

B. Constant region of heavy chains

C. Variable regions of light and heavy chains

D. Constant regions of light and heavy chains

Ans. D.

145. Complement system can be activated by binding of antigen to

A. IgA

B. IgD

C. IgE

D. IgM

Ans. D.

146. C1 component of classical complement pathway is made up of

A. Complements 1q and 1r

B. Complements 1q and 1s

C. Complements 1r and 1s

D. Complements 1q, 1r and 1s

Ans. D.

147. The components of complement system are activated by

A. Microsomal hydroxylation

B. Phosphorylation

C. Glycosylation

D. Proteloysis

Ans. D.

148. The component system forms a membrane attack complex made up of

A. Complements 1q, 1r and 1s

B. Complements 1, 2, 3 and 4

C. Complements 5b, 6, 7 and 8

D. Factors B and D

Ans. D.

149. Factors B and D are required in

A. The classical pathway of complement fixation

B. The alternate complement pathway

C. Both (A) and (B)

D. None of these

Ans. B.

150. The alternate complement pathway doesn't involve

A. Antigen-antibody complex
B. Complement 3
C. Factors B and D
D. Membrane attack unit

Ans. A.

151. Antibody diversity arises from

A. Gene amplification
B. Gene re-arrangement
C. Alternative splicing
D. All of these

Ans. D.

152. A light chain gene is constructed from the following segments:

A. Variable and constant segments
B. Variable, joining and constant segments
C. Variable, diversity and constant segments
D. Variable, joining, diversity and constant segments

Ans. B.

153. In metabolic point of view, amino acids are classified as

A. Glycogenic
B. Ketogenic
C. Glycogenic or Ketogenic
D. All of these

Ans. D.

154. Diversity segments are present in

A. Light chain genes
B. Heavy chain genes
C. Light and heavy chain genes
D. None of these

Ans. B.

155. Constant segments of heavy chains are of

A. Five types
B. Six types
C. Seven types
D. Eight types

Ans. D.

156. Gamma heavy chains are of

A. Two types
B. Three types
C. Four types
D. Five types

Ans. C.

157. Gamma heavy chains are present in

A. IgA
B. IgG
C. IgM
D. IgD

Ans. B.

158. Heavy chains in IgD are of following type:

A. Alpha B. Gamma

C. Delta D. Epsilon

Ans. C.

159. On exposure to any antigen, the first antibody to be formed is of the following class:

A. IgA B. IgG

C. IgM D. IgE

Ans. C.

160. Cell-mediated immunity is the function of

A. B lymphocytes B. T lymphocytes

C. Plasma cells D. Basophils

Ans. B.

161. The most abundant T cells are

A. Cytotoxic T cells B. Helper T cells

C. Suppressor T cells D. Memory T cells

Ans. B.

162. T cells can recognise

A. Free antigens B. Antigens bound to cells

C. Antigens bound to antibodies D. Antigens bound to MHC proteins

Ans. D.

163. MHC proteins are unique to

A. Each cell B. Each organ

C. Each individual D. Each species

Ans. C.

164. MHC class I proteins are present on the surface of

A. B cells only B. T cells only

C. Macrophages only D. All cells

Ans. D.

165. MHC class I proteins, in conjunction with antigens are recognised by

A. Cytotoxic T cells B. Helper T cells

C. Suppressor T cells D. Memory T cells

Ans. A.

166. MHC class II proteins are present on the surface of

A. All cells
B. B lymphocytes only
C. Macrophages only
D. Macrophages and B lymphocytes

Ans. D.

167. MHC Class II proteins, in conjunction with antigens, are recognized by

A. Cytotoxic T cells
B. Helper T cells
C. Suppressor T cells
D. Memory T cells

Ans. B.

168. CD 8 is a transmembrane glycoprotein present in

A. Cytotoxic T cells
B. Helper T cells
C. Suppressor T cells
D. Memory T cells

Ans. A.

169. CD 4 is a transmembrane glycoprotein present in

A. Cytotoxic T cells
B. Helper T cells
C. Suppressor T cells
D. Memory T cells

Ans. B.

170. Cytotoxic T cells release

A. Perforins
B. Interleukins
C. Colony stimulating factors
D. Tumour necrosis factor

Ans. B.

171. Helper T cells release

A. Interleukins
B. Colony stimulating factors
C. Tumour necrosis factor
D. All of these

Ans. B.

172. MHC Class III proteins include

A. Immunoglobulins
B. Components of complement system
C. T cells receptors
D. CD4 and CD8 proteins

Ans. D.

173. Human immunodeficiency virus destroys

A. Cytotoxic T cells
B. Helper T cells
C. B cells
D. Plasma cells

Ans. B.

174. In allergic diseases, the concentration of the following is increased in plasma:
A. IgA B. IgG
C. IgD D. IgE

Ans. D.

175. IgE has a tendency to attach to
A. Basophils B. Mast cells
C. Both (A) and (B) D. None of these

Ans. C.

176. Reaginic antibody is
A. IgA B. IgG
C. IgD D. IgE

Ans. D.

177. Active immunity can be produced by administration of
A. Killed bacteria or viruses B. Live attenuated bacteria or viruses
C. Toxoids D. All of these

Ans. D.

178. Passive immunity can be produced by administration of
A. Pure antigens B. Immunoglobulins
C. Toxoids D. Killed bacteria or viruses

Ans. B.

179. Helper T cells release all the following except
A. Interleukins B. Colony stimulating factors
C. Perforins D. Tumour necrosis factor

Ans. C.

180. IgG cleaved by papain into
A. Two light and two heavy chains
B. Two Fab and one Fc fragments
C. Two pairs of one light and one heavy chain each
D. One Fab and two Fc fragments

Ans. B.

181. Bence-Jones protein is
A. An immunoglobulin
B. A dimer of heavy chains
C. A dimer of light chains
D. A dimer of one heavy and one light chains

Ans. C.

182. Bence-Jones proteins possess all the following properties except

A. They are dimers of light chains

B. Their amino acids sequences are identical

C. Their N-terminal halves have variable amino acid sequences

D. Their C-terminal halves have constant amino acid sequences

Ans. B.

183. Immunoglobulins are characterized by their

A. Heavy chains
B. Molecular weight
C. Light chains
D. Electrophoretic behavior

Ans. A.

184. The half-life of antibody protein is about

A. 4 weeks
B. 3 weeks
C. 2 weeks
D. 1 week

Ans. C.

185. Lymphocytes are responsible for the formation of

A. Serum
B. Plasma
C. Antibody
D. Calcium

Ans. C.

186. Platelets contain an enzyme which has important role in clotting in blood. This enzyme is known as

A. Cholinesterase
B. Transaminase
C. Decarboxylase
D. Thrombokinase

Ans. D.

187. The immunoglobulins are differentiated and also named on the basis of

A. Electrophoretic mobility

B. Heat stability

C. Molecular weight

D. Sedimentaiton coefficient like 7 S, 19 S etc.

Ans. D.

188. The immunoglobulins are classified on the basis of

A. Light chains
B. Heavy chains
C. Carbohydrate content
D. Electrophoretic mobility

Ans. B.

189. All immunoglobulins contain

A. 4 L chains
B. 4 H chains
C. 3 L chains
D. 2 L chains and 2 H chains

Ans. D.

190. An immunoglobulin molecule always contains

A. 1 κ and 3 λ type of chains
B. 2 κ and 1 λ type of chains
C. 3 κ and 1λ type of chains
D. 2 κ and 2 λ chains

Ans. D.

191. The number of types of H chains identified in human is

A. 2
B. 3
C. 4
D. 5

Ans. D.

192. The number of hypervariable region in L chain is

A. 1
B. 2
C. 3
D. 4

Ans. C.

193. The number of hypervariable region in H chain is

A. 1
B. 2
C. 3
D. 4

Ans. D.

194. Type γ H chain is present in

A. Ig G
B. Ig A
C. Ig M
D. Ig D

Ans. A.

195. Type α H chain is present in

A. Ig E
B. Ig A
C. Ig M
D. Ig D

Ans. B.

196. Type μ H chain is present in

A. Ig G
B. Ig A
C. Ig M
D. Ig D

Ans. C.

197. Type δ H chain is present in

A. Ig G
B. Ig A
C. Ig M
D. Ig D

Ans. D.

198. Type ε H chain is present in

A. Ig A
B. Ig M
C. Ig D
D. Ig E

Ans. D.

199. A 'J' chain is present in

A. Ig D
B. Ig M
C. Ig G
D. Ig E

Ans. B.

200. A secretory protein T chain (T protein) is present in

A. Ig A
B. Ig M
C. Ig D
D. Ig E

Ans. A.

201. A pentamer immunoglobulin is

A. Ig G
B. Ig A
C. Ig M
D. Ig E

Ans. C.

202. The portion of the immunoglobulin molecule that binds the specific antigen is formed by

A. Variable regions of H and L chains
B. Constant region of H chain
C. Constant region of L chain
D. Hinge region

Ans. A.

203. The class specific function of the different immunoglobulin molecules is constituted by

A. Variable region of L chain
B. Constant region of H chain
C. Variable region of H chain
D. Constant region particularly CH2 and CH3 of H chain

Ans. D.

204. Hinge region, the region of Ig molecule which is flexible and more exposed to enzymes is the

A. Region between first and second constant regions of H chain (domains CH1 and CH2)

B. Region between second and third constant regions of H chain (CH2 and CH3)

C. Variable regions of H chain

D. Variable regions of L chain

Ans. A.

205. The smallest immunoglobulin is

A. Ig G B. Ig E

C. Ig D D. Ig A

Ans. A.

206. The number of sub classes of Ig G is

A. 2 B. 3

C. 4 D. 8

Ans. C.

207. Most abundant Ig G subclass in the serum is

A. Ig G1 B. Ig G2

C. Ig G3 D. Ig G4

Ans. A.

208. The immunoglobulin which can cross the placenta is

A. Ig A B. Ig M

C. Ig G D. Ig D

Ans. C.

209. The immunoglobulin possessing lowest concentration of carbohydrate is

A. Ig A B. Ig E

C. Ig M D. Ig G

Ans. D.

210. The normal serum level of Ig G is

A. 1200 mg% B. 500 mg%

C. 300 mg% D. 200 mg%

Ans. A.

211. The half life of Ig G is

A. 2–8 days
B. 1–4 days
C. 19–24 days
D. 6 days

Ans. C.

212. Most heat labile immunoglobulin is

A. Ig G
B. Ig A
C. Ig M
D. Ig D

Ans. D.

213. The immunoglobulin possessing highest concentration of carbohydrate is

A. Ig G
B. Ig M
C. Ig A
D. Ig D

Ans. D.

214. The normal serum level of Ig D is

A. 1 mg%
B. 2 mg%
C. 3 mg%
D. 5 mg%

Ans. C.

215. The half life of Ig D is

A. 1 day
B. 2–8 days
C. 10–15 days
D. 20–24 days

Ans. B.

216. The carbohydrate content of Ig M is about

A. 2.8%
B. 6.4%
C. 8.0%
D. 10.2%

Ans. D.

217. The immunoglobulin having highest sedimentation coefficient is

A. Ig G
B. Ig A
C. Ig M
D. Ig D

Ans. C.

218. The immunoglobulin having highest molecular weight is

A. Ig G
B. Ig M
C. Ig E
D. Ig A

Ans. B.

219. The half life of IgM is

A. 2 days
B. 4 days
C. 5 days
D. 8 days

Ans. C.

220. The normal serum level of Ig M is

A. 50 mg%
B. 120 mg%
C. 200 mg%
D. 300 mg%

Ans. B.

221. The immunoglobulin associated with reaginic antibody is

A. Ig E
B. Ig D
C. Ig M
D. Ig A

Ans. A.

222. The immunoglobulin having least concentration in serum is

A. Ig A
B. Ig M
C. Ig D
D. Ig E

Ans. D.

223. The half life of Ig E protein is

A. 1–6 days
B. 2–8 days
C. 10 days
D. 20 days

Ans. A.

224. The immunoglobulin which provides highest antiviral activity is

A. Ig D
B. Ig E
C. Ig A
D. Ig G

Ans. C.

225. The half life of Ig A is

A. 6 days
B. 2–4 days
C. 5–10 days
D. 12–20 days

Ans. A.

226. The normal serum level of Ig A is

A. 100 mg%
B. 200 mg%
C. 300 mg%
D. 400 mg%

Ans. B.

227. Variable regions are present in

A. Immunoglobulins
B. α-Chains of T cell receptors
C. β-Chains of T cell receptors
D. All of these

Ans. D.

228. MHC proteins of cells

A. Display antigens of self and non self origin
B. Interact with B and T cells
C. Activate and deactivate antibody production
D. Switch on and off interferon production
E. A & B
F. C & D.

Ans. E.

229. Which of those immunoglobulin classes is mainly found in external secretions?

A. Ig A
B. Ig D
C. Ig M
D. IgE

Ans. A.

230. Cleavage of an IgG molecule by a specific protease can produce

A. An antigen-binding site and two constant regions
B. Two heavy chain-light chain dimers
C. An inactive mixture of oligopeptides
D. Two Fab fragments and one Fc fragment

Ans. D.

231. Papain digest IgG into

A. Two fab fragments and one fc fragment
B. Three fab fragments and two fc fragments
C. Two fab fragments and two fc fragments
D. Three fab fragments and three fc fragments

Ans. A.

232. Antibodies can be used

A. For the localization of proteins in the cell
B. For protein purification
C. To catalyze chemical reactions
D. All of the above

Ans. D.

233. Type A blood

A. Can be used to donate to type AB individuals

B. Can be used to donate to type B individuals

C. Contains type B antigens on the surface of red blood cells

D. Can always be used to donate to an Rh^+ individual

Ans. A.

234. Which of the following are responsible for immune specificity?

A. Antigens
B. Antibodies
C. T lymphocytes
D. Macrophage

Ans. B.

235. Which species lack immunoglobulin light chains?

A. Camels
B. Humans
C. cows
D. Buffalo

Ans. A.

236. Monoclonal refers to

A. A single clone of antibody-producing cells

B. All the antibody molecules which are identical

C. The binding with same antigenic site with identical binding affinities

D. All of the above

Ans. D.

237. β-Lymphocytes are often called simply

A. B cells
B. T cells
C. T Lymphocytes
D. None of these

Ans. A.

238. IgE provides

A. Immunity against some parasites

B. Complement killings of the cells and phagocytosis

C. Secretions in the body

D. All of the above

Ans. A.

239. Fab fragment has

A. One antigen binding site
B. Two antigen binding site
C. One antibody binding site
D. Two antibody binding site

Ans. A.

240. The main function of antibodies is to

A. Kill all the foreign bodies

B. Generate antigens, thus conferring immunization

C. Protect the circulatory system

D. Chemically combine with the antigen which induces it, inactivate the antigen and protect the body from disease

Ans. D.

241. Alum is an effective adjuvant because it

A. Disaggregates the antigen.

B. Is immunogenic for stem cells

C. Is immunogenic for T cells

D. Slows the release of antigen

Ans. C.

242. A secondary antibody is an antibody that

A. Has been used in prior experiments

B. Is synthetically produced

C. Binds to another antibody

D. Is produced in boostered animals

Ans. C.

243. The immunoglobulin fold is

A. Found only in IgG molecules

B. A β-barrel composed of a three- and a four-stranded antiparallel β-sheet

C. Both (a) and (b)

D. Found six times in the IgG molecule

Ans. B.

244. Antibodies of the IgG class

A. Consist of four subunits

B. Are glycoproteins

C. Are secreted into the bloodstream

D. All of the above

Ans. D.

245. Each IgA antibody molecule consists of

A. Four polypeptide chain and has two antigen binding site

B. Two polypeptide chain and has one antigen binding site

C. Three polypeptide chain and has two antigen binding site

D. Two polypeptide chain and has two antigen binding site

Ans. A.

246. Antibodies in the human immune system can identify approximately 10^8 different molecules. Which one of the following is correct?

A. This diversity is generated from 10^8 different immunoglobulin genes

B. Many of these molecules are self-antigens

C. Most of these antibodies recognize proteins

D. Most of these antibodies recognize small organic molecules

Ans. **C.**

247. Monoclonal antibodies were first produced by

A. Georges Kohler and Cesar Milstein

B. Sarkar and Sommer

C. Selman Waksman

D. Edward Jenner and Louis Pasteur

Ans. **A.**

248. A polyclonal antibody response

A. Is produced only in response to polymeric antigens

B. Is produced by several B cells recognizing different epitopes on the same antigen

C. Occurs during the lag phase of the immune response

D. Violates clonal selection

Ans. **B.**

249. Structures of anti-PCP antibody shows that the tight binding of PCP to the antibody is primarily due to

A. Hydrophobic forces B. Electrostatic forces

C. Van der Waals forces D. None of these

Ans. **A.**

250. Antigenic determinants bind to which portions of an antibody?

A. Variable regions B. Constant regions

C. Only light chains D. Only heavy chains

Ans. **A.**

251. The humoral immune response relies on the production of soluble proteins called

A. Antibodies B. Macromolecules

C. Lymphocytes D. None of these

Ans. **A.**

252. The human IgG class of antibodies is divided into

A. Five IgG classes
B. Two IgG classes
C. Three IgG classes
D. Four IgG classes

Ans. D.

253. For specific antigen recognition by T cells,

A. Antigen is bound by a T cell membrane antibody
B. Denaturation of antigen does not reduce epitope recognition
C. MHC molecules are not required
D. Antigen exposure during T cell maturation is required

Ans. B.

254. Antigen, when injected in the body activates its specific lymphocytes in the

A. Blood circulation
B. Draining lymph nodes
C. MALT (mucosa associated
D. Spleen lymphoid tissue

Ans. B.

255. A molecule that can be covalently linked to a non-immunogenic antigen to make it an immunogen is called a (n)

A. Adjuvant
B. Carrier
C. Hapten
D. Mitogen

Ans. B.

256. Which of the following is incorrect with regard to antigen epitopes?

A. An epitope may be shared by two different antigens
B. A protein molecule usually contains multiple epitopes
C. B cells bind only processed antigen epitopes
D. Epitopes may be linear or assembled

Ans. C.

257. Very low doses of antigen may induce

A. Hypersensitivity
B. Immunological ignorance
C. Low zone tolerance
D. Low zone immunity

Ans. C.

258. During the lag period between antigen contact and detection of adaptive immunity,

A. Antigen is hidden from the immune system in macrophages
B. Innate immune effectors are eliminating antigen
C. Innate immunity blocks the activation of adaptive immune effector cells
D. New B and T cells with the appropriate antigen specificity must be produced in the bone marrow

Ans. B.

259. Lymphocytes are activated by antigen in the

A. Blood stream
B. Bone marrow
C. Liver
D. Lymph nodes

Ans. D.

260. A pathogen can be a (n)

A. Agent that causes a disease
B. Virus
C. Bacteria
D. All of these

Ans. D.

261. CD antigens

A. Allow leukocytes to recognize antigen
B. Are each expressed on only one cell type
C. Are expressed on immune cells to mark them for separation
D. Function as receptors for cytokine and CAMs

Ans. D.

262. A virus vaccine that can activate cytotoxic T cells must contain

A. A high dose of virus particles
B. An adjuvant to stimulate T cell division
C. Live virus
D. Virus peptides

Ans. C.

263. The ability of an antigen to induce an immune response does not depend on the antigen's

A. Ability to enter the thyroid
B. Degree of aggregation
C. Dose
D. Size

Ans. A.

264. The antibiotic penicillin is a small molecule that does not induce antibody formation. However, penicillin binds to serum proteins and forms a complex that in some people induces antibody formation resulting in an allergic reaction. Penicillin is therefore

A. An antigen
B. A hapten
C. An immunogen
D. Both an antigen and a hapten

Ans. D.

265. Lack of reaction to our own human leukocyte antigens (HLAs) is known as?

A. Autoimmunity
B. Complement system
C. Clonal selection
D. Tolerance

Ans. D.

266. Which of the following components of the vertebrate immune response occurs first upon invasion by a virus or bacterium?

A. Activation of killer T lymphocytes

B. Activation of B lymphocytes

C. The inflammatory response

D. Mobilization of complement proteins

Ans. C.

267. Which of the following white blood cells act as scavengers when they engulf and digest pathogens?

A. Macrophages B. T cells

C. B cells D. Lymphocytes

Ans. A.

268. A cell which defends against body cells in which viruses are reproducing is

A. Exotoxin B. Cytotoxic T cell

C. Endotoxin D. Suppressor T cell

Ans. B.

269. Which of the following is most likely to produce anaphylaxis in a susceptible individual?

A. Pollen B. Mold

C. Dust D. Bee sting

Ans. D.

270. What type of B cell remains dormant in the body, but can respond rapidly if the same antigen appears again?

A. T cells B. Memory cells

C. Plasma cells D. Macrophages

Ans. B.

271. The maturation of T cells and the production of particular T cell receptors occurs in the

A. Thyroid gland B. Thymus gland

C. Testes D. All of these

Ans. B.

272. Which of the following provide specific defense against viruses and bacteria?

A. T cells B. B cells

C. Complement D. Inflammation

Ans. B.

273. Which of these is a type of specific defence against pathogens?

A. Lymphocytes
B. Macrophages
C. Phagocytes
D. Leukocytes

Ans. A.

274. In animals, blood clots serve the function of

A. Consuming invading organisms
B. Helping them match the background coloration of the habitat
C. Stimulating production of killer T lymphocytes
D. Repairing damage to the body wall

Ans. D.

275. What is the result of invasion of a body by pathogens?

A. Infection
B. Inflammation
C. Swelling
D. Pus

Ans. A.

276. What is the behavior in which T cells and B cells constantly travel throughout the body seeking out and destroying foreign substances?

A. Antibody-mediated immune response
B. Immune surveillance
C. Cell-mediated immune response
D. Vaccination

Ans. B.

277. In a fetus, where are lymphocytes produced?

A. In the spleen
B. In the bone marrow
C. In the liver
D. In the heart

Ans. C.

278. Which of the following produces the antibodies employed in the specific immune response of vertebrates?

A. B lymphocytes
B. T lymphocytes
C. Neutrophils
D. Macrophages

Ans. A.

279. Which of the following is not part of the vertebrate immune system?

A. Lymphocytes
B. Antibodies
C. Cardiac glycosides
D. Lymph nodes

Ans. C.

280. The protein, produced by B cells that binds to a specific antigen is

A. Phagocyte B. Leukocyte

C. Vaccine D. Antibody

Ans. D.

281. Which of the following characteristics are common in lymphocytes, macrophages, and neutrophils?

A. They are all part of the nonspecific immune response in vertebrates

B. They are all part of the specific immune response in vertebrates

C. They are all part of the internal defenses of nonvertebrates

D. They are all types of white blood cells

Ans. D.

282. Which of the following blood proteins can destroy pathogens?

A. Major histocompatibility complex B. Platelets

C. Fibrinogen D. Complement system

Ans. D.

283. Which of these is part of the lymphoid system in humans?

A. Liver B. Stomach

C. Tonsils D. Kidneys

Ans. C.

284. What type of B cell is like a tiny factory that produces antibodies identical to the B cell receptor that bind to the original antigen?

A. T cells B. Memory cells

C. Plasma cells D. Macrophages

Ans. C.

285. Which of the following immune cells would have an especially low count in a patient with advanced AIDS?

A. Killer T lymphocytes B. Helper T lymphocyte

C. B lymphocytes D. None of these

Ans. B.

286. In cellular immunity, T lymphocytes are responsible for the recognition and killing of foreign invaders. The cells are

A. Cytotoxic T lymphocytes (CTL) B. Killer T cells

C. Both (a) and (b) D. None of the above

Ans. C.

287. Plasma cells produce thousands of—— that are released into the bloodstream

A. Antigens B. Antibodies

C. Helper T cells D. Virus fragments

Ans. B.

288. If a person is vaccinated against a disease sometime in the past, which of the following is currently in your body?

A. The disease organism itself and antigens for the disease organism

B. A very high level of antibodies against the disease antigens

C. Memory B lymphocytes for the antigen of this disease organism

D. All of the above

Ans. D.

289. What is a protein produced by host cells infected by viruses?

A. Interferon B. Histamine

C. Antiserum D. Vaccine

Ans. A.

290. Polysaccharides on the surface of infecting microorganisms can also activate complement directly in the absence of

A. Antibody via the alternative pathway

B. Antigen via the alternative pathway

C. Antibody via metabolic pathway

D. None of the above

Ans. A.

291. Antibodies bound to an invading microorganism activate the complement system via

A. Classical pathway B. Metabolic pathway

C. Embden Meyerhof pathway D. Entner-Doudoroff pathway

Ans. A.

292. The immune response to a booster vaccine is called a(n)

A. Cellular response B. Innate response

C. Primary response D. Secondary response

Ans. D.

293. Immunological memory is due to

A. Short lived macrophage that can recognize specific pathogens

B. Long lived B cells that secrete a specific antibody

C. Long lived B cells that secrete a specific antigen

D. Short lived helper T cells that signal macrophage to divide

Ans. B.

294. What is the result of an abnormal response of the immune system to part of a person's own body?

A. Passive immunity
B. Cancer
C. An allergic response
D. An autoimmune disease

Ans. D.

295. What are the solutions prepared from weakened or dead microorganisms, viruses, or toxins that provide some immunity from diseases?

A. Vaccines
B. Histamines
C. Drugs
D. Antibiotics

Ans. A.

296. During exposure to a foreign invader, there are more ——— present in the vertebrate body than before exposure

A. Antibodies
B. Lymphocytes
C. Macrophages and antigens
D. All of these

Ans. D.

297. To elicit the best antibodies to mouse MHC I, it should be injected into a

A. Goat
B. Mouse of the same genetic background (strain)
C. Mouse of a different strain
D. Rat

Ans. A.

298. To detect a humoral immune response to influenza virus, it is possible to measure

A. Cytotoxicity of virus-infected cells in tissue culture
B. Dividing T cells in the draining lymph nodes
C. Plasma cytokine levels
D. Serum antibody titer

Ans. D.

299. Which of the following is in the lymph nodes of a person battling a cold virus ?

A. Huge numbers of white blood cells
B. Trapped viruses that have been roaming the body
C. Lymph ducts that enter and exit the nodes and Lymph fluid
D. All of the above

Ans. D.

300. Immunogenicity

A. Depends on the ability of the native antigen to be presented by MHC

B. Is usually a property of self antigens such as eye tissue

C. Is not a property of antibodies

D. Is not a property of haptens

Ans. D.

301. The HIV virus infects primarily

A. Brain cells

B. Cells in the immune system

C. Red blood cells

D. Liver cells

Ans. B.

302. Chronic granulomatous disease results from a failure to perform oxidative burst. This deficiency would be most likely to interfere with

A. CTL killing of viruses

B. Dendritic cell activation to become a mature APC

C. Infected cell processing of virus peptides

D. Macrophage intracellular killing of bacteria

Ans. D.

303. Difficulties with somatic gene therapy arise from all of the following except

A. GVHD caused by mature T cells in the transplanted cells

B. Inserting a gene so that it will function properly

C. Limited life span of more mature hematopoietic cells

D. Transducing genetic material into stem cells

Ans. A.

304. A monoclonal antibody (mAb) specific for the 2,4-dinitrophenyl (DNP) hapten might also bind

A. Leu or Ileu

B. His or Pro

C. Tyr or Phe

D. Ser or Thr

Ans. C.

305. Retinoblastoma is due to a mutation in a

A. Kinase

B. Tumor supressor

C. Cyclin

D. Viral gene

Ans. B.

306. An autoimmune disease is

A. AIDS
B. Measles
C. Lupus
D. Mumps

Ans. C.

307. If Class II MHC is not expressed in the thymus, the resulting immune deficiencies would include all of the following except reduced

A. Alternative complement activation.
B. CD8 T cell-mediated cytotoxicity
C. Macrophage activation to vesicular pathogens
D. IgG synthesis

Ans. A.

308. To treat HIV infections using drugs, the major problem is that

A. The drugs that are good inhibitors cannot by synthesized
B. The drugs interfere with normal digestion
C. The virus particles with altered (mutant) proteases arise
D. The drugs are rapidly degraded

Ans. C.

309. The primary reason for AIDS, a deadly disease is that it

A. Is caused by a virus
B. Is caused by a bacterium
C. Destroys key components of the body's internal defense system
D. Causes a breakdown of the body's inflammatory response

Ans. C.

310. A selective IgA deficiency would be expected to result in problems with

A. Bacterial infections
B. Infections following dental work due to bacteria entering the bloodstream
C. Mucosal pathogens
D. Pathogens which can survive inside macrophages

Ans. C.

311. Combined cellular and humoral immune deficiencies result from lack of all of the following except

A. A thymus
B. Class II MHC
C. HIV infection of $CD4^+$ T cells
D. Transporter of antigen peptides (TAP)

Ans. D.

312. An example of an immunodeficiency disorder is

A. Thyroiditis B. Rheumatic fever

C. Systemic lupus erythematosus D. AIDS

Ans. D.

313. Bone marrow given to an infant with SCID must

A. Be irradiated to eliminate GVHD

B. Contain mature T cells that can begin making immune responses immediately

C. Come from a donor that shares some MHC alleles with the recipient

D. Come from one of the child's parents

Ans. C.

314. X-linked hyper IgM syndrome, resulting in high levels of serum IgM and low levels of serum IgG, is caused by a defect in CD40L expression. The specific immune event that would be prevented by a defective CD40L would be

A. Activation of B cells by T-independent antigens

B. Failure of B cells to provide co-stimulation for Th2 activation

C. Failure of Th2 cells to provide co-stimulation for B cell isotype switching

D. Failure of Th2 cells to provide co-stimulation for B cell proliferation

Ans. C.

315. DiGeorge's syndrome is characterized by the lack of a thymus. The mouse model closest to this human disease would be a

A. Knock-out mouse for RAG-1 and RAG-2

B. Knock-out mouse for a thymus

C. Nude mouse

D. Recombinant mouse for CD3

Ans. C.

316. Which of the Rous sarcoma virus has a homologous cellular protein ?

A. C-src B. V-src

C. V-ha-src D. V-ha-ras

Ans. A.

317. Infants are most susceptible to bacterial infection due to low circulating levels of IgG

A. In utero (before birth) B. At 0-3 months of age

C. At 3-12 months of age D. At 12-24 months of age

Ans. C.

318. The chemical, typically released by the body in an allergic response is

A. Histamine
B. Allergens
C. Antihistamines
D. Perforins

Ans. A.

319. An organism's first line of defense against attack by an invader such as a virus or bacterium is usually

A. To flee or hide
B. Its body wall
C. A specific immune response
D. A nonspecific immune response

Ans. B.

320. Which of the following are responsible for causing the diseases?

A. Pathogens
B. T cells
C. Lymphocytes
D. Macrophages

Ans. A.

321. In Rocket Immunodiffusion the length of the rocket is

A. Proportional to the amount of antibody placed in each well
B. Inversely proportional to the amount of antibody placed in each well
C. Inversely proportional to the amount of antigen placed in each well
D. Proportional to the amount of antigen placed in each well

Ans. D.

322. Radial Immunodiffusion is similar to

A. Double-diffusion
B. Gel diffusion
C. Ouchterloney technique
D. All of these

Ans. A.

323. Agarose a porous matrix used in various molecular biology technique is made by repetitive units of

A. Maltose
B. Agarobiose
C. Agar
D. None of these

Ans. B.

324. Rocket Immunodiffusion is also known as

A. Gel diffusion
B. Electroimmunodiffusion
C. Double-diffusion
D. None of these

Ans. B.

325. What would happen if serum is omitted from the ELISA, but all other steps remain same?

A. Anti-human Ig-conjugate would not bind and be washed away

B. The OD values would be nearly the same as the assay control

C. Both (a) and (b)

D. Anti-human Ig-conjugate would bind non-specifically to the ELISA plate

Ans. C.

326. RAST test (radio allergosorbent test) is often used to detect

A. Antibodies associated with allergies (IgE)

B. Antigen associated with allergies (IgE)

C. Bacteriophages

D. None of the above

Ans. A.

327. What would happen if the anti-human Ig-conjugate is not washed free of the well before the substrate is added?

A. The ELISA would not develop when the substrate was added

B. The ELISA would develop normally

C. All wells would show uniform over-development due to unbound and excess anti-human Ig enzyme conjugate

D. None of the above

Ans. C.

328. An antigen preparation and an antibody preparation are tested by immunodiffusion. Three bands are found, indicating that

A. There was more than one antigen

B. The antibody was impure

C. The temperature was too high

D. There was one antibody and one antigen

Ans. A.

329. Immunoelectrophoresis techniques are designed to separate the mixture components from each other by using electrophoresis

A. Prior to reaction with antibody

B. Prior to reaction with antigen

C. After reaction with antibody

D. After reaction with antigen

Ans. A.

330. Which of the following is an immunoelectrophoresis technique?

A. Two-dimensional immunoelectrophoresis

B. Counterimmunoelectrophoresis

C. Coimmunoelectrophoresis

D. Both (a) and (b)

Ans. D.

331. Which of those immunoglobulin classes is mainly found in external secretions?

A. Ig A B. Ig D

C. Ig M D. IgE

Ans. A.

332. Cleavage of an IgG molecule by a specific protease can produce

A. An antigen-binding site and two constant regions

B. Two heavy chain-light chain dimers

C. An inactive mixture of oligopeptides

D. Two Fab fragments and one Fc fragment

Ans. D.

333. Papain digest IgG into

A. Two fab fragments and one fc fragment

B. Three fab fragments and two fc fragments

C. Two fab fragments and two fc fragments

D. Three fab fragments and three fc fragments

Ans. A.

334. Antibodies can be used

A. For the localization of proteins in the cell

B. For protein purification

C. To catalyze chemical reactions

D. All of the above

Ans. D.

335. Type A blood

A. Can be used to donate to type AB individuals

B. Can be used to donate to type B individuals

C. Contains type B antigens on the surface of red blood cells

D. Can always be used to donate to an Rh^+ individual

Ans. A.

336. Which of the following are responsible for immune specificity?

A. Antigens B. Antibodies

C. T lymphocytes D. Macrophage

Ans. B.

337. Which species lack immunoglobulin light chains?

A. Camels
B. Humans
C. Cows
D. Buffalo

Ans. A.

338. Monoclonal refers to

A. A single clone of antibody-producing cells
B. All the antibody molecules which are identical
C. The binding with same antigenic site with identical binding affinities
D. All of the above

Ans. D.

339. β-Lymphocytes are often called simply

A. B cells
B. T cells
C. T Lymphocytes
D. None of these

Ans. A.

340. IgE provides

A. Immunity against some parasites
B. Complement killings of the cells and phagocytosis
C. Secretions in the body
D. All of the above

Ans. A.

341. Fab fragment has

A. One antigen binding site
B. Two antigen binding site
C. One antibody binding site
D. Two antibody binding site

Ans. A.

342. The main function of antibodies is to

A. Kill all the foreign bodies
B. Generate antigens, thus conferring immunization
C. Protect the circulatory system
D. Chemically combine with the antigen which induces it, inactivate the antigen and protect the body from disease

Ans. D.

343. Alum is an effective adjuvant because it

A. Disaggregates the antigen. B. Is immunogenic for stem cells

C. Is immunogenic for T cells D. Slows the release of antigen

Ans. C.

344. A secondary antibody is an antibody that

A. Has been used in prior experiments

B. Is synthetically produced

C. Binds to another antibody

D. Is produced in boostered animals

Ans. C.

345. The immunoglobulin fold is

A. Found only in IgG molecules

B. A β-barrel composed of a three- and a four-stranded antiparallel β-sheet

C. Both A and B

D. Found six times in the IgG molecule

Ans. B.

346. Antibodies of the IgG class

A. Consist of four subunits B. Are glycoproteins

C. Are secreted into the bloodstream D. All of the above

Ans. D.

347. Each IgA antibody molecule consists of

A. Four polypeptide chain and has two antigen binding site

B. Two polypeptide chain and has one antigen binding site

C. Three polypeptide chain and has two antigen binding site

D. Two polypeptide chain and has two antigen binding site

Ans. A.

348. Antibodies in the human immune system can identify approximately 10^8 different molecules. Which one of the following is correct?

A. This diversity is generated from 10^8 different immunoglobin genes

B. Many of these molecules are self-antigens

C. Most of these antibodies recognize proteins

D. Most of these antibodies recognize small organic molecules

Ans. C.

349. Monoclonal antibodies were first produced by

A. Georges Kohler and Cesar Milstein

B. Sarkar and Sommer

C. Selman Waksman

D. Edward Jenner and Louis Pasteur

Ans. A.

350. A polyclonal antibody response

A. Is produced only in response to polymeric antigens

B. Is produced by several B cells recognizing different epitopes on the same antigen

C. Occurs during the lag phase of the immune response

D. Violates clonal selection

Ans. B.

351. Structures of anti-PCP antibody shows that the tight binding of PCP to the antibody is primarily due to

A. Hydrophobic forces B. Electrostatic forces.

C. Van der Waals forces. D. None of these

Ans. A.

352. Antigenic determinants bind to which portions of an antibody?

A. Variable regions B. Constant regions

C. Only light chains D. Only heavy chains

Ans. A.

353. The humoral immune response relies on the production of soluble proteins called

A. Antibodies B. Macromolecules

C. Lymphocytes D. None of these

Ans. A.

354. The human IgG class of antibodies is divided into

A. Five IgG classes B. Two IgG classes

C. Three IgG classes D. Four IgG classes

Ans. D.

355. Unpaired H-bond donors and acceptors are found in the hydrophobic core of a protein

A. Only at the ends of a-helices B. Only at the turns connecting p-strands

C. Only on Pro residues D. Rarely

Ans. D.

356. For the unfolding reaction of Protein G, $\Delta H^\circ = 210.6$ kJ/mol, this means that

A. Unfolding is favored enthalpically

B. Folding is favoured enthalpically

C. The entropy is positive at all temperatures

D. The entropy is negative at all temperatures

Ans. B.

357. Attractive Vander Waals forces occur between

A. Apolar molecules in the liquid state

B. Any pair of nearby atoms

C. Polar molecules in the solid state

D. Only if other forces are less favourable

Ans. B.

358. Which of the following forces is the most favourable for protein folding?

A. Conformational entropy
B. Hydrophobic Interactions
C. Vander Waals interactions
D. Hydrogen bonds

Ans. B.

359. Which of the following is the most correct?

A. Charged amino acids are never buried in the interior of a protein

B. Charged amino acids are seldom buried in the interior of a protein

C. All hydrophobic amino acids are buried when a protein folds

D. Tyrosine is only found in the interior of proteins

Ans. B.

360. Which of the following forces is the most unfavourable for protein folding?

A. Conformational entropy
B. Hydrophobic interactions
C. Vander Waals interactions
D. Electrostatic interactions

Ans. A.

361. The correlation between free energy ΔG transfer between the aqueous/organic phases and the surface area of amino acid residues

A. Reflects the reduction in solvent-accessible area during protein folding

B. Is only meaningful for the polar amino acids

C. Ignores the important contribution of the peptide bond

D. Is similar to effects seen with SDS denaturation

Ans. A.

362. If the egg white protein, ovalbumin, is denatured in a hard-boiled egg, then which of the following is least affected?

A. The primary structure of ovalbumin

B. The secondary structure of ovalbumin

C. The tertiary structure of ovalbumin

D. The quaternary structure of ovalbumin

Ans. A.

363. Buried hydrophobic side chains in a globular protein fit into a hole formed by the side chains of

A. 1-3 other amino acids
B. 5-7 other amino acids

C. 9-12 other amino acids
D. 13-15 other amino acids

Ans. B.

364. For specific antigen recognition by T cells,

A. Antigen is bound by a T cell membrane antibody

B. Denaturation of antigen does not reduce epitope recognition

C. MHC molecules are not required

D. Antigen exposure during T cell maturation is required

Ans. B.

365. Antigen, when injected in the body activates its specific lymphocytes in the

A. Blood circulation
B. Draining lymph nodes

C. MALT (mucosa associated)
D. Spleen lymphoid tissue

Ans. B.

366. A molecule that can be covalently linked to a non-immunogenic antigen to make it an immunogen is called a (n)

A. Adjuvant
B. Carrier

C. Hapten
D. Mitogen

Ans. B.

367. Which of the following is incorrect with regard to antigen epitopes?

A. An epitope may be shared by two different antigens

B. A protein molecule usually contains multiple epitopes

C. B cells bind only processed antigen epitopes

D. Epitopes may be linear or assembled

Ans. C.

368. Very low doses of antigen may induce

A. Hypersensitivity B. Immunological ignorance

C. Low zone tolerance D. Low zone immunity

Ans. C.

369. During the lag period between antigen contact and detection of adaptive immunity,

A. Antigen is hidden from the immune system in macrophages

B. Innate immune effectors are eliminating antigen

C. Innate immunity blocks the activation of adaptive immune effector cells

D. New B and T cells with the appropriate antigen specificity must be produced in the bone marrow

Ans. B.

370. Lymphocytes are activated by antigen in the

A. Blood stream B. Bone marrow

C. Liver D. Lymph nodes

Ans. D.

371. A pathogen can be a (n)

A. Agent that causes a disease B. Virus

C. Bacteria D. All of these

Ans. D.

372. CD antigens

A. Allow leukocytes to recognize antigen

B. Are each expressed on only one cell type

C. Are expressed on immune cells to mark them for separation

D. Function as receptors for cytokine and CAMs

Ans. D.

373. A virus vaccine that can activate cytotoxic T cells must contain

A. A high dose of virus particles B. An adjuvant to stimulate T cell division

C. Live virus D. Virus peptides

Ans. C.

374. The ability of an antigen to induce an immune response does not depend on the antigen's

A. Ability to enter the thyroid B. Degree of aggregation

C. Dose D. Size

Ans. A.

375. The antibiotic penicillin is a small molecule that does not induce antibody formation. However, penicillin binds to serum proteins and forms a complex that in some people induces antibody formation resulting in an allergic reaction. Penicillin is therefore

A. An antigen
B. A hapten
C. An immunogen
D. Both an antigen and a hapten

Ans. D.

376. Enzyme-driven metabolic pathways can be made more efficient by

A. Concentrating enzymes within specific cellular compartments
B. Grouping enzymes into free-floating, multienzyme complexes
C. Fixing enzymes into membranes so that they are adjacent to each other
D. All of the above

Ans. D.

377. Which of the following (s) is/are serine proteases?

A. Chymotrypsin
B. Trypsin
C. Elastase
D. All of these

Ans. D.

378. Which of the following statements about enzymes or their function is true?

A. Enzymes do not alter the overall change in free energy for a reaction
B. Enzymes are proteins whose three-dimensional form is key to their function
C. Enzymes speed up reactions by lowering activation energy
D. All of the above

Ans. D.

379. Tryprotophan synthetase of E.coli, a typical bifunctional oligomeric enzyme consist of

A. A protein designated A
B. Two proteins designated A and B
C. A protein A and one-subunit a
D. A protein designated B

Ans. B.

380. Lack of reaction to our own human leukocyte antigens (HLAs) is known as?

A. Autoimmunity
B. Complement system
C. Clonal selection
D. Tolerance

Ans. D.

381. Which of the following components of the vertebrate immune response occurs first upon invasion by a virus or bacterium?

A. Activation of killer T lymphocytes

B. Activation of B lymphocytes

C. The inflammatory response

D. Mobilization of complement proteins

Ans. C.

382. Which of the following white blood cells act as scavengers when they engulf and digest pathogens?

A. Macrophages B. T cells

C. B cells D. Lymphocytes

Ans. A.

383. A cell which defends against body cells in which viruses are reproducing is

A. Exotoxin B. Cytotoxic T cell

C. Endotoxin D. Suppressor T cell

Ans. B.

384. Which of the following is most likely to produce anaphylaxis in a susceptible individual?

A. Pollen B. Mold

C. Dust D. Bee sting

Ans. D.

385. What type of B cell remains dormant in the body, but can respond rapidly if the same antigen appears again?

A. T cells B. Memory cells

C. Plasma cells D. Macrophages

Ans. B.

386. The maturation of T cells and the production of particular T cell receptors occurs in the

A. Thyroid gland B. Thymus gland

C. Testes D. All of these

Ans. B.

387. Which of the following provide specific defense against viruses and bacteria?

A. T cells B. B cells

C. Complement D. Inflammation

Ans. B.

388. Which of these is a type of specific defense against pathogens?

A. Lymphocytes B. Macrophages

C. Phagocytes D. Leukocytes

Ans. A.

389. In animals, blood clots serve the function of

A. Consuming invading organisms

B. Helping them match the background coloration of the habitat

C. Stimulating production of killer T lymphocytes

D. Repairing damage to the body wall

Ans. D.

390. What is the result of invasion of a body by pathogens?

A. Infection B. Inflammation

C. Swelling D. Pus

Ans. A.

391. What is the behaviour in which T cells and B cells constantly travel throughout the body seeking out and destroying foreign substances?

A. Antibody-mediated immune response

B. Immune surveillance

C. Cell-mediated immune response

D. Vaccination

Ans. B.

392. In a foetus, where are lymphocytes produced?

A. In the spleen B. In the bone marrow

C. In the liver D. In the heart

Ans. C.

393. Which of the following produces the antibodies employed in the specific immune response of vertebrates?

A. B lymphocytes B. T lymphocytes

C. Neutrophils D. Macrophages

Ans. A.

394. Which of the following is not part of the vertebrate immune system?

A. Lymphocytes B. Antibodies

C. Cardiac glycosides D. Lymph nodes

Ans. C.

395. The protein, produced by B cells that binds to a specific antigen is

A. Phagocyte B. Leukocyte

C. Vaccine D. Antibody

Ans. D.

396. Which of the following characteristics are common in lymphocytes, macrophages, and neutrophils?

A. They are all part of the nonspecific immune response in vertebrates

B. They are all part of the specific immune response in vertebrates

C. They are all part of the internal defenses of nonvertebrates

D. They are all types of white blood cells

Ans. D.

397. Which of the following blood proteins can destroy pathogens?

A. Major histocompatibility complex B. Platelets

C. Fibrinogen D. Complement system

Ans. D.

398. Which of these is part of the lymphoid system in humans?

A. Liver B. Stomach

C. Tonsils D. Kidneys

Ans. C.

399. What type of B cell is like a tiny factory that produces antibodies identical to the B cell receptor that bind to the original antigen?

A. T cells B. Memory cells

C. Plasma cells D. Macrophages

Ans. C.

400. Which of the following immune cells would have an especially low count in a patient with advanced AIDS?

A. Killer T lymphocytes B. Helper T lymphocyte

C. B lymphocytes D. None of these

Ans. B.

401. In cellular immunity, T lymphocytes are responsible for the recognition and killing of foreign invaders. The cells are

A. Cytotoxic T lymphocytes (CTL) B. Killer T cells

C. Both (a) and (b) D. None of the above

Ans. C.

402. Plasma cells produce thousands of ———— that are released into the bloodstream

A. Antigens
B. Antibodies
C. Helper T cells
D. Virus fragments

Ans. B.

403. If a person is vaccinated against a disease sometime in the past, which of the following is currently in your body?

A. The disease organism itself and antigens for the disease organism
B. A very high level of antibodies against the disease antigens
C. Memory B lymphocytes for the antigen of this disease organism
D. All of the above

Ans. D.

404. What is a protein produced by host cells infected by viruses?

A. Interferon
B. Histamine
C. Antiserum
D. Vaccine

Ans. A.

405. Polysaccharides on the surface of infecting microorganisms can also activate complement directly in the absence of

A. Antibody via the alternative pathway
B. Antigen via the alternative pathway
C. Antibody via metabolic pathway
D. None of the above

Ans. A.

406. Antibodies bound to an invading microorganism activate the complement system via

A. Classical pathway
B. Metabolic pathway
C. Embden Meyerhof pathway
D. Entner-Doudoroff pathway

Ans. A.

407. The immune response to a booster vaccine is called a(n)

A. Cellular response
B. Innate response
C. Primary response
D. Secondary response

Ans. D.

408. Immunological memory is due to

A. Short lived macrophage that can recognize specific pathogens

B. Long lived B cells that secrete a specific antibody

C. Long lived B cells that secrete a specific antigen

D. Short lived helper T cells that signal macrophage to divide

Ans. B.

409. What is the result of an abnormal response of the immune system to part of a person's own body?

A. Passive immunity B. Cancer

C. An allergic response D. An autoimmune disease

Ans. D.

410. What are the solutions prepared from weakened or dead microorganisms, viruses, or toxins that provide some immunity from diseases?

A. Vaccines B. Histamines

C. Drugs D. Antibiotics

Ans. A.

411. During exposure to a foreign invader, there are more ———— present in the vertebrate body than before exposure

A. Antibodies B. Lymphocytes

C. Macrophages and antigens D. All of these

Ans. D.

412. To elicit the best antibodies to mouse MHC I, it should be injected into a

A. Goat

B. Mouse of the same genetic background (strain)

C. Mouse of a different strain

D. Rat

Ans. A.

413. To detect a humoral immune response to influenza virus, it is possible to measure

A. Cytotoxicity of virus-infected cells in tissue culture

B. Dividing t cells in the draining lymph nodes

C. Plasma cytokine levels

D. Serum antibody titer

Ans. D.

414. Which of the following is in the lymph nodes of a person battling a cold virus?
   A. Huge numbers of white blood cells
   B. Trapped viruses that have been roaming the body
   C. Lymph ducts that enter and exit the nodes and Lymph fluid
   D. All of the above

Ans. D.

415. Immunogenicity
   A. Depends on the ability of the native antigen to be presented by MHC
   B. Is usually a property of self antigens such as eye tissue
   C. Is not a property of antibodies
   D. Is not a property of haptens

Ans. D.

416. The HIV virus infects primarily
   A. Brain cells
   B. Cells in the immune system
   C. Red blood cells
   D. Liver cells

Ans. B.

417. Chronic granulomatous disease results from a failure to perform oxidative burst. This deficiency would be most likely to interfere with
   A. CTL killing of viruses
   B. Dendritic cell activation to become a mature APC
   C. Infected cell processing of virus peptides
   D. Macrophage intracellular killing of bacteria

Ans. D.

418. Difficulties with somatic gene therapy arise from all of the following except
   A. GVHD caused by mature T cells in the transplanted cells
   B. Inserting a gene so that it will function properly
   C. Limited life span of more mature hematopoietic cells
   D. Transducing genetic material into stem cells

Ans. A.

419. A monoclonal antibody (mAb) specific for the 2,4-dinitrophenyl (DNP) hapten might also bind
   A. Leu or Ileu
   B. His or Pro
   C. Tyr or Phe
   D. Ser or Thr

Ans. C.

420. Retinoblastoma is due to a mutation in a

A. Kinase
B. Tumor supressor
C. Cyclin
D. Viral gene

Ans. B.

421. An autoimmune disease is

A. AIDS
B. Measles
C. Lupus
D. Mumps

Ans. C.

422. If Class IIMHC is not expressed in the thymus, the resulting immune deficiencies would include all of the following except reduced

A. Alternative complement activation.
B. CD8 T cell-mediated cytotoxicity
C. Macrophage activation to vesicular pathogens
D. IgG synthesis

Ans. A.

423. Specific translocations are associated with

A. Colon cancer
B. Breast cancer
C. Pancreatic cancer
D. Some leukemias

Ans. D.

424. To treat HIV infections using drugs, the major problem is that

A. The drugs that are good inhibitors cannot by synthesized
B. The drugs interfere with normal digestion
C. The virus particles with altered (mutant) proteases arise
D. The drugs are rapidly degraded

Ans. C.

425. The primary reason for AIDS, a deadly disease is that it

A. Is caused by a virus
B. Is caused by a bacterium
C. Destroys key components of the body's internal defense system
D. Causes a breakdown of the body's inflammatory response

Ans. C.

426. A selective IgA deficiency would be expected to result in problems with

A. Bacterial infections

B. Infections following dental work due to bacteria entering the bloodstream

C. Mucosal pathogens

D. Pathogens which can survive inside macrophages

Ans. C.

427. Combined cellular and humoral immune deficiencies result from lack of all of the following except

A. A thymus

B. Class II MHC

C. HIV infection of $CD4^+$ T cells

D. Transporter of antigen peptides (TAP)

Ans. D.

428. An example of an immunodeficiency disorder is

A. Thyroiditis

B. Rheumatic fever

C. Systemic lupus erythematosus

D. AIDS

Ans. D.

429. Bone marrow given to an infant with SCID must

A. Be irradiated to eliminate GVHD

B. Contain mature T cells that can begin making immune responses immediately

C. Come from a donor that shares some MHC alleles with the recipient

D. Come from one of the child's parents

Ans. C.

430. X-linked hyper IgM syndrome, resulting in high levels of serum IgM and low levels of serum IgG, is caused by a defect in CD40L expression. The specific immune event that would be prevented by a defective CD40L would be

A. Activation of B cells by T-independent antigens

B. Failure of B cells to provide co-stimulation for Th2 activation

C. Failure of Th2 cells to provide co-stimulation for B cell isotype switching

D. Failure of Th2 cells to provide co-stimulation for B cell proliferation

Ans. C.

431. DiGeorge's syndrome is characterized by the lack of a thymus. The mouse model closest to this human disease would be a

A. Knock-out mouse for RAG-1 and RAG-2

B. Knock-out mouse for a thymus

C. Nude mouse

D. Recombinant mouse for CD3

Ans. C.

432. Which of the Rous sarcoma virus has a homologous cellular protein?

A. C-src B. V-src

C. V-ha-src D. V-ha-ras

Ans. A.

433. Infants are most susceptible to bacterial infection due to low circulating levels of IgG

A. In utero (before birth) B. At 0-3 months of age

C. At 3-12 months of age D. At 12-24 months of age

Ans. C.

434. The chemical, typically released by the body in an allergic response is

A. Histamine B. Allergens

C. Antihistamines D. Perforins

Ans. A.

435. The competitive immunoassay can be used

A. To detect very small amounts of antigen

B. To detect antibody associated with allergies (IgE)

C. Both A and B

D. Commonly to detect trace amounts of drugs.

Ans. C.

436. Which of the following is an immunodiffusion test?

A. Double-diffusion B. Gel diffusion

C. Ouchterloney technique D. All of these

Ans. D.

437. Which of the following lymphokine (s) is secreted by delayed-type-hypersensitivity cells?

A. Macrophage stimulating factor B. Migration inhibiting factor

C. Macrophage activating factor D. All of the above

Ans. D.

438. Which of the following is an example of autoimmune disease ?

A. Rheumatoid arthritis B. Systemic lupus erythematosus

C. Polyarteritis nodosa D. All of the above

Ans. D.

439. Immunosuppressive agent(s) is/are

A. Cyclosporine B. Methotrexate

C. Anti-lymphocyte serum D. All of these

Ans. D.

440. Induction of tolerance mechanism(s) is/are

A. Suppression B. Clonal deletion

C. Clonal anergy D. All of these

Ans. D.

441. Lens antigens of the eye are

A. Cross reacting antigens B. Sequestrated antigens

C. Neoantigens D. None of these

Ans. B.

442. Negative phase is observed in

A. Secondary humoral response B. Primary humoral response

C. Both A and B D. None of these

Ans. A.

443. Method (s) that can be used to detect CMI is/are

A. Migration inhibition

B. Target cell destruction factor test

C. Skin test for delayed hypersensitivity

D. All of the above

Ans. D.

444. In which of the following cell mediated immunity (CMI) participates?

A. Delayed hypersensitivity reaction B. Graft versus host reaction

C. Allograft rejection D. All of the above

Ans. D.

445. Over activity of T_h cells may result into

A. Autoimmunity B. Optimal antibody response

C. Optimal cell mediated response D. None of the above

Ans. A.

446. VDRL test is an example of

A. Tube test B. Ring test

C. Slide test D. None of these

Ans. C.

447. Weil-Felix reaction is based on sharing of antigens between

A. Sheep RBCs and EB virus

B. Mycoplasma and human O group RBCs

C. Rickettsial antigens and antigens of certain strains of Proteus

D. None of these

Ans. C.

448. Agglutination reaction is more sensitive than precipitation for the detection of

A. Antigens

B. Antibodies

C. Complement

D. Antigen-antibody complexes

Ans. A.

449. Precipitation reaction is relatively less sensitive for the detection of

A. Antigens

B. Antigen-antibody complexes

C. Antibodies

D. Complement

Ans. C.

450. In which of the following case a large lattice is formed?

A. Antibody is in excess

B. Antigens and antibodies are in optimal proportion

C. Antigen is in excess

D. None of these

Ans. B.

451. Ring test is used for

A. C reactive protein test

B. Ascoli's thermoprecipitation test

C. typing of Streptococci and Pneumococci

D. All of the above

Ans. D.

452. Precipitation reaction can be converted into agglutination reaction by coating soluble antigen onto

A. Bentonite particles

B. RBCs

C. Latex particles

D. All of these

Ans. D.

453. Commercially available ELISA kits are used for the detection of

A. Rotavirus B. Hepatitis B surface antigen

C. Anti-HIV antibodies D. All of these

Ans. D.

454. Monoclonal antibody production requires

A. Mouse splenic lymphocytes B. Mouse myeloma cells

C. Both A and B D. None of these

Ans. C.

455. Quellung reaction is used for typing of

A. Klebsiella pneumoniae B. Streptococcus pneumoniae

C. Both A and B D. None of these

Ans. C.

456. Fluorescent treponemal antibody test is an example of

A. Indirect immunofluorescence B. Direct immunofluorescence

C. Both A and B D. None of these

Ans. A.

457. Counter-immunoelectrophoresis is used for the detection of

A. Meningococcal antigen B. Hepatitis B surface antigen

C. Alpha-fetoprotein D. All of these

Ans. D.

458. The test (s) based on the principle of toxin neutralization is/are

A. Nagler's reaction B. Schick test

C. Both A and B D. None of these

Ans. C.

459. Slide agglutination reaction is/are useful for the identification of the culture(s) of

A. Shigella B. Vibrio Cholerae

C. Salmonella D. All of these

Ans. D.

460. Amount of various immunoglobulin classes can be measured by

A. Double diffusion in one dimension

B. Single diffusion in two dimensions

C. Single diffusion in one dimension

D. Double diffusion in two dimensions

Ans. B.

461. Which type of interferon is produced by T lymphocytes?

A. α B. β

C. γ D. γ and β

Ans. C.

462. Lack of reaction to our own human leukocyte antigens (HLAs) is known as?

A. Complement system B. Autoimmunity

C. Tolerance D. Clonal selection

Ans. C.

7

Industrial Microbiology

1. The best medium for the production of Penicillin is

   A. Nutrient agar B. Corn steep liquor

   C. Sulfite waste liquor D. Whey

Ans. B.

2. Industrially important antibiotic producing organisms shall be isolated by

   A. Disk plate method B. Direct plate method

   C. Serial dilution method D. Crowded plate method

Ans. D.

3. Industrial alcohol will be produced by using starter culture

   A. Top yeast B. Middle yeast

   C. Bottom yeast D. Feeder yeast

Ans. C.

4. Pyruvate decarboxylase acetaldehyde + CO2 = This reaction is specially observed in

   A. Lactic acid fermentors B. Ethanol fermentors

   C. Algae D. Plants

Ans. B.

5. The pyruvate, dehydrogenase ® multienzyme complex does not occur in

   A. Aerobic bacteria B. Microphilic bacteria

   C. Facultative anaerobic bacteria D. Strictly anaerobic bacteria

Ans. B.

6. A major ingredient of penicillin production media is

   A. Corn meal B. Corn steep liquor

   C. Cane steep liquor D. None of these

Ans. B.

7. The outstanding example of traditional microbial fermentation product is

A. Vinegar B. Penicillin

C. Citric acid D. Tetracyclin

Ans. A.

8. Which of the following involves the formation of nitrate from ammonia

A. Ammonification B. Denitrification

C. Nitrification D. Nitrogen fixation

Ans. C.

9. In alcoholic fermentation, CO2 is evolved during

A. Decarboxylation of pyruvic acid B. Formation of acetaldehyde

C. Oxidation of acetaldehyde D. Both a and b

Ans. D.

10. In the industrial production of streptomycin, the secondary metabolite or by products is

A. Vitamin – B12 B. Vitamin – C

C. Vitamin – B6 D. Ethanol

Ans. A.

11. Tobacco and tea leaves are fermented to give flavour and taste. This type of fermentation is known as

A. Alcohol fermentation B. Curing

C. Degradation D. Lactic acid fermentation

Ans. B.

12. Vinegar fermentation involves

A. Yeasts only B. Yeasts with lactic bacteria

C. Yeasts with acetic acid bacteria D. Yeasts with butyric acid bacteria

Ans. C.

13. By-product of acetone-butanol fermentation include

A. Riboflavin B. Penicillin

C. Isopropanol D. All of these

Ans. A.

14. Thermo resistant bacteria are important in the preservation of foods by

A. Freezing B. Canning

C. Chemicals D. Irradiation

Ans. B.

15. The fungus used in the industrial production of citric acid:

A. Rhizopus Oryzac B. Fusarium moniliformae

C. Rhizopus nigricans D. Aspergillus nigricans

Ans. D.

16. Penicillin is commercially produced by

A. P. notatum B. P. chrysogenum

C. P. citrinum D. P. roquefortii

Ans. B.

17. The most commonly used microorganism in alcohol fermentation is

A. Aspergilus niger B. Bacillus subtilis

C. Sacharomyces cerevisiae D. Escherichia coli

Ans. A.

18. Vitamin B12 can be estimated and determined by using organism

A. Lactobacillus sps B. Lactobacillus leichmannii

C. Bacillus subtilis D. E. coli

Ans. B.

19. Batch fermentation is also called

A. Closed system B. Open system

C. Fed-Batch system D. Sub-merger system

Ans. A.

20. To differentiate lactose and non-lactose fermentors the medium used is

A. Mac Conkey's medium B. Stuart's medium

C. Sugar medium D. Citrate medium

Ans. A.

21. The micro-organism useful for fermentation are

A. Bacteria B. Yeast

C. Fungi D. None of these

Ans. B.

22. Industrial microbiology, mainly depends on the phenomenon

A. Pasteurisation B. Fermentation

C. Vaccination D. Both b and c

Ans. B.

23. Streptokinase is also termed as

A. Fibrionolysin
B. Catalase
C. Coagulase
D. Hyaluronidase

Ans. A.

24. Streptokinase is produced by

A. Staphylococcus aureus
B. Streptococcus pneumoniae
C. Str. faecalis
D. Str. Pyogenes

Ans. D.

25. Large vessel containing all the parts and condition necessary for the growth of desired microorganisms is called

A. Bio reactor
B. Auto reactor
C. Impeller
D. None of these

Ans. A.

26. For thorough mixing of medium and inoculum the part of fermentor useful is

A. Shaft
B. Headspace
C. Impeller
D. Sparger

Ans. C.

27. In fermentor the top portion left without broth is called

A. Shaft
B. Head space
C. Impeller
D. Sparger

Ans. B.

28. Over heating of fermentor during fermentation is controlled by

A. Cooling jacket
B. Steam
C. Cool air
D. None of these

Ans. A.

29. Antifoam agent is

A. Silicon compounds
B. Corn oil
C. Soyabean oil
D. All of these

Ans. D.

30. The capacity of laboratory fermentors is

A. 12–15 liters
B. 2000 gallons
C. 500 liters
D. 10000 gallons

Ans. A.

31. L. lysine is produced from

A. Corynebacterium glutamicum
B. Corynebacterium sps.
C. Mycobacterium sps.
D. None of these

Ans. A.

32. Methods used to get immobilized enzymes:

A. Adsorption
B. Encapsulation
C. Covalent bonding
D. All of these

Ans. D.

33. Microorganisms used for alcohol production

A. Saccharomyces cerevisiae
B. Bacillus subtilis
C. Penicillium chrysogenum
D. None of these

Ans. A.

34. For streptomycin production the microorganisms required are

A. Streptomyces griseus
B. Streptomyces niger
C. Saccharomyces cereviceae
D. All of these

Ans. A.

35. The by-product during streptomycin production is

A. Vitamin A
B. Proline
C. Vitamin B12
D. None of these

Ans. C.

36. For acetic acid production the methods followed are

A. Orleans process
B. Rapid process
C. Submerged process
D. All of these

Ans. D.

37. For amylase production the micro organism required is

A. B. subtilis
B. S. cerevisiae
C. A. niger
D. None of these

Ans. A.

38. Pectinase is industrially produced from

A. S. cerevisiae
B. Trichoderma Koningi
C. A. nigar
D. None of these

Ans. C.

39. Cellulose are produced from

A. S. cerevisiae
B. Trichoderma koningii
C. A. nigar
D. None of these

Ans. B.

40. Industrial production of Vitamin-B12 is from

A. Propionibacterium sps.
B. Pseudomonas sps.
C. Both a and b
D. None of these

Ans. C.

41. Clostridium acetobutylicum is used for the production of

A. Acetone - Butanol
B. Ethanol
C. Vitamin-B12
D. None of these

Ans. B.

42. In the production of ethanol industrially the yeast used is

A. K. pneumoniae
B. Kluyreromyces fragilis
C. S. cerevisiae
D. Both b and c

Ans. D.

43. Citric acid is used as

A. Flavouring agent in food
B. As an antioxident
C. As preservative
D. All of the above

Ans. D.

44. Citric acid is produced in aerobic conditions by the fungi

A. Aspergillus
B. Penicillin
C. Mucor
D. All of these

Ans. D.

45. The raw material for citric acid production is

A. Corn
B. Molasses
C. Starch
D. None of these

Ans. A.

46. Aspergillus niger is used generally for the production of

A. Ethanol
B. Penicillin
C. Citric acid
D. Lactic acid

Ans. C.

47. In the citric acid production, the pH to be maintained in the fermentor is

A. 7.0 B. 5.0 to 6.0

C. 8.0 to 9.0 D. 1.0 to 6.0

Ans. B.

48. The required temperature for the production of citric acid is

A. 10°C – 80°C B. 30°C – 50°C

C. 20°C – 50°C D. 25°C – 30°C

Ans. D.

49. The penicillin produced in large scale submerged fermentations are

A. Penicillin-A B. Penicillin-D

C. Penicillin-G D. None of these

Ans. C.

50. The strain of fungi used for the large scale production of penicillin is

A. Penicillium chrysogenum B. P. notatum

C. Streptomyces aurecus D. Saccharomyces sps

Ans. A.

51. 6-amino penicillanic acid is prepared from Penicillin by

A. Acylase B. Penicillin G acylase

C. Penicillinone D. None of these

Ans. B.

52. The pH, to be maintained for the production of penicillin is

A. 7.5 B. 6.5

C. 8.0 D. 5.0

Ans. B.

53. First Pasteur conducted fermentation experiments in

A. Milk B. Food material

C. Fruit juices D. Both a and c

Ans. C.

54. Which one of the following is called as ‘brewers yeast’

A. Saccharomyces ludwigi B. Saccharomyces cerevisiae

C. Saccharomyces boulardii D. Saccharomyces pastorianus

Ans. B.

55. Butanol is obtained by fermenting molasses by
A. Clostridium butyricum and Cl. acetobutylicum
B. Clostridium butyricum and Cl. tetani
C. Clostridium butyricum and lactobacillus
D. Clostridium butyricum and Cl. oceanicm

Ans. A.

56. Which of the following is the source of Vit A ?
A. Streptococcus
B. Rhodotorula gracilis
C. Both A and B
D. Yeast

Ans. B.

57. Yeast cells are good source of
A. Vitamin A & B
B. Vitamin A & D
C. Vitamin B & D
D. All of these

Ans. C.

58. Roquefort cheese is ripened by
A. Penicillium roqueforti
B. Penicillium camemberti
C. All Penicillium sp.
D. Penicillium rhizogenes

Ans. A.

59. Penicillum camemberti is used for ripening of
A. Roqueforti cheese
B. Camembert cheese
C. All cheese
D. Fruits

Ans. B.

60. Unicelled microbes grown as source of proteins are called
A. Microbial proteins
B. Single cell protein
C. Unicelled proteins
D. None of these

Ans. B.

61. Which of the following are rich source of protein
A. Spirulina and Chlorella
B. Chlorella and Scenedesmus
C. Scenedesmus
D. All the above

Ans. D.

62. Zymase is obtained from
A. Saccharomyces ludwigi
B. Saccharomyces cerevisiae
C. Saccharomyces boulardii
D. None of the above

Ans. B.

63. Glucose oxidase is obtained from

A. Saccharomyces cerevisiae B. Aspergillus niger

C. Spirulina D. Penicillium sp.

Ans. B.

64. Pectinase is obtained from

A. Saccharomyces cerevisiae B. Aspergillus sp.

C. Spirulina D. Penicillium sp.

Ans. D.

65. Bacillus thuringiensis is used as

A. Insecticide B. Fungicide

C. Microbial agent D. Rodenticide

Ans. A.

66. Petroleum degrading species include

A. Nocardia B. Micrococcus

C. Penicillium D. All of the above

Ans. D.

67. Kojic acid is obtained from

A. Nocardia B. Micrococcus

C. Penicillium D. Aspergillus

Ans. D.

68. Fumaric acid is obtained from

A. Saccharomyces cerevisiae B. Aspergillus niger

C. Rhizopus stolonifer D. Penicillium sp.

Ans. C.

69. The most commonly used microorganism in alcohol fermentation is

A. Aspergillus niger B. Bacillus subtilis

C. Saccharomyces cerevisiae D. E. coli

Ans. A.

70. Vit B 12 can be estimated and determined by using organism

A. Lactobacillus sp. B. L. leichmanni

C. Bacillus subtilis D. E. coli

Ans. B.

71. Batch fermentation is also called

A. Closed system
B. Open system
C. Fed-batch system
D. Submerger system

Ans. A.

72. To differentiate lactose and nonlactose fermentors the medium used is

A. Mc Conkey's medium
B. Stuart's medium
C. Sugar medium
D. Citrate medium

Ans. A.

73. The microorganism useful for fermentation are

A. Bacteria
B. Yeast
C. Fungi
D. None of these

Ans. B.

74. Industrial microbiology mainly depends on the phenomenon

A. Pasteurization
B. Fermentation
C. Vaccination
D. Both B and C

Ans. B.

75. Streptokinase is also termed as

A. Fibrinolysin
B. Catalase
C. Coagulase
D. Hyaluronidase

Ans. A.

76. Streptokinase is produced by

A. Staphylococcus aureus
B. Streptococcus pneumoniase
C. Str. faecalis
D. Str. pyogenes

Ans. D.

77. Large vessel containing all the parts and condition necessary for the growth of desired microorganisms is called

A. Bioreactor
B. Autoreactor
C. Impeller
D. None of these

Ans. A.

78. Basic principle in industrial microbiology is

A. Suitable growth conditions
B. Fermentation
C. Providing aspectic conditions
D. All of these

Ans. B.

79. Considering fermentation at industrial level, microorganism Aspergillus is used to form

A. Formic acid
B. Acrylic acid
C. Glycerol
D. Ethanol

Ans. A.

80. Glycerol ($C_3H_8O_3$) is used at industry level for the

A. Production of plastics
B. Leather treatment
C. Production of vinegar
D. Production of cosmetics

Ans. D.

81. Most common example of fermented cereal product is

A. Pickles
B. Bread
C. Yogurt
D. Cheese

Ans. B.

82. Technique of SCP is introduced by

A. Gregor Mendel
B. Louis Pasteur
C. Professor Scrimshaw
D. Ian Wilmot

Ans. C.

83. Fermentation which is carried by yeast is called

A. Pyruvic fermentation
B. Acrylic fermentation
C. Lactic acid fermentation
D. Alcoholic fermentation

Ans. C.

84. Process through which glucose molecules ($C_6H_{12}O_6$) release energy is called

A. Oxidation-reduction
B. Nitrogen reduction
C. Oxygen reduction
D. Nitrogen oxidation

Ans. A.

85. Carbon dioxide (CO_2) is removed in alcoholic fermentation from

A. Pyruvic acid
B. Nitric acid
C. Sulphuric acid
D. Hydrochloric acid

Ans. A.

86. Production of different products by using mass culture of microorganisms is classified as

A. Bacillus production
B. Reproduction
C. Fermentation
D. Pollination

Ans. C.

87. Applications of fermentation includes

A. Cereal products
B. Dairy products
C. Beverage products
D. All of above

Ans. D.

88. By using single-cell protein, amount of protein that can be produced by algae grown in ponds(per acre) is

A. 20 tons
B. 30 tons
C. 40 tons
D. 50 tons

Ans. A.

89. Fermentation which is carried by bacteria is called

A. Lactic acid fermentation
B. Alcoholic fermentation
C. Pyruvic fermentation
D. Acrylic fermentation

Ans. A.

90. Considering fermentation at industrial level, microorganism Saccharomyces is used to form

A. Glycerol
B. Ethanol
C. Formic acid
D. Both A and B

Ans. D.

91. Considering bread production, fermentation is caused by

A. Carbolic acid
B. Carbon dioxide
C. Methane
D. Ethane

Ans. B.

92. Pyruvic acid in alcoholic fermentation reduced to acetaldehyde which further reduced into

A. Carbon dioxide
B. Methanol
C. Ethanol
D. Methane

Ans. C.

93. Pyruvic acid in alcoholic fermentation leads to

A. Glucose
B. Lactose
C. Lactic acid
D. Acetaldehyde

Ans. D.

8

Miscellaneous

1. In the first months of life, babies often develop resistance to specific pathogenic micro-organisms by inheriting it from their mother. Which of the following terms is used to describe this condition?

   A. Acquired immunity B. Dead vaccine
   C. Live vaccine D. Natural immunity
   E. Passive immunity

Ans. E.

2. The two strands of DNA are joined noncovalently by

   A. Ionic bonds B. Covalent bonds
   C. Hydrogen bonds between bases D. Polar charges

Ans. C.

3. The bases Adenine and Thymine are paired with

   A. Double hydrogen bonds B. Single hydrogen bonds
   C. Triple hydrogen bonds D. Both b and c

Ans. A.

4. The no. of hydrogen bonds existing between Guanine and Cytosine are

   A. 5 B. 2
   C. 3 D. None of these

Ans. C.

5. The length of each coil in DNA strand is

   A. 15 A° B. 34 A°
   C. 30 A° D. 5 A°

Ans. B.

6. Nucleic acids are highly charged polymers due to

A. There is phosphodiester bond between 5'-hydroxyl of one ribose and 3'–hydroxyl of next ribose

B. They have positive and negative ends

C. Nucleotides are charged structures

D. Nitrogenous bases are highly ionized compounds

Ans. A.

7. What are the structural units of nucleic acids?

A. N-bases B. Nucleosides

C. Nucleotides D. Histones

Ans. C.

8. In Electron Microscope source of electrons is from

A. Mercury lamp B. Tungsten metal

C. Both a and b D. None of these

Ans. B.

9. The resolution power of the compound microscope is

A. 0.2 micron B. 0.2 millimeter

C. 0.2 Angstrom units D. 0.2 centimeter

Ans. A.

10. Electron microscope gives magnification upto

A. 100 X B. 2000 X

C. 50,000 X D. 2,00,000 X

Ans. D.

11. Eye cannot resolve any image less than

A. 1μ B. 2 μ

C. 7 μ D. 5 μ

Ans. D.

12. Compound Microscope was discovered by

A. A.V. Leeuwenhoek B. Pasteur

C. Janssen and Hans D. None of these

Ans. C.

13. Magnification range of light microscope is

A. 1000x – 5000x B. 1000x – 2000x

C. 500x – 1000x D. None of these

Ans. B.

14. Condensation of light in light Microscope is by

A. Objective B. Condensor

C. Ocular D. All of these

Ans. B.

15. Light gathering capacity of Microscope is called

A. Numerical aperture B. Angular aperture

C. Both a and b D. None of these

Ans. A.

16. If 10x and 40x objectives are used (air is the medium), the numerical aperture is

A. 1.5 B. 2.0

C. 1.0 D. 1.8

Ans. C.

17. The ability of Microscope to distinguish two objects into two separate objects, is called

A. Resolving power B. Wave length

C. N.A. D. None of these

Ans. A.

18. Source of light in fluorescence microscopy is from

A. Mercury lamp B. Sunlight

C. Both a and b D. None of these

Ans. A.

19. The magnification power of electron microscope developed by Knoll and Ruska is

A. 10,000x B. 12,000x

C. 15,000x D. 20,000x

Ans. B.

20. In electron microscope source of electrons is from

A. Mercury lamp B. Tungsten metal

C. Both a and b D. None of these

Ans. B.

21. The electron passed out from the specimen are called

A. Primary electrons B. Secondary electrons

C. Tertiary electrons D. None of these

Ans. B.

22. Fluorescent substance used in fluorescent microscopy are

A. Quinine sulphate B. Auramine

C. All of these D. None of these

Ans. C.

23. Light yellowish color seen in cow's milk is due to the presence of———.

A. Carotene B. Curcumin

C. Cyanophycin D. Riboflavin

Ans. A.

24. Three domain system of classification of organism is based on

A. rRNA sequence B. cyt-C sequence

C. rRNA and cyt-C sequence D. Morphology and rRNA sequence

Ans. A.

25. Which type of interferon is produced by T lymphocytes?

A. α B. β

C. γ D. γ and β

Ans. C.

26. Which of the following is semi-continuous (diploid) cell line?

A. Hela B. Hep-2

C. WI-38 D. KB

Ans. C.

27. In cell culture, measles may lead to

A. Nuclear pyknosis B. Transforming of cells

C. Syncytium formation D. Rounding & aggregation of cells

Ans. C.

28. The repressor protein, since the cell is resistant to lysis from externally infecting phage, is also called

A. Immunity repressor B. Immunity operon

C. Operon repressor D. None of these

Ans. A.

29. In the process of freeze drying, a dense cell suspension is placed in small vials and is frozen at

A. -60 to -78°C B. -20 to -30°C

C. -30 to -48°C D. -48 to -58°C

Ans. A.

30. The average human body contains approximately —— cells, —— bacteria and —— virus.

Ans. 10^{13}, 10^{14} and 10^{15}.

31. Conventional fluorescent microscopy has a resolution of —— nm and single molecule localization microscopy has resolution of —— nm.

Ans. 200-500 nm ; Less than 1 nm.

32. High throughput sequencing methods are ———, ——— and ———.

Ans. 454, Illumina, SoLid (Sequencing by oligonucleotide ligation and detection).

33. Eukaryotic cells produce ——— to ——— virus particles per cell.

Ans. 1000 to 10,000.

34. Which of the following methods would be most appropriate for sterilizing an antibiotic solution?

A. Dry heat sterilization
B. Microfiltration
C. Autoclaving
D. Desiccation

Ans. B.

35. Plastic implants can pose a serious nosocomial infection problem because

A. Phagocytes have trouble moving on the plastic surface
B. Phagocytes have trouble engulfing bacteria embedded in a biofilm
C. Infected implants usually have to be surgically removed
D. All of the above

Ans. D.

36. Which of the following may account for the small size of the cells ?

A. The rate of diffusion
B. The surface area/volume ratio
C. The number of mRNAs that can be produced by the nucleus
D. All of these

Ans. D.

37. Which of the following structures is the smallest ?

A. Viroid
B. Hydrogen atom
C. Bacterium
D. Mitochondria

Ans. B.

38. The matrix of blood is known as

A. Plasma B. Serum

C. RBC and WBC D. WBC & platelets

Ans. A.

39. The percentage of formed elements in the blood is

A. 45% B. 50%

C. 55% D. 65%

Ans. A.

40. The life span of RBC is

A. 100 days B. 110 days

C. 120 days D. 130 days

Ans. C.

41. The ratio of WBC and RBC is

A. 1:60 B. 1:600

C. 1:6000 D. 1:60000

Ans. B.

42. During blood coagulation, thromboplastin is released by

A. RBC B. Blood plasma

C. Leucocytes D. Clumped platelets and damaged tissues

Ans. D.

43. The life span of WBC is approximately

A. Less than 10 days B. Between 20-30 days

C. Between 2-3 months D. More than 3 months

Ans. B.

44. Which of these term is not related to microbiology

A. Environmental B. Super

C. Medical

Ans. B.

45. What is full form of MHA ?

A. Multiple Hazy Agar B. Multiple Husk Agar

C. Muller Hinton Agar

Ans. C.

46. Who is the father of modern microbiology ?

A. Jenner B. Louis Pasteur

C. Leuwenhoek D. Lister

Ans. B.

47. Stain for Rickettsia is

A. Methylene blue B. Giemsa strain

C. Gram's stain

Ans. C.

48. The polymerase chain reaction or PCR is a technique that

A. Was used to demonstrate DNA as the genetic material

B. Is used to determine the content of mineral

C. Uses short DNA primers and a thermostable DNA polymerase to replicate specific DNA sequences in vitro

D. Measures the ribosome transfer rate during translation

Ans. C.

49. Who discovered blood circulation ?

A. J.J. Baird B. Galileo

C. William Harvey D. Louis Pasteur

Ans. C.

50. Who discovered bacteria, protozoa ?

A. Nicholas Copernicus B. Leeuwenhoek

C. John Gutenberg D. Louis Pasteur

Ans. B.

51. Which of the following materials is used as a bioplastic ?

A. Polystyrene B. Polypropylene

C. Polyhydroxybutyrate D. Dextran

Ans. C.

52. A trickling filter is used for

A. Antibiotic production B. Beer production

C. Citric acid manufacturing D. Waste water treatment

Ans. D.

53. A double spiral heat exchanger is a

A. Direct heat exchanger B. Indirect heat exchanger

C. A temperature control device D. Thermostat

Ans. B.

54. The importance of yeast extract in the industrial fermenter is

A. Acts as vitamin and micronutrient source

B. Acts as nitrogen source

C. Acts as carbon source

D. Acts as carbon and vitamin source

Ans. A.

55. A fed batch process is a

A. Closed system B. Continuous system

C. Intermittently fed system D. Biphasic system

Ans. C.

56. Soy meal, peptone and tryptone are used as the source of

A. Carbon source B. Carbon and nitrogen source

C. Nitrogen source D. Mineral source

Ans. C.

57. An air lift fermenter uses

A. An impeller for mixing

B. Air bubbles for mixing the contents

C. Differential density for mixing purpose

D. A sparger for mixing the contents

Ans. C.

58. Batch sterilization cycle time consists of

A. Two phases B. Three phases

C. Four phases D. Five phases

Ans. B.

59. A spray dryer works on the principle of

A. Contact drying B. Sublimation

C. Lyophilisation D. Adiabatic drying

Ans. D.

60. Protected fermentation uses

A. Sterilized media B. Pasteurized media

C. Pasteurized media with low pH D. unsterilized media

Ans. C.

61. Molasses and corn steep liquor are usually used as

A. Carbon source for large scale industrial fermentation process

B. Carbon source for small scale industrial fermentation process

C. Mineral source for large scale industrial fermentation process

D. Mineral source for small scale industrial fermentation process

Ans. A.

62. The importance of tryptone in microbiology is

A. To produce lysogeny broth for microbes

B. To produce metabolic broth for microbes

C. To stimulate beta galactosidase production

D. For the artificial stimulation of lac operon

Ans. A.

63. Marmite – an important commercial product is a

A. Fermentation main product B. Fermentation by product

C. Partially fermented sugar D. Completely fermented sugar

Ans. B.

64. The phenomenon of production of ethanol by yeast cells under high concentration of glucose rather than producing biomass by TCA cycle is described as

A. Warburg effect B. Simpson's effect

C. Crabtree effect D. Olivosky's effect

Ans. C.

65. A bioreactor to which fresh medium is continuously added, while culture liquid containing leftover nutrients, metabolic end products and microorganisms are continuously removed at the same rate is called

A. Cryostat B. Chemostat

C. Fed batch fermenter D. Continuous fermenter

Ans. B.

66. The first antibody to contact invading microorganism is

A. IgG B. IgA

C. IgM D. IgD

Ans. C.

67. The feeling of general discomfort is called as

A. Arthritis B. Symptom

C. Malaise D. Pain

Ans. C.

68. The utilization of elemental carbon by microbes during bio-geochemical cycle is called

A. Dissimilation B. Immobilization

C. Mineralization D. Neutralization

Ans. B.

69. Which of the following is a sexual spore of fungi ?

A. Conidiospore B. Ascospore

C. Teliospore D. Sporangiospore

Ans. B.

70. Kuru disease in human is caused by

A. Virus B. Virioids

C. Prions D. Prions and Virioids

Ans. C.

71. Chondroid of some bacteria are better known as

A. Bacterial mitochondria B. Mesosomes

C. Bacterial plastids D. Bacterial plasmids

Ans. B.

72. The resolving power of an optical microscope is

A. 0.2 μm B. 0.2A°

C. 0.2 nm D. 0.2 mm

Ans. A.

73. The reduction of virulence of a microorganism is known as

A. Attenuation B. Exaltation

C. Inactivation D. Hibernation

Ans. A.

74. The process of enhancement of virulence of a microorganism is called

A. Activation B. Hyperactivation

C. Exaltation D. Tyndalization

Ans. C.

75. Which of the following structure is absent in Gram positive bacteria ?

A. Cell wall
B. Teichoic acid
C. Murein
D. Outer membrane

Ans. D.

76. Which of the following process is not possible to do by a eukaryotic organism ?

A. Decomposition
B. Nitrogen fixation
C. Anaerobic respiration
D. Causing disease

Ans. B.

77. Bacteria with a tuft of flagella found at one of the cell pole is called

A. Monotrichus
B. Lophotrichous
C. Peritrichous
D. Polotrichous

Ans. B.

78. The transfer of plasmid from one bacteria to a different strain is a best example for

A. Horizontal gene transfer
B. Vertical gene transfer
C. Homozygous gene transfer
D. Heterozygous gene transfer

Ans. A.

79. The process in which all living cells, spores and viruses are completely destroyed from an object is called

A. Disinfection
B. Pasteurization
C. Sterilization
D. Antisepsis

Ans. C.

80. UHT sterilization involved high temperature exposure of objects for ———.

A. 1-3 sec
B. 1-3 min
C. 1-3 hours
D. 10-30 hours

Ans. A.

81. ——— is an antiseptic.

A. Chlorine
B. Copper sulphate
C. Ozone
D. 70% ethanol

Ans. D.

82. Error rate of Taq DNA polymerase

A. 10^{-4}
B. 10^{-14}
C. 10^{-24}
D. 10^{-40}

Ans. A.

83. The best form of DNA to transform E. coli is ————.

A. Linear B. Covalently closed

C. Nicked circles D. Nicked linear

Ans. B.

84. ———— phage is widely used for phage display technique

A. M13 B. φ

C. λ phage D. T7 phage

Ans. A.

85. ———— RNA polymerase has a single subunit.

A. E.coli B. B.subtilis

C. T7 D. λ phage

Ans. C.

86. Same DNA may code for more than one protein by ————.

A. Gene splitting B. RNA splitting

C. Alternative splicing of RNA D. None

Ans. C.

87. Bacterial cells can be stained with ———— to reveal the presence of lipid inclusions.

A. Saffranin B. Methylene blue

C. Trypan blue D. Sudan dyes

Ans. D.

88. Glucose that is taken in by a bacterial cell is made to stay within the cell by ————.

A. Attaching to membranes B. Immediate utilization

C. Phosphorylation D. Conversion to fructose

Ans. C.

89. Magnetosomes are inclusions of ———— in certain bacteria.

A. Iron oxide B. Iron phosphate

C. Iron nitrate D. Iron chloride

Ans. A.

90. In a population of $1X\ 10^8$ bacterial cells, if there is 50% killing ———— number of cells would remain viable

A. $0.5X\ 10^8$ B. $1X\ 10^4$

C. 50 D. $0.2X10^8$

Ans. A.

91. ———-- is a predator bacteria that infects other gram negative bacteria.

A. Haemophilus influenza B. Pseudomonas putida

C. Proteus mirabilis D. Bdellovibrio

Ans. D.

92. ———— are prokaryotic, but have the ability to carry out oxygenic photosynthesis.

A. Photorhizobium B. Cyanobacteria

C. Chlorobium D. Rhodospirillum

Ans. B.

93. ———— is the only bacterial genus where sterols are present in the cell membrane.

A. Escherichia B. Mycoplasma

C. Chlamydia D. Vibrio

Ans. B.

94. Who discovered Endoplasmic reticulum ?

Ans. Keith Porter in 1945.

95. Who discovered ribosome ?

Ans. George Emil Palade in 1950.

96. Who discovered chloroplast ?

Ans. Konstantin Mereschkowski in 1905.

97. Who discovered Golgi apparatus ?

Ans. Camillo Golgi in 1898.

98. Who discovered Mitochondria ?

Ans. Carl Benda in 1898.

99. Who discovered lysosome ?

Ans. Christian de Duve in 1955.

100. Who discovered peroxisome ?

Ans. J. Rhodin in 1954.

101. Who discovered nucleolus ?

Ans. John Gurdon and Donald Brown in 1964.

102. Which of the following amino acid is sweet in taste ?

A. Glycine B. Alanine

C. Glutamic acid D. None of these

Ans. A.

103. Which of the following amino acid act as inhibitory neurotransmitter ?

A. Glycine
B. Alanine
C. GABA
D. All of these
E. None of these

Ans. D. Inhibitory amino acid neurotransmitters (IAA) : GABA, alanine, beta alanine, Taurine

Excitatory amino acid neurotransmitters (EAA) : L-glutamate, L-Aspartate, L-Cysteine, L-Homocysteine.

104. The amino acid commonly used as an ingredient in the buffers of SDS-PAGE ?

A. Lysine
B. Glutamic acid
C. Glycine
D. Aspartic acid and Lysine together

Ans. C.

105. Which of the following amino acid will be absent in alpha helix structure of protein?

A. Glycine
B. Galine
C. Glutamic acid
D. Proline

Ans. D.

106. Amino acid used in the 'stripping' of Western blotting experiment is

A. Glutamic acid
B. Phenyl alanine
C. Alanine
D. Glycine

Ans. D.

107. Total number of proteinogenic (protein building) amino acids in the living world is

A. 20
B. 21
C. 22
D. 23

Ans. C. There are a total of 22 protein coding amino acids, among these 20 are coded by standard genetic code (standard amino acids). The remaining two amino acids (Selenocysteine and Pyrrolysine) are coded by two stop codons. The 1st one is coded by UGA and 2nd one by UAG.

108. Which of the following is a glucogenic amino acid ?

A. Glycine
B. Proline
C. Alanine
D. Both A & B
E. All of these

Ans. E. Glucogenic amino acids are those amino acids which are converted into glucose by glucogenesis during fasting and starvation. Except Leucine and Lysine all amino acids are glucogenic.

Ketogenic amino acids are directly converted into Acetyl CoA through ketogenesis and enters into Kreb's cycle for energy release. Leucine and Lysine are exclusively ketogenic amino acids. Some amino acids are both glucogenic and ketogenic such as isoleucine, threonine, phenylalanine, tyrosine and tryptophan.

109. Which of the following amino acid act as excitatory neurotransmitter ?

A. Glutamate
B. Aspartate
C. Cysteine
D. All of these
E. None of these

Ans. D.

110. Which amino acid act as the precursor of nucleotide biosysnthesis ?

A. Aspartate
B. Glycine
C. Glutamine
D. Both A and B
E. All of these

Ans. E.

111. Bacteria prefer to use the codon CGA instead of AGA to code for Arginine. This is an example for ———.

A. second genetic code
B. Nullomers
C. Transcriptional decoding
D. Allomers

Ans. B.

112. Which one of the following is an example of bioplastic ?

A. Polyaspartate
B. Polyglutamate
C. Poly-L-Lysine
D. All of these

Ans. A.

113. Histone is rich in

A. Lysine
B. Arginine
C. Histidine
D. Lysine and Arginine

Ans. D.

114. Single letter code of pyrrolysine is ———.

A. B
B. J
C. O
D. U

Ans. C.

115. Which of the following is not an essential amino acid ?

A. Proline
B. Histidine
C. Leucine
D. Methionine

Ans. A.

116. What is the molecular weight of Glycine ?

A. 75 gmol-1 B. 80 gmol-1

C. 90 gmol-1 D. 95 gmol-1

Ans. A.

117. Among the 20 standard proteins coding amino acids, which one is least occurs in proteins ?

A. Glycine B. Alanine

C. Tryptophan D. Methionine

Ans. C.

118. Which amino acid among the 20 standard protein coding amino acids, is most abundantly occurs in proteins ?

A. Glycine B. Methionine

C. Serine D. Leucine

Ans. D.

119. Which of the following amino acid is having more polarity ?

A. Lysine B. Arginine

C. Histidine D. Aspartate

Ans. B.

120. Majority of enzyme's active site usually contain one or more ——— residues ?

A. Glycine B. Tryptophan

C. Histidine D. Arginine

Ans. C.

121. The following is the amino acid sequence of an alien polypeptide. AGQHIKXSKPW. The X in the sequence represent

A. Asparagine B. Isoleucine

C. An ambiguous amino acid D. An unknown amino acid

Ans. D.

122. Amino acid acting as a defensive molecule in plant

A. Canavanine B. Concanavalin

C. Proline D. All of these

Ans. A.

123. Which amino acid act as the precursor for the synthesis of the neurotransmitter serotonin

A. Tyrosine B. Tryptophan

C. Glycine D. Arginine

Ans. B.

124. ———-- is an exclusively ketogenic amino acid in human ?

A. Valine B. Methionine

C. Leucine D. Proline

Ans. C.

125. pI of ——— is nearer to physiological pH.

A. Lysine B. Histidine

C. Arginine D. Glutamic acid

Ans. B.

126. Which amino acid act as the precursor of dopamine ?

A. Glycine B. Aspartate

C. Valine D. Tyrosine

Ans. D.

127. Amino acid which act as the precursor of IAA (Indole -3 –acetic acid) biosynthesis in plants is ———-.

A. Tyrosine B. Phenylalanine

C. Tryptophan D. Methionine

Ans. C.

128. Amino acid involved in urea cycle ———-—.

A. Ornithine B. Citruline

C. Arginine D. Both A & B

E. All of these

Ans. E.

129. Which of the amino acid has the buffering capacity at physiological pH ?

A. Lysine B. Arginine

C. Histidine D. Aspartic acid

Ans. C.

130. Amino acid which act as the precursor of epinephrine synthesis is ———.

A. Glycine B. Aspartate

C. Tyrosine D. Valine

Ans. C.

131. Which amino acid act as the precursor of nitric oxide biosynthesis in animals ?

A. Phenyl alanine B. Arginine

C. Aspartate D. Ornithine

Ans. B.

132. Which of the following is an essential amino acid ?

A. Aspartic acid
B. Alanine
C. Leucine
D. All of these

Ans. C.

133. Which of the following is an non-essential amino acid ?

A. Alanine
B. Histidine
C. Lysine
D. Methionine
E. All of these

Ans. A.

134. Which of the following amino acid is coded by a single codon ?

A. Lysine
B. Arginine
C. Tryptophan
D. Phenylalanine

Ans. C.

135. First discovered amino acid is ————.

A. Asparagine
B. Aspartate
C. Glutamate
D. Glutamine

Ans. B. It was discovered by Plisson in 1827.

136. Last discovered amino acid is ————.

A. Leucine
B. Isoleucine
C. Threonine
D. Serine

Ans. C. It was discovered by William Cumming Rose in 1930.

137. The vitreous humor of eye is composed of————.

A. Heparin
B. Hyaluronic acid
C. Keratan sulphate
D. Chondroitin sulphate

Ans. B.

138. Sulbactum is a ————.

A. Beta lactam antibiotic
B. Beta lactamase
C. Beta lactamase inhibitor
D. A class of penicillin

Ans. C.

139. Which of the following is not a sugar molecule of the O antigen of gram negative bacteria ?

A. Tyvelose
B. Abequose
C. 2 Keto- 3 deoxyoctanoate
D. Teichoic acid

Ans. D.

140. Which of the following is a sugar alcohol ?

A. Arabitol B. Manitol

C. Sorbitol D. All of these

Ans. D.

141. Reserve food material of fungi is ———.

A. Glucose B. Starch

C. Laminarin D. Glycogen

Ans. D.

142. Which of the following is a non-reducing sugar ?

A. Maltose B. Lactose

C. Trehalose D. Cellobiose

Ans. C.

143. Which of the following sugar do not form cyclic structure ?

A. Erythrulose B. Dihydroxy acetone

C. Both A & B D. Erythrose

Ans. C.

144. Which of the following sequence correctly represent the sweetness of glucose, sucrose and fructose

A. Glucose < Sucrose <Fructose B. Sucrose <Glucose < Fructose

C. Glucose < Fructose <Sucrose D. Glucose > Fructose > Sucrose

Ans. A.

145. Which of the following commonly acts as the precursor for the synthesis of Vit C in plants ?

A. Fructose B. Ribose

C. Glucose D. Ribulose

Ans. C.

146. An autoimmune disease that affects the thyroid gland is ———.

A. Tay-Sachs disease B. Addition's disease

C. Graves' disease D. Behcet's disease

Ans. C. Tay-Sachs disease : a fatal autosomal recessive genetic disorder of deterioration of nerve cells in the early childhood. The disease is caused by the abnormal accumulation of gangliosides (a membrane lipid) in the nerve cells of brain. Addition's disease : An autoimmune disorder of endocrine system where the adrenal glands do not produce steroid hormone glucocorticoids and mineralocorticoids. Behcet's disease : An autoimmune disease of blood vessels leading to mucous membrane ulceration and ocular problems.

147. The reserve food material of green algae is

A. Laminarin B. Chrysolaminarin

C. Floridian starch D. Starch

Ans. D. Laminarin : reserve food material of brown algae. Chrysolaminarin : reserve food material of diatoms. Floridian starch : reserve food material of red algae.

148. The only carbohydrate which is not having any chiral carbon atom is

A. Gluteraldehyde B. Erythrose

C. Dihydroxyacetone D. Erythrulose

Ans. C.

149. A pentose sugar reported to be present in heart cells

A. Xylose B. Arabinose

C. Lyxose D. Xylulose

Ans. C.

150. Which of the following is an alpha lactone ?

A. Vit C B. Vit D

C. Vit A D. Vit K

Ans. A.

151. A sweetner used in sugar less gums and candies

A. Ribitol B. Xylitol

C. Inositol D. Mannitol

Ans. B.

152. Carbohydrate are organic compounds made up of

A. Carbon, hydrogen

B. Carbon, hydrogen and oxygen

C. carbon, hydrogen, oxygen and nitrogen

D. carbon and oxygen

Ans. B.

153. The most common monomer of carbohydrate is

A. Nucleotides B. Glucose

C. Amino acids D. Maltose

Ans. B.

154. Monosaccharides are

A. Aldoses B. Ketoses

C. Both A & B D. None of these

Ans. C.

155. The minimum number of carbon in a monosaccharide is

A. 1 B. 2

C. 3 D. 4

Ans. C.

156. All the following are monosaccharides except

A. Glucose B. Fructose

C. Maltose D. Galactose

Ans. C.

157. Two monosaccharides are joined by

A. Peptide bond B. Phosphodiester bond

C. Glycosidic bond D. Hydrogen bond

Ans. C.

158. All the following are reducing sugars except

A. Glucose B. Maltose

C. Sucrose D. Lactose

Ans. C.

159. All the following are storage polysaccharides except

A. Starch B. Cellulose

C. Glycogen D. Dextran

Ans. B.

160. Carbohydrates occur naturally in

A. D form B. L form

C. Both the above D. None of the above

Ans. A.

161. A lipid is formed by the condensation reactions between

A. Carbon and hydrogen B. Fatty acids and alcohol

C. Fatty acids and amino acids D. Fatty acids and amines

Ans. B.

162. Which of the following statement is wrong regarding lipids

A. Lipids are insoluble in water B. Lipids are insoluble in ethanol

C. Lipids are soluble in benzene D. Lipids are insoluble in chloroform

Ans. B.

163. Lipids are important constitutents of

A. Nucleus B. Ribosome

C. Both A & B D. Biological membranes

Ans. D.

164. Which of the following is a derived lipid ?

A. Fats B. Oils

C. Steroids D. Waxes

Ans. C.

165. Fats consist of

A. Alcohol linked by ester bonds to 3 fatty acids

B. Glycerol molecules linked by ester bonds to 3 fatty acids

C. Glycerol molecules linked by ester bonds to a fatty acids

D. Glycerol molecules linked by ester bonds to 4 fatty acids

Ans. B.

166. Compounds with carbohydrates along with fatty acids are called

A. Simple lipids B. Waxes

C. Glycolipids D. Phospholipids

Ans. C.

167. Cardiolipin is a

A. Glycolipids B. Phospholipids

C. Simple lipids D. None of these

Ans. B.

168. Cerebrosides are glycoplipids that are important constituent of

A. Biological membrane B. Lung

C. Brain D. Bones

Ans. C.

169. Phytoesterol include

A. Ergosterol B. Stigmasterol

C. Both A and B D. Cholesterol

Ans. C.

170. Which of the following is not a derivative of cholesterol

A. Steroid hormones B. Vitamin E

C. Bile salts D. Vitamin D

Ans. B.

171. Sickle cell anaemia is due to

A. Change in beta chain of haemoglobin

B. Change in alpha chain of haemoglobin

C. Change in gammachain of haemoglobin

D. None of these

Ans. A.

172. Huntington's chorea is characterized by

A. Incongruent muscle movement

B. Inability to speak

C. Disordered muscle movement and mental deterioration

D. Weak eye sight and hearing power

Ans. C.

173. Individual with Turner's syndrome is

A. Normal female

B. Normal male

C. A male with rudimentary testes and underdeveloped penis

D. A female with rudimentary ovaries and underdeveloped breasts

Ans. C.

174. Queen Victoria was carrier of hemophilia a sex linked disease. What is true ?

A. Hempphilia would have ocurred more in her male than female descendants

B. Queen's father must have had hemophilia

C. All of her sons would have had haemophilia

D. All of her daughters would have had haemophilia

Ans. A.

175. Duchenne's muscular dystrophy is a

A. Dominant sex linked disorder

B. Dominant autosomal disorder

C. Recessive sex linked disorder

D. Recessive autosomal disorder

Ans. C.

176. AIDS is an emerging disease?

A. True

B. False

Ans. A.

177. Which year was ebola recognized ?

A. 1892

B. 1976

C. 1977

Ans. C.

178. What was recognized in 2003 as an emerging disease ?

A. AIDS
B. Lyme
C. SARS
D. Ebola

Ans. C.

179. In 1992, there was evolution of a new strain of bacteria namely———.

Ans. Cholera

180. Which is the animal symbol of WWF (World Wildlife Fund) ?

A. Red Panda
B. Giant Panda
C. Tiger
D. Kangaroo

Ans. B.

181. The most important human activity leading to the extinction of wildlife is

A. Pollution of wildlife
B. Hunting of valuable wildlife products
C. Introduction of alien species
D. Alternation and destruction of the natural habitats

Ans. D.

182. If we uncover half of the forest, covering of the earth what crisis will be produced at most and at first ?

A. Some species will become extinct
B. Population and ecological imbalance will rise up
C. Energy crisis will occur
D. Rest half forests will maintain this imbalance

Ans. A.

183. When is the World Wildlife week ?

A. 1st week of September
B. Last week of September
C. 1st week of October
D. Last week of October

Ans. C.

184. Red data book provides data on

A. Red flowered plants
B. Red colored fishes
C. Lists of plants and animals
D. Endangered plants and animals

Ans. D.

185. Wildlife is continuously decreasing. What is the main reason of this ?

A. Predation
B. Cutting down of forest
C. Destruction of habitat
D. Hunting

Ans. C.

186. Viable material of endangered species can be preserved by

A. Gene bank B. Gene library

C. Gene pool D. Herbarium

Ans. A.

187. The first person to discover vitamin was

A. Jenner B. Funk

C. Calvin D. Mellanby

Ans. B.

188. Scurvy occurs due to deficiency of

A. Vitamin A B. Vitamin B

C. Vitamin C D. Vitamin D

Ans. C.

189. Osteomalacia in adults is caused due to deficiency of

A. Vitamin A B. Vitamin B

C. Vitamin C D. Vitamin D

Ans. C.

190. Xerophthalmia in man is caused by the deficiency of

A. Vitamin K B. Vitamin A

C. Vitamin D D. Vitamin C

Ans. B.

191. Cobalt containing vitamin is

A. Vitamin B1 B. Vitamin B2

C. Vitamin B6 D. Vitamin B12

Ans. D.

192. Which of the following pairs is not correctly matched ?

A. Vitamin B4- Pellagra B. Vitamin B12-Pernicious anaemia

C. Vitamin C – Scurvy D. Vitamin B6- Beriberi

Ans. D.

193. Vitamins often act as

A. Apoenzyme B. Holoenzymes

C. Cofactors D. Coenzymes

Ans. D.

194. Castle intrinsic factor is connected with internal absorption of

A. Pyridoxine B. Riboflavin

C. Thiamine D. Cobalamine

Ans. D.

195. A steroid vitamin is

A. A B. D.

C. E D. K

Ans. D.

196. Vitamin E prevents

A. Formation of Vitamin D in skin B. Secretion of superfluous enzymes

C. Keratinisation of epidermal cells D. Absorption of hrmful enzymes

Ans. C.

197. Pepsin is secreted by

A. Zymogen cells of stomach B. Zymogen cells of duodenum

C. Paneth cells D. None of the above

Ans. A.

198. The deficiency marasmus in children is caused by due to the deficiency of

A. Fats B. Carbohydrates

C. Proteins D. Vitamins

Ans. C.

199. Starch is converted to maltase by

A. Invertase B. Amylase

C. Sucrase D. Maltase

Ans. B.

200. The enzyme trypsin is found in

A. Pancreatic juice B. Saliva

C. Bile juice D. Intestinal juice

Ans. A.

201. Crypts of Lieberkuhn is an example of

A. Simple tubular gland B. Coiled tubular gland

C. Simple alveolar gland D. Compound alveolar gland

Ans. A.

202. During fasting the sequence by which the organic compounds are used up by the body

A. Fats, next carbohydrate and then protein

B. Carbohydrate, protein, lipid

C. Protein, lipid, carbohydrate

D. Carbohydrate, fat, protein

Ans. D.

203. The principal action of enteropeptidase is only to activate —— of the pancreatic juice

A. Amino peptidase
B. Trypsinogen

C. Trypsin
D. Chymotrypsin

Ans. B.

204. Due to protein deficiency if symptoms of thin limbs, retarded growth of body and brain, edema, diarrhoea develop, the condition is called

A. Pellegra
B. Kwashiorkor

C. Marasmus
D. Megaloblastic anaemia

Ans. B.

205. Brunner's glands are found in

A. Stomach
B. Ileum

C. Duodenum
D. Oesophagus

Ans. C.

206. Dental formula of man is

A. 1223, 1223
B. 2132, 2132

C. 2123, 2123
D. 3212, 3212

Ans. C.

207. Kuffer cells are found in

A. Kidney
B. Liver

C. Blood
D. Heart

Ans. B.

208. Stomach of camel does not have

A. Rumen
B. Reticulum

C. Omasum
D. Abomasum

Ans. C.

209. The digestion of carbohydrate is completed in

A. Mouth B. Duodenum

C. Ileum D. Stomach

Ans. B.

210. The unique properties of each amino acid are determined by its particular

A. Amino group

B. R group

C. Kinds of peptide bonds

D. Presence of hydrogen

E. Number of bonds to other amino acids

Ans. B.

211. Which of the following amino acids is most compatible with alpha helical structure?

A. Proline B. Alanine

C. Lysine D. Cysteine

E. Glycine

Ans. B.

212. The greatest buffering capacity at physiological pH would be provided by a protein rich in which of the following amino acids.

A. Lysine B. Valine

C. Leucine D. Histidine

E. Histamine

Ans. D.

213. The highest concentration of cystine can be found in

A. Melanin B. Chondroitin sulphate

C. Myosin D. Keratin

E. Collagen

Ans. D.

214. A peptide bond

A. Has a partial double bond character

B. Is ionized at physiological ph

C. Is cleaved by agents that denature proteins, such as organic solvents and high concentration of urea

D. It is ound in fatty acids

E. Is stable to heating in strong acids

Ans. A.

215. Which of the following statements is correct ?

A. The alpha helix can be composed of more than one popypeptide chain

B. Beta sheets exists only in the antiparrallel form

C. Beta bends often contain proline

D. Motifs are a type of secondary structure

E. The alpha helix is stalized primarily by ionic interactions between the side chains of amino acids

Ans. C.

216. Amino acids are mostly synthesized from

A. Mineral salts

B. Fatty acids

C. Volatile acids

D. Monosaccharides

E. Alpha ketoglutaric acid

Ans. E.

217. What are the most diverse molecules in the cell ?

A. Lipids

B. Carbohydrates

C. Proteins

D. Minerals

E. Vitamins

Ans. C.

218. The structure of a protein can be denatured by

A. Heat

B. The presence of oxygen gas

C. The presence of carbon dioxide gas

D. The polar bonds of water molecules

E. All of the above

Ans. A.

219. Which one of the following statements about protein structure is correct?

A. Proteins consisting of one polypeptide can have quaternary structure

B. The formation of a disulphide bond in a protein requires that the two participating cysteine residues be adjacent to each other in the primary sequence of the protein

C. The stability of quaternary structure in proteins is mainly due to covalent bonds among the subunits

D. The information required for the correct folding of a protein is contained in the specific sequences of amino acids along the polypeptide chain

E. The denaturation of proteins always leads to irreversible loss of secondary and tertiary structure

Ans. D.

220. Lysosomes are

A. Store house of genetic material

B. Interconnected channels in the cytoplasm

C. Bags of hydrolytic enzymes

D. Power house of the cell

Ans. C.

221. All of the following activities are taking place inside the mitochondria, except:

A. Electron transport chain (ETC) B. Beta oxidation of fatty acid

C. De novo fatty acid synthesis D. Citric acid cycle

Ans. C.

222. All of the following lipids are present in the plasma membrane, except:

A. Chloesterol B. Triacylglycerol

C. Lecithin D. Sphingomyelin

Ans. B.

223. Which of the following are features of endocytosis ?

A. LDL uptake is by endocytosis

B. Heparin helps in this mechanism

C. Plasma membrane is invaginated to form vesicles

D. Cytoplasmic side of vesicle is coated by clathrin filaments

Ans. B.

224. Galactosyl transferase is a marker enzyme of

A. Plasma membrane B. Mitochondria

C. Golgi complex D. Lysosome

Ans. C.

225. Which of the following cellular organelle can cause autodigestion?

A. Lysosomes B. Microsomes

C. Peroxisomes D. Golgi bodies

Ans. A.

226. Peroxisomes are

A. The site of biological oxidation

B. Involved in the production of free radicals

C. Concerned with drug detoxification

D. The site of post translational modifications

Ans. B.

227. Which of the following are not synthesised in the endoplasmic reticulum ?
A. RNA B. Lipoproteins
C. Ganglioside D. Glycoproteins

Ans. C.

228. Fluidity of plasma membrane depends on
A. Membrane pumps B. Concentration of proteins
C. Glycosylation of proteins D. Nature of fatty acids

Ans. D.

229. Golgi bodies are
A. Concerned with disposal of waste products
B. Engaged in transport of molecules into mitochondria
C. Involved in phagocytosis
D. Temporary storage sites for secretory products

Ans. D.

230. A lipid is formed by the condensation reactions between
A. Carbon and hydrogen B. Fatty acids and alcohol
C. Fatty acids and amino acids D. Fatty acids and amines

Ans. B.

231. Which of the following statement is wrong about lipid ?
A. Lipids are insoluble in water B. Lipids are insoluble in ethanol
C. Lipids are soluble in benzene D. Lipids are insoluble in chloroform

Ans. B.

232. Lipids are important constituents of
A. Nucleus B. Ribosome
C. Both a and b D. Biological membranes

Ans. D.

233. Which of the following is a derived lipid ?
A. Fats B. Oils
C. Steroids D. Waxes

Ans. C.

234. Fats consists of
A. Alcohol linked by ester bonds to 3 fatty acids
B. Glycerol molecule linked by ester bonds to 3 fatty acids
C. Glycerol molecule linked by ester bonds to a fatty acids
D. Glycerol molecule linked by ester bonds to 4 fatty acids

Ans. B.

235. Compounds with carbohydrates along with fatty acids are called

A. Simple lipids
B. Waxes
C. Glycolipids
D. Phospholipids

Ans. C.

236. Cardiolipin is a

A. Glycolipids
B. Phospholipids
C. Simple lipids
D. None of these

Ans. B.

237. Cerebrosides are glycolipids that are important constituent of

A. Biological membrane
B. Lung
C. Brain
D. Bones

Ans. C.

238. Phytosterol include

A. Ergosterol
B. Stigmasterol
C. Both A & B
D. Cholesterol

Ans. C.

239. Which of the following is not a derivative of cholesterol ?

A. Steroid hormones
B. Vitamin E
C. Bile salts
D. Vitamin D.

Ans. B.

240. Which of the following cell organelle can be viewed by a light microscope ?

A. Ribosome
B. Endoplasmic Reticulum
C. Golgi
D. Mitochondria

Ans. D.

241. Which of the following statement about mitochondria is not true ?

A. Size and shape of mitochondria varies in a cell
B. Mitochondria in the cell can fuse with one another
C. Large mitochondria in the cell can split into two
D. In all cells, one mitochondria will be exceptionally larger than others

Ans. D.

242. Mitochondria in the human sperm cell are occupied at ———.

A. Sperm head
B. Mid piece
C. Sperm tail
D. No mitochondria in the sperms

Ans. B.

243. Which of the following statement is true regarding the membrane system of mitochondria ?

A. Chemical composition of both inner and outer membrane of mitochondria are same

B. Outer membrane contain more proteins/lipid ratio (by weight) than inner membrane

C. Inner membrane contain more proteins /lipid ratio (by weight) than outer membrane

D. Phospholipids are completely absent on the outer membrane of mitochondria

Ans. C.

244. Which of the following membrane lipid constituent can be considered as the lipid marker of inner mitochondrial membrane ?

A. Lecithin B. Cardiolipin

C. Ceramide D. Sphingo-ceramide

Ans. B.

245. The only other place where cardiolipin can be found naturally other than mitochondrial inner membrane is———.

A. Inner membrane of mitochondria

B. Apoptosome

C. Bacterial plasma membrane

D. Membrane of glyoxysome

Ans. C.

246. The cellular organelle(s) involved in the regulation of Ca+2 level in the cell

A. Mitochondria

B. Endoplasmic reticulum

C. Endoplasmic reticulum and Mitochondria

D. Mitochondria and vesicles

Ans. C.

247. BUN is:

A. A blood test for kidney function B. A urine test for kidney function

C. A blood test for liver function D. A urine test of kidney and liver function

E. Something to eat at dinner

Ans. A.

248. The term antibiotic was coined by

A. Selman Waksman
B. Louis Pasteur
C. Edward Jenner
D. Alexander Fleming

Ans. A.

249. Carcinoma refers to

A. Malignant tumours of the colon
B. Malignant tumours of the skin or mucous membrane
C. Benign tumours of the connective tissue
D. Benign tumours of the connective tissue

Ans. B.

250. The organism which causes pneumonia in human beings is

A. Amphitrichous
B. Monotrichous
C. Atrichous
D. Peritrichous

Ans. C.

251. The incubation period of Hepatitis 'B' virus is:

A. 42-56 days
B. 30-180 days
C. 15-20 days
D. One week

Ans. B.

252. Which of the following birth control measure can be considered as the safest?

A. Termination of unwanted pregnancy
B. The use of physical barriers
C. The rhythm method
D. Sterilization techniques

Ans. D.

253. A localized inflammatory response appears at the site of infection causes redness, swelling, pain and heat due to certain chemical, they are

A. Histamine and prostaglandins
B. Prostaglandins and cerumen
C. Histamine and cerumen
D. Cerumen and mucus

Ans. A.

254. Antivenom is used for the treatment of snake bite. The treatment of snake bite by antivenom is an example of

A. Naturally acquired passive immunity
B. Artificially acquired active immunity
C. Artificially acquired passive immunity
D. Specific natural immunity

Ans. C.

255. Zygote with three copies chromosome 21 is known to cause

A. Hays fever B. Scurvy

C. Parkinson Disease D. Downs syndrome

Ans. D.

256. In amylose chain, glucose molecules are linked through

A. 1→3 bond B. 1→4 bond

C. 2→2 bond D. 2→4 bond

Ans. B.

257. Word "Saccharide" refers to

A. Many B. Sweet

C. Water D. None of above

Ans. B.

258. Sugar transports in plants is

A. Glucose B. Sucrose

C. Maltose D. Fructose

Ans. B.

259. Joining of two monosaccharides take place through

A. Glyosidic bond B. Condensation

C. Oxidation D. Cellular respiration

Ans. B.

260. Pentose includes

A. Fructose B. Glucose

C. Deoxyribose D. Galactose

Ans. C.

261. Adenosine Triphosphate (ATP) is formed by the

A. ADP B. Phosphate

C. Monosaccharides D. All of above

Ans. D.

262. Amylose is formed by condensation between

A. α-glucose molecules

B. β-fructose molecules

C. Between α-glucose and β-fructose molecules

D. None of above

Ans. A.

263. Industrially produced polymers are included

A. Polythene B. Polyester

C. Nylon D. All of above

Ans. D.

264. In shops, Sugar is commonly in form of

A. Glucose B. Sucrose

C. Maltose D. Fructose

Ans. B.

265. Most common element in living organisms is

A. Hydrogen B. Carbon

C. Oxygen D. Nitrogen

Ans. A.

266. Molecular structure of amylopectin is

A. Longer than amylose B. Shorter than amylose

C. Do not branch D. Are formed through 1,2 linkages

Ans. B.

267. Which Carbon atom number is not part of ring in $C_6H_{12}O_6$

A. 1 B. 3

C. 5 D. 6

Ans. C.

268. Lactose is formed by combining glucose with

A. Glucose B. Fructose

C. Galactose D. None of above

Ans. C.

269. Least common element in living organisms is

A. Hydrogen B. Carbon

C. Oxygen D. Nitrogen

Ans. D.

270. Molecules which do not act as building block of life is/are

A. Ethane B. Propane

C. Butane D. All of above

Ans. D.

271. Subunits which are similar or identical to one another are called as

A. Polymers B. Monomers

C. Peptides D. All of above

Ans. B.

272. Galactose is an example of

A. Triose B. Pentose

C. Hexose D. None of above

Ans. C.

273. Addition of water occurs in

A. Condensation B. Hydrolysis

C. Transpiration D. Osmoregulation

Ans. B.

274. Which statement is incorrect? chemical reaction of reduction is

A. Carried out by reducing sugars

B. Carried out by sucrose-like sugars

C. Reducing sugars are oxidized in process

D. Can be carried out through Benedict's solution

Ans. B.

275. Long chains or ring structures are formed by atoms of

A. Hydrogen B. Carbon

C. Oxygen D. Nitrogen

Ans. B.

276. All is true for glucose but

A. It is a non reactive molecule

B. It interferes with cell chemistry

C. It can make cell contents too concentrated

D. It is main source of energy for cells

Ans. A.

277. Plants may not store

A. Glucose itself B. Starch

C. Cellulose D. Protoplasm

Ans. B.

278. Monomer of nucleic acid is

A. Amino acid B. Peptides

C. Nucleotide D. Lipid

Ans. C.

279. Sum of all biochemical reactions in body are referred to as

A. Biochemistry B. Metabolism

C. Molecular biology D. Condensation

Ans. B.

280. Carbon-based monomers is/are

A. Nylon B. PVC

C. Both A and B D. None of above

Ans. C.

281. Benedict's solution is not

A. An alkaline solution B. An acidic solution

C. Made up of Copper Sulphate D. Used for starch test

Ans. A.

282. Hydroxyl ions in $C_6H_{12}O_6$ are

A. 1 B. 3

C. 5 D. 7

Ans. C.

283. A Pentose includes

A. Glucose B. Galactose

C. Fructose D. Ribose

Ans. D.

284. An Isomer refers to

A. Two forms of same chemicals B. Same molecule switching two forms

C. Both A and B D. None of above

Ans. C.

285. RNA is made of Polymerization through

A. Trioses B. Pentoses

C. Hexoses D. Starch

Ans. B.

286. Autosomal recessive traits are

A. Albinism, phenylketonuria and infantile amaurotic idiocy

B. Albinism, phenylketonuria and haemophilia

C. Phenylketonuria, red green colour blindness and muscular dystrophy

D. Huntington's chorea, polydactyly and albinism

Ans. A.

287. Duchenne's muscular dystrophy is a

A. dominant sex linked disorder

B. Dominant autosomal disorder

C. Recessive sex linked disorder

D. Recessive autosomal disorder

Ans. C.

288. In Tay Sach's disease

A. child is born normal

B. There is no cure

C. Child develops severe CNS damage and dies in 3-4 years

D. All of these

Ans. D.

289. Congenital diseases are

A. Disease present in birth

B. Deficiency diseases

C. Spread from one individual to another

D. Occur during life

Ans. A.

290. A late acting dominant disorder is

A. Polydactyly

B. Phenylketonuria

C. Tay Sach's disease

D. Huntington's chorea

Ans. D.

291. Turner's syndrome does not occur in males (44+y) because

A. An ovum is seldom devoid of X chromosome

B. Foetus with 44+ Y complement dies

C. A male sperm doe not penetr4ate X deficient ovum

D. Unexplained

Ans. B.

292. Genetic code consists of

A. 2 letters

B. 3 letters

C. 4 letters

D. 5 letters

Ans. B.

293. The initiator AUG in prokaryotes codes for

A. Valine
B. Methionine
C. Phenylalanine
D. Formyl methionine

Ans. D.

294. Genetic code is not

A. Overlapping
B. Degenerate
C. Universal
D. With commas

Ans. D.

295. UAA is known as

A. Opal
B. Amber
C. Ochre
D. None of these

Ans. C.

296. Amber is

A. AAA
B. GGG
C. UAG
D. UGA

Ans. C.

297. Which one of the following is known as Opal

A. AUG
B. GUG
C. UAG
D. UGA

Ans. D.

298. If methionine comes as an intermediate amino acid in protein synthesis, the codon which codes it is

A. AUG
B. GUG
C. UUU
D. AGG

Ans. A.

299. Glycine is coded by

A. GGG
B. CCC
C. AAA
D. UAA

Ans. A.

300. Which one of the following is not a mRNA codon ?

A. UUG
B. UCU
C. TAG
D. UUU

Ans. C.

301. Wobble hypothesis was proposed by

A. Watson B. Crick

C. Nirenberg D. Holley

Ans. B.

302. Oncogenes are specific sequences in DNA

A. That code for reverse transcriptase B. When expressed produce cancer

C. Which are tumour markers D. Trigger off differentiation process

Ans. D.

303. All are oncogene products except

A. Growth factors B. Tyrosine kinase

C. Tumour necrosis factor D. Interleukin 2

Ans. D.

304. Oncogenes may be activated by all except

A. Promoter insertion B. Viral infection

C. Reverse transcriptase D. Mutation in proto-oncogene

Ans. C.

305. Which is an anticancer drug ?

A. Allopurinol B. Acyclovir

C. 6 Mercaptopurine D. Zidovudine

Ans. C.

306. All the following are tumour markers except

A. Alpha 1 antitrypsin

B. Alpha fetoprotein

C. Tartarate labile acid phosphatise

D. Regan isozyme of alkaline phosphatase

Ans. A.

307. Which malignancy results from the deletion of oncosuppressor gene ?

A. Multiple myeloma B. Retinoblastoma

C. Lymphosarcoma D. Bronchogenic carcinoma

Ans. B.

308. All the following viruses are reported to be carcinogenic except

A. Varicella B. Human papilloma virus

C. Hepatitis B virus D. Epstein Barr virus

Ans. A.

309. Which is true with regard to p53 ?

A. It is an oncosuppressor gene product

B. It is an inducer of heme synthesis

C. It is an oncogene

D. None of these

Ans. A.

311. All are correct with src oncogene except

A. Oncogene product is localized in membrane

B. Src product is a protein kinase that phosphorylates tyrosine

C. Srv DNA is seen in tumour tissue not in normal cells

D. Src gene is part of Rous Sarcoma RNA virus

Ans. C.

312. Ozone in stratosphere extends

A. 10-20 km B. 20-25 km

C. 25-35 km D. 35-45 km

Ans. B.

313. According to Kyoto Protocol the major nations abide to reduce concentration of green house gases by

A. 2008 B. 2010

C. 2012 D. 2018

Ans. C.

314. Which of the following group of gases cause photochemical smog ?

A. O3, PAN and CO B. O2, PAN and NO2

C. O3, PAN and NO2 D. HC, PAN and NO

Ans. C.

315. Bioindicators are used for

A. O2 demand B. Air pollution

C. Mineral present D. All of these

Ans. D.

316. Gaseous pollutants can be controlled by

A. Arrestors B. Electrostatic precipitators

C. Incineration D. Adsorption

Ans. D.

3117. It is estimated that out of the total global warming the relative contribution of CO_2, CH_4, CFCs and N_2O are found respectively

A. 60%, 20%, 14% and 6%
B. 6%, 20%, 14% and 6%
C. 14%, 20%, 6% and 6%
D. 20%, 20%, 14% and 6%

Ans. A.

318. Which of the following is not an air pollutant ?

A. Pollen from plants
B. Hydrocarbons
C. Sulphur dioxide
D. Phosphates

Ans. D.

319. Which of the following is not a renewable exhaustible natural resource ?

A. Water
B. Wildlife
C. Minerals
D. Animals

Ans. C.

320. Which one of the following is a most efficient device to eliminate particulate matters from industrial emissions ?

A. Pyrolysis
B. Cyclonic separators
C. Electrostatic precipitator
D. Trajectory separators

Ans. C.

321. Which of the following is true ?

i. Benzene hexachloride a nonbiodegradable pollutant
ii. CO_2 is a primary air pollutant
iii. SO_2 causes brown air effect during traffic congestion in cities
iv. anthropogenic air pollutants are natural in origin

A. i &ii
B. ii &iii
C. i & iv
D. i & iii

Ans. A.

322. Genital herpes are caused by the herpes simplex viruses

A. HTLV-1
B. HIV, HSV-1, HSV-2
C. HSV-1 & HSV-II
D. HPV, HSV-1 & HSV-2

Ans. C.

323. Women are at greater risk for HPV genital infections because

A. Of the frequency of their menstrual cycle
B. Of their hormonal make up
C. They have a larger mucosal surface area exposed in the genital area
D. They are often the passive partner in the sexual act

Ans. C.

324. Lymphadenopathy refers to

A. Shrunken lymph nodes
B. Swollen or enlarged lymph nodes
C. Cancer of the lymph nodes
D. Infected lymph nodes

Ans. B.

328. Syphilis is a complex systemic sexually transmitted infection caused by

A. The spirochete
B. A virus
C. A helminth
D. A fungus

Ans. A.

325. Chlamydia is a leading cause of preventable blindness in the new born

A. True
B. False

Ans. A.

326. For genital warts cryotherapy is contraindicated in pregnancy

A. True
B. False

Ans. B.

327. Bacterial vaginosis is the most common cause of vaginal infection in women of reproductive age

A. True
B. False

Ans. A.

328. Dyspareunia refers to difficulty in achieving and sustaining an erection

A. True
B. False

Ans. B.

329. As Chlamydia is often asymptomatic, treatment is often commenced on a presumptive basis

A. True
B. False

Ans. A.

330. Gonorrhoea is a rare communicable disease

A. True
B. False

Ans. B.

331. If not treated appropriately, syphilis can lead to blindness, paralysis, psychiatric illness, cardiovascular damage and death

A. True
B. False

Ans. A.

332. Syphilis is generally characterised by two clinical stages

A. True
B. False

Ans. B.

333. Older women between the ages of 60 and 70 years are most at risk of pelvic inflammatory disease

A. True B. False

Ans. A.

334. Viruses replicate in

A. Soil B. Dead tissue

C. Living tissue D. Culture medium

Ans. C.

335. Prophase refers to

A. Viral genome outside the host cell

B. Viral genome that integrates with the bacterial genome

C. Viral genome in the culture medium

D. Newly synthesized viral genome within the host cell

Ans. B.

336. Longest known virus is

A. øX174 B. T 1 phage

C. TMV D. Citrus tristeza

Ans. D.

337. Who crystallised and isolated viruses for the first time

A. W. M. Stanley B. F. C. Bawden

C. K.M. smith D. D. Ivanowski

Ans. A.

338. Which of the following plant virus has DNA in it ?

A. Tobacco mosaic virus B. Potato mosaic virus

C. Tomato mosaic virus D. Cauliflower mosaic virus

Ans. D.

339. The bacteriophage contains an enzyme

A. Dehydrogenase B. Urease

C. Protease D. Lysozyme

Ans. D.

340. Virion is

A. Nucleic acid of virus

B. Protein of virus

C. Antiviral agent

D. Completely assembled virus outside the host

Ans. D.

341. Which of the following pair of disease is caused by virus ?

A. Measles, rabies
B. Typhoid, Tetanus
C. Cholera, Tuberculosis
D. AIDS, Syphilis

Ans. A.

342. Viral diseases have no cure because

A. Viruses have no cell wall
B. Presence of capsid
C. Virus possess no cytoplasm
D. Virus can multiply repeatedly within the host cell

Ans. D.

343. AIDS virus has effect upon

A. Leucocytes
B. Lymphocytes
C. Erythrocytes
D. Thrombocytes

Ans. B.

344. Which protein has been produced generating a transgenic sheep that is used for replacement therapy for individuals at risk from emphysema ?

A. Plasminogenic activator
B. Alpha antitrypsin
C. Casein
D. Amyloid precursor proteins

Ans. B.

345. Which of the following is the word used to describe what happens when the nucleus of a sperm joins with the nucleus of an egg cell ?

A. Sex
B. Fertilization
C. Intercourse
D. Reproduction

Ans. B.

346. DNA in fish is injected into

A. Pronuclei
B. Cytoplasm
C. Both A & B
D. None of these

Ans. B.

347. Transgenic goats have been used to produce which of the following protein that is used for dissolving blood clots?

A. Amyloid precursor protein
B. α_1-anti trypsin (AAT)
C. Casein
D. A variant of human tissue-type plasminogen activator

Ans. D.

348. Transfection refers to which of the following?

A. Synthesis of mRNA from DNA template

B. Synthesis of protein based on mRNA sequence

C. Introduction of foreign gene in to a cell

D. The process by which a cell become malignant

Ans. C.

349. Chromosomes may be isolated from metaphase cells by

A. Hypertonic lysis

B. Hypertonic lysis

C. Both A & B

D. Isotonic lysis

Ans. B.

350. Superovulation is primarily the result of

A. Decreased atresia in medium and large follicles (>1.7 mm)

B. Increased atresia in medium and large follicles (>1.7 mm)

C. Increased atresia in the small follicles (<1.7 mm)

D. Decreased atresia in small follicles (<1.7 mm)

Ans. A.

351. Genetic change can occur only in

A. one way

B. Two ways

C. Three ways

D. Four ways

Ans. D.

352. Which of these carries the thousands of genes needed to allow animal and plant cells to pass on inherited characteristics?

A. Chromosomes

B. Chromatogram

C. Chromatography

D. Chromium

Ans. A.

353. Animal pharming can be defined as

A. Growing animals for farming

B. Programming animals to produce novel products

C. Generating transgenic animals for farming

D. None of the above

Ans. B.

354. When a fertilized egg cell develops into an embryo, the entropy of the living system

A. Decreases B. Increases

C. Remains constant D. None of these

Ans. A.

355. For the transfer of whole individual chromosomes, they are isolated from the cells at

A. Prophase B. Metaphase

C. Telophase D. Anaphase

Ans. B.

356. Fusion of karyoplast with the enucleated cell is achieved in presence of

A. Cytochalasin B B. Polyethylene glycol

C. Both A & B D. Alcohol

Ans. B.

357. Which of the following statements best describes a clone?

A. An artificial life form

B. An offspring where all of the genetic material in every cell is identical to that of both parents

C. An offspring where all of the genetic material in every cell is identical to that of one of its parents

D. A type of sheep

Ans. C.

358. In transgenic fish, the genes are introduced by

A. Microinjection in fish B. Viruses

C. Transfer of whole nuclei D. All of these

Ans. A.

359. Production of transgenic animals require transfections of

A. Eggs or embryos B. Stem cells

C. Red blood cells D. All of these

Ans. A.

360. Which of the following statement is correct?

A. Variation is caused by genes

B. Variation is caused by the environment

C. Variation can be caused by both genes and the environment

D. None of these

Ans. A.

361. Which of the following gene have been introduced into the transgenic fish?

A. Human or rat gene for growth hormone

B. Chicken gene for delta crystalline protein

C. E.coli gene for β-galactosidase

D. All of the above

Ans. D.

362. Cloning is a method by which numbers of genetically identical organisms are derived from a single organism by

A. Vegetative propagation

B. Vegetative initiation

C. Vegetative termination

D. None of these

Ans. A.

363. Which of the following is/are the method of transfection for making transgenic animals?

A. Transfer of whole nuclei

B. Transfer of whole individual chromosomes or fragment

C. Transfer of DNA

D. All of the above

Ans. D.

364. DNA microinjection into the egg has been used to produce which of the following transgenic animals?

A. Mice

B. Chicken

C. Pigs

D. All of these

Ans. D.

365. Transgenic goats produce a variant of human tissue type plasminogen activator protein in

A. Blood

B. Urine

C. Milk

D. Muscles

Ans. C.

366. For the rapid genetic progress, embryo transfer (ET)

A. Will be as potent a tool as AI (artificial insemination)

B. Will not be as potent a tool as AI (artificial insemination)

C. ET can't be used at all

D. Will be a superior tool than AI

Ans. B.

367. Enucleation of the cells can be achieved by treating the cells with

A. Polyethylene glycol
B. Cytochalasin B
C. Both A & B
D. Alcohol

Ans. B.

368. When the cells are enucleated and centrifuged, nuclei

A. Detach from cell and settle at the bottom
B. Detach from cell and remain in the supernatant
C. Nuclei remain attached to the cell
D. None of the above

Ans. A.

369. Superovulation is an

A. Increased ovulatory response by external hormonal therapy
B. Decreased ovulatory response by external hormonal therapy
C. Decreased ovulatory response by internal hormonal therapy
D. Increased ovulatory response by internal hormonal therapy

Ans. A.

370. Which of the following best describes artificial insemination?

A. Transplanting an embryo into the uterus
B. Fertilization of an egg in a test tube
C. Selectively breeding healthy animals
D. Taking the sperm and placing it directly

Ans. D.

371. Which part of a cell carries the information that is passed from one generation to the next?

A. Cell
B. Nucleus
C. Cytoplasm
D. Chloroplast

Ans. B.

372. DNA is microinfected into the fertilized egg

A. After the fusion of male and female nuclei
B. Before the fusion of male and female nuclei
C. At the time of fusion of male and female nuclei
D. Any time, it can be infected

Ans. B.

373. In which year, Dolly the first mammalian clone was born?

A. 1995 B. 1997

C. 1996 D. 1998

Ans. C.

374. Which of the following statements is false?

A. Continuous variation produces a spread of variation within a population

B. Discontinuous variation is the result of genetics alone

C. Blood group is an example of discontinuous variation

D. Discontinuous variation is influenced by the environment

Ans. D.

375. Embryo transfer (ET) refers to the technique by which fertilized ova are collected from the reproductive tract of a genetically

A. Superior female and transferred to the inferior

B. Inferior female and transferred to the superior

C. Balanced female

D. None of these

Ans. A.

376. The number of follicles at any particular stage is governed by

A. The rate of entry of dormant follicles

B. The rate of growth of follicles

C. The rate of loss of follicles

D. All the above

Ans. D.

377. The nucleous of mature unfertilized ovum may be removed by

A. Irradiation B. Surgery

C. Both A & B D. Neutralization and homogenization

Ans. C.

378. Karyotplast is

A. Cell devoid of cell wall

B. Nuclei

C. Nuclei with only some residual plasma membrane

D. Cell with nucleus

Ans. C.

379. The success of embryo transplantation depends upon the ability to obtain an increased number of embryos from animals of superior genetic merit, which can be achieved by the use of

A. Exogenous gonadatrophic hormones

B. Endogenous gonadatrophic hormones

C. Both A & B

D. FSH

Ans. A.

380. Multiple ovulation and embryo transfer (MOET)

A. Can increase the rate of progress in dairy cattle

B. Allows progeny testing of males

C. Allows progeny testing of females

D. All the above

Ans. D.

381. The technique, mainly used for the diagnosing birth defects in the foetus by means of needle, is called

A. Amniocentesis b. Ectogensis

C. Transplantation D. All the above

Ans. A.

382. Which of these established cell lines originate from a mouse embryo ?

A. 3T3 B. BHK-21

C. HeLa D. BTK

Ans. A.

383. Which of the following has been confirmed on sugarcane genotypes ?

A. Bacilliform virus B. Cytomegalovirus

C. Varicella-zoster virus D. Erythrovirus

Ans. A.

384. Human serum albumin has been synthesized by

A. Transgenic potato and tobacco plants

B. Transgenic maize plants

C. Transgenic wheat plants

D. Any of the above

Ans. A.

385. Avermectins (AVM) are macrocyclic lactones which have potent antihelmintic and insecticidal action. They are generally derived from the mycelia of

A. Streptomyces avermitilis
B. B. thrunigiensis
C. P. flourescens
D. L. Peruvianum

Ans. A.

386. The tumor phenotype, which can be maintained indefinitely in tissue culture, results from the expression of genes on the

A. T-DNA
B. c-DNA
C. r-DNA
D. m-RNA

Ans. A.

387. Somaclonal variation method refers to

A. Heritable changes
B. Genetic isolation
C. Small number of species having limited commercial potential
D. Large number of plant cells

Ans. A.

388. α and β cyclodextrins are produced by

A. Transgenic tomato
B. Transgenic maize
C. Transgenic potato
D. Transgenic wheat

Ans. C.

389. α and β cyclodextrins are used for

A. Pharmaceutical delivery system
B. Flavour and odour enhancement in foods
C. Removal of undesired compounds like caffeine from foods
D. All of the above

Ans. D.

390. Microinjection technique of introducing NA is a

A. Physical method
B. Biological method
C. Combination of physical and biological method
D. Chemical method

Ans. A.

391. MS medium, is found essential for initial morphogenesis of the immature embryos and to enhance callus development, when supplemented with

A. GA_3 B. GA_3 and coconut milk

C. Adenine D. Adenine and kinetin

Ans. B.

392. Antibiotics are

A. Carbohydrate in nature B. Protein in nature

C. Fats D. Vitamins in nature

Ans. B.

393. Catalytic hydrogenation of vegetable oils convert them in to

A. Vegetable ghee B. Vitamins

C. Proteins D. Carbohydrates

Ans. A.

394. Layer of fat under mammalian skin acts as an

A. Electric insulator B. Thermal insulator

C. Protection from germs D. Protection from viruses

Ans. B.

395. Amino acids which are not synthesized by human body are called

A. Essential amino acids B. Non essential amino acids

C. Simple amino acids D. Complex amino acids

Ans. B.

396. Linkage which joins two amino acid units is called

A. Peptide bond B. Covalent bond

C. Ionic bond D. Hydrogen bond

Ans. A.

397. Vitamin D activates enzymes

A. Less than 100 B. More than 100

C. 50 D. 25

Ans. B.

398. Monosaccharides can contain

A. 4 to 5 carbon atoms B. 1 to 5 carbon atoms

C. 7 to 9 carbon atoms D. 3 to 6 carbon atoms

Ans. D.

399. Strands of DNA are held together by

A. Covalent bond B. Ionic bond

C. Hydrogen bond D. Dipole dipole interaction

Ans. C.

400. Cholesterol comes from

A. Animal products B. Vegetable products

C. Fruit products D. Insect products

Ans. A.

401. Vitamin which is fat soluble is

A. Vitamin B B. Vitamin C

C. Vitamin D D. Vitamin F

Ans. C.

402. Building blocks of all proteins are

A. Hydroxyl group B. Carbonyl group

C. Amino acids D. Simple sugars

Ans. C.

403. Proteins work in body to

A. Transport and store oxygen and nutrients

B. Speed up reactions

C. Regulate important systems

D. All of above

Ans. D.

404. Gelatin is used in production of

A. Industrial items B. Ropes

C. Curry D. Bakery items

Ans. D.

405. Human body can synthesize only

A. 12 amino acids B. 10 amino acids

C. 15 amino acids D. 5 amino acids

Ans. B.

406. Lipids include

A. Sucrose B. Maltose

C. Fats and oils D. Thymine

Ans. C.

407. Enzymes are protein in nature and are used as

A. Biological catalyst
B. Chemical catalyst
C. Reaction inhibitor
D. Reaction stopper

Ans. A.

408. Source of Butyric acid is

A. Butter
B. Palm oil
C. Beef fat
D. Olive oil

Ans. A.

409. Lipid which is solid at room temperature is called

A. Oil
B. Protein
C. Sugar
D. Fat

Ans. D.

410. Maltose is obtained from

A. Sugarcane
B. Fruits
C. Cereals
D. Plants

Ans. C.

411. RNA (Ribonucleic Acid) is made up of

A. Ribose sugar
B. Phosphate unit
C. Nitrogen base
D. All of above

Ans. D.

412. General formula for monosaccharides is

A. CH_2O
B. $(CH_2O)_n$
C. CH_n
D. C_nH_n

Ans. B.

413. 1g of glucose ($C_6H_{12}O_6$) provides energy

A. 10J
B. 160KJ
C. 15.6KJ
D. 80KJ

Ans. C.

414. Vitamin which helps in antioxidation is

A. Vitamin E
B. Vitamin K
C. Vitamin A
D. Vitamin D

Ans. A.

415. Monosaccharides (simple sugars) have

A. Oxidizing nature B. Reducing nature

C. Redox nature D. Neutralizing nature

Ans. B.

416. Vitamin which helps in chemical transmission of images from eye to brain is

A. Vitamin A B. Vitamin B

C. Vitamin C D. Vitamin D

Ans. A.

417. Our bodies cannot produce

A. Minerals B. Proteins

C. Vitamins D. Carbohydrates

Ans. C.

418. Glucose ($C_6H_{12}O_6$) and fructose ($C_6H_{12}O_6$) are

A. Simple sugars B. Simple salts

C. Simple acids D. Complex sugars

Ans. A.

419. By help of fermentation, starch is converted to

A. Rectified spirit B. Dextrin

C. Cellulose D. Sucrose

Ans. A.

420. A DNA (Deoxyribonucleic Acid) can store and transmit the

A. Genetic information B. Cell information

C. Blood D. Nerves

Ans. A.

421. Upon hydrolysis oligosaccharides form

A. 1 to 8 molecules of simple sugars B. 10 to 12 molecules of simple sugars

C. 5 to 8 molecules of simple sugars D. 2 to 9 molecules of simple sugars

Ans. D.

422. Starch and cellulose are

A. Crystalline solids B. Amorphous solids

C. Liquids D. Gasses

Ans. B.

423. Important sources of proteins are

A. Meat B. Eggs

C. Cheese D. All of above

Ans. D.

424. Nuclei of cells consists of

A. Proteins B. Carbohydrates

C. Nucleic acids D. Vitamins

Ans. C.

425. Key to ability of DNA to pass and store genetic information is

A. Its hydrogen bonding B. Its double stranded structure

C. Its deoxyribose sugar D. Its nitrogen base

Ans. B.

426. Nucleotides consists of

A. Nitrogenous base B. Pentose sugar

C. Phosphate group D. All of above

Ans. D.

427. RNA (Ribonucleic Acid) exists in form of

A. Solid B. Gas

C. Double strand D. Single strand

Ans. D.

428. A component of plant or animal tissue insoluble in water is called

A. Protein B. Carbohydrate

C. Vitamin D. Lipids

Ans. D.

429. Plants convert glucose ($C_6H_{12}O_6$) in to

A. Starch B. Cellulose

C. Both A and B D. Sucrose

Ans. C.

430. Long chain carboxylic acids are named as

A. Lipids B. Fatty acids

C. Phospholipids D. Cholesterol

Ans. B.

431. Sugars which rotate plane of polarized light in clockwise direction are called

A. Lactose sugars B. Complex sugars

C. Dextrose sugars D. Simple sugars

Ans. C.

432. Term hardware is referred to

A. Software B. Data

C. Machinery D. Procedure

Ans. C.

433. Temporary memory of computer is

A. ROM B. Secondary memory

C. Both A and B D. RAM

Ans. D.

434. Glass fibers have thickness equal to

A. Test tube B. Capillary tube

C. Hair D. Half inch ribbon

Ans. C.

435. Number of operating computers on internet is

A. Nearly 10 million B. Nearly 20 million

C. More than 50 million D. 30 million

Ans. C.

436. Cassettes are based on

A. Electricity B. Magnetism

C. Electromagnetism D. Waves

Ans. B.

437. First use of pure microbiological process in an industrial procedure was made by Chaim Weizmann in

A. 1921 B. 1925

C. 1917 D. 1907

Ans. C.

438. Application of biotechnology procedures in medical processes is classified as

A. White biotechnology B. Red biotechnology

C. Blue biotechnology D. Green biotechnology

Ans. B.

439. Field of biotechnology which is applied to industrial processes is known as

A. Blue biotechnology B. Green biotechnology

C. White biotechnology D. Red biotechnology

Ans. C.

440. Example of green biotechnology is

A. Industrial antibiotics B. Industrial chemicals

C. Industrial catalysts D. BT corn and pesticides

Ans. D.

441. Application of biotechnology procedures in agricultural field is classified as

A. White biotechnology B. Red biotechnology

C. Blue biotechnology D. Green biotechnology

Ans. D.

442. Process of using natural bacteria in mining industry is known as

A. Biodegradation B. Biogenomics

C. Bioremediation D. Bioleaching

Ans. D.

443. First use of pure microbiological process in an industrial procedure was made by

A. Alexander Fleming B. Louis Pasteur

C. Charles Darwin D. Chaim Weizmann

Ans. D.

444. Mold Pencillium was discovered by Alexander Fleming in

A. 1931 B. 1928

C. 1935 D. 1939

Ans. B.

445. Example of red biotechnology is

A. Antibiotics B. Pesticides

C. Industrial catalysts D. Bt corn

Ans. A.

446. Term of biotechnology used to describe aquatic and marine applications is known as

A. Blue biotechnology B. Green biotechnology

C. White biotechnology D. Red biotechnology

Ans. A.

447. Example of white biotechnology is

A. Bt corn
B. Use of enzymes in industry
C. Use of pesticides
D. Use of antibiotics

Ans. B.

448. Economic output and investment of different types of biotechnologies is known as

A. Bioremediation
B. Biodegradation
C. Bioeconomic
D. Bioleaching

Ans. C.

449. Mold Pencillium was discovered by

A. Alexander Fleming
B. Louis Pasteur
C. Charles Darwin
D. Chaim Weizmann

Ans. A.

450. Process of using living organisms to develop products is known as

A. Genome engineering
B. Medical engineering
C. Biotechnology
D. Bioengineering

Ans. C.

451. First use of biotechnology to convert food source into other form was made by

A. Alexander Fleming
B. Louis Pasteur
C. Charles Darwin
D. Chaim Weizmann

Ans. B.

452. Interdisciplinary field of biotechnology to address biological problems using computation techniques is known as

A. Bioremediation
B. Bioleaching
C. Bioinformatics
D. Biodegradation

Ans. C.

453. Genetic testing identifies changes in

A. Genes
B. Proteins
C. Chromosomes
D. All of above

Ans. D.

454. Of 10,000 tones of annual global opium production, used in medicine is

A. 400 tones
B. 300 tones
C. 600 tones
D. 700 tones

Ans. A.

455. All is true for local anaesthesia, but,

A. That it causes local numbness

B. It causes a loss of sensation in area being injected

C. Contains Cocaine

D. Cause gastric ulcers

Ans. D.

456. To induce sleep, narcotic drugs taken may include

A. Heroin

B. Morphine

C. Opium

D. All of these

Ans. D.

457. According to surveys, most young people smoke in order to

A. Overcome jealousy

B. Cover for their failures and weaknesses

C. Give an impression of adulthood and maturity

D. Give an impression of happiness and success

Ans. B.

458. If drug of an addicted person is withheld, person experiences

A. Insomnia

B. Sleep and stupor

C. With drawl symptoms

D. Death

Ans. C.

459. Wheat, wheat bran and molasses together form the

A. Penicillin

B. Alcohol

C. Postum

D. Sebum

Ans. C.

460. Morphine is a type of

A. Cannabis

B. Amphetamines

C. Narcotic drugs

D. Depressant drugs

Ans. C.

461. Postum is a replacement of

A. Nicotine

B. Caffeine

C. Alcohol

D. Penicillin

Ans. B.

462. Chronic Obstructive lung disease occurs due to

A. Emphysema B. Depressant drugs

C. Amphetamines D. Cocaine

Ans. A.

463. Alkaloids found in opium do not include

A. Morphine B. Codeine

C. Cocaine D. Opium

Ans. C.

464. AIDS stands for

A. Acquired Iodine deficiency syndrome

B. Acquired inherited defective syndrome

C. Acquired immune deficiency syndrome

D. Acquired immune deflated sensations

Ans. C.

465. Excess mucus is produced causing smokers cough due to

A. Nicotine B. Tar

C. Irritants D. Morphine

Ans. C.

466. Nicotine ($C_{10}H_{14}N_2$)

A. Is a carcinogenic substance B. Makes blood clot easily

C. Makes blood dilute D. Helps in lumen becoming narrower

Ans. B.

467. Prolonged alcohol ($C_nH_{2n+1}OH$) consumption

A. Helps overcome fatigue B. Causes loss of appetite

C. Cirrhosis D. Gastric ulcers

Ans. C.

468. Bacterial diseases are treated with drug containing

A. Erythromycin B. Aspirin

C. Paludrine D. Morphine

Ans. A.

469. Smoking is no longer regarded as

A. Unsafe B. Prohibited

C. Socially accepted D. Socially unaccepted

Ans. C.

470. Examples of stimulant drugs are

A. Barbiturates B. Marijuana

C. Morphine D. Cocaine

Ans. D.

471. Rate of heartbeat and blood pressures increases due to

A. Tar B. Nicotine

C. Cocaine D. Morphine

Ans. B.

472. Nicotine ($C_{10}H_{14}N_2$) is a

A. Socially accepted drug B. Drug of abuse

C. Traditional medicine D. Recent medicinal discover

Ans. B.

473. Opium, morphine and heroin are examples of

A. Opiates B. Cocaine

C. Depressant drugs D. Cannabis

Ans. A.

474. Cilia can not remove air and dust particles from lungs and trachea due to

A. Nicotine B. Carbon monoxide

C. Irritants D. Tar

Ans. D.

475. Number of alkaloids in opium are at least

A. 20 B. 25

C. 30 D. 35

Ans. B.

476. Outcomes of long term alcohol ($C_nH_{2n+1}OH$) consumption includes

A. Liver cirrhosis B. Gastric ulcers

C. Intestinal injuries D. Both A and B

Ans. D.

477. Drugs useful against bacteria resistant to penicillin include

A. Cephalosporin B. Erythromycins

C. Augmentin D. Both A and B

Ans. D.

478. If taken in large amount, gastric ulcers may be caused by

A. Cocaine B. Aspirin

C. Cephalosporin D. Tetracycline

Ans. B.

479. Malarial parasites are treated with drug containing

A. Penicillin B. Paludrine

C. Aspirin D. Morphine

Ans. B.

480. Long term effect of alcohol disturbs the

A. Nervous system B. Digestive system

C. Cardio-vascular system D. All of these

Ans. B.

481. Adrenaline production is stimulated due to

A. Carbon monoxide B. Tar

C. Nicotine D. Cocaine

Ans. C.

482. Too much caffeine can damage the

A. Heart B. Kidneys

C. Pancreas D. Both A and B

Ans. D.

483. With drawl symptoms from a narcotic drug includes

A. Hallucinations B. Insomnia

C. Excess hunger D. Sweating

Ans. A.

484. Due to tar, an over multiplication of cells in lungs causes

A. Atherosclerosis B. Insomnia

C. Blood clotting D. Cancer

Ans. D.

485. Broad-spectrum antibiotics are _______.

A. Erythromycins B. Cephalosporin

C. Tetacyclines D. Penicillin

Ans. C.

486. Chronic Obstructive lung disease occurs because of

A. Chronic bronchitis B. Emphysema

C. Asthma D. Both A and B

Ans. D.

487. Active ingredient causing thinning of blood in aspirin is

A. Benzoic acid B. Picric acid

C. Hydrochloric acid D. Salicylic acid

Ans. D.

488. Postum dates back to

A. 1893 B. 2700 BC

C. 1000 years D. 1975

Ans. A.

489. Aspirin lowers risk of

A. Heart attack B. Coma

C. Diabetes D. Migraines

Ans. A.

490. Ability of red blood cells (RBCs) to carry oxygen (O_2) is reduced due to

A. Salicylic acid in lungs B. Carboxy acids

C. Carbon monoxide D. Distortion in hemoglobin structure

Ans. C.

491. LSD stands for

A. Lysergic ethylaminate B. Lysergic acid diethylamide

C. Lysergic acid dillusionaminates D. Lysergic saturated dichloromethane

Ans. B.

492. Few enlarged alveoli vs. many minute alveoli pose risk of

A. Production of mucus in air passages

B. Inefficient exchange of gases

C. Blood clotting

D. Dull and insensitive brain

Ans. B.

493. An uncontrolled abnormal division of cells is called as

A. Substance abuse B. Growth

C. Maturation D. Cancer

Ans. D.

494. Drug is
   A. Produced by endocrine glands
   B. Produced by exocrine glands
   C. Secreted through pituitary gland
   D. Externally administered chemical substances

Ans. D.

495. Example of analgesics include
   A. Caffeine B. Cocaine
   C. Novocain D. Aspirin

Ans. D.

496. Due to irritants in cigarettes, many minute alveoli coalesce to form
   A. Lumps of cells B. Cancer
   C. Blood clot D. Enlarged alveoli

Ans. D.

497. Carbon monoxide (CO) causes
   A. Numbness of brain B. Secretion of adrenaline
   C. Weakens wall of alveoli D. Risk of atherosclerosis

Ans. D.

498. Caffeine is found in
   A. Tea B. Coffee
   C. Coke D. All of these

Ans. D.

499. Illusions, hallucinations and distorted images are caused by
   A. Depressant drugs B. Opiates
   C. Cannabis D. Amphetamines

Ans. C.

500. Friends teasing that non-smoker is not sporting enough and lively turns into
   A. Teasing pressure B. Community-pressure
   C. Moral-pressure D. Peer group pressure

Ans. D.

501. In a healthy lung, air spaces or air sacs
   A. Are few B. Are in form of large air sacs
   C. Are too fine to be visible D. May become carcinogenic

Ans. C.

502. Short term effect of alcohol disturbs the

A. Nervous system B. Digestive system

C. Cardio-vascular system D. All of these

Ans. A.

503. Due to smoking, narrow arteries bringing blood to fetus cause

A. Child born prematurely

B. Reduction in amount of food reaching fetus

C. Brain development affected

D. Risk of miscarriage

Ans. B.

504. Cigarette smokers become addicted to

A. Caffeine B. Nicotine

C. Paludrine D. All of these

Ans. B.

505. Insomnia and epilepsy can be treated through

A. Caffeine B. Cocaine

C. Marijuana D. Nicotine

Ans. C.

506. Formation of essential components of bacterium cell wall is inhibited by

A. Tetracycline B. Erythromycins

C. Penicillin D. Both A and B

Ans. D.

507. Liver cells become damaged due to

A. Excess of adrenaline B. Excess of alcohol

C. Excess of toxins like benzoic acid D. Excess of salicylic acid

Ans. B.

508. Atherosclerosis causes

A. Fatty deposits on inner wall of arteries

B. Lumen becoming narrower

C. Blockage in blood vessels

D. All of these

Ans. D.

509. Stimulant drugs are not used to treat

A. depression B. fatigue
C. insomnia D. induce sleep

Ans. C.

510. Cilia lining air passage is paralyzed due to

A. Tar B. Irritants
C. Nicotine D. Both A and B

Ans. D.

511. Heroin is several times more powerful than

A. Opium B. Cannabis
C. Morphine D. Barbiturates

Ans. C.

512. Division of bacteria is inhibited through the

A. Cephalosporins B. Tetracyclines
C. Erythromycins D. All of these

Ans. A.

513. In cirrhosis, damaged liver cells are replaced by

A. Toxins like benzoic acid B. Large amount of peptones
C. Fibrous tissues D. All of these

Ans. C.

514. Barbiturates are often prescribed for treatment of

A. Epilepsy B. Depression
C. Excess hunger D. All of these

Ans. A.

515. Largest and only legal producer of opium is

A. Singapore B. India
C. Afghanistan D. USA

Ans. B.

516. AIDS is caused due to

A. Sharing injection needles
B. Transmission of immunodeficiency virus
C. Unsterilized injection needles
D. All of these

Ans. D.

517. Heart attack or stroke results due to

A. Blood made diluted
B. Blood clotting made easy
C. Lack of sleep
D. Feeling hungry all time

Ans. B.

518. At same time, smoking can not provide stimulation and

A. Reduce aging
B. Reduce tension
C. Induce sensation
D. Induce sleep

Ans. B.

519. Examples of depressant drugs include

A. Marijuana
B. Cocaine
C. Barbiturates
D. Morphine

Ans. C.

520. Local numbness and loss of sensation is caused by

A. Anesthetics
B. Analgesics
C. Anemia
D. Diarrhea

Ans. A.

521. Carbon dioxide (CO_2) and water (H_2O) are produced as output when

A. Oxidation of glucose occurs
B. When oxidation does not occur at all
C. When oxidation is accompanied with cell division
D. When oxidation is accompanied with water

Ans. A.

522. Hydrogen peroxide (H_2O_2)

A. Helps line up cell proteins
B. Is poisonous to tissues
C. Is often needed as a catalyst
D. Aids in oxidation of glucose

Ans. B.

523. More hydrogen peroxide (H_2O_2) in urine, the

A. Lighter color of strip
B. Acidic urine be
C. Darker color of strip
D. More healthier a person be

Ans. C.

524. Amylase becomes denatured at a alkaline pH of

A. 6
B. 7
C. 8
D. 9

Ans. D.

525. Nature of rennin is slightly

A. Acidic B. Alkaline

C. Water based D. Mineral based

Ans. A.

526. While cutting big molecules to smaller molecules, enzymes may be called as

A. Molecular knife B. Molecular lancet

C. Molecular fork D. Molecular scissors

Ans. D.

527. At a pH 7 to 4.5, activity of amylase

A. Stops B. Slows

C. Expedites D. Ends

Ans. B.

528. Proteases is commonly found in

A. Pineapple B. Pomegranate

C. Papaya D. Paprika

Ans. C.

529. One of most common essential component of many co-enzymes is

A. Vitamin D12 B. Vitamin K

C. Vitamin E D. Vitamin B complex

Ans. D.

530. Most reactions in living cells are

A. Reversible B. Irreversible

C. Static D. Redox

Ans. A.

531. Conversion of amino acid in useful proteins is carried out by

A. Centriole B. Cytoplasm

C. Protoplasm D. Nucleoplasm

Ans. B.

532. Enzymes catalyze biochemical processes occurring in living cells over

A. On strong heating B. At room temperature

C. In freezing cold D. Very narrow temperature range

Ans. D.

533. Digestive enzymes are used in

A. House paints
B. Washing powder
C. Dying fabrics
D. Car wash

Ans. B.

534. Digestion does not involve

A. Breaking of particles in starch
B. Simpler substances
C. Water soluble substances
D. Substances diffusible through cell membranes

Ans. A.

535. In mammals, catalase is common in

A. Liver
B. Blood
C. Pancreas
D. Both A and B

Ans. D.

536. pH value of above 7 indicates

A. Pure water
B. Pure enzyme
C. Pure alkaline
D. Pure acidic

Ans. C.

537. Substance which can alter or speed up chemical reaction without itself being chemically unchanged is

A. Saliva
B. Pathology
C. Catalyst
D. Influenza

Ans. C.

538. Denatured protein enzymes are but

A. More soluble
B. Low coagulation
C. Easily affected by acids and alkaline substances
D. Sparingly insoluble

Ans. C.

539. In order to increase rate of reaction,

A. Limiting factor shall increase
B. Limiting factor shall decrease
C. Substrate concentration shall be increased
D. Enzyme concentration shall be increased

Ans. B.

540. Lipases digests

A. Lipids
B. Carbohydrates
C. Proteins
D. Liver juices

Ans. A.

541. Enzymes are largely

A. Fat-based
B. Carbohydrates-based
C. Protein-based
D. Minerals-based

Ans. C.

542. Enzymes are

A. Produced regularly
B. Only when they are needed
C. Same for plants and animals
D. Are commonly found in blood

Ans. B.

543. To expedite heating potassium chlorate ($KClO_3$) to get oxygen (O_2) and potassium chloride (KCl), suitable catalyst may be

A. Silver
B. Chlorine
C. Manganese Oxide
D. Citric acid

Ans. C.

544. When potassium chlorate ($KClO_3$) is heated, products include

A. Potassium chloroform and water
B. Potassium chloride and water
C. Potassium chloride and enzymes
D. Potassium carbonate and oxygen

Ans. B.

545. Amylase works optimally at a pH of

A. 4
B. 4.5
C. 7
D. 9

Ans. C.

546. Beyond optimum temperature, enzyme

A. Becomes flat
B. Becomes hyperactive
C. Divides to form smaller enzymes
D. Becomes denatured

Ans. D.

547. While testing presence of sugar in urine, strip colour changes due to amount of

A. Glucose oxidase
B. Peroxidase
C. Hydrogen per oxide
D. Hydrogen bicarbide

Ans. C.

548. Sucrose is broken down into glucose ($C_6H_{12}O_6$) and fructose ($C_6H_{12}O_6$) through enzyme

A. Salivary amylase B. Salicylate

C. Sucrase D. Sucral

Ans. C.

549. Organic catalysts called enzymes are mainly made up of

A. Carbohydrates B. Fats

C. Potassium D. Proteins

Ans. D.

550. Many food substances taken in by animals are

A. Soluble in water B. Insoluble in water

C. Can be digested without enzymes D. Are digested through fats

Ans. B.

551. Salivary and pancreatic amylase help digest

A. Proteins B. Starch

C. Fats D. Minerals

Ans. B.

552. At a pH 7 to 9, activity of amylase

A. Stops B. Slows

C. Expedites D. Ends

Ans. B.

553. Binding of enzyme and substrate on active site is explained through

A. Hide and seek hypothesis B. Lock and hide hypothesis

C. Lock and run hypothesis D. Lock and key hypothesis

Ans. D.

554. In fish, large molecules are normally made up of

A. Proteins and fats B. Proteins and carbohydrates

C. Minerals and proteins D. Minerals and Fats

Ans. A.

555. Using manganese oxide as a catalyst, in heating potassium chlorate ($KClO_3$), manganese oxide (Mn_xO_y)

A. Evaporates B. Melts

C. Remains unchanged D. Becomes magnesium carbonate

Ans. C.

556. Mammals do not produce

A. Salivary amylase B. Catalase

C. Pancreatic amylase D. Cellulose

Ans. D.

557. Extreme changes in acidity or alkalinity of solutions

A. Produce more hydrogen per oxide

B. More enzymes are needed

C. Enzymes may become denatured

D. Foods gets digested earlier

Ans. C.

558. Lipids are a form of

A. Carbohydrates B. Proteins

C. Fats D. Minerals

Ans. C.

559. Nature of pepsin is slightly

A. Acidic B. Alkaline

C. Water based D. Mineral based

Ans. A.

560. Denatured enzyme

A. Looses its concave structure

B. Looses its active sites

C. Gets divided into many smaller enzymes

D. Becomes even more quicker in chemical reactions

Ans. B.

561. Enzyme pepsin has been named by

A. Substance upon which it acts like pepsin

B. Byproduct it produces like peptic acid

C. Person who isolated it from plants body

D. Person who discovered it

Ans. D.

562. Nature of most intestinal enzymes is

A. Acidic B. Alkaline

C. Water based D. Mineral based

Ans. B.

563. Neutral point like water (H_2O) has a pH of

A. 5 B. 6

C. 7 D. 10

Ans. C.

564. Chemical reaction of digestion is called as

A. Hydrolysis B. Oxidation

C. Hydrolases D. Formation of ATP

Ans. C.

565. Organic catalysts may also be called as

A. Chemical Catalysts B. Biological catalysts

C. Physical catalysts D. Situational Catalysts

Ans. B.

566. pH value of below 7 indicates

A. Pure water B. Pure enzyme

C. Pure alkaline D. Pure acidic

Ans. D.

567. Enzyme activity can also be charted through the

A. Rate of digestion B. Rate of reaction

C. Level of pH D. Number of active sites

Ans. B.

568. Catalase is common in

A. Plants B. Animals

C. Insects D. Both A and B

Ans. D.

569. Most of co-enzymes are

A. Protein based B. Water based

C. Easily denatured D. Non-protein based

Ans. D.

570. For most enzymes optimum temperature is

A. 30-40 °C B. 40-50 °C

C. 40-45 °C D. 45-50 °C

Ans. C.

571. Pepsin helps in digestion of

A. Peptic acid B. Proteins

C. Water soluble substances D. Fats

Ans. B.

572. Steapsin is found in

A. Salivary amylase B. Pancreatic amylase

C. Pancreatic juice D. Protoplasm

Ans. C.

573. Foam rubber is produced when latex is combined with

A. Papain B. Catalase

C. Proteases D. Lipases

Ans. B.

574. Starch $(C_6H_{10}O_5)_n$ is a form of

A. Proteins B. Fats

C. Minerals D. Carbohydrate

Ans. D.

575. Plants do not produce

A. Cellulose B. Lignin

C. Cellulase D. Amylase

Ans. D.

576. Amylase becomes denatured at a acidic pH of

A. 4 B. 5

C. 6 D. 7

Ans. A.

577. Papain is found in

A. Papaya B. Proteases

C. Pepsin D. Pancreatic amylase

Ans. A.

578. Conversion of hydrogen peroxide (H_2O_2) to water (H_2O) and oxygen (O_2) is carried out by

A. Catalysis B. Catalase

C. Bile D. Fructose

Ans. B.

579. In plants, enzymes become denatured above

A. 40 °C B. 50 °C

C. 60 °C D. 70 °C

Ans. C.

580. Food oxidation during cellular respiration is carried out through

A. Lipases B. Cellulose

C. Oxidation-reduction enzymes D. Production of hydrogen bioxide

Ans. C.

581. Pepsin is a type of

A. Salivary amylase B. Pancreatic amylase

C. Cellulose D. Proteases

Ans. D.

582. Enzyme action depends upon

A. Active site B. Available site

C. Recognizable site D. Detachable site

Ans. A.

583. Substances on which enzymes act are called as

A. Prostrate B. Hydrate

C. Glucate D. Substrate

Ans. D.

584. Building up and breaking down reactions can be called as

A. Substrate and hydrate reactions

B. Synthesis and hydratic reactions

C. Synthesis and hydrolysis reactions

D. Synchronizing and hyperactive reactions

Ans. C.

585. Pepsin and rennin enzymes are found in the

A. Liver B. Intestine

C. Gall bladder D. Stomach

Ans. D.

586. Very low temperatures make enzyme

A. Hyperactive B. Freeze

C. Dissolve in water D. Inactive

Ans. D.

587. Glucose oxidase and peroxidase aid in

A. Making chocolates

B. Dying leather

C. Detecting presence of sugar in urine

D. Making sweets

Ans. C.

588. Papain found in papaya becomes denatured above

A. 45 °C B. 55 °C

C. 65 °C D. 75 °C

Ans. C.

589. If malaria is not treated, outcomes could include

A. Death B. Anaemia

C. Heart failure D. Both A and B

Ans. D.

590. Mosquito larvae and pupae can be exterminated through small fish like

A. Guppies B. Gold fish

C. Tubifax worms D. Seahorse

Ans. A.

591. Inside mosquitoes, plasmodium reproduces

A. Sexually B. Asexually

C. Unisexually D. Bisexually

Ans. C.

592. Transference of food from one trophic level to next is

A. Accompanied with an energy gain

B. Accompanied with energy loss

C. Accompanied with macronutrients only

D. Accompanied with micronutrients only

Ans. B.

593. Water where fresh and sea water mix is known as

A. Brackish water B. Blackish water

C. Intermingling water D. Stagnant water

Ans. A.

594. In a community, food chains are linked together to form

A. Ecological niche
B. Food niche
C. Food web
D. All of these

Ans. C.

595. Sea water is alkaline with a pH of

A. less than 8
B. 8
C. 9
D. 10

Ans. B.

596. Interaction of living things and non-living things is known as

A. Ecological niche
B. Ecological community
C. Ecosystem
D. Ecology

Ans. C.

597. Type of energy trapped in dead bodies is in form of

A. Physical energy
B. Radiant energy
C. Chemical energy
D. All of these

Ans. C.

598. Energy pyramid is broader at base and narrower at apex, as energy

A. Increases along food chain
B. Decreases along food chain
C. Remains same along food chain
D. May increase or decrease along food chain

Ans. B.

599. Seldom fatal disease is known as

A. Malignant
B. Benign
C. Tertian malaria
D. Anaemia

Ans. B.

600. Carbon dioxide (CO_2) is released in atmosphere through

A. Respiration
B. Combustion
C. Decay
D. All of these

Ans. D.

601. Hydrophytes may be

A. Partially submerged
B. Fully submerged
C. Free floating
D. All of above

Ans. D.

602. In order to float, water weeds have

A. Poorly developed vascular bundles

B. Poorly developed supporting tissues

C. Air spaces to help plant float

D. Small base area

Ans. C.

603. Due to osmotic pressure in marine fish, kidneys

A. Excretes salts
B. Excretes small amount of water

C. Produce concentrated urine
D. All of these

Ans. D.

604. Xerophytes

A. Does not shed leaves in periods of drought

B. Develop fleshy stems

C. Have no mechanism to store water

D. Rely solely on leaves for photosynthesis

Ans. B.

605. Animals living in sea water tend to loose water through

A. Osmosis
B. Active transport

C. Gills
D. Diffusion

Ans. A.

606. Internodes of plants growing in light are

A. Tall
B. Short

C. Herbaceous
D. All three depending on type of plant

Ans. B.

607. Ultrafiltration retains

A. Study of interaction among organisms

B. Combination of community and physical and chemical factors making up non-living environment.

C. Number of population trees

D. Community of population

Ans. B.

608. In order to reduce water loss, plants may

A. Shed leaves

B. Depend on peripheral layer of root

C. Will show cell division in shoot apex

D. Get rid of stomata

Ans. A.

609. Severe and fatal diseases are called

A. Malignant b. Benign

C. Tertian malaria D. Typhoid

Ans. A.

610. Simplest form of nutrients are

A. Organic compounds B. Inorganic nutrients

C. Organic nutrients D. Organic macromolecules

Ans. B.

611. Starfish and corals can be found in

A. Fresh water only B. In oceans and seas only

C. Stream only D. Lakes and ponds

Ans. B.

612. More energy is available if man feeds

A. Directly on plants B. On cattle

C. On meat D. On quaternary consumers

Ans. A.

613. In carbon cycle, flow of energy is

A. Linear B. Cyclical

C. Reversible D. Irreversible

Ans. A.

614. Larvae breath through

A. Feeding brushes B. Pair of air floats

C. Pair of spiracles D. Pair of gills

Ans. C.

615. When decomposers respire,

A. Carbon dioxide is produced B. Carbon dioxide is reduced

C. Carbon monoxide is produced D. Carbon monoxide is reduced

Ans. A.

616. An ecosystem does not need

A. Solar energy
B. Materials from outside
C. Chemical energy
D. Food energy

Ans. A.

617. Abiotic environment does not concern

A. Living things
B. Light
C. Water
D. Oxygen

Ans. A.

618. Plasmodium resides in mosquito's

A. Proboscis
B. Liver
C. Stomach
D. All of these

Ans. C.

619. Disease that is always present to some extent is called

A. Endemic
B. Epidemic
C. Exodemic
D. Ectodemic

Ans. A.

620. Problem of water loss from cells and salt gain is faced by

A. Freshwater bony fish
B. Marine bony fish
C. Marine boneless fish
D. All three

Ans. B.

621. Density can be measured through

A. Number of individuals per square meter
B. Number of individuals per unit area
C. Number of total population in a mile
D. Volume per unit mass

Ans. B.

622. Biomass is the

A. Total mass of living matter at each trophic level
B. Total mass of living things in a biosphere
C. Total number of living organisms in a given area
D. Total energy transferred to each trophic level

Ans. A.

623. In any ecosystem, ultimate source of energy is

A. Plants as primary consumers B. Sun as radiant energy

C. Secondary consumer D. Heterotroph

Ans. B.

624. All parts of Earth where life can be found are called

A. Populations B. Ecosystems

C. Biosphere D. Communities

Ans. C.

625. Interaction and interdependence of plants and animals in a certain place is known as

A. Ecological niche B. Ecological community

C. Ecological habitat D. Both A and B

Ans. D.

626. During night, fresh water is made more acidic due to

A. Onset of photosynthesis B. Caesura of photosynthesis

C. Onset of respiration D. Onset of transpiration

Ans. B.

627. In any ecosystem, form of energy that can not be recycled is

A. Light energy B. Chemical energy

C. Heat energy D. Mechanical energy

Ans. C.

628. Group of organisms of same species living in defined areas called

A. Population B. Community

C. Kingdom D. Phylum

Ans. A.

629. In strong day light, fresh water (H_2O)

A. Can be more alkaline B. Can be more acidic

C. Is neutral D. Is salty

Ans. A.

630. Special breeding roots in mangrove plants are called as

A. Hydro pores B. Hydrilla

C. Hypha D. Pneumatophores

Ans. D.

631. Survival of aquatic organisms only in their environment is an example of

A. High specialization B. Less specialization

C. Adaptation D. Metabolism

Ans. A.

632. Lives of organisms are greatly affected by

A. Producers B. Consumers

C. Decomposers D. All of these

Ans. A.

633. In an ecological community, change in one member

A. Affects other population of community

B. Does not affect other populations

C. Affects other ecosystems

D. Affects other communities

Ans. A.

634. Ecological niche refers to the

A. How an organism fits in environment

B. How an organism depends on various organisms

C. How an organism adapts a new environment

D. Both A and B

Ans. D.

635. Fats, amino acids and proteins are formed through

A. Glucose B. Water

C. Glycogen D. Cellulose

Ans. A.

636. Primary consumers are

A. Plants B. Herbivores

C. Carnivores D. Cat family

Ans. B.

637. Fungi and bacteria act as

A. Primary consumers B. Secondary consumers

C. Decomposers D. Detritivores

Ans. C.

638. Hookworms live inside intestines and

A. Help in milk formation in mammals

B. Help in digestion of cellulose

C. Suck blood

D. Consume faeces

Ans. C.

639. Many freshwater fish

A. Can live in oceans B. Cannot live in oceans

C. Cannot live in river D. Cannot live in streams

Ans. B.

640. In any community, various populations live

A. Interdependently B. Independently

C. Dependently D. Interdependently

Ans. A.

641. Avicennia is an example of

A. Hydrophytes B. Xerophytes

C. Saprophytes D. Spectophyte

Ans. A.

642. Larvae changes into pupa in

A. 2 days B. 4 days

C. 6 days D. 1 week

Ans. D.

643. Ability to withstand fluctuations in salt concentration is more in

A. Fresh water organisms B. Sea water organisms

C. Brackish water organisms D. Muddy water organisms

Ans. C.

644. Both abiotic and biotic factors operating in an environment are called as

A. Ecological niche B. Ecological community

C. Ecosystem D. Ecology

Ans. C.

645. Cycling of carbon (C), nitrogen (N_2), oxygen (O_2) and water (H_2O) is brought about by

A. Chemical processes B. Physical processes

C. Biological processes D. All of these

Ans. D.

646. Mosquito egg remain afloat due to

A. Water vapours around them
B. Air floats around them
C. Air sacs around them
D. Higher density of it compared to water

Ans. B.

647. Coal, natural gas and oil are forms of

A. Fossil fuels
B. Carbon compounds
C. Nitrogen compounds
D. Both A and B

Ans. D.

648. Seed formation occurs

A. When flowering season starts
B. When environment is suitable for growth
C. On approach of unfavourable season
D. When fruit turns lumpy

Ans. C.

649. Due to salt concentrations, aquatic animals are confronted with

A. Feeding problems
B. Breathing problems
C. Excretory problems
D. Osmotic problems

Ans. D.

650. For most types of fresh water organisms, best water

A. Has a pH above 8
B. Has a pH below 8
C. Has a pH almost 7
D. Is salty one

Ans. C.

651. Fall in temperature may result in a

A. Animals accustomed to dark
B. Increase in metabolic activities to produce heat
C. Decrease in metabolic activities of animals
D. All of these

Ans. C.

652. Living organisms can not use

A. Light energy
B. Chemical energy
C. Heat energy
D. Mechanical energy

Ans. C.

653. Balancing of nutrients in nature is

A. Random B. Crude

C. Little D. Delicate

Ans. D.

654. Organisms capable to convert radiant energy in chemical energy are

A. Plants B. Animals

C. Microbes D. All of these

Ans. A.

655. Chemical energy trapped in dead bodies is released in form of

A. Light energy B. Kinetic energy

C. Heat energy D. Chemical energy

Ans. C.

656. Fish inability of survival in another habitat is an example of

A. Less differentiation B. High differentiation

C. Less integration D. High integration

Ans. B.

657. Two or more food chains may be interlinked through

A. Food web B. Food cycle

C. Carbon cycle D. Nitrogen cycle

Ans. A.

658. Excess water entering in body cells accompanied with a loss of salts is faced by

A. Freshwater bony fish B. Marine bony fish

C. Marine boneless fish D. All three

Ans. A.

659. Energy released as heat to environment

A. Returns to same system

B. Returns to same organisms that produced it

C. Is non-cyclical in nature

D. Is converted to light

Ans. C.

660. Ecological niche defines the

A. Function of an organism in its habitat

B. Diet of an organism

C. Food chain

D. Population of an organism

Ans. A.

661. Pupa survives through
A. Feeding through water
B. Feeding through proboscis
C. Food accumulated in larva stage
D. Caudal flaps

Ans. C.

662. Highly concentrated urine is produced by
A. Freshwater bony fish
B. Marine bony fish
C. Marine boneless fish
D. All three

Ans. B.

663. More selective reabsorption of water is carried out in kidneys of
A. Marine boneless fish
B. Freshwater bony fish
C. Marine bony fish
D. All three

Ans. B.

664. Slimy scaly skin helps
A. To glide swiftly in water
B. To respire
C. Helps in osmosis
D. Helps to reduce rate of water loss

Ans. D.

665. Series of energy transference in form of food is called a
A. Food pyramid
B. Food chain
C. Ecological niche
D. Food cycle

Ans. B.

666. More energy is available in a
A. Shorter food chain
B. Longer food chain
C. Smaller food cycle
D. Larger food cycle

Ans. A.

667. In night, cease of photosynthesis makes water
A. More acidic
B. More alkaline
C. Neutral
D. Salty

Ans. A.

668. Vector transfers malarial parasite
A. From a healthy person to an infected person
B. From an infected person to a mosquitoes
C. From an infected person to a healthy person
D. From a healthy person to a mosquito

Ans. C.

669. Food chain and food web is made up of
A. Trophic levels
B. Ecological niche
C. Ecological community
D. Community

Ans. A.

670. All energy that enters biotic part of ecosystem is lost as
A. Light energy
B. Kinetic energy
C. Heat energy
D. Chemical energy

Ans. C.

671. During respiration, carbon dioxide (CO_2) is
A. Produced
B. Released in environment
C. Absorbed
D. Depleted

Ans. B.

672. Malaria is caused by parasitic protozoan called as
A. Anopheles
B. Plasmodium
C. Plasmolysis
D. Anophelysis

Ans. B.

673. Greatest amount of energy is lost while
A. Moving from producers to pri-consumers
B. Moving from pri-consumers to sec-consumers
C. Moving from sec-consumers to tertiary consumers
D. Heat is lost during respiration

Ans. A.

674. Pupa swims in water through
A. Caudal flaps
B. Wriggles in water
C. Air floats
D. Ripples and waves

Ans. A.

675. Each stage in food chain is called a/an
A. Photon level
B. Phantom level
C. Trophic level
D. Energy level

Ans. C.

676. In a food chain, organisms
A. Feed on preceding one
B. Provides food for succeeding organisms
C. Provide more energy for next trophic level
D. Both A and B

Ans. D.

677. Trophic level refers to the

A. Axis around earth
B. Stage in an ecological niche
C. Stage in a food chain
D. Energy level in a food web

Ans. C.

678. Balance between producers and consumers forms the

A. Food web
B. Food chain
C. Food cycle
D. Carbon cycle

Ans. A.

679. Damage, diseases and death may be caused by the

A. Symbiotic relationship
B. Parasitic relationship
C. Saprophytic relationship
D. Neutral relationship

Ans. B.

680. Malarial preventive drugs include

A. Quinine
B. Chloroquine
C. Paludrine
D. Penicillin

Ans. C.

681. Chemical energy trapped in dead bodies is released through the

A. Decomposition
B. Fungi and bacteria
C. Virus
D. Both A and B

Ans. D.

682. If plants absorb carbon dioxide (CO_2) in water (H_2O), water becomes

A. Alkaline
B. Acidic
C. Neutral
D. Salty

Ans. B.

683. Any part of Earth where life can exist is called a

A. Populations
B. Community
C. Ecosystem
D. Biosphere

Ans. D.

684. Tertian malaria can be

A. Benign
B. Malignant
C. Deadly
D. Both A and B

Ans. D.

685. Carbon dioxide (CO_2) is one of end products of decomposition and its nature is

A. Organic
B. Inorganic
C. Artificial
D. Replicative

Ans. B.

686. Due to osmotic problems in freshwater bony fish, kidneys

A. Have to produce concentrated urine
B. Have to reabsorb water
C. Have to produce dilute urine
D. Have to release water

Ans. C.

687. Mosquito eggs hatch out in larvae in

A. 2 days
B. 4 days
C. 6 days
D. 1 week

Ans. A.

688. Large amount of dilute urine is produced in

A. Freshwater bony fish
B. Marine bony fish
C. Marine boneless fish
D. All three

Ans. A.

689. pH (power of Hydrogen) of about 8 is characteristic of

A. Sea water
B. Fresh water
C. Stagnant water
D. Lime water

Ans. A.

690. Fish can come to water for air breathing in waters of

A. Low oxygen concentration
B. High oxygen concentration
C. Low hydrogen concentration
D. High hydrogen concentration

Ans. A.

691. Plants capable to survive conditions of extreme drought are

A. Xerophytes
B. Hydrophytes
C. Cortex
D. Herbaceous

Ans. A.

692. Pneumatophores grow

A. Downward in water
B. Downward in soil
C. Upward in water
D. Upward in soil

Ans. C.

693. Glucose ($C_6H_{12}O_6$) is formed during photosynthesis, by
   A. Getting water through roots
   B. By carbon dioxide entering through stomata
   C. Minerals obtained through fertilizers
   D. By oxygen being used in respiration

Ans. B.

694. Along food chain, total energy level
   A. Increases progressively B. Decreases progressively
   C. Increases aggressively D. Decreases aggressively

Ans. B.

695. In marram grass, water loss is reduced through
   A. Fewer leaves B. Enlarged stomata
   C. Stomata covered by tiny hairs D. Lenticels

Ans. C.

696. If organism of one trophic level is parasite, the
   A. Pyramid number gets higher B. Pyramid number gets inverted
   C. Pyramid of number gets lower D. Pyramid of number gets infected

Ans. B.

697. Highly branched chains of glucose units result in
   A. Starch B. Glycogen
   C. Cellulose D. Galactose

Ans. B.

698. Prevention of heat is attributed to the
   A. Rate of digestion B. Rate of reaction
   C. Rate of heat production D. Rate of heat gained

Ans. C.

699. Diabetic people need to
   A. Increase water intake B. Reduce water intake
   C. Eliminate any physical activity D. Enhance any physical activity

Ans. A.

700. Condensation of glucose molecules ($C_6H_{12}O_6$) results in
   A. Starch B. Cellulose
   C. Glycogen D. Glucagon

Ans. D.

701. Rich sources of Vitamin B are

A. Liver
B. Fresh liver oils
C. Green leafy vegetables
D. Egg yolk

Ans. A.

702. Fats act as

A. Insulating material
B. A constituent of protoplasm
C. Restricts water loss
D. All of these

Ans. D.

703. Minerals do not include

A. Iodine
B. Calcium
C. Sodium
D. Iron

Ans. A.

704. General feeling of irritability and tiredness may be due to lack of

A. Proteins
B. Carbohydrates
C. Fats
D. Vitamins

Ans. D.

705. Linkage of amino acids is called a

A. Condensation reaction
B. Oxidation reaction
C. Hydrolysis reaction
D. Reduction reaction

Ans. A.

706. $C_{12}H_{22}O_{11}$ is general formula of

A. Monosaccharide
B. Polysaccharides
C. Disaccharides
D. Trisaccharide

Ans. C.

707. In ethanol (C_2H_5OH) emulsion test, resulting emulsion is of

A. Sky blue colour
B. Cloudy white colour
C. Cranberry pink colour
D. Violet colour

Ans. B.

708. Structural component of haemoglobin is

A. Manganese
B. Zinc
C. Iron
D. Chorine

Ans. C.

709. Thyroxin is secreted from

A. Thiamine deficiency
B. Theological inheritance
C. Thyroid glands
D. Muscles used for breathing

Ans. C.

710. Most of animal fats are

A. Saturated fats
B. Unsaturated fats
C. Monounsaturated fats
D. Monosaturated fats

Ans. A.

711. Symptoms of kwashiorkor include

A. Cracked and scaly skin
B. Loss of appetite
C. Excess sweating
D. Itching

Ans. A.

712. Stored energy found in most foods is called as

A. Potential kinetic energy
B. Potential physical energy
C. Potential chemical energy
D. Adenosine triphosphate

Ans. C.

713. An average polypeptide chain may contain up to

A. 300 amino acids
B. 400 amino acids
C. 500 amino acids
D. More than 500 amino acids

Ans. C.

714. Lack of dietary fibre causes

A. Kwashiorkor
B. Rickets
C. Dysentery
D. Constipation

Ans. D.

715. Fructose ($C_6H_{12}O_6$) is very uncommon in

A. Animals
B. Plants
C. Herbs
D. Ferns

Ans. A.

716. Starch $(C_6H_{10}O_5)_n$ is broken down to form glucose ($C_6H_{12}O_6$) units when hydrolyzed by

A. Alkaline base
B. Acidic base
C. Neutral base
D. Salty base

Ans. B.

717. All are characteristics of energy, but,

A. Energy can not be created

B. Energy can not be destroyed

C. Energy can be converted from one form to other

D. Energy is never lost

Ans. D.

718. Bulk of undigested matter is made up of

A. Glycogen B. Cellulose

C. Galactose D. Stearic acid

Ans. B.

719. Muscles are mostly made up of

A. Proteins B. Starch

C. Fiber D. Cellulose

Ans. A.

720. In Malaysia and Singapore, average daily energy requirements of boys compared to girls is

A. More for boys and lesser for girls B. More for girls and lesser for boys

C. Same for both gender D. Cannot be estimated

Ans. A.

721. Amino acids are joined to form

A. Proteins B. Lipids

C. Unsaturated fats D. Cytoplasm

Ans. A.

722. Energy balance refers to the

A. Equation of rate of oxidation

B. Amount of starch in take

C. Equilibrium between energy intake and energy expenditures

D. Equilibrium of rate of reduction

Ans. C.

723. Vegetables fats are

A. Saturated fats B. Unsaturated fats

C. Monounsaturated fats D. Disaturated fats

Ans. B.

724. Ability to do work is defined as

A. Activity
B. Engagement
C. Locomotion
D. Energy

Ans. D.

725. Test of proteins is known as

A. Iodine Test
B. Biuret test
C. Ethanol emulsion test
D. Benedict Test

Ans. B.

726. All is true for Voodoo lily, but,

A. Flies stay away due to rotten fresh smell
B. Its helps plant in reproduce
C. More smelling compounds are vaporized due to heat
D. Insects are attracted for pollination

Ans. A.

727. Anaemia is caused due to

A. Deficiency of proteins
B. Deficiency of starch
C. Deficiency of iron
D. Over-nutrition

Ans. C.

728. Breakage of hydrogen bonds in protein coils results in

A. Activation of enzymes
B. Denaturation of proteins
C. Expedites digestive system
D. Inactivation of protein molecules

Ans. B.

729. Water-soluble vitamins are

A. Stored in body
B. Excreted by body
C. Released by body muscles
D. Released by bone-marrow

Ans. B.

730. Glucose ($C_6H_{12}O_6$) and fructose ($C_6H_{12}O_6$) can be obtained if sucrose ($C_{12}H_{22}O_{11}$) is heated in presence of

A. Dilute hydrogen sulphide
B. Dilute hydrogen peroxide
C. Dilute hydrochloric acid
D. Dilute sulphuric acid

Ans. C.

731. If iodine is applied to glycogen-rich food, resulting colour will be

A. Violet
B. Blue-black
C. Red
D. Brown

Ans. D.

732. Water insolubility of glycogen makes it excellent for

A. Polymerization
B. Suitable for storage materials
C. Late digestion
D. Weight loss

Ans. B.

733. Obesity results if

A. Energy intake is lesser than energy expenditure
B. Umber of enzymes become more than food
C. Energy expenditure is less than energy intake
D. Energy expenditure is more than energy intake

Ans. C.

734. Lack of vitamin B may result in

A. Poor eye sight
B. Dull skin
C. Tooth decay
D. Poor cellular respiration

Ans. D.

735. Lactose ($C_{12}H_{22}O_{11}$) can be hydrolyzed to glucose ($C_6H_{12}O_6$) and galactose ($C_6H_{12}O_6$) in presence of enzyme

A. Lactase
B. Maltase
C. Sucrose
D. Lipases

Ans. A.

736. Hair cover is no longer an efficient insulator in

A. Strong winds
B. Water
C. Arctic pole
D. Alaska

Ans. B.

737. In respiratory system, dust particles are trapped due to

A. Nucleic acids
B. Nectar
C. Amino acids
D. Mucus

Ans. D.

738. Very high protein intake is

A. Good for health
B. Good for kidneys and liver
C. Dangerous for kidneys and liver
D. Helps in weight loss

Ans. C.

739. In cold climate, more energy is required to

A. Maintain locomotion
B. Maintain ones weight
C. Maintain social relationships
D. Maintain body temperature

Ans. D.

740. Protein molecules are but

A. Water soluble

B. Very large to pass through living membranes

C. Need to by hydrolyzed to get digested

D. Produce amino acids as final product

Ans. A.

741. Type of energy produced during movement is called

A. Catalytic energy B. Physical energy

C. Chemical energy D. Kinetic energy

Ans. D.

742. Energy reserves are normally stored as

A. Glycogen B. Simple sugars

C. Complex sugars D. All of these

Ans. A.

743. To hydrolyze Tristearin, enzyme used is

A. Sucrose B. Lipase

C. Maltase D. Amylase

Ans. B.

744. In hydrolysis, larger molecules are broken down into smaller molecules by addition of

A. Amino acids B. Water

C. Grape sugar D. Sucrose

Ans. B.

745. Polar bear liver contains an enormous amount of

A. Vitamin B complex B. Vitamin E

C. Vitamin D D. Folic acid

Ans. C.

746. During weight loss, an increased protein diet

A. Is good for health

B. Helps build muscles and cuts fats

C. Is necessary for vital processes

D. May increase amount of nitrogen in body

Ans. D.

747. Healthy consumption of fats is

A. Unsaturated fats
B. Saturated fats
C. Blubber
D. Glycogen

Ans. B.

748. Vitamins

A. Do not provide energy
B. Are inorganic in nature
C. Can not be hydrolyzed
D. Need special enzymes to be digested

Ans. A.

749. In protein structure, a hydrocarbon side chain is denoted through

A. P
B. Q
C. R
D. S

Ans. C.

750. Disadvantage of fats is

A. Efficient source of energy
B. Effective insulative material
C. Reduction in rate of heat loss
D. Solvent for vitamins

Ans. C.

751. Fat-soluble vitamins helps in all but

A. Formation of teeth
B. Formation of bones
C. Increased tooth decay
D. Knock knees

Ans. C.

752. Amino acid chain in a protein molecule is

A. Straight
B. Coiled
C. Curved
D. Concave

Ans. B.

753. Sources of vitamin may include

A. Plant foods
B. Microorganisms living in gut
C. Meat and eggs
D. Both A and B

Ans. C.

754. Bread and cereal group is rich in

A. Minerals
B. Carbohydrates
C. Fats
D. Vitamins

Ans. B.

755. An overactive thyroid gland may

A. Slow metabolic rate B. Expedite metabolic rate

C. May denature metabolic enzymes D. May increase pH from 7 to 9 approx.

Ans. B.

756. Lactose can also be called as

A. Milk sugar B. Malt sugar

C. Cane sugar D. Grape sugar

Ans. A.

757. Dietary imbalances cause

A. Malnutrition B. Starvation

C. Eating only proteins D. High cholesterol

Ans. A.

758. Starch is commonly formed and stored in

A. Animals B. Plants

C. Fish D. Insects

Ans. B.

759. As compared to carbohydrates, fats are lower in proportion of

A. Hydrogen B. Oxygen

C. Carbon D. All of these

Ans. B.

760. All are types of complex sugars, but,

A. Maltose B. Lactose

C. Fructose D. Sucrose

Ans. C.

761. When one gram of carbohydrates ($C_nH_{2m}O_m$) completely burnt, released energy is

A. 12 kilojoules B. 14kilojoules

C. 16 kilojoules D. 18 kilojoules

Ans. C.

762. Amount of energy requires depends upon the

A. Number of fast food chains visited annually

B. Number of hours a person sleeps

C. Body size

D. All of these

Ans. C.

763. Damage to nervous system and limb paralysis is caused due to

A. Rickets B. Beriberi

C. Diabetes D. Scurvy

Ans. B.

764. Basal metabolic rate shall be measured while a person is

A. Jogging B. Going to work

C. Resting D. Sweating

Ans. C.

765. Fish rich in fat include

A. Herring-like fish B. Sharks

C. Trout D. All of these

Ans. A.

766. Prevention of heat loss is more efficient in

A. Women B. Men

C. Children D. People doing very heavy work

Ans. A.

767. Philodendron flowers temperature may exceed

A. 30 °C B. 36 °C

C. 40 °C D. 46 °C

Ans. D.

768. Elements of carbon (C), hydrogen (H_2) and oxygen (O_2) are present in

A. Fats B. Carbohydrates

C. Vitamins D. Both A and B

Ans. D.

769. All is true for resting organisms, but,

A. No energy is lost in sleep

B. Sleeping requires food

C. Organisms continue growth in sleep

D. Organisms' medulla keeps working even in sleep

Ans. A.

770. Vitamin D can be created from a natural substance under skin called as

A. Estrogen B. Ergosterol

C. Pellagra D. Pernicious

Ans. B.

771. Commonly found inside liver of fish is

A. Proteins
B. Fibre
C. Vitamins
D. Fats

Ans. D.

772. Cereals, potatoes and tapioca are common sources of

A. Simple sugars
B. Complex sugars
C. Polysaccharides
D. Monosaccharides

Ans. C.

773. Vitamin D can also be called

A. Ascorbic acid
B. Calciferol
C. Phytomenadione
D. Absisic acid

Ans. B.

774. Loss of equilibrium in energy intake and energy expenditure results in

A. Malnutrition
B. Over-nutrition
C. Kwashiorker
D. Both A and B

Ans. C.

775. Starch $(C_6H_{10}O_5)_n$ is a most common storage form of

A. Lipids
B. Fats
C. Amino acids
D. Carbohydrates

Ans. D.

776. Condensation reaction always results in formation of complex sugar (disaccharide or polysaccharide) and

A. Amino acids
B. Lipids
C. Water
D. Maltose

Ans. C.

777. Average adult protein requirement is

A. 40 to 50 g
B. 50 to 70 g
C. 50-100 g
D. 70-100 g

Ans. C.

778. Blue black colour is produced when substance containing starch is mixed with

A. Biuret solution
B. Benedict solution
C. Iodine
D. Alcohol

Ans. C.

779. Process of condensing many small molecules to form one large molecule is called

A. Polymerization B. Condensation

C. Hydrolysis D. Oxidation

Ans. A.

780. Element that is not a part of minerals is

A. Manganese B. Chlorine

C. Phosphorous D. Iron

Ans. A.

781. Enzyme to digest starch $(C_6H_{10}O_5)_n$ to sugar maltose $(C_{12}H_{22}O_{11})$ is

A. Protease B. Amylase

C. Pepsin D. Maltase

Ans. B.

782. Glycogen $(C_6H_{10}O_5)_n$ is

A. Soluble in water B. A form of fats

C. Insoluble in water D. A form of protein

Ans. C.

783. If Biuret solution is added to egg white, resulting colour will be

A. Blue B. Black

C. Red D. Violet

Ans. D.

784. In Healthy Diet Pyramid, fruits and vegetables are at the

A. Level 1 B. Level 2

C. Level 3 D. Level 4

Ans. B.

785. An average daily intake of carbohydrates $(C_nH_{2m}O_m)$ shall be

A. 10% B. 15%

C. 25% D. 60%

Ans. D.

786. Tristearin can be hydrolyzed to form

A. Stearic acid B. Glycerol

C. Glycogen D. Both A and B

Ans. D.

787. Cellulose $(C_6H_{10}O_5)_n$ is a form of

A. Monosaccharide
B. Disaccharides
C. Polymerization
D. Polysaccharides

Ans. D.

788. Basal metabolic rate measures

A. How fast chemical reactions occur
B. Time lapse between eating and passing stool
C. Number of enzymes required
D. Number of active sites

Ans. A.

789. Enzyme causing breakdown of sucrose into simple sugar $(C_6H_{12}O_6)$ is

A. Pepsin
B. Protease
C. Saliva amylase
D. Sucrase

Ans. D.

790. In order to digest proteins, it is converted into

A. Glucose
B. Fibre
C. Polypeptides
D. Casein

Ans. C.

791. Butter, cheese and nuts are a source of

A. Proteins
B. Fibre
C. Vitamins
D. Fats

Ans. D.

792. According to healthy diet pyramid, fat, salt and sugar shall be

A. Eaten more often
B. Shall be eliminated to avoid cholesterol, blood pressure and diabetes
C. Shall be eaten only sometimes
D. Shall be eaten least

Ans. D.

793. Minerals are

A. Water insoluble
B. Inorganic compounds
C. Organic compounds
D. Fat-soluble

Ans. B.

794. In Healthy Diet Pyramid, meat and alternatives are at the

A. Level 1 B. Level 2

C. Level 3 D. Level 4

Ans. C.

795. All are organic nutrients, but,

A. Fats B. Proteins

C. Fibre D. Minerals

Ans. D.

796. In order to get glucose ($C_6H_{12}O_6$), enzyme maltase shall be applied to

A. Maltose B. Starch

C. Galactose D. Glycogen

Ans. A.

797. Sucrose ($C_{12}H_{22}O_{11}$) may be called as

A. Reducing sugars B. Non-reducing sugars

C. Inorganic nutrient D. Polysaccharides

Ans. B.

798. Fats are present in protoplasm especially in the

A. Cell sap B. Protoplasmic membranes

C. Cytoplasm D. Centrioles

Ans. B.

799. Carbohydrates ($C_nH_{2m}O_m$) include all but

A. Chitin of arthropods B. Sugar

C. Cellulose D. Dietary fiber

Ans. D.

800. Rickets is caused due to deficiency of

A. Vitamin B complex B. Vitamin E

C. Vitamin K D. Vitamin D

Ans. D.

801. Lack of fat soluble vitamins causes

A. Internal bleeding of gums B. Loosening of teeth

C. Painful swollen joints D. Multiple fractures

Ans. D.

802. If generalized formulae of carbohydrates is $C_nH_{2m}O_m$, n and m for glucose are

A. n=3 and m=3 respectively
B. n=3 and m=6 respectively
C. n=6 and m=6 respectively
D. n=12 and m=12 respectively

Ans. C.

803. Balanced diet for one person may be suitable for

A. Growing children
B. All other persons
C. Pregnant women
D. No other person

Ans. D.

804. Cellulose $(C_6H_{10}O_5)_n$ can be digested in herbivores through

A. Fungi
B. Amoeba
C. Bacteria
D. Pathological traces

Ans. C.

805. To test presence of reducing sugars in food, test conducted is

A. Benedict Test
B. Iodine Test
C. Biuret Test
D. Bromine Test

Ans. A.

806. When one gram of fats is completely burnt, amount of energy released is

A. 20-25 kilojoules
B. 26-30 kilojoules
C. 31-35 kilojoules
D. 36-40 kilojoules

Ans. D.

807. Sugar results after hydrolysis of

A. Peptones
B. Carbohydrates
C. Trace elements
D. Fats

Ans. B.

808. Basal metabolic rate of a child is ———— than an old person.

A. Higher
B. Lower
C. Same
D. All of these

Ans. A.

809. Liver and muscles are common places of storage of

A. Glycogen
B. Amino acids
C. Lipids
D. Galactose

Ans. A.

810. Combination of glucose ($C_6H_{12}O_6$) and fructose ($C_6H_{12}O_6$) molecules result in

A. Maltose B. Sucrose

C. Galactose D. Lactose

Ans. B.

811. In order to digest polypeptides, they are converted into

A. Glucose B. Fibre

C. Amino acids D. Polypeptides

Ans. C.

812. Peptone means bond between

A. 2 or more amino acids B. 3 or more amino acids

C. 4 or more amino acids D. 5 or more amino acids

Ans. B.

813. Cellulose can not be digested by

A. Plants B. Fish and mammals

C. Herbivores D. Fungi

Ans. B.

814. People experiencing muscle wasting are a case of

A. Mal nutrition B. Starvation

C. Over-eating D. Over nutrition

Ans. B.

815. Hydrolysis can not be carried out without

A. Water B. Amino acids

C. Peptides D. Mitochondria

Ans. A.

816. When needed glycogen $(C_6H_{10}O_5)_n$ can be easily hydrolyzed to

A. Starch B. Galactose

C. Glucose D. Lactose

Ans. C.

817. Unsaturated fatty acid chains bend at places of

A. Carbon molecules B. Hydrogen molecules

C. Oxygen molecules D. All of these

Ans. B.

818. Lactose ($C_{12}H_{22}O_{11}$) is largely obtained from

A. Malt sugar B. Grape sugar

C. Milk sugar D. Cane sugar

Ans. C.

819. Trace elements do not include

A. Iodine B. Zinc

C. Manganese D. Calcium

Ans. D.

820. Age, Gender, Body size and climate determine the

A. Growth rate of an individual B. Basal metabolic rate

C. Basal hydrolysis rate D. Pressure influence on growth rate

Ans. C.

821. Across age, basal metabolic rate

A. Changes B. Remains constant

C. Increases D. Decreases

Ans. D.

822. One way of managing a balanced diet is through

A. Eating less of very thing B. Avoiding ice creams

C. Often skip meals D. A healthy pyramid way

Ans. D.

823. Peptide bond is formed between

A. Two starch molecules B. Two amino acids

C. Two galactose molecules D. Two fat molecules

Ans. B.

824. In Malaysia and Singapore, average daily energy requirements of women compared to men

A. Is more for men and lesser for women

B. Is more for women and lesser for men

C. Is alike for both

D. Cannot be estimated

Ans. A.

825. In case of malnutrition, basic body needs are met through consumption of stored

A. Fats and glucose B. Fats and glycogen

C. Starch and cellulose D. Peptones

Ans. B.

826. In starvation, first thing to be consumed to keep vital processes is

A. Fats and glucose B. Fats and glycogen

C. Fats and amino acids D. Fats and cellulose

Ans. B.

827. Despite keeping a check on weight, an increase in weight may be due to more

A. Sodium in diet B. Potassium in diet

C. Chlorine in diet D. Manganese in diet

Ans. A.

828. Most fish and white meat are

A. Starch-free B. Calorie-free

C. Fat-free D. Glycogen-free

Ans. C.

829. Function of myoglobin is to

A. Prevent swollen joints B. Aid in muscular contraction

C. Aid in blood clotting D. Keeps retina intact

Ans. B.

830. Softening of bones results in

A. Kwashiorkor B. Rickets

C. Osteomalacia D. Arthritis

Ans. C.

831. Unequal food distribution results in

A. Mal nutrition B. Starvation

C. Over eating D. All of these

Ans. D.

832. Most of vital activities are performed when we are

A. Awake B. Asleep

C. Snoring D. Eating a lot

Ans. B.

833. Simple and complex sugars may be called as

A. Reducing sugars
B. Non-reducing sugars
C. Inorganic nutrient
D. Polysaccharides

Ans. A.

834. Liver produces urea to remove

A. Excess hydrogen
B. Excess hydrogen peroxide
C. Excess nitrogen
D. Excess starch

Ans. C.

835. Calcification of kidneys is caused due to

A. Lack of dietary fibre
B. Excess of sugar
C. Excess of starch
D. Excess of fat-soluble vitamins

Ans. D.

836. Functions of carbohydrates ($C_nH_{2m}O_m$) include all but

A. Production of amino acids
B. Production of fats
C. Production of cellulose cell wall
D. Formation of antibodies to combat disease

Ans. D.

837. Glucose ($C_6H_{12}O_6$) can also be called as

A. Cane sugar
B. Cranberry sugar
C. Grape sugar
D. Malt sugar

Ans. C.

838. Diseases like rickets, scurvy and beriberi occur due to deficiency of

A. Amino acids
B. Carbohydrates
C. Lipids
D. Vitamins

Ans. D.

839. To keep heart running

A. Energy is required
B. No energy is required
C. Heart beat occurs automatically
D. Depends on asleep or awake

Ans. A.

840. On boiling with Benedict solution, reducing sugar will form a precipitate of

A. Green colour
B. Red colour
C. Blue-black colour
D. Violet colour

Ans. B.

841. Basal metabolism refers to amount of energy required

A. To eat dinner | B. To carry out all vital processes
C. For running a marathon | D. To keep heart beating

Ans. B.

842. Galactose ($C_6H_{12}O_6$) and lactose ($C_{12}H_{22}O_{11}$) are commonly found in

A. Animals other than mammals | B. Mammals
C. Microscopic organisms | D. Plants

Ans. B.

843. Peristalsis prevents

A. Movement of undigested food in large intestine
B. Signs of constipation
C. Wavelike muscular movements
D. Use of too much water

Ans. B.

844. Deficiency of ascorbic acid causes

A. Rickets | B. Beriberi
C. Scurvy | D. All of these

Ans. C.

845. An average daily intake of fats shall be

A. 10% | B. 15%
C. 25% | D. 60%

Ans. C.

846. As compared to constituent glucose molecules ($C_6H_{12}O_6$), glycogen $(C_6H_{10}O_5)_n$ occupies

A. More space | B. Less space
C. Become concave | D. Becomes convex

Ans. B.

847. Rate of heat lost depends upon the

A. Amount of fatty issues in a body
B. Amount of muscular tissue in body
C. Number of sweat glands under skin
D. Amount of heavy work done

Ans. A.

848. Rate of evaporation is decreased through the

A. Sebaceous glands B. Protoplasm

C. Thick layer of blubber D. Hair follicles

Ans. A.

849. Rich source of vitamins include

A. Fresh raw vegetables B. Fresh boiled vegetables

C. Fried potatoes D. Processed cheese

Ans. A.

850. Rickets is caused due to deficiency of

A. Sodium B. Chlorine

C. Iodine D. Calcium

Ans. D.

851. Function of trace elements is to

A. Trace benefits of minerals B. Trace benefit of vitamins

C. Trace benefits of proteins D. None of above

Ans. D.

852. Basic building block of protoplasm is

A. Lipids B. Amino acids

C. Unsaturated fats D. Cytoplasm

Ans. B.

853. Disease arising due to vitamin C deficiency is called

A. Scurvy B. Beriberi

C. Rickets D. Kwashiorkor

Ans. A.

854. Basal metabolism, physical activity and heat- all collectively determine the

A. Energy intake B. Energy expenditures

C. Energy in heart beat D. Energy required to stay emotionally well

Ans. B.

855. Term "fats" can be used to refer to

A. Solid animal fats B. Liquid animal fats

C. Plant fats D. All of these

Ans. D.

856. Physically tiring jobs may result in basal metabolic rate of

A. 480 kJ B. 850kJ

C. 1500kJ D. 2050kJ

Ans. D.

857. Beriberi disease is caused due to constant use of

A. White rice and fish B. White rice and chicken

C. Brown rice and fish D. Brown rice and mutton

Ans. B.

858. Galactose ($C_6H_{12}O_6$) is a components of

A. Glucose B. Lactose

C. Sucrose D. Fructose

Ans. B.

859. Types of amino acids present in proteins are

A. 22 B. 32

C. 42 D. 52

Ans. A.

860. Lactose ($C_{12}H_{22}O_{11}$) can be commonly found in

A. Sugar cane B. Sugar beet

C. Cereals D. Mammals milk

Ans. D.

861. If generalized formulae of carbohydrates is $C_nH_{2m}O_m$, n and m for sucrose is

A. n=12 and m=10 B. n=10 and m=11

C. n=12 and m=11 D. n=10 and m=10

Ans. C.

862. Average daily intake of iron for adults is

A. About 0.02 grams B. About .06 grams

C. About 0.08 grams D. About 1 gram

Ans. A.

863. Proteins are but

A. Essential to replace worn-out protoplasm

B. Helps in hydrolysis of enzymes

C. A source of energy

D. Help to develop antibodies to combat diseases

Ans. B.

864. After fats and glycogen ($C_{24}H_{42}O_{21}$) are consumed in case of starvation, next nutrient to be consumed is

A. Proteins B. Starch

C. Cellulose D. Adrenosine triphosphate

Ans. A.

865. An extreme case of muscle wasting is damage to

A. Brain B. Liver

C. Stomach D. Heart

Ans. D.

866. Weight reduction program should be based on

A. Low intake of dietary fiber B. Low intake of vitamins

C. Low intake of fats D. All of these

Ans. C.

867. Very few organisms can digest

A. Glycogen B. Cellulose

C. Galactose D. Stearic acid

Ans. B.

868. Term used to describe all of chemical reactions occurring inside any organism

A. Condensation B. Oxidation

C. Polymerization D. Metabolism

Ans. D.

869. Mucus is made through

A. Fats B. Lipids

C. Carbohydrates D. Amino acids

Ans. C.

870. Heat, acids (H^+) or alkalis (OH^-) easily break the

A. Coils in proteins structure B. Glucose into galactose

C. Saturated fats in cholesterol D. Cellulose into glucose

Ans. A.

871. Peristalsis is enabled through

A. Minerals B. Vitamins

C. Trace elements D. Dietary fibre

Ans. D.

872. Energy is measured in units called

A. Horsepower's B. Watts

C. Calories D. Joules

Ans. D.

873. Highest energy value is provided by

A. Lipids B. Fats

C. Starch D. Glucose

Ans. B.

874. All are compounds of carbon, but,

A. Mineral salts B. Fats

C. Vitamins D. Fiber

Ans. A.

875. In order to break starch $(C_6H_{10}O_5)_n$ to form glucose $(C_6H_{12}O_6)$ units, starch needs to be

A. Hydrolyzed B. Condensed

C. Oxidized D. Polymerized

Ans. A.

876. An excess of fat-soluble vitamins can cause

A. Demineralization of bones B. Calcification of soft tissues

C. Ulcers in digestive tract and liver D. Both A and B

Ans. D.

877. Water-soluble vitamins need to be supplied

A. Daily

B. Weekly

C. Fortnightly

D. Can easily be stored in body for later use

Ans. A.

878. Common fat to cause heart attack is

A. Unsaturated fats B. Cholesterol

C. Monounsaturated fat D. Bisaturated fat

Ans. B.

879. By nature, Vitamins are

A. Fibre B. Minerals

C. Organic compounds D. Inorganic compounds

Ans. C.

880. All are types of polysaccharides, but,

A. Starch B. Glucose

C. Galactose D. Cellulose

Ans. C.

881. Processed foods generally lack

A. Fiber B. Minerals

C. Starch D. Vitamins

Ans. D.

882. If sucrose ($C_{12}H_{22}O_{11}$) is heated in presence of enzymes or catalysts, output will be

A. Glucose B. Lactose

C. Maltose D. Galactose

Ans. A.

883. Weight reduction program shall not

A. Increase protein intake B. Increase water intake

C. Increase intake of citrus fruits D. Increase intake of leafy vegetables

Ans. A.

884. Number of glucose ($C_6H_{12}O_6$) units in a starch $(C_6H_{10}O_5)_n$ molecule may be up to

A. 100 B. 200

C. 220 D. 300

Ans. B.

885. Fibre is important for proper functioning of

A. Liver B. Large intestine

C. Kidneys D. Small intestine

Ans. B.

886. Essential constituent of protoplasm is

A. Water B. Vacuoles

C. Centrioles D. Tonoplast

Ans. A.

887. Glycogen ($C_{24}H_{42}O_{21}$) is a type of

A. Monosaccharide B. Disaccharides

C. ATPs D. Polysaccharides

Ans. D.

888. Persons lower metabolic rate may be due to

A. Fact that he is a child
B. A decrease in saliva amylase
C. Fact he lives in tropic climate
D. Low production of thyroxin

Ans. D.

889. Calcium (Ca) and phosphorus (P_4) are essential for

A. Internal skeleton
B. Exoskeleton
C. Tissues
D. Cartilage

Ans. A.

890. Function of thyroxin is to

A. Regulate breathing rate
B. Regulate metabolic rate
C. Regulate sweat glands
D. Regulate prevention of heat loss

Ans. B.

891. Common name of glycogen ($C_{24}H_{42}O_{21}$) is

A. Plant starch
B. Animal starch
C. Fungal starch
D. All of these

Ans. B.

892. Protein deficiency in children is called as

A. Beriberi
B. Scurvy
C. Diabetes
D. Kwashiorkor

Ans. D.

893. In animals and fungi, glycogen ($C_{24}H_{42}O_{21}$) is stored in form of

A. Lipids
B. Amino acids
C. Carbohydrates
D. Sugars

Ans. C.

894. Energy reserves are normally stored as

A. Lactose
B. Glucose
C. Fat
D. All of these

Ans. C.

895. Saturated fatty acids chains are

A. Straight
B. Curved
C. Twisted
D. Compressed

Ans. A.

896. Lactose ($C_{12}H_{22}O_{11}$) can be hydrolyzed producing

A. Glucose
B. Galactose
C. Fructose
D. Both A and B

Ans. D.

897. Coiled chains of proteins are linked through weaker bonds of

A. Carbon atoms
B. Hydrogen atoms
C. Oxygen atoms
D. All of these

Ans. B.

898. Fats acts as a solvent for

A. Protoplasm
B. Fat-soluble vitamins
C. Insulating materials
D. Mineral ions (Ca^{+2}, Na^{+}, K^{+}, Mg^{+2})

Ans. B.

899. Nutritional anaemia often occurs due to lack of

A. Calcium
B. Iron
C. Iodine
D. Sodium

Ans. B.

900. Average daily intake of calcium for growing children is

A. About 0.02 grams
B. About .06 grams
C. About 0.08 grams
D. About 1 gram

Ans. D.

901. Light-sensitive pigment in retina is created by

A. Vitamin A
B. Vitamin E
C. Vitamin D
D. Vitamin B complex

Ans. A.

902. Animals store carbohydrates mainly in form of

A. Cellulose
B. Starch
C. Galactose
D. Glycogen

Ans. D.

903. Hydrolysis of polypeptides result in

A. Amino acids
B. Fatty acids
C. Amylase
D. Small amount of sodium

Ans. A.

904. Vitamin A is not found in

A. Fresh liver oils
B. Green leafy vegetables
C. Citrus fruits
D. Egg yolk

Ans. C.

905. Thyroid gland is found in the

A. Joints
B. Liver
C. pancreas
D. Neck

Ans. D.

906. Complete digestion of one gram of proteins results in

A. 14 kilojoules of energy
B. 15 kilojoules of energy
C. 16kilojoules of energy
D. 17 kilojoules of energy

Ans. D.

907. Sulfur (S_8) and phosphorus (P_4) are often present in

A. Proteins
B. Fats
C. Carbohydrates
D. Glucose

Ans. A.

908. Condensation reaction is reverse of

A. Lock and key hypothesis
B. Oxidation
C. Hydrolysis
D. Glycogen formation

Ans. C.

909. Glucose, fructose and galactose ($C_6H_{12}O_6$) are

A. Simple sugars
B. Polymer sugar
C. Complex sugar
D. Compound sugar

Ans. A.

910. Heart has to work harder to pump blood round body of

A. An embryo
B. An infant
C. An obese person
D. An athlete

Ans. C.

911. In hot climates, average water consumption must be

A. 3 Liters
B. 4 Liters
C. 8 gallons
D. 4 gallons

Ans. A.

912. Common test for starch presence is

A. Benedict Test
B. Iodine test
C. Biuret Test
D. Bromine Test

Ans. B.

913. In Healthy Diet Pyramid, bread and cereals are at the

A. Level 1
B. Level 2
C. Level 3
D. Level 4

Ans. A.

914. Maltose, lactose and sucrose ($C_{12}H_{22}O_{11}$) belong to which class of carbohydrates

A. Monosaccharide
B. Disaccharides
C. ATPs
D. Polysaccharides

Ans. B.

915. Over-consumption of Vitamins may result in

A. Scurvy
B. Beriberi
C. Rickets
D. Death

Ans. D.

916. Water acts as a reactant in

A. Polymerization
B. Condensation
C. Oxidation
D. Hydrolysis

Ans. D.

917. Deficiency of calciferol causes

A. Rickets
B. Beriberi
C. Scurvy
D. All of these

Ans. A.

918. Most complicated food molecules are of

A. Proteins
B. Fats
C. Carbohydrates
D. Glucose

Ans. A.

919. Internal skeleton is made up of bones and cartilage in

A. Mammals
B. Nematodes
C. Arthropods
D. Echinodermata

Ans. A.

920. People with gallstones in gall bladder shall avoid

A. Proteins B. Fibre

C. Vitamins D. Fats

Ans. D.

921. Obesity is a case of

A. Over-nutrition B. Under-nutrition

C. Starvation D. Under eating

Ans. A.

922. One of simplest carbohydrates is

A. Maltose B. Sugar glucose

C. Fructose D. Galactose

Ans. B.

923. Synthesis of new protoplasm largely depends upon

A. Proteins B. Starch

C. Cellulose D. Cytoplasm

Ans. A.

924. Fatty acids and glycerol ($C_3H_8O_3$) are produced after hydrolysis of

A. Amino acids B. Fats

C. Starch D. Cellulose

Ans. B.

925. In mammals, bones and cartilage result in

A. Exoskeleton B. Internal skeleton

C. Epidermis D. Endodermis

Ans. B.

926. Sucrose ($C_{12}H_{22}O_{11}$) is not found in

A. Sugar beets B. Carrots

C. Mammals D. Sweet fruits

Ans. C.

927. In carbohydrates ($C_nH_{2m}O_m$), ratio of hydrogen (H_2) and oxygen (O_2) is

A. 2:01 B. 3:01

C. 2:02 D. 1:01

Ans. A.

928. If fatty acids can take in no more of hydrogen atoms (H), it is called as

A. Saturated fats
B. Unsaturated fats
C. Monosaturated fats
D. Biunsaturated fats

Ans. A.

929. Water soluble vitamins are characterized by all but

A. Resistant to heat and high temperatures
B. Obtained from citrus fruits
C. Obtained from green vegetables
D. Obtained from fresh juices

Ans. A.

930. To grow, repair and reproduce, more and more

A. Cytoplasm is needed
B. Protoplasm is needed
C. Centrioles are needed
D. Chromatins are needed

Ans. B.

931. Fructose ($C_{12}H_{22}O_{11}$) is commonly found in

A. Animals
B. Plants
C. Insects
D. Fish

Ans. B.

932. Joules contributed to understanding of

A. Energy development
B. Energy conversion
C. Energy crisis
D. Organic energy

Ans. B.

933. Carbohydrate and protein, when combined, form

A. Amino acids
B. Fibre
C. Mucus
D. Nucleic acids

Ans. C.

934. Age, activities and life style determines the

A. Peristalsis
B. Rate of reaction
C. Amount of food materials
D. Sleep time

Ans. C.

935. From person to person amount of food materials

A. Remain alike
B. Decrease
C. Varies
D. Increase

Ans. C.

936. Lack of ascorbic acid causes

A. Tooth decay
B. Demineralization of bones
C. Calcification of soft tissues
D. Poor healing of wounds

Ans. D.

937. Starvation, mal-nutrition and over-nutrition are caused due to

A. Obese eating all food
B. Food is too expensive to buy
C. People do not what to eat and what to avoid
D. Unequal food distribution

Ans. D.

938. Beriberi diseases originated in

A. France
B. England
C. China
D. Sweden

Ans. C.

939. Carbohydrates, fats, proteins, vitamins and minerals are form of

A. Water soluble solvents
B. May be stored in body
C. Are forms of nutrients
D. Shall not be eaten by an obese person

Ans. C.

940. Fat-soluble vitamins need to be supplied

A. Daily
B. Weekly
C. Fortnightly
D. Can easily be stored in body for later use

Ans. D.

941. Muscle wasting includes

A. Skeletal muscles
B. Cardiac muscles
C. Organic muscles
D. Both A and B

Ans. C.

942. An average daily intake of proteins shall be

A. 10%
B. 15%
C. 25%
D. 60%

Ans. B.

943. Combination of glucose ($C_6H_{12}O_6$) and galactose ($C_6H_{12}O_6$) molecules result in

A. Maltose B. Galactose

C. Lactose D. Sucrose

Ans. C.

944. Disaccharides ($C_{12}H_{22}O_{11}$) are also called as

A. Simple sugars B. Polymer sugar

C. Complex sugar D. Compound sugar

Ans. C.

945. Cold climate vs. tropics, basal metabolic rate is

A. Higher B. Lower

C. Constant D. Changes with day and night

Ans. A.

946. Inorganic nutrients include

A. Water B. Vitamins

C. Fibre D. Carbohydrates

Ans. A.

947. It is believed that vitamin C deficiency can be avoided by consuming

A. Limes B. Lentils

C. Proteins D. Potatoes

Ans. A.

948. How many species of bacteria are present inside the human's mouth ?

Ans. Bacteria can be found virtually everywhere, from volcanic springs to arctic regions. The human mouth is home to more than 500 species of bacteria. Each square centimeter of human's skin averages about 100,000 bacteria.

949. Which bacteria can withstand radiation ?

Ans. Deinococcus radiodurans withstand blasts of radiation 1,000 times greater than that would kill a human being.

950. Which one is the largest bacterium ?

Ans. The largest bacteria found so far can actually be seen without the use of a microscope (Thiomargarita namibiensis and Epulopiscium fischelsoni). Thiomargarita namibiensis which means "sulfur pearl of Namibia" is a single celled giant bacteria that lives in the ocean.

951. Which one is the largest tapeworm ?

Ans. Beef tapeworm (Taenia saginata) is the largest parasite (which causes taeniasis in human), which can easily grow 7½ meters or 25 feet long that lives in human's guts.

952. What is the example of smallest bacteria ?

Ans. The smallest known bacteria are so tiny that they were once thought to be viruses (Mycoplasmas).

953. What is the quantum of O2 generated by microbes ?

Ans. Microbes generate at least half the oxygen we breathe.

954. Which of the following characteristic differentiate lysosome from other organelles?

A. Lysosome is a micro organelle

B. Lysosome is a single membrane bounded organelle

C. Lysosome present only in plants

D. All the above

Ans. B.

955. The main function of carotenoid in photosynthesis is

A. Light absorption

B. Prevention of photooxidation of chlorophyll

C. Acts as light absorbing centre

D. Acts as the source of electrons

Ans. B.

956. Most essential features required to maintain a plasmid in a host cell is

A. Ability to transfect cells

B. Antibiotic resistance

C. Origin of replication and marker for selection

D. Capacity to insert into the host genome

Ans. C.

957. Which of the following is a softwood tree ?

A. Mahogony B. Sal tree

C. Rosewood D. Cyperus

Ans. D.

958. In Pisum sativum, the pair of contrasting characters studied by Mendel was actually located on

A. One chromosome B. Two chromosome

C. Four chromosome D. Seven chromosome

Ans. C.

959. The exact reason for Mendel's law of independent assortment is

A. Linkage B. Crossing over

C. Disjunction D. Nondisjunction

Ans. C.

960. The number of linkage groups in an organism will be equal to

A. Number of autosomes B. Number of haploid set

C. Number of diploid set D. 2X number of diploid set

Ans. B.

961. Abzymes are

A. Zymogens B. Inactive proteinases

C. Antibody with catalytic activity D. RNA with catalytic activity

Ans. C.

962. Which of the following organelle is absent in plants ?

A. Mitochondria B. Peroxisomes

C. Glyoxysomes D. Lysosomes

Ans. D.

963. Cytoplast is a

A. Enucleated protoplast B. A cytoplasmic hybrid

C. A cell without cell wall D. A cell without vacuole

Ans. A.

964. Individuals of a species inhabiting the same geographical area are called

A. Allopatric B. Sympatric

C. Parapatric D. Metapatric

Ans. B.

965. Microtubules are the main components of

A. Spindle apparatus B. Muscle network

C. Nuclear membrane complex D. Actin network

Ans. A.

966. Antibody is present in the saliva is

A. IgA B. IgG

C. IgM D. IgD

Ans. A.

967. In an ant colony, the male individuals will be

A. Haploid B. Diploid

C. Triploid D. Polyploid

Ans. A.

968. The important characteristic of a housekeeping gene

A. They are all inducible genes

B. They are permanently kept inactive in somatic cells

C. All expressed in all cells

D. They are positively regulated genes

Ans. C.

969. What is the molecular weight of water ?

A. 10g/mol B. 15 g/mol

C. 18g/mol D. 20g/mol

Ans. C.

970. What is the H+ ion concentration in pure water ?

A. $1X10^{-7}m$ B. $1X10^{7}m$

C. $1X10^{-14}m$ D. $1X10^{14}m$

Ans. A.

971. The equilibrium constant of ionization reaction of pure water is

A. $1.8X10^{-14}m$ B. $1.8X10^{-16}m$

C. $1.8X10^{-7}m$ D. $1.8X10^{-8}m$

Ans. B.

972. The pH of pure water is neutral. The best explanation for this is

A. The pH of pure water is 7

B. In pure water the concentration of H+ and OH- are same

C. Water do not contain free H+ and OH- ions

D. Water will never ionize

Ans. B.

973. As the pKa of an acid increases, the acid will be

A. More weaker B. More stronger

C. Converted to neutral solution D. Converted to basic solution

Ans. A.

974. Buffers are mixtures of

A. Strong acid and strong base

B. Strong acid and weak base

C. Weak acid and their conjugate base

D. Weak base and their conjugate acid

Ans. C.

975. If a solution has to be a buffer, its pH should be

A. At its pKa value
B. At its Ka value

C. At 7
D. At 14

Ans. A.

976. The most important peculiarity of water when compared to other solvents is that water has

A. High boiling point, high melting point and high heat of vaporization

B. High boiling point, low melting point and low heat of vaporization

C. Low boiling point, high melting point and low heat of vaporization

D. Low boiling point, low melting point and low heat of vaporization

Ans. A.

977. Normal pH of human blood is

A. 7.0
B. 7.2

C. 7.3
D. 7.4

Ans. D.

978. The water level in the human body is regulated by the hormone ————.

A. ACTH
B. Oxytocin

C. FSH
D. Epinephrine

Ans. B.

979. The polarity of water molecule is due to

A. Difference in electronegativity of oxygen and hydrogen atoms in water

B. The readily ionizing behaviour of water

C. The positive charge of water molecule

D. The negative charge of water molecule

Ans. A.

980. The van der Waals radius of hydrogen atom in water molecule is

A. 1.2 A°
B. 1.4 A°

C. 1.6 A°
D. 1.8 A°

Ans. A.

981. Papain found in papaya becomes denatured above

A. 45 °C B. 55 °C

C. 65 °C D. 75 °C

Ans. C.

982. It is believed that vitamin C deficiency can be avoided by consuming

A. Limes B. Lentils

C. Proteins D. Potatoes

Ans. A.

983. Relatively denser protoplasm is called as

A. Cytoplasm B. Nucleoplasm

C. Cell sap D. Mitochondrion

Ans. B.

984. Disaccharides ($C_{12}H_{22}O_{11}$) are also called as

A. Simple sugars B. Polymer sugar

C. Complex sugar D. Compound sugar

Ans. C.

985. Digestive systems do not exist in

A. Animals B. Plants

C. Mammals D. All of these

Ans. B.

986. Glycogen ($C_{24}H_{42}O_{21}$) is converted to glucose ($C_6H_{12}O_6$) through enzyme called as

A. Rennin B. Mucin

C. Glycogen phosphorylase D. Erepsin

Ans. C.

987. White matter

A. Makes up nerve fibres B. Forms central part of brain

C. Forms outer part of brain D. Is found in PNS

Ans. B.

988. Red colour in arteries is attributed to

A. Hemoglobin B. Oxyhaemoglobin

C. Aplastic anemia D. Carboxyhemoglobin

Ans. B.

989. An average daily intake of proteins shall be

A. 10% B. 15%

C. 25% D. 60%

Ans. B.

990. Pulmonary arteries carry

A. Red oxygenated blood

B. Bluish red deoxygenated blood

C. Deoxygenated blood from heart to lungs

D. Oxygenated blood from lungs to heart

Ans. C.

991. Pepsin and rennin enzymes are found in the

A. Liver B. Intestine

C. Gall bladder D. Stomach

Ans. D.

992. Fat-soluble vitamins need to be supplied

A. Daily

B. Weekly

C. Fortnightly

D. Can easily be stored in body for later use

Ans. D.

993. Angina pectoris literally means

A. Chest pains B. Narrowing of lumen

C. Dilatation of arteries D. Abnormal deposits of fatty materials

Ans. A.

994. The earth originated

A. 4.6 million years ago B. 8.5 billion years ago

C. 2.6 billion years ago D. 1.2 billion years ago

Ans. A.

995. The first living cell originated

A. 4.6 million years ago B. 3.8 billion years ago

C. 2.6 billion years ago D. 1.2 billion years ago

Ans. B.

996. The first formed cells were

A. Photoautotrophs B. Saprotrophs

C. Chemoautotrophs D. Chemoheretotrophs

Ans. C.

997. The first formed photosynthetic organisms were

A. Algae B. Cyanobacteria

C. Mycoplasmas D. Bryophytes

Ans. B.

998. The first formed organisms were

A. Unicellular eukaryotes B. Multicellular simple eukaryotes

C. Unicellular prokaryotes D. Multicellular prokaryotes

Ans. C.

999. The scientifically suggested reason for the extinction of dinosaurs is

A. Volcanic eruption B. Massive storm

C. Massive asteroid hit D. Massive flood

Ans. C.

1000. The atmosphere or primitive earth was

A. CO_2 rich B. O_2 rich

C. Both A and B D. CO_2 rich and free O_2 was absent

Ans. D.

1001. Which of the following is the widely accepted theory regarding origin of life on earth ?

A. Cosmozoic theory B. Theory of spontaneous generation

C. Theory of chemical evolution D. Theory of special creation

Ans. C.

1002. Evolution may be defined as

A. Continuous genetic variation B. Discontinuous genetic variation

C. Inheritance of acquired characters D. All of these

Ans. A.

1003. The most important requirement for evolution is

A. Mutation B. Natural selection

C. Variations D. Continuity of germplasm

Ans. C.

1004. The economy of Pakistan is based on

A. Agriculture B. Industry

C. Mineral resources D. None of these

Ans. A.

1005. Which one of the following is major export commodity of Pakistan ?

A. Wheat B. Cotton

C. Sugar D. Rice

E. None of these

Ans. B.

1006. Sahiwal is a breed of

A. Buffalo B. Cow

C. Sheep D. Goat

Ans. B.

1007. Vertebrate pests of crops include

A. Insects B. Wild boar

C. Spiders D. None of these

Ans. B.

1008. Sericulture means

A. Rearing of honey bees B. Rearing of silk worms

C. Both of these D. None of these

Ans. B.

1009. Gossypium Hirsutism is the botanical name of

A. Sugarcane B. Wheat

C. American cotton D. Maize

Ans. C.

1010. Kharif crop includes

A. Wheat B. Cotton

C. None of these D. Both A & B

Ans. B.

1011. Genetically modified organism (GMO) is the term used for the organism produced through the application of

A. Genetic engineering B. Mendelian genetics

C. None of these

Ans. A.

1012. The term bioinformatics was coined by

A. J.D.Watson
B. Margaret Dayhoff
C. Puling Hogeweg
D. Frederic Sanger

Ans. C.

1013. Margaret Dayhoff developed the first protein sequence database called

A. SWISS PROT
B. PDB
C. Atlas of protein sequence and structure
D. Protein sequence databank

Ans. C.

1014. Stepwise method for solving problems in computer science is called

A. Flowchart
B. Sequential design
C. Procedure
D. Algorithm

Ans. D.

1015. The first completed gene sequence was of

A. M13 phage
B. T4 phage
C. ØX174
D. Lambda phage

Ans. C.

1016. The term used to refer something 'performed on computer or computer simulation'

A. Dry lab
B. Web lab
C. In vitro
D. In silico

Ans. D.

1017. Laboratory work using chemicals, drugs etc using water is referred as

A. Dry lab
B. Web lab
C. Wet lab
D. In silico

Ans. C.

1018. Laboratory work using computer generated models generally offline is referred as

A. Dry lab
B. Web lab
C. Wet lab
D. In silico

Ans. A.

1019. Laboratory work using computers and associated web based analysis generally online is referred as

A. Dry lab
B. Web lab
C. Wet lab
D. In silico

Ans. B.

1020. "In vitro" in latin means

A. Within the glass
B. Within the lab
C. Outside the lab
D. Outside the glass

Ans. A.

1021. NCBI was established in

A. 1988
B. 1989
C. 1990
D. 1991

Ans. A.

1022. Application of bioinformatics include

A. Data storage and management
B. Drug designing
C. Understand relationships between organisms
D. All of the above

Ans. D.

1023. The computational methodology that tries to find the best matching between two molecule, a receptor and ligand is called

A. Molecular matching
B. Molecular docking
C. Molecular fitting
D. Molecule affinity checking

Ans. B.

1024. Proteomics is the study of

A. Set of proteins
B. Set of proteins in a specific region of the cell
C. Entire set of expressed proteins in a cell
D. None of these

Ans. C.

1025. The process of finding relative location of genes on a chromosome is called

A. Gene tracing
B. Genome mapping
C. Genome walking
D. Chromosome walking

Ans. B.

1026. A compound that has desirable properties to become a drug is called

A. Lead
B. Find
C. Fit drug
D. Fit compound

Ans. A.

1027. What is the term used for the automated in vitro testing of large numbers of compounds using genetically modified cells ?

A. Robotic testing
B. High throughput screening
C. Multiscreening
D. Nanotechnology

Ans. B.

1028. Which source has been particularly fruitful in finding novel antitumour agents such as

A. Marine sources
B. Venom and toxins
C. Combinatorial chemistry
D. Animals

Ans. A.

1029. Which of the following drugs was not isolated from a natural source ?

A. Quinine
B. Morphine
C. Isoniazid
D. Artemisinin

Ans. C.

1030. What is the term used for drugs that are similar in structure to a known drug and which are used for the same purpose

A. Copycat drugs
B. Me-too drugs
C. Derivative drugs
D. Analogue drugs

Ans. B.

1031. Natural products are often used as lead compounds in the design and synthesis of novel drugs. Which of the following general characteristics of a natural product is most likely to be a disadvantage in synthesizing analogues ?

A. Novel of structure
B. Complexity of structure
C. Level of activity
D. Availability

Ans. B.

1032. Which of the following statements is not true of herbal medicines ?

A. Herbal medicines may contain a range of active principles acting together to produce beneficial effect

B. Herbal medicines have no side effects compared to conventional medicines

C. It is more difficult to receive an overdose of an active drug if it is present in a herbal medicine rather than as a purre medicine

D. Certain compounds in herbal medicines may enhance the activity of the active principle

Ans. B.

1033. Which of the following is not an endogenous compound ?

A. Dopamine
B. Endorphins
C. Noradrenaline
D. Desipramine

Ans. D.

1034. Bt cotton is not

A. A GM plant
B. Insect resistant
C. A bacterial gene expressing system
D. Resistant to all pesticides

Ans. D.

1035. C-peptide of human insulin is

A. A part of mature insulin molecule
B. Responsible for formation of disulphide bridges
C. Removed during maturation of proinsulin to insulin
D. Responsible for its biological activity

Ans. C.

1036. GEAC stands for

A. Genome Engineering Action Committee
B. Ground Environment Action Committee
C. Genome Engineering Approval Committee
D. Genetic and Environment Approval Committee

Ans. C.

1037. α-1 antitrypsin is

A. An antacid
B. An enzyme
C. Used to treat arthritis
D. Used to treat emphysema

Ans. D.

1038. A probe which is a molecule used to locate specific sequence in a mixture of DNA or RNA molecules could be

A. A single stranded RNA
B. A single stranded DNA
C. Either RNA or DNA
D. Can be ssDNA but not ssRNA

Ans. C.

1039. Choose the correct option regarding retrovirus

A. An RNA virus that can synthesise DNA during infection

B. A DNA virus that can synthesise RNA during infection

C. A ssDNA virus

D. A dsRNA virus

Ans. A.

1040. The site of production of ADA in the body is

A. Bone marrow
B. Lymphocytes
C. Blood plasma
D. Monocytes

Ans. B.

1041. The protoxin is

A. A primitive toxin
B. A denatured toxin
C. Toxin produced by protozoa
D. Inactive toxin

Ans. D.

1042. Pathophysiology is the

A. Study of physiology of pathogen

B. Study of normal physiology of host

C. Study of altered physiology of host

D. None of the above

Ans. D.

1043. The trigger for activation of toxin of Bacillus thuringiensis is

A. Acidic pH of stomach
B. High temperature
C. Alkaline pH of gut
D. Mechanical action in the insect gut

Ans. C.

1044. Golden rice is

A. A variety of rice grown along the yellow river in china

B. Long stored rice having yellow colour tint

C. A transgenic rice having gene for carotene

D. Wild variety of rice with yellow coloured grains

Ans. C.

1045. In RNAi genes are silenced using

A. ssDNA
B. dsDNA
C. dsRNA
D. ssRNA

Ans. C.

1046. What is the full form ADA ?

A. Adenosine deoxyaminase B. Adenosine deaminase

C. Aspartate deaminase D. Arginine deaminase

Ans. B.

1047. The first clinical gene therapy was done for the treatment of

A. AIDS B. Cancer

C. Cystic fibrosis D. SCID resulting from deficiency of ADA

Ans. D.

1048. Silencing of a gene could be achieved through the use of

A. A short interfering RNA (RNAi) B. Antisense RNA

C. Both the above D. None of the above

Ans. C.

1049. Yeast are most likely to grow in frozen fruits during

A. Slow thawing B. Refrigeration

C. Ambient temperature D. None of these

Ans. A.

1050. Watery soft rot is found mostly in

A. Fruits B. Vegetables

C. Cereals D. All of these

Ans. B.

1051. Black mold rot is caused by

A. A. Flavus B. A. Niger

C. Trichoderma D. Trichothecium roseum

Ans. B.

1052. Concentrate of fruits and vegetable juices

A. Favours the growth of A.Niger and A.flavus species

B. Favours the growth of yeast and of acid and sugar tolerant Leuconostoc and lactobacillus species

C. None of the above

Ans. B.

1053. The predominant micro-organisms in frozen foods are

A. Bacteria B. Micrococcus

C. Yeast and moulds D. None of these

Ans. C.

1054. Anthracnose is a defect which can be observed as

A. Spotting of leaves
B. Spotting of seedpods
C. Spotting of fruits
D. All of these

Ans. D.

1055. Stem and rots caused by species of molds involve

A. Leaves of fruits
B. Stem ends of fruits
C. Spotting on vegetables
D. Spotting on fruits

Ans. B.

1056. Species of ———— are predominant on thawing vegetables like sweet corn and peas when the temperature of thawing is fairly low

A. Streptococcus
B. Micrococcus
C. Both A & B
D. None of these

Ans. B.

1057. Under what conditions food poisoning bacteria may grow and produce toxins in vegetables?

A. When thawed vegetables are held at refrigerated temperature for any considerable period
B. When thawed vegetables are held at room temperature for any considerable period
C. When thawed vegetables are held below refrigerated temperature for any considerable period
D. None of these

Ans. B.

1058. Bacterial soft rot is caused due to

A. Fermentation of pectin
B. Fermentation of sugars
C. Formation of ketones
D. Formation of amino acids

Ans. A.

1059. Saprophytic bacteria cause

A. Sliminess or souring in piled, wet and heating vegetables
B. Brown rot in vegetables
C. Black rot in fruits
D. Bacterial soft rot

Ans. A.

1060. The micro-organism which is present in both fresh and frozen juices is

A. E. coli
B. Enterobacter aerogenes
C. P. Chrysogenum
D. None of these

Ans. B.

1061. The technique first described to determine the incipient spoilage in meat was

A. Homogenate extract volume (HEV) B. Agar Plate Count (APC)

C. Extract Release Volume (ERV) D. None of the above

Ans. C.

1062. Which of the following is responsible for a musty or earthy flavor?

A. Actinomycetes B. Flavobacterium

C. Both A & B D. Pseudomonas syncyanea

Ans. A.

1063. Molds causing spoilage of eggs include species of

A. Cladosporium B. Mucor

C. Thamnidium D. All of these

Ans. D.

1064. Vacuum packaged meats are spoiled by

A. B.thermosphacta B. Lactobacilli

C. Both (a) and (b) D. None of these

Ans. C.

1065. More spoilage of eggs is caused by

A. Bacteria than molds B. Molds than bacteria

C. Synergistically D. None of these

Ans. A.

1066. The growth of Streptomyces on straw or elsewhere near the egg may produce

A. Musty or earthy flavours B. Hay odour

C. Fishy flavour D. Cabbage-water flavour

Ans. A.

1067. Unopened, sliced bacon, packaged in material somewhat highly resistant to oxygen permeability, is spoiled mostly by

A. Lactobacilli B. Micrococci

C. Fecal Streptococci D. Molds

Ans. A.

1068. Pink rots in eggs is caused by the strains of

A. Pseudomonas

B. Pseudomonas fluorescens

C. Species of Micrococcus or Bacillus

D. None of the above

Ans. A.

1069. Beef hams are made spongy by species of

A. Rhodotorula B. Bacillus

C. Pseudomonas D. Red Bacillus

Ans. B.

1070. The red color of meat, called its bloom, may be changed to shades of green, brown or grey as a result of production of oxidizing compounds by bacteria. Which of the following species are reported to cause the greening of sausage?

A. Lactobacillus B. Leuconostoc

C. Both A & B D. Pseudomonas

Ans. C.

1071. Yellow discolorations in meat are caused by bacteria with yellow pigments, usually species of

A. Micrococcus B. Flavobacterium

C. Both (a) and (b) D. Pseudomonas syncyanea

Ans. C.

1072. Which of the following (s) is/are responsible for the green patches on the surface of meats under aerobic conditions?

A. P. expansum B. P. asperulum

C. P. oxalicum D. All of these

Ans. D.

1073. Which of the following microorganisms grow in beef at a temperature of 15°C and above?

A. Micrococci B. Psudomonas

C. Both A & B D. Lactobacillus

Ans. C.

1074. Green rots in eggs is chiefly caused by

A. Pseudomonas fluorescens B. Micrococcus or Bacillus species

C. Molds or yeasts D. All of the above

Ans. A.

1075. Black rots in eggs is most commonly caused by

A. Species of Proteus B. Species of Micrococcus or Bacillus

C. Molds or yeasts D. All of these

Ans. A.

1076. In storage atmospheres of high humidity variety of molds may cause

A. Superficial fungal spoilage B. Bacterial spoilage

C. Both A & B D. None of these

Ans. **A.**

1077. Which of the following microorganism spoil poultry in polyethylene bags?

A. Pseudomonas achromobacter B. Pseudomonas alcaligenes

C. Hetero-fermentative species D. Catalase negative bacteria

Ans. **A.**

1078. Black spots in meat are produced mainly by

A. Cladosporium B. Thamnidium

C. Mucor D. Rhizopus

Ans. **A.**

1079. Which of the cause(s) has/have been suggested for the chill rings in sausage?

A. Oxidation

B. Production of organic acids or reducing substances by bacteria

C. Excessive water

D. All of the above

Ans. **D.**

1080. Lactic acid bacteria in meats may be responsible for

A. Slime formation at the surface or within especially in presence of sucrose

B. Production of green discoloration

C. Souring

D. All of the above

Ans. **D.**

1081. Colourless rots in eggs is caused by

A. Pseudomonas alcaligenes

B. Pseudomonas fluorescens

C. Both A & B

D. None of these

Ans. **A.**

1082. The greening of sausage may appear as a green ring not far from the casing, a green core, or a green surface. The cause of greening is the production of hydrogen peroxide by

A. Hetero-fermentative species B. Catalase negative bacteria

C. Both A & B D. None of these

Ans. **C.**

1083. Iced, cut up poultry often develops a slime i.e. accompanied by an odour describe as tainted, acid, sour or dishraggy. This defect is chiefly by the species of

A. Pseudomonas B. Pseudomonas alcaligens

C. Hetero-fermentative species D. Catalase negative bacteria

Ans. A.

1084. Which of the following is recommended for the improvement in flavor during ageing of beef under controlled conditions?

A. Thamnidium B. Rhizopus

C. T. elegans D. M. mucedo

Ans. A.

1085. The spoilage of eggs by fungi goes through stages of mold growth that give the defects their names. Very early mold growth is termed

A. Pin-spot molding B. Fungal rotting

C. Superficial fungal spoilage D. Any of these

Ans. A.

1086. 'White spot in meat is formed due to presence of

A. P. expansum B. Sporotrichum carnis

C. Both A & B D. P. oxalicum

Ans. B.

1087. The number of members of the division Phaeophyta that live in freshwater habitats

A. Is greater than the number of members of the division Chloro-phyta that live in freshwater habitats

B. Is lesser than the number of members of the division Chlorophyta that live in freshwater habitats

C. Is equal to the number of members of the division Chlorophyta that live in freshwater habitats

D. None of the above

Ans. B.

1088. Bioluminescence is a phenomenon associated with

A. Chrysophyta B. Phaeophyta

C. Pyrrophyta D. Chlorophyta

Ans. C.

1089. Which of the following algal divisions is characterized by possession of chlorophylls A and B, starch as the energy storage material, cellulosic cell walls and live in freshwater and marine habitats?

A. Chlorophyta B. Chrysophyta

C. Phaeophyta D. Pyrrophyta

Ans. A.

1090. Which algal division is divided up into three main groups consisting of the golden-brown algae, the yellow-green algae and the diatoms?

A. Chlorophyta B. Chrysophyta
C. Phaeophyta D. Pyrrophyta

Ans. B.

1091. Zooxanthellae are algal symbiont that live within coral reef animals. These algae belong to

A. Chlorophyta B. Chrysophyta
C. Pyrrophyta D. Rhodophyta

Ans. C.

1092. All algae possess

A. Nuclei B. Chloroplasts
C. Both A & B D. None of these

Ans. C.

1093. Algae is a nonvalid taxinomic term that refers to

A. Eukaryotic organisms that have chlorophyll A and produce O_2
B. Well developed cellular structure including a conducting system
C. Both A & b
D. None of these

Ans. A.

1094. Which of the following algal divisions is characterized by possession of chlorophylls A and B, paramylon as the energy storage material, and the presence of a pellical instead of a cell wall?

A. Chlorophyta B. Euglenophyta
C. Pyrrophyta D. Chrysophyta

Ans. B.

1095. Laminarin is an energy storage material characteristic of

A. Chlorophyta B. Chrysophyta
C. Phaeophyta D. Pyrrophyta

Ans. C.

1096. Chlamydomonas and Volvox are similar because

A. They both are motile B. They are members of the Chlorophyta
C. Both A & B D. None of these

Ans. C.

1097. Characteristics used to place algae into divisions include all of the following except

A. Form of storage material

B. Flagella number and location

C. Accessor pigments used in photosynthesis

D. All of the above

Ans. D.

1098. Which algal division never produces motile, flagellated cells among any of its members?

A. Chlorophyta B. Chrysophyta

C. Phaeophyta D. Rhodophyta

Ans. D.

1099. Starch is an energy storage material characteristic of

A. Chlorophyta B. Chrysophyta

C. Phaeophyta D. Rhodophyta

Ans. D.

1100. Number of flagella produced by motile cells in

A. Members of the phaeophyta is greater than members of the Oomycota

B. Members of the Oomycota is greater than members of the Phaeophyta

C. Members of the Phaeophyta is approximately equal to members of the Oomycota

D. None of the above

Ans. C.

1101. The algae Chlamydomonas demonstrates a complex life cycle that switches between haploid and diploid forms. This life cycle is called

A. The sexual-asexual exchange B. The transposition cycle

C. An alternation of generations D. Algal transformation

Ans. C.

1102. The number of flagella produced by motile cells in

A. Members of the Rhodophyta is greater than members of the Phaeophyta

B. Members of the Phaeophyta is greater than members of the Rhodophyta

C. Members of the Rhodophyta is exactly or approximately equal to members of the Phaeophyta

D. None of the above

Ans. B.

1103. Algae are classified into 6 groups, technically known as

A. Categories B. Divisions
C. Genera D. Domains

Ans. B.

1104. The ———— is the vegetative body of algae.

A. Mycelium B. Plasmodium
C. Pseudoplasmodium D. Thallus

Ans. D.

1105. Agar, which is the solidifying agent in many bacterial culture media, is part of the cell wall of

A. Chlorophyta B. Chrysophyta
C. Pyrrophyta D. Rhodophyta

Ans. D.

1106. The kelps are algae found in

A. Chlorophyta B. Chrysophyta
C. Phaeophyta D. Rhodophyta

Ans. C.

1107. Frustules made of silica are characteristic of

A. Euglenoids B. Diatoms
C. Desmids D. Seaweeds

Ans. B.

1108. Algae are found in all of the following places except

A. Oceans B. Soils
C. Lakes and streams D. Associates with fungi

Ans. B.

1109. Which of the following best describes the algae known as diatoms?

A. Cells have intricate shells of silicon dioxide with two halves
B. Cells are encased in rigid walls composed of cellulose coated with silicon
C. Cells have flagella and a light-detecting eye spot
D. Cells contain carotenoid pigments as well as chlorophyll A and B

Ans. A.

1110. Chrysolaminarin is an energy storage material characteristic of

A. Chlorophyta B. Chrysophyta
C. Plaeophyta D. Rhodophyta

Ans. B.

1111. Non bacterial ropiness or sliminess in milk and milk products may be due to the

A. Stringiness caused by mastitis and in particular by fibrin and leucocytes from the cow's blood

B. Sliminess resulting from the thickness of the cream

C. Stringiness due to thin films of casein or lactalbumin during cooling

D. All of the above

Ans. D.

1112. The yoghurt is made from

A. Lactobacillus bulgaricus B. Streptococcus thermophilus

C. S. Cremoris D. Mixed culture of A and B

Ans. D.

1113. Cheese cancer of Swiss and similar cheese is caused by

A. Oospora Crustacea B. Oospora caseovorans

C. Oospora aurianticum D. None of these

Ans. B.

1114. Swelling of the can is caused primarily by

A. Gas forming, anaerobic spore formers

B. Gas forming, aerobic spore formers

C. Both (a) and (b)

D. None of these

Ans. A.

1115. Bulgarian butter milk is made with the help of

A. Lactobacillus bulgaricus B. Streptococcus lactis

C. Streptococcus thermophilus D. S. Cremoris

Ans. A.

1116. Ropiness caused by Enterobacter usually is

A. Worse at the middle of the milk B. Worse at the bottom of the milk

C. Worse near the top of the milk D. All of these

Ans. C.

1117. A brown colour in milk may result from

A. Pseudomonas putrefaciens

B. The enzymatic oxidation of tyrosine by P. fluorescens

C. Both A and B

D. S. marcescens

Ans. C.

1118. Which of the following species of Clostridium is responsible for formation of dark green to black colours in cheese?

A. Clostridium tyrobutyricum
B. Clostridium sporogenes
C. Clostridium herbarum
D. None of these

Ans. C.

1119. Certain strains of Streptococcus lactis var. maltigenes may produce

A. Bitter flavour
B. Acid flavour
C. Burnt or caramel flavour
D. None of these

Ans. C.

1120. The acidity may be described as "aromatic" when

A. Lactic streptococci and aroma forming Leuconostoc species are growing together
B. Streptococcus lactis and other lactis are growing together
C. Appreciable amounts of volatile fatty acids are produced by Coliform bacteria
D. All of the above

Ans. A.

1121. Surface taint in butter which is blamed on Pseudomonas putrefaciens is also called as

A. Rabbito
B. Putridity
C. Both A and B
D. None of these

Ans. C.

1122. Cheese with too low an acidity because of the addition of cream or the failure of the starter often is made gelatinous or slimy by

A. Pseudomonas
B. P. fragi
C. Alcaligenes metalcaligenes
D. All of these

Ans. D.

1123. Pseudomonas syncyanea produces a

A. Bluish gray to brownish colour in milk in its pure form
B. Brownish colour to bluish gray in milk in its pure form
C. Gray to brownish colour in milk
D. Yellow colour in milk

Ans. A.

1124. Pseudomonas nigrifaciens in mildly salted butter may cause

A. Black smudge
B. Greenish areas
C. Pink colour
D. None of these

Ans. A.

1125. Esters like flavors in butter are resulted from the action of

A. P. mephitica B. Aeromonas hydrophila

C. P. fragi D. Pseudomonas synxantha

Ans. C.

1126. Acidophilus milk which is used for its therapeutic properties in intestinal disorders requires for its manufacture a pure culture of

A. Lactobacillus bulgaricus B. Streptococcus thermophilics

C. Lactobacillus acidophilus D. None of the above

Ans. C.

1127. A yellow color in the creamy layer of milk may be caused by

A. Pseudomonas synxantha B. Pseudomonas syncyanea

C. Both A and B D. S. marcescens

Ans. A.

1128. An alkaline reaction in milk is caused by the alkali formers bacteria as

A. Pseudomonas fluorescens B. A. viscolactis

C. Both A & B D. none of these

Ans. C.

1129. Bacterial ropiness in milk is caused by

A. Slimy capsular material from the cells usually gums or mucins

B. Slimy capsular material from the cells usually proteins

C. Slimy capsular material from the cells usually lipids

D. All of the above

Ans. A.

1130. Fishiness in butter is caused by

A. Aeromonas hydrophila B. Pseudomonas synxantha

C. Pseudomonas syncyanea D. none of these

Ans. A.

1131. The chief type of spoilage in sweetened condensed milk may be

A. Gas formation by sucrose fermenting yeasts

B. Thickening caused by micrococci

C. Mold colonies growing on the surface

D. All of the above

Ans. D.

1132. Which of the following strain(s), that grow in the jellies and candid fruits, are able to grow in sugar concentration upto 67.5%?

A. Aspergillus
B. Penicillium
C. Citromyces
D. All of these

Ans. D.

1133. The ability of B.coagulans to grow in tomato juice depends upon the

A. Number of spores present
B. The availability of oxygen
C. The pH of the juice
D. All of these

Ans. D.

1134. Flat sour spoilage of acid foods is caused by

A. B.coagulans
B. B.pepo
C. Both A and B
D. B.stearothermophillus

Ans. A.

1135. The most important kind of chemical spoilage of canned foods is the hydrogen swell which is favoured by

A. Increasing acidities of foods
B. Increasing temperature of storage
C. Imperfection in the tinning and lacquering
D. All of these

Ans. D.

1136. The presence of viable non-spore forming bacteria in heat process canned foods indicates leakage of the container. Which of the following is responsible for the spoilage of leaky cans?

A. Plant equipment
B. Cooling water
C. Highly acidic medium
D. High sugar content

Ans. B.

1137. Sulphur stinker spoilage, is uncommonly found in

A. Low acid foods
B. Medium acid foods
C. High acid foods
D. Any of these

Ans. A.

1138. Medium acid foods with a pH between 5.3 and 4.5 are likely to undergo

A. Flat sour spoilage
B. Putrefaction
C. Both A & B
D. T A spoilage

Ans. D.

1139. Canned sweetened condensed milk may become thickened by

A. Bacillus species
B. Clostridium species
C. Micrococcus species
D. Saccharomyces species

Ans. C.

1140. The canned acid foods such as pineapple, tomatoes and pears have been found spoiled by C.pasteurianum. Such spoilage is more likely when the pH of the food is

A. >4.5
B. <4.5
C >5.3
D. <5.3

Ans. A.

1141. Which of the following species can cause bitterness, acidity and curdling in canned milk, cream and evaporated milk?

A. Bacillus
B. Clostridium
C. Both A and B
D. Saccharomyces

Ans. A.

1142. Acid foods with a pH between 4.5 and 3.7 usually are spoiled by

A. B.coagulans
B. Saccharolytic anaerobe
C. Both A and B
D. None of these

Ans. C.

1143. The butyric acid type of fermentation in acid or medium acid foods, with swelling of the container by the carbon dioxide and hydrogen gas is caused by

A. C.butyricum
B. C.pasteurianum
C. Both A and B
D. C.pasteurianum

Ans. C.

1144. Which of the following(s) is/are proteolytic or putrefactive decomposing proteins with the production of malodorous compounds such as H_2S, mercaptans, ammonia, indole and skatole?

A. C.sporogenes
B. C.putrifaciens
C. Both A and B
D. C.butyricum

Ans. C.

1145. Canned poultry is more often spoiled by

A. Putrefactive than by Saccharolytic Clostridia
B. Saccharolytic Clostridia than by putrefactive
C. Saccharomyces species
D. Micrococcus species

Ans. A.

1146. Canned meat and fish exhibit spoilage by

A. Bacillus sp. B. Clostridiumsp.

C. Both A and B D. Saccharomyces

Ans. C.

1147. High acid foods with a pH < 3.7 undergo spoilage by

A. Saccharolytic anaerobe

B. B.coagulans

C. Both A and B

D. Do not undergo spoilage by microorganisms

Ans. B.

1148. The putrefactive anaerobes grow best in the

A. Low acid canned foods B. Medium acid canned foods

C. High acid canned foods D. Any of these

Ans. A.

1149. High acid foods with a pH above 5.3 are especially subjected to

A. Flat sour spoilage B. Putrefaction

C. Both A and B D. TA spoilage

Ans. C.

1150. Which of the following toxin causing botulism is less toxic to human beings?

A. Type A B. Type B

C. Type C D. None of these

Ans. B.

1151. Which of the following is a food infection?

A. Salmonellosis B. Botulism

C. Staphylococcal intoxication D. None of these

Ans. A.

1152. The staphylococcal intoxication refers to presence of

A. An enterotoxin B. Neurotoxin

C. Mycotoxin D. All the above

Ans. A.

1153. A bacterial food intoxication refers to

A. Illness caused by presence of pathogens

B. Food borne illness caused by the presence of a bacterial toxin formed in food

C. Both A and B

D. None of the above

Ans. B.

1154. The method of successful treatment of botulism prior to appearance of botulism symptoms involve administration of

A. Antibiotic
B. Analgesic
C. Antitoxin
D. Antipyretic

Ans. C.

1155. Botulism is caused by the presence of toxin developed by

A. Clostridium tyrobutyricum
B. Clostridium sporogenes
C. Clostridium botulinum
D. None of these

Ans. C.

1156. Which of the following is true to prevent botulism from smoked fish?

A. The fish should be heated at its coolest part to at least 82°C for 30 min during or after smoking
B. Fish should be immediately frozen after packaging and kept frozen
C. Good sanitation should be maintained throughout production and handling
D. All of the above

Ans. D.

1157. Salmonellois is caused by the

A. Enterotoxin of Salmonella spp
B. Endotoxin of Salmonella spp
C. Neurotoxin of Salmonella spp
D. Exoenterotoxin of Salmonella spp

Ans. B.

1158. Group I C. botulinum strains generally includes in

A. All types of strains (proteolytic) A, B and F
B. All types of strains (non-proteolytic) E and F
C. All types of strains (proteolytic) C, D and F
D. None of the above

Ans. A.

1159. The application of Gamma rays destroys botulism toxin. The dose of gamma rays required for this purpose is

A. 73 Gy
B. 73 Rad
C. 7.3 M rad
D. 173 Rad

Ans. C.

1160. Arrange the potencies of toxin in descending order of the following canned foods

A. Peas>string bean>spinach>corn
B. Corn> string bean>peas>spinach
C. Corn> spinach> peas>string beans
D. Corn> peas>string beans>spinach

Ans. D.

1161. The milk streptococci produce acetoin that gets spontaneously oxidized yielding a flavorings agent (responsible for aroma of butter) that is

A. Acetone B. Acetyl CoA

C. Butyric acid D. Diacetyl

Ans. D.

1162. The botulism intoxication occurs due to

A. An enterotoxin B. Neurotoxin

C. Mycotoxin D. All of these

Ans. B.

1163. The Bacillus cereus causes gastroenteritis by the production of an exoenterotoxin which is released in food as a result of

A. Cell growth B. Cell autolysis

C. Cell permeation D. Cell damage

Ans. B.

1164. Staphylococcal intoxication is caused by the toxin in the food from

A. Staphylococcus aureus B. S. Cerevisiae

C. S. Thermophillus D. None these

Ans. A.

1165. The most important organism involved in manufacture of Koji is

A. Aspergillus oryzae B. Aspergillus soyae

C. Both a & B D. Lactobacillus lactis

Ans. C.

1166. The most commonly used medium for the build up of cultures and the production of baker's yeast consist of

A. Molasses and minerals B. Molasses, minerals and salts

C. Molasses D. Molasses, lactose

Ans. B.

1167. The manufacture of baker's yeast involve

A. S. Cerevisiae B. S. Thermophillus

C. Bacillus subtilis D. None of the above

Ans. A.

1168. Which of the following organism is found at the initial stages in the batter of Idli?

A. Leuconostoc mesentroides B. Aspergillus niger

C. Bacillus nation D. None of these

Ans. A.

1169. Grains spoiled by molds are a potential animal or human health hazard as well as a great economic loss. Which is/are the common species of molds in the spoilage of stored grains by molds?

A. Aspergillus
B. Penicillium
C. Fusarium
D. All of these

Ans. D.

1170. Ropiness in bread is caused by

A. Bacillus subtilis
B. A.Niger
C. R. nigricans
D. P. expansum

Ans. A.

1171. Which of the following (s) is/are the major spoilage of soft drinks from the marked growth of yeasts and bacteria?

A. Cloudiness and ropiness
B. Flat sour spoilage
C. Superficial fungal spoilage
D. Pin-spot molding

Ans. A.

1172. Mined salt has been reported to contain about

A. 50% Micrococcus, 10% Coryneforms and 14% Bacillus
B. 60% Micrococcus, 20% Coryneforms and 14% Bacillus
C. 70% Micrococcus, 20% Coryneforms and 4% Bacillus
D. 70% Micrococcus, 20% Coryneforms and 10% Bacillus

Ans. C.

1173. Which of the following characteristic of the Rotavirus was important for the construction of the Rotashield vaccine?

A. The possession of a segmented RNA genome
B. A limited number of capsule types
C. The ability of monkey Rotavirus strains to cause serious illness (diarrhoea) in human beings
D. The ability of the Rotavirus to be transmitted faster

Ans. A.

1174. Plastic implants can pose a serious nosocomial infection problem because

A. Phagocytes have trouble moving on the plastic surface
B. Phagocytes have trouble engulfing bacteria embedded in a biofilm
C. Infected implants usually have to be surgically removed
D. All the above

Ans. D.

1175. A major difference between EHEC and EPEC is

A. EHEC secretes a Shiga-like toxin and EPEC does not

B. EHEC possesses a type III secretion system and EPEC does not

C. EPEC rearranges host cell actin and EHEC does not

D. EPEC passes through the placenta to infect the fetus and EHEC does not

Ans. A.

1176. The nature of the poliovirus gives for oral vaccination (Sabin vaccine) as part of the eradication programme is

A. Heat killed virus

B. Live attenuated strains of all three immunological types

C. Small dosage of wild-type live viruses

D. Formalin-inactivated viruses

Ans. B.

1177. Which of the following is true regarding anthrax?

A. Anthrax is caused by a virus

B. Anthrax is highly contagious

C. Inhalation anthrax and cutaneous anthrax are caused by separate strains of Bacillus anthracis

D. Inhalation Anthrax requires infection with a large number of spores

Ans. D.

1178. The toxins produced by bacteria

A. Kill viruses

B. Encourage bacterial reproduction

C. Interfere with physiological processes in the body

D. All of the above

Ans. C.

1179. Pseudomembraneous colitis is

A. Precipitated by the use of certain antibiotics

B. Caused by a gram-positive bacterium

C. Caused by a spore-forming bacterium

D. All of the above

Ans. D.

1180. Both Mycobacterium tuberculosis and Streptococcus pneumonia

A. Are Acquired By Inhalation

B. Have Cell Walls That Contain A High Content Of Mycolic Acids

C. Have Polysaccharide Capsules

D. Stay in the lung and rarely, if ever, enter the bloodstream

Ans. A.

1181. Cholera toxin is an A-B type toxin in which the B portions bind to a receptor on a host cell and the A portion enters the cell to cause

A. ADP ribosylation of adenylate cyclase that stops production of cAMP

B. ADP ribosylation of a G protein that locks it into an active form that stimulates adenylate cyclase to make cAMP

C. Cleavage of rRNA that results in disruption of ribosome function

D. ADP ribosylation of guanylate cyclase that stimulates production of cGMP

Ans. B.

1182. Mucus helps in protecting against pathogens by

A. Lowering the pH

B. Facilitating the growth of normal flora

C. Blocking access and attachment of pathogens to mucosal surfaces

D. Sequestering Iron

Ans. C.

1183. Type III secretion systems are used to inject "effector" proteins directly into a host cell. Salmonella uses a type III secretion system to help the pathogen to

A. Survive the acid pH of the stomach

B. Secrete LT (heat labile toxin) and ST (heat stable toxin) into the lumen of the intestine

C. Survive within macrophages

D. Activate T cells to proliferate and secrete cytokines

Ans. C.

1184. Which of these cytokines is also known under the name cachectin?

A. Interferon gamma

B. Interleukin 2

C. Tumor necrosis factor (TNF)

D. None of the above

Ans. C.

1185. Which is not a major defense mechanism in the stomach?

A. Proteolytic enzymes B. Low pH
C. Dense normal flora D. All of these

Ans. C.

1186. The agent responsible for causing mad cow disease is thought to be a

A. Fungus B. Protozoa
C. Prion D. Virus

Ans. C.

1187. The "A" subunit of diphtheria toxin

A. Binds host cell receptors found on heart cells
B. Cause ADP ribosylation of a factor involved in protein synthesis
C. Forms cAMP that leads to fluid accumulation
D. Lysis macrophages with the release of cytokines

Ans. B.

1188. Coxsackie virus B3, a subgroup of enteroviruses, commonly causes

A. Acute hemorrhagic conjunctivitis B. Muscular dystrophy
C. Myocarditis D. Gastroenteritis

Ans. C.

1189. Prontosil is

A. An effective antibacterial when used in animals
B. An effective antibacterial when used in in-vitro cultures
C. An effective antibacterial both in animals as well as in in-vitro cultures
D. Not used as an antibacterial agent

Ans. C.

1190. All infections do not cause fever and all fevers are not due to infections which of the following is an example of non-infectious cause of fever?

A. Typhoid B. Chicken pox
C. Rheumatic disease D. Malaria

Ans. C.

1191. Immunization with which of the following toxoid induces high titer serum antibody, but does not protect from the corresponding disease?

A. Tetanus B. Botulism
C. Diphtheria D. Shigellosis

Ans. B.

1192. Which of the following statements is not true regarding Mycobacterium tuberculosis and/or the disease it causes?

A. The pathogen contains mycolic acid in its cell wall

B. The pathogen can live inside macrophages

C. Antibodies to the pathogen are protective

D. None of these

Ans. C.

1193. An important host defence of human beings is a dense resident microbiota associated with

A. Lungs B. Bladder

C. Uterus D. Vagina

Ans. D.

1194. Lactoferrin helps to protect against pathogens by

A. Sequestering iron B. Blocking sebum production

C. Lowering the pH D. Facilitating the growth of normal flora

Ans. A.

1195. The influenza vaccine is administered each year because

A. Mutations in the viral hemagglutinin may allow the virus to evade the immune response elicited by previous vaccines

B. It is a polysaccharide vaccine that does not confer long-term protection

C. The vaccine is sufficiently toxic to make it necessary to administer only a small amount at any one time

D. None of these

Ans. A.

1196. Which of the following disease is caused by DNA viruses?

A. Polio B. Yellow fever

C. Measles D. Smallpox

Ans. D.

1197. Which of the following is common in the disease caused by Corynebacterium diphtheriae and Bacillus anthracis?

A. Both organisms are gram-positive spore formers

B. Diphtheria toxin and edema toxin are ADP ribosylating toxins

C. The most serious disease symptoms are the direct result of toxin action

D. Both organisms cause skin and respiratory tract infections

Ans. C.

1198. Fatalities following influenza infection are usually due to the

A. Dehydration B. Bacterial superinfection

C. Damage to the heart muscle D. Formation of granulomas in the lung

Ans. B.

1199. Which of the following disease is not caused by microbial protein toxin?

A. Botulism B. Diphtheria

C. Shigella dysentery D. Tuberculosis

Ans. D.

1200. In the human disease cholera, what is it that actually ends up killing the victim?

A. Faulty carrier proteins

B. Dehydration and loss of nutrients

C. Too little water in the food stream

D. The toxin produced by the bacterium

Ans. B.

1201. Each of the 3 virulence factors of Bacillus anthracis i.e.the capsule, edema toxin and lethal toxin can affect the activity of

A. B cells B. Macrophages

C. Ciliated epithelial cells D. M cells

Ans. B.

1202. The chief spoilage organisms on smoked fish are

A. Molds B. Bacteria

C. Both A & B D. Fungi

Ans. A.

1203. A musty or muddy odor of the fish is attributed to

A. The growth of Streptomyces species in the mud at the bottom of the body of water

B. The mud at the bottom of the body of water

C. The growth of Pseudomonas species in the mud at the bottom of the body of water

D. None of the above

Ans. A.

1204. In chilled shrimp——— is chiefly responsible for spoilage

A. Achromobacter B. Pseudomonas

C. Micrococcus or Bacillus species D. Molds or yeasts

Ans. A.

1205. Marinated (sour pickled) fish should not have spoilage problems unless

A. The acid content is very high
B. The acid content is low enough
C. The acid content is moderate
D. None of the above

Ans. B.

1206. The predominant kind of bacteria causing spoilage in fish at chilling temperature is

A. Pseudomonas sp.
B. Micrococcus
C. Bacillus
D. None of the above

Ans. A.

1207. The bacteria most often involved in the spoilage of fish are

A. Part of the natural flora of the external slime of fishes and their intestinal contents
B. Part of the natural flora of the internal slime of fishes only
C. Both A & B
D. None of the above

Ans. A.

1208. The red or pink color of the fish is generally caused from the growth of

A. Sarcina
B. Micrococcus or Bacillus sp.
C. Molds or yeasts
D. All of these

Ans. D.

1209. At higher temperatures, the souring of Oysters may be the result of the fermentation of sugars by

A. Coliform bacteria
B. Streptococci
C. Lactobacilli and yeast
D. All of these

Ans. D.

1210. Normally, due to the holding of the chilled fish

A. Pseudomonas increase in numbers
B. Achromobacters decrease
C. Flavobacteria increase temporarily and then decrease
D. All of the above

Ans. D.

1211. All of the following species are considered coliforms except

A. Enterobacter aerogenes
B. Klebsiella pneumonia
C. Salmonella typhi
D. Escherichia coli

Ans. C.

1212. The sulphur pearl of Namibia, Thiomargarita namibiensis

A. Is the world's largest bacterium

B. Stores high concentrations of nitrate in a huge internal vacuole which takes up 98% of the organisms volume

C. Both A and B

D. Is the world's smallest bacterium

Ans. C.

1213. Which of the following is correct?

A. Ultramicrobacteria or nanobacteria are the dominant bacteria in marine systems

B. Ultramicrobacteria or nanobacteria are so numerous that they are a major food source for heterotrophic flagellates

C. Both A and B

D. None of the above

Ans. A.

1214. Coliforms are used as indicator organisms because

A. They are present wherever enteric pathogens are present

B. A testing procedure with great specificity is easy to perform

C. Both A and B

D. None of the above

Ans. C.

1215. Which of the following species in water reveal the presence of faecal pollution of human or animal origin?

A. E.coli

B. Faecal Streptococci

C. Clostridium perfringens

D. All of these

Ans. D.

1216. The concept of putting microbes to help clean up the environment is called

A. Pasteurization

B. Bioremediation

C. Fermentation

D. Biolistics

Ans. B.

1217. Some cyanobacteria produce potent neurotoxins that, if ingested, will kill humans. These cyanobacteria are most likely to contaminate

A. Water rich in organic carbon wastes but poor in phosphate

B. Water that are anoxic

C. Water rich in phosphate wastes but poor in organic carbon

D. None of the above

Ans. C.

1218. The biogas production process takes place at the temperature

A. Lesser than 25°C
B. 25-40°C
C. 45-60°C
D. All of these

Ans. D.

1219. Treatment of municipal water supplies is based upon

A. Coagulation, filtration, chlorination
B. Chlorination, coagulation, filtration
C. Filtration, coagulation, chlorination
D. Coagulation, chlorination, filtration

Ans. A.

1220. The use of microbes to break down synthetic waste products such as polychlorinated biphenyls is called

A. Bioinformatics
B. Biolistics
C. Biotechnology
D. Bioremediation

Ans. D.

1221. Activated sludge contains large number of

A. Bacteria
B. Yeasts and molds
C. Protozoa
D. All of these

Ans. D.

1222. Iron bacteria can produce

A. Slime
B. Undesirable odors and tastes
C. Both A & B
D. None of the above

Ans. C.

1223. Which of the following statement is not correct?

A. The use of 25-40°C temperatures allows the biogas production to be more stable
B. The use of 25-40°C temperatures does not destroy potentially harmful bacteria
C. The use of 25-40°C temperatures destroys potentially harmful bacteria
D. None of the above

Ans. C.

1224. Oxidation ponds are shallow ponds, generally designed at the depth of

A. 2 to 40 feet
B. 4 to 6 feet
C. 1 to 3 feet
D. 5 to 8 feet

Ans. A.

1225. The acetate-utilizing methanogens are responsible for

A. 20% of methane produced in a biogas reactor

B. 50% of methane produced in a biogas reactor

C. 70% of methane produced in a biogas reactor

D. 85% of methane produced in a biogas reactor

Ans. C.

1226. Which of the following is responsible for the corrosion problem?

A. Iron bacteria B. Sulphur bacteria

C. Slime forming bacteria D. All of these

Ans. B.

1227. Water testing relies on the detection of certain indicator organisms known as

A. Acid fast bacteria B. Bacteroids

C. Coliforms D. Dinoflagellates

Ans. C.

1228. Which of the following is a drug that interferes with the process of DNA production in the virus that causes genital herpes?

A. Erythromycin B. Vancomycin

C. Amantadine D. Acyclovir

Ans. D.

1229. Which of the antibiotic is not used as a food preservative ?

A. Pimaricin B. Nisin

C. Tylosin D. Beta lactam antibiotic

Ans. D.

1230. The most selective antibiotics are those that interfere with the synthesis of

A. Bacterial DNA B. Bacterial RNA

C. Bacterial cell walls D. Bacterial plasma membrane

Ans. C.

1231. Cycloserine inhibits

A. Alanine racemase B. D-alanyl - D-alanine synthetase

C. Both A & B D. Amidase

Ans. C.

1232. Which antibiotic has a beta-lactam ring?

A. Cephalosporin B. Penicillin

C. Tetracycline D. Streptomycin

Ans. B.

1233. Chemotherapeutic agents must

A. Prevent/destroy the activity of a parasite

B. Leave unaltered the host's natural defence mechanisms

C. Be able to come in contact with the parasite by penetrating the cells

D. All of the above

Ans. D.

1234. Novobiocin can be used against

A. Gram +ve Staphylococci B. Gram -ve Meningococci & Gonococci

C. Haemophilus D. All of these

Ans. D.

1235. Interference mechanism of ciprofloxacin and norfloxacin is due to their action on

A. Cell wall synthesis B. Cell membrane function

C. DNA function D. Protein synthesis

Ans. C.

1236. By which of the following means antifungal chemotherapeutic agents may affect fungi?

A. Interfere with nuclear division by preventing the aggregation of microtubules needed for mitosis

B. Interfere with normal nucleic acid synthesis

C. Interfere with ergosterol biosynthesis and thus alter the structure of the cytoplasmic membrane as well as the function of several membrane-bound enzymes like those involved in nutrient transport and chitin synthesis

D. all the above

Ans. D.

1237. Which of the following methods would be most appropriate for sterilizing an antibiotic solution?

A. Dry heat sterilization B. Microfiltration

C. Autoclaving D. Desiccation

Ans. B.

1238. Which of the following drugs involves modification of the drug by enzymatic modification or degradation of its active element to alter its/their resistance?

A. Penicillins B. Chloramphenicol

C. Aminoglycosides D. All of these

Ans. D.

1239. Who developed the concept of specific toxicity?

A. Pasteur B. Fleming
C. Watson D. Ehrlich

Ans. D.

1240. When using alcohol as an antiseptic, which concentration is considered most effective?

A. 95% B. 50%
C. 70% D. 25%

Ans. C.

1241. Fluoroquinolones are antibiotics which inhibit

A. DNA polymerase B. RNA polymerase
C. DNA gyrase D. Cross linking of peptidoglycan

Ans. C.

1242. Which of the following is used only in life-threatening situations when no other drug is adequate?

A. Penicillins B. Tetracycline
C. Chloramphenicol D. Streptomycin

Ans. C.

1243. The susceptibility of a microorganism to antibiotics and other chemotherapeutic agents can be determined by using

A. Tube dilution technique B. Paper disk plate
C. Both A & B D. None of these

Ans. C.

1244. Most antibiotics are isolated from

A. Viruses B. Aquatic microorganisms
C. Soil microorganisms D. Plants

Ans. C.

1245. Which of the following group is not the carbohydrate containing antibiotic?

A. Streptomycin & Streptothricin B. Vancomycin & Moenomycin
C. Everninomycin & Nogirimycin D. Erythromycin & candicidin

Ans. D.

1246. The penicillin stable in gastric acid and suitable for oral administration is

A. Methicillin B. Carbenicillin
C. Closacillin D. Pencillin-G

Ans. C.

1247. Which of the following is not an example of potent antitumer agents?

A. Anthramycin B. Sibromycin

C. Neothramycin D. Erythromycin

Ans. D.

1248. More promising chemotherapeutic agents for treating viral diseases is

A. Leukocytic interferon B. Fibroblast interferon

C. Interferon D. Nystatin

Ans. C.

1249. A parenteral route of drug administration refers to

A. Oral B. Nonoral

C. Intravenously D. Intramuscularly

Ans. B.

1250. Which of the following antibiotics can't be used for treatment of infections with β-lactamase-producing Staphylococcus aureus?

A. Vancomycin B. Ampicillin/sulbactam

C. Cephalothin D. Piperacillin

Ans. D.

1251. Which of the following is not an aminoglycoside antibiotic?

A. Streptomycin B. Neomycin

C. Kanamycin D. Cephalosporin

Ans. D.

1252. The nitrofurans differ from the antibiotics in that they

A. Do not occur naturally B. Occur naturally

C. Are antimicrobial drugs D. All of these

Ans. A.

1253. Quinolones are

A. Antimetabolites B. Penicillin derivatives

C. Bacteriostatic D. Broad-spectrum

Ans. D.

1254. Which of the following is not a semi synthetic chemotherapeutic agent?

A. Ampicillin B. Carbenicillin

C. Penicillin D. Sulfonamide

Ans. C.

1255. Which of the following tests is used to determine the minimal lethal concentration?

A. Broth dilution test
B. Agar dilution test
C. Dilution susceptibility tests
D. All of these

Ans. D.

1256. The mode of action of polymyxin is to

A. Inhibit protein synthesis
B. Inhibit DNA synthesis
C. Injury to the plasma membrane
D. Inhibit folic acid synthesis

Ans. C.

1257. Polyene antibiotics are

A. Large ring structures
B. β-lactam - thiazolidine ring
C. Small ring structures
D. Any of these

Ans. A.

1258. Which of the following may cause resistance to penicillin?

A. Impermeability of cell envelope
B. Production of β-lactamases by bacteria
C. Alteration or lack of penicillin-binding proteins
D. All of the above

Ans. D.

1259. The third generation cephalosporin agents is

A. Cefotaxime
B. Cefoxitin
C. Cephalothin
D. Cephalexin

Ans. A.

1260. The penicillin resistant to β-lactamases is

A. Carbenicillin
B. Closacillin
C. Penicillin-G
D. Ampicillin

Ans. B.

1261. The antibiotics not clinically useful for Pseudomonas aeruginosa infection is

A. Aminoglycosides
B. Ceftazidime
C. Piperacillin
D. Trimethoprim-sulphamethoxazole

Ans. D.

1262. Which of the following drugs may show plasmid-mediated resistance?

A. Nalidixic acid
B. Ampicillin
C. Rifampicin
D. Methicillin

Ans. B.

1263. The scientist who first discovered the substance penicillin was

A. Joseph Lister B. Alexander Fleming

C. Paul Ehrlich D. None of these

Ans. B.

1264. The larger the ————–, the better the chemotherapeutic agent.

A. Therapeutic index B. Therapeutic dose

C. Selective toxicity D. Spectrum

Ans. A.

1265. Chelate forming peptide antibiotic are/is

A. Bleomycins B. Sideromycins

C. Both A & B D. Vancomycin

Ans. C.

1266. With which of the following aminoglycosides interfere ?

A. Protein synthesis B. DNA function

C. Cell wall synthesis D. Cell membrane function

Ans. A.

1267. Which of the following protein synthesis mechanisms may be affected by particular drugs?

A. Peptide bond formation B. mRNA translocation

C. Aminoacyl-tRNA binding D. All of these

Ans. D.

1268. The antibiotics not having good activity against Enterobacteriaceae is

A. Clindamycin B. Cefoxitin

C. Trimethoprim-sulphamethoxazole D. Ciprofloxacin

Ans. A.

1269. Quinones and related antibiotics are

A. Tetracyclines B. Actinorhodin

C. Mitomycin D. All of these

Ans. D.

1270. Both penicillin and fluoroquinolones

A. Bind to and inactivate a bacterial protein

B. Inhibit the cross-linking of peptidoglycan

C. Are inactivated by β-lactamase

D. Must be transported into the cytoplasm in order to act

Ans. A.

1271. A broad-spectrum antibiotic such as chloramphenicol is one that

A. Kills both gram positive and gram negative bacteria

B. Kills all bacteria

C. Kills numerous types of microbes

D. Kills all microorganisms

Ans. C.

1272. Vancomycin inhibits peptidoglycan synthesis by binding

A. D-alanyl - D-alanine B. Alanine racemase

C. D-alanyl - D-alanine synthetase D. Amidase

Ans. A.

1273. Nystatin is a drug used for treatment of diseases caused by

A. Gram negative bacterium B. Gram positive bacterium

C. Yeast D. Protozoan

Ans. C.

1274. Which is not an amino acid and peptide antibiotic?

A. Penicillin B. Actinomycin

C. Bacitracin D. Tetranactin

Ans. D.

1275. Cephalosporins and Penicillins interfere with which of the following?

A. Protein synthesis B. DNA function

C. Cell membrane function D. Cell wall synthesis

Ans. D.

1276. Bacterial cells susceptible to penicillium can be protected from destruction if the medium in which they are exposed is of

A. High osmotic pressure B. Low osmotic pressure

C. Moderate osmotic pressure D. High surface tension

Ans. A.

1277. The compound(s) which act(s) as metabolic antagonist is/are

A. Trimethoprim B. Sulphonamides

C. Both A & B D. None of these

Ans. C.

1278. Amphotericin B and polymyxin interfere with

A. Cell wall synthesis B. Protein synthesis

C. Cell membrane function D. DNA function

Ans. C.

1279. Which of the following is not β-lactamase-resistant penicillin?

A. Oxacillin B. Nafcillin

C. Carbenicillin D. Methicillin

Ans. C.

1280. The antibiotics which affords a broad spectrum of antimicrobial coverage against aerobic and anaerobic bacteria, rickettsiae, chlamydiae, and mycoplasmas is

A. Gentamicin B. Tetracycline

C. Metronidazole D. Vancomycin

Ans. B.

1281. Which of the following when used in proper concentration stimulates the Ascomycetes fermentation of vitamin B_{12} and can be used to counteract toxicity of iron in Candida species?

A. Co B. Ni

C. Zn D. Ca

Ans. A.

1282. Pectinase, an enzyme used for increasing yield and for clarifying juice is obtained by

A. A.Oryzae B. A.Niger

C. A.flavus D. All of these

Ans. D.

1283. The 95% ethanol is equivalent to

A. 190 proof B. 110 proof

C. 170 proof D. 120 proof

Ans. A.

1284. Which species from the followings is resistant to methyl tryptophan?

A. Candida utilis B. E.coli

C. B.subtilis D. Hansenula anomala

Ans. C.

1285. Which of the following substance is employed to neutralize the lactic acid as it is produced (because lactic acid bacteria do not tolerate high concentrations of acid?

A. $CaCO_3$ B. $(NH_4)_2 HPO_4$

C. $MgSO_4$ D. Na_2SO_4

Ans. A.

1286. Alcohol production from starch and raw sugar utilizes selected strains of

A. Saccharomyces cerevisiae
B. Candida pseudotropicalis
C. Candida utilis
D. None of these

Ans. A.

1287. Fungal amylases using stationary culture with wheat bran utilizes

A. A.Oryzae
B. A.Niger
C. A.Flavus
D. S. Cerevisiae

Ans. A.

1288. Why high concentration of sugars are not employed in the fermentation medium?

A. Calcium lactate is not produced
B. Calcium lactate crystallizes from the medium and slows down the process of fermentation
C. High sugar concentration itself crystallizes
D. None of the above

Ans. B.

1289. Which of the following organism produces enzyme taka diastase?

A. A.Oryzae
B. B.subtilis
C. A.Niger
D. S. Cerevisiae

Ans. A.

1290. Which of the following is not an industrial product made by the fungus Aspergillus niger?

A. Galactosidase
B. Citric acid
C. Gluconic acid
D. Lysine

Ans. D.

1291. The biotin level in obtaining L-gluatmic acid by fermentation using Micrococcus glutamicus is critical because

A. Too low level prevents growths, hence L-glutamic acid production
B. Too high level prevents L-glutamic acid production
C. Both A & B
D. None of these

Ans. C.

1292. Most productive species among the different vitamin B_{12} producing Pseudomonads is

A. P. denitrificans
B. P. ovalis
C. P. aureofaciens
D. None of these

Ans. A.

1293. The enzyme which converts optically active isomers of lactic acid to the optically inactive racemic mixture is

A. Isomerise B. Racemase

C. Dehydrogenase D. Invertase

Ans. B.

1294. The sugar concentration of molasses used in fermentation should be

A. 10-18% B. 20-30%

C. 4-5% D. 30-38%

Ans. A.

1295. Bacitracin, an antibiotic similar to penicillin, is produced by

A. Bacillus polymyxa B. Streptomyces erythreus

C. Bacillus licheniformis D. Aspergillus fumigates

Ans. C.

1296. Which of the following Ascomycetes are used for riboflavin production?

A. Eremnothecium ashbyii B. Ashbya gossypii

C. Candida guilliermondia D. Both A and B

Ans. D.

1297. B. flavum strain can be used for the production of

A. L-Threonine B. L-Proline

C. L-Isoleucine and L-Histidine D. All the above

Ans. D.

1298. A major organism used in commercial bioleaching for copper recovery is

A. Desulfovibrio desulfuricans B. Pseudomonas aeruginosa

C. Aspergillus niger D. Thiobacillus ferrooxidans

Ans. D.

1299. During fermentation, pyruvic acid is converted into organic products such as

A. Glucose and fructose B. Starch and cellulose

C. Ethyl alcohol and lactic acid D. Citric acid and isocitric acid

Ans. C.

1300. Which of the following are true for the heterofermentative microorganism producing lactic acid?

A. Only trace amounts of end products other than lactic acid

B. Some lactic acid with carbon dioxide, ethyl alcohol, acetic acid and trace amount of few other products

C. They are used for commercial lactic acid production

D. none of the above

Ans. B.

1301. The submerged fermentation of vinegar utilizes special fermentor designs known as

A. Acetator B. Cavitator

C. Packed vinegar generator D. Both A and B

Ans. D.

1302. The major organism used in the microbial production of citric acid is

A. Penicillin notatum B. Rhizopus nigrificins

C. Aspergillus niger D. Lactobacillis delbrueckii

Ans. C.

1303. Which of the following organism is utilized for the production of D-L-alanine?

A. Microbacterium ammoniaphilum B. Brevibacterium flavum

C. Arthrobacter paraffineus D. C.glutamicum

Ans. A.

1304. The aerated submerged bacterial fermentation to produce vitamin B_{12} employs strains of

A. Propionibacterium B. Pseudomonas

C. Acetobacter D. Both A and B

Ans. D.

1305. Which of the following is a heterofermentative micro-organism ?

A. Leuconostoc mesenteroides B. Lactobacillus delbrueckii

C. Lactobacillus bulgaricus D. Lactobacillus pentosus

Ans. B.

1306. Riboflavin is a by-product of——— fermentation carried out by Clostridium spp.

A. Citric acid B. Acetone butanol

C. Streptomycin D. Ethanol

Ans. B.

1307. Rickes et al. recovered active crystalline vitamin B_{12} from the culture of

A. Streptomyces griseus B. Bacillus megaterium

C. Streptomyces olivaceus D. Streptomyces lactis

Ans. A.

1308. The rapid process of microbial oxidation developed to produce acetic acid from ethanol at Schutzenbach, Germany is also known as

A. Packed generator B. Trickle method

C. Orleans process D. Both A & B

Ans. D.

1309. Which of the following micro organism utilizes lactose as a carbon source in production of lactic acid from whey media?

A. Lactobacillus bulgaricus
B. Lactobacillus delbrueckii
C. Lactobacillus pentosus
D. Leuconostoc mesenteroides

Ans. A.

1310. The organism which utilizes the pentose of sulphite waste liquor for lactic acid production is

A. Streptomyces lactis
B. Lactobacillus bulgaricus
C. Lactobacillus casei
D. Leuconostoc pentosus

Ans. D.

1311. Chlorotetracycline a broad spectrum antibiotic is produced by

A. Streptomyces aureofaciens
B. Streptomyces rimosus
C. Streptomyces venezuelae
D. Streptomyces erythreus

Ans. A.

1312. The production of acetic acid from ethanol is an

A. Anaerobic process
B. Aerobic process
C. A combination of both
D. None of the above

Ans. B.

1313. Which of the following agents involve biosensors linking with electronic circuit?

A. Microorganisms
B. Microbially derived enzymes
C. Either microorganisms or microbially derived enzymes
D. Neither microorganisms nor microbially derived enzymes

Ans. B.

1314. β-carotene is also known as

A. Vitamin A
B. provitamin A
C. Vitamin C
D. Vitamin D

Ans. B.

1315. Vinegar is a fermentation derived food product containing not less than

A. 4% acetic acid
B. 15% acetic acid
C. 25% acetic acid
D. 6% acetic acid

Ans. A.

1316. The maximum concentration of ethanol that is achieved by successive distillation of fermentation broth in continuous stills is

A. 60% B. 95%

C. 70% D. 99%

Ans. B.

1317. The strain C.glutamicum can be used for the production of

A. L-ornithine B. L-phenylalanine

C. L-glutamine D. All of these

Ans. D.

1318. Which of the following is known for greater stability of the riboflavin producing capacity?

A. Eremothecium ashbyii B. Ashbya gossypii

C. Candida flareri D. None of these

Ans. B.

1319. Species of the genus Streptomyces are known for

A. The production of antibiotics B. The production of beer

C. The production of cheese D. Nitrification

Ans. A.

1320. The organism used to produce L-glutamic acid is

A. Micrococcus glutamicus B. Brevibacterium aminogenes

C. Arthrobacter globiformis D. All of these

Ans. D.

1321. The species of Acetobacter which produces cellulosic strands to hold the cells in lime layer is

A. Acetobacter curvum B. Accetobacter orleanense

C. Acetobacter xylinum D. Acetobacter schuetzenbachii

Ans. C.

1322. The commonly used media for submerged bacterial fermentation at commercial scale is

A. Beet molasses B. Liver extract

C. Germinated seed D. None of these

Ans. A.

1323. Which of the following microorganism produces only L(+) - lactic acid without further racemization ?

A. Leuconostoc mesenteroides B. Lactobacillus delbrueckii

C. Rhizopus oryzae D. Lactobacillus bulgaricus

Ans. C.

1324. The recovery of vitamin from fermentation broth is carried out prior to

A. Acidification
B. Alcohol treatment
C. Autolysis
D. None of these

Ans. C.

1325. Naringinase, an enzyme commonly used for removal of bitter taste from citrus juice is obtained from

A. A. niger
B. A. flavus
C. A. oryzae
D. S. cerevisiae

Ans. A.

1326. Protease, which is used for flavouring of sake and haze removal in sake is produced by

A. A. oryzae
B. A. flavus
C. B. cereus
D. A. niger

Ans. A.

1327. The organism B.brevis can be used commercially for the production of

A. Gramicidin A
B. Tyrothricin (bacitracin tyrocidin complex)
C. Tyrocidin
D. All of the above

Ans. D.

1328. The early assay employed for measuring penicillin activity were based upon the quantity required to prevent growth of S. aureus over

A. 20 mm diameter zone using the cylinder plate method of assay
B. 24 mm diameter zone using the cylinder plate method of assay
C. 200 mm diameter zone using the cylinder plate method of assay
D. None of the above

Ans. B.

1329. Penicillin G is also known as

A. Hydroxy benzyl penicillin
B. Phenoxy methyl penicillin
C. Benzyl penicillin
D. 2-pentenyl penicillin

Ans. C.

1330. A major organic acid produced by a microbial process used in foods is

A. Sulphuric acid
B. Citric acid
C. Oxalic acid
D. Uric acid

Ans. B.

1331. Sarcina sickness of beer is caused by

A. Saccharomyces cerevisiae
B. Pedicoccus cerevisiae
C. S. carlsbergensis
D. Zygomonas anaeroium

Ans. B.

1332. The Sarcina sickness of beer, caused by Pedicoccus cerevisiae, is characterized by

A. Sourness
B. Turbidity
C. Popiness
D. All of these

Ans. D.

1333. Parsnip like odour and taste in beer is caused by

A. Flavobacterium proteus
B. Zygomonas anaeroium
C. Lactobacillus patorianus
D. S. carlsbergensis

Ans. A.

1334. A special beer yeast of the bottom type is

A. S. cerevisiae
B. S. carlsbergensis
C. S. thermophillus
D. None of the above

Ans. B.

1335. When the fermentation of fructose results in the bitter product mannitol, the fermentation is sometime termed as

A. Mannkic
B. Mannitic
C. Amertume
D. None of these

Ans. B.

1336. Heavy, thick, slimy film of bacteria in the slow process of vinegar manufacture reduces

A. The rate of hydrogenation
B. The rate of acetification
C. The rate of esterification
D. The rate of purification

Ans. B.

1337. Which of the following beer is of Japanese origin with an alcohol content of 14 to 17%?

A. Sake
B. Pulpue
C. Sonti
D. Lager

Ans. A.

1338. The crushed grapes used for wine manufacturing are also known as

A. Wort
B. Must
C. Hop
D. Pilsener

Ans. B.

1339. The potential spoilage organism in beer is

A. Saccharomyces diastaticus
B. S. carlsbergensis
C. S. cerevisiae
D. S. lactis

Ans. A.

1340. The spoilage most commonly occurring in wine is tourne which refers to

A. Acid formation from aldehyde and ketones
B. Acid formation from sugars, glucose and fructose
C. Both A & B
D. None of the above

Ans. B.

1341. The fermentation of wine can be carried out using the strains of

A. Saccharomyces cerevisiae
B. Saccharomyces carlsbergenesis
C. Bacillus subtilis
D. Pedicoccus cerevisiae

Ans. A.

1342. Acetic acid bacteria spoiling musts and wines are inhibited by

A. 5-7% alcohol by volume
B. 14-15% alcohol by volume
C. 24-25% alcohol by volume
D. 30-35% alcohol by volume

Ans. B.

1343. The micro-organisms causing wine spoilage are

A. Wild yeast
B. Moulds
C. Bacteria
D. All of these

Ans. D.

1344. Most important species of vinegar bacteria causing sliminess is

A. Acetobacter aceti
B. Saccharomyces carlsbergiensis
C. Lactobacillus lactis
D. None of the above

Ans. A.

1345. S. patorianns can cause

A. Coudiness in beer
B. Ester like taste in beer
C. Stringent taste in beer
D. Bitter taste

Ans. A.

1346. Which of the following lymphokine (s) is secreted by delayed-type-hypersensitivity cells?

A. Macrophage stimulating factor B. Migration inhibiting factor

C. Macrophage activating factor D. All of the above

Ans. D.

1347. Which of the following is an example of autoimmune disease ?

A. Rheumatoid arthritis B. Systemic lupus erythematosus

C. Polyarteritis nodosa D. All of the above

Ans. A.

1348. Immunosuppressive agent(s) is/are

A. Cyclosporine B. Methotrexate

C. Anti-lymphocytic serum D. All of these

Ans. D.

1349. Induction of tolerance mechanism(s) is/are

A. Suppression B. Clonal deletion

C. Clonal anergy D. All of these

Ans. D.

1350. Lens antigens of the eye are

A. Cross reacting antigens B. Sequestrated antigens

C. Neoantigens D. None of these

Ans. B.

1351. Negative phase is observed in

A. Secondary humoral response B. Primary humoral response

C. Both A & B D. None of the above

Ans. A.

1352. Method(s) that can be used to detect CMI is/are

A. Migration inhibition

B. Target cell destruction factor test

C. Skin test for delayed hypersensitivity

D. All of the above

Ans. D.

1353. In which of the following cell mediated immunity (CMI) participates?

A. Delayed hypersensitivity reaction B. Graft versus host reaction

C. Allograft rejection D. All of the above

Ans. D.

1354. Overactivity of Th cells may result into

A. Autoimmunity B. Optimal antibody response

C. Optimal cell-mediated response D. None of the above

Ans. A.

1355. The bacteria which is novobiocin resistant is

A. Staphylococcus aureus B. S epidermidis

C. S saprophyticus D. None of these

Ans. C.

1356. The bacteria which are inhibited on crystal violet (1:500,000) blood agar, is/are

A. Streptococci B. Staphylococci

C. Both A & B D. None of these

Ans. B.

1357. Which of the following Staphylococcal haemolysins does not possess leucocidal activity?

A. α haemolysin B. γ haemolysin

C. β haemolysin D. δ haemolysin

Ans. C.

1358. The genus/genera that belongs to the family Micrococcaceae is

A. Micrococcus B. Staphylococcus

C. Planococcus D. All of these

Ans. D.

1359. Identify the bacteria which is oxidase-negative and catalase-positive?

A. Staphylococcus B. Streptococcus

C. Neisseria D. Pseudomonas

Ans. A.

1360. Coagulase-reacting factor is necessary for

A. Slide coagulase test B. Tube coagulase test

C. Tube coagulase test D. None of these

Ans. B.

1361. Bacteria which produces coagulase is

A. S epidermidis
B. S saprophyticus
C. S aureus
D. S hominis

Ans. C.

1362. Staphylococcal food poisoning usually manifests itself following ingestion of contaminated food after

A. 2-6 hours
B. 8-12 hours
C. 12-18 hours
D. 18-36 hours

Ans. A.

1363. Which of the following Staphylococcal haemolysins does not cause lysis of human RBCs?

A. β haemolysin
B. γ haemolysin
C. α haemolysin
D. δ haemolysin

Ans. C.

1364. The toxin of Staphylococcus aureus that may result into scalded skin syndrome is

A. Enterotoxin
B. Leucocidin
C. Epidermolytic toxin
D. Haemolysin

Ans. C.

1365. The bacteria which can ferment mannitol anaerobically is

A. Staphylococcus aureus
B. S epidermidis
C. S saprophyticus
D. None of these

Ans. A.

1366. Protein A is found in cell wall of

A. Coagulase-negative staphylococci
B. Staphylococcus aureus
C. Micrococci
D. None of these

Ans. B.

1367. The most common cause of cystitis (after Escherichia coli) in healthy sexually active women is

A. Staphylococcus saprophyticus
B. Proteus mirabilis
C. Pseudomonas aeruginosa
D. Klebsiella pneumonia

Ans. A.

1368. Which of the following can be used to detect clumping factor?

A. Tube coagulase test
B. Slide coagulase test
C. Precipitation test
D. None of these

Ans. B.

1369. Most strains of Staphylococcus aureus indicate

A. Phosphatase production B. A golden-yellow pigment

C. β-haemolysis on sheep blood agar D. All of the above

Ans. D.

1370. McFadyean's reaction is employed for the presumptive diagnosis of

A. Anthrax B. Tetanus

C. Typhoid D. All of these

Ans. A.

1371. The bacteria, used to examine the efficacy of autoclave, is

A. B polymyxa B. B. brevis

C. Bacillus stearothermophilus D. B. megaterium

Ans. C.

1372. Antibodies to which of the following antigens of Bacillus anthracis are protective?

A. Capsular polypeptide B. Somatic polysaccharide

C. Anthrax toxin D. None of these

Ans. C.

1373. The test(s) which can be used to differentiate anthrax bacilli from anthracoid bacilli is/are

A. Presence of medusa-head colony B. Presence of capsule

C. Susceptibility to gamma phage D. All of these

Ans. D.

1374. Medusa head appearance of the colonies may be due to

A. Bacillus anthracis B. Proteus mirabilis

C. Clostridium tetani D. Pseudomonas aeruginosa

Ans. A.

1375. Food most often associated with emetic type of food poisoning caused by Bacillus cereus, is

A. Meat B. Rice

C. Milk D. Eggs

Ans. B.

1376. Koch's postulates were satisfied for the first time with

A. Clostridium tetani B. Corynebacterium diphtheria

C. Bacillus anthracis D. Salmonella typhi

Ans. C.

1377. Ascoli's thermoprecipition test helps in confirming the laboratory diagnosis of

A. Tetanus
B. Anthrax
C. Typhoid
D. Cholera

Ans. B.

1378. Which of the following serotypes of Salmonella does not produce H_2S ?

A. S choleraesuis
B. S paratyphi A
C. Both A & B
D. None of these

Ans. C.

1379. Which of the following is the commonest species of Salmonella for causing zoonotic disease?

A. S. Indiana
B. S. Newport
C. S. typhimurium
D. S. enteritidis

Ans. C.

1380. Which of the following media is selective for Salmonella?

A. Thiosulphate citrate bile salt agar
B. Wilson and Blair's brilliant-green bismuth sulphite agar medium
C. Bile salt agar
D. All of the above

Ans. B.

1381. Xylose lysine deoxycholate (XLD) agar is better selective medium than the deoxycholate citrate agar (DCA) because

A. It is selective
B. It imparts better growth
C. It contains high salt concentration
D. It is less inhibitory to S. dysentriae and S. flexneri

Ans. D.

1382. Which of the following property(ies) is/are seen in the members of family Enterobacteriaceae?

A. They are catalase-positive
B. They are oxidase-negative
C. They ferment glucose
D. They reduce nitrates to nitrites

Ans. B.

1383. Dysentery may be caused by

A. Enteropathogenic Escherichia coli
B. Enteroinvasive E.coli
C. Enterotoxigenic E.coli
D. Verotoxigenic E.coli

Ans. C.

1384. Which of the following(s) bacteria belong to the family Entero-bacteriaceae ?

A. Yersinia
B. Shigella
C. Salmonella
D. All of these

Ans. D.

1385. Transmission of bubonic plague is by

A. Rat flea
B. Inhalation
C. Ingestion
D. All of these

Ans. A.

1386. The bacteria, which is more resistant to adverse environmental conditions, is

A. S sonnei
B. S dysenteriae
C. S flexneri
D. S boydii

Ans. A.

1387. The reaction(s) that is/are usually positive in Escherichia coli, is/ are

A. Glucose fermentation
B. Indole reaction
C. Mehtyl red reaction
D. All of these

Ans. D.

1388. An enrichment medium for the isolation of Shigella is

A. Alkaline peptone water
B. Terathionate broth
C. Selenite F broth
D. None of these

Ans. C.

1389. In Widal test the significant titres for H agglutinins is

A. 1:50 or more
B. 1 : 100 or more
C. 1 : 200 or more
D. 1: 400 or more

Ans. C.

1390. Heat-labile enterotoxin of Escherichia coli activates

A. Guanylate cyclase
B. Adenylate cyclase
C. Both A and B
D. None of thee

Ans. B.

1391. The bacteria that is negative for fermentation of mannitol is

A. S flexneri
B. S boydii
C. S dysenteriae
D. S sonnei

Ans. C.

1392. Transmission of pneumonic plague from man to man is through

A. Inoculation B. Ingestion

C. Droplet infection D. All of these

Ans. C.

1393. Which of the following genus belongs to family Spirochaetaceae?

A. Treponema B. Spirochaeta

C. Borrelia D. All of these

Ans. D.

1394. Which of the following bacteria is/are known as coliform bacilli?

A. Escherichia B. Klebsiella

C. Enterobacter D. All of these

Ans. D.

1395. The agent(s) which can cause plague is/are

A. Yersinia pestis B. Proteus mirabilis

C. Pseudomonas aeruginosa D. All of these

Ans. A.

1396. Salmonellae can also be killed by

A. Pasteurization B. Chlorination

C. Boiling D. All of these

Ans. D.

1397. Sereny test is used for the detection of

A. Enteropathogenic Escherichia coli B. Enterotoxigenic E.coli

C. Enteroinvasive E.coli D. Verotoxigenic E.coli

Ans. C.

1398. Prodigiosin (red pigment) is produced by members of genus

A. Hafnia B. Enterobacter

C. Serratia D. Cirobacter

Ans. C.

1399. Which of the following serotypes of Salmonella can cause gastroenteritis?

A. S. enteritidis B. S Newport

C. S typhimurium D. All of these

Ans. D.

1400. Sylvatic plague occurs in

A. Mice B. Squirrels

C. Chipmunks D. All of these

Ans. D.

1401. Verotoxin 1 of E.coli is similar to

A. Cholera toxin B. Shiga toxin

C. Heat stable enterotoxin of E.coli D. Heat labile enterotoxin of E.coli

Ans. B.

1402. Which of the following determine the pathogenicity of Yersinia pestis?

A. V and W antigens

B. F1 envelope antigen

C. Production of pigmented colonies on haemin containing media

D. All of these

Ans. D.

1403. Enterobacter can be differentiated from Klebsiella by

A. Ornithine B. Motility

C. Both A & B D. None of these

Ans. C.

1404. In Yersinia pestis, capsule is best demonstrated in cultures grown at

A. 25°C B. 29°C

C. 37°C D. 45°C

Ans. C.

1405. Which of the following can readily kill Salmonellae?

A. Moist heat at 55°C for 20 min B. Moist heat at 55°C for 10 min

C. Moist heat at 55°C for 30 min D. Moist heat at 55°C for 1 h

Ans. D.

1406. Traveller's diarrhea is caused by

A. Enteropathogenic Escherichia coli (EPEC)

B. Enteroinvasive E.coli (EIEC)

C. Enterotoxigenic E. coli (ETEC)

D. Entero haemorrhagic E. coli (EHEC)

Ans. C.

1407. Which of the following disease is caused by Yersinia enterocolitica in man?

A. Gastroenteritis
B. Mesenteric lymphadenitis
C. Septicaemia
D. All of these

Ans. D.

1408. The most common cause of urinary tract infection in the community is

A. Klebsiella pneumonia
B. Proteus vulgaris
C. Escherichia coli
D. Citrobacter freundii

Ans. C.

1409. Bipolar staining is characteristic of

A. Yersinia pestis
B. Proteus mirabilis
C. Pseudomonas aeruginosa
D. All of these

Ans. A.

1410. Spirochaetes exhibit

A. Corkscrew-like rotatory movement
B. Flexion and extension motility
C. Translatory motion
D. All of the above

Ans. D.

1411. Species of Shigella which is predominant in India is

A. S. sonnei
B. S. dysenteriae
C. S. boydii
D. S. flexneri

Ans. D.

1412. Which of the following species/subspecies of Klebsiella produce indole?

A. K pneumoniae subspecies rhinoscleromatis
B. K pneumoniae subspecies aerogenes
C. K pneumoniae subspecies pneumonia
D. K oxytoca

Ans. D.

1413. Primarily human pathogenic bacteria is/are

A. Salmonella typhi
B. S paratyphi A
C. S paratyphi B
D. all of these

Ans. D.

1414. The bacteria which produce(s) β-galactosidase is/are

A. Citrobacter
B. Enterobacter
C. Serratia
D. All of these

Ans. D.

1415. Which of the following property(ies), shown by the organisms belong(s) to the family Enterobacteriaceae?

A. They are catalase-positive
B. They are oxidase-negative
C. They ferment glucose
D. All of these

Ans. D.

1416. In Widal test, the significant titre for O agglutinins is generally

A. 1:50 or more
B. 1:100 or more
C. 1:150 or more
D. 1:200 or more

Ans. B.

1417. Selective media for the isolation of Shigella is

A. Hektoen enteric agar
B. Salmonella-Shigella agar
C. Xylose lysine deoxycholate agar
D. All of these

Ans. D.

1418. The technique(s), used for the assay of heat-labile enterotoxin produced by Escherichia coli, is/are

A. Steroid production in Yl mouse adrenal cell culture
B. Morphological changes in Chinese hamster ovary
C. Enzyme-linked immunosorbent assay
D. All of these

Ans. D.

1419. Yersinia enterocolitica and Y. pestis can be differentiated on the basis of which of the following tests?

A. Decarboxylation of ornithine
B. Fermentation of sucrose and cellobiose
C. Motility at 22°C
D. All of these

Ans. D.

1420. Example of the pathogenic bacteria is/are

A. L. Biflexa
B. L. Parva
C. Leptospira interrogans
D. All of these

Ans. C.

1421. The media which serve(s) as enrichment media for Salmonella is/are

A. Tetrathionate broth
B. Brilliant green tetrathionate broth
C. Selenite-F broth
D. All of these

Ans. D.

1422. Human pathogenic bacteria is/are

A. B pseudomallei
B. Burkholderia mallei
C. Pseudomonas aeruginosa
D. All of these

Ans. D.

1423. Which of the following biochemical reaction is characteristic of Pseudomonas aeruginosa?

A. Production of pyocyanin
B. Oxidative utilization of glucose
C. Oxidase production
D. All of these

Ans. D.

1424. Pseudomonas aeruginosa can be diagnosed from the pigment, known as

A. Pyocyanin
B. Pyoverdin
C. Pyomelanin
D. Pyorubrin

Ans. A.

1425. The most popular method for typing of Pseudomonas aeruginosa is

A. Antibiogram
B. Serotyping
C. Bacteriophage
D. Pyocin

Ans. D.

1426. Which of the following infection(s) can be caused by Pseudomonas aeruginosa ?

A. Urinary tract infection
B. Wound and burn infection
C. Respiratory tract infection
D. All of these

Ans. D.

1427. The substance(s) which can be produced by strains of Pseudomonas aeruginosa is/are

A. Exotoxins A and S
B. Elastase
C. Haemolysins
D. All of these

Ans. D.

1428. Balanced growth is defined as

A. Cultures undergoing balanced growth while maintaining a constant chemical composition
B. Balancing the growth while controlling the pH
C. Balancing the growth while controlling the temperature
D. Balancing the growth while changing the nutrient composition

Ans. A.

1429. Semi-solid media, prepared with agar at concentrations of 0.5% or less are useful for the cultivation of

A. Microaerophillic bacteria
B. Lactobacilli
C. E.coli
D. All of these

Ans. A.

1430. The cell mass can be measured optically by determining the amount of light scattered by a suspension of cells. The measurements are usually at a wavelength of

A. 300-400 nm
B. 400-500nm
C. 500-600nm
D. 600-700nm

Ans. D.

1431. Which of the following is not an indirect method for the measurement of cell mass ?

A. Nutrient composition
B. Cell dry weight
C. Viscosity
D. Heat evolution

Ans. B.

1432. Callus cultures are amorphous cell aggregates arising from the unorganized growth of explants on an

A. Liquid medium
B. Solid nutrient medium
C. Aseptic solid nutrient medium
D. Solid or liquid medium

Ans. C.

1433. The protoplast can be used to

A. Modify genetic information
B. Create plant hybrid
C. Study plant viral infections
D. All of these

Ans. D.

1434. Which of the following is incorrect ?

A. Mammalian cells are larger and more complex than microorganisms
B. Their growth rate is very fast compared to microorganisms
C. Mammalian cells are fragile
D. Most animal cells only grow when attached to surface

Ans. B.

1435. The size of a single plant cell is usually within the range of

A. 10-20 μm in diameter and 25-100 μm long
B. 20-40 μm in diameter and 100-200 μm long
C. 40-60 μm in diameter and 200-300 μm long
D. 60-80 μm in diameter and 300-400 μm long

Ans. B.

1436. Which of the following is incorrect ?

A. Plant cells are larger than the bacterial or fungus cells

B. Plant cells tend to grow in clumps

C. Plant cells are less sensitive to shear than microbial cells

D. Plant cells are more genetically unstable than microbial cells

Ans. C.

1437. The archaebacterium Halobacterium, an extreme halophile, and Sulfolobus, a thermoacidophile, can be cultured in the presence of antibiotics such as streptomycin and chloramphenicol because

A. They contain ether-linked isoprenoids in their plasma membrane

B. They lack murein in their cell wall

C. They contain 80S, as opposed to 70S, ribosomes

D. All of the above

Ans. B.

1438. The isolation of the gonorrhoea - causing organisms, Neisseria gonorrhoeae,from a clinical specimen is facilitated by the use of media containing

A. Cellulose B. Certain antibiotics

C. Succinate D. None of these

Ans. B.

1439. Anchorage -dependent cells require

A. Wettable surface for growth B. Dry surface for growth

C. Either A & B D. Nothing to do with surface

Ans. A.

1440. Stringent anaerobes can be grown in a media by taking special measure as

A. Boiling the media for several minutes

B. Addition of cysteine

C. Passing through oxygen-free nitrogen

D. Any of these

Ans. D.

1441. Radical shifts in pH can be prevented by incorporating

A. A buffer B. An oxidizing agent

C. A reducing agent D. Any of these

Ans. A.

1442. Lactobacilli grow best under

A. Strict anaerobic conditions

B. Microaerophilic conditions in presence of 5% CO_2 and pH6

C. Microaerophilic conditions in presence of 3% CO_2 and pH5

D. Microaerophilic conditions in presence of 2% CO_2 and pH4

Ans. B.

1443. Which of the following genera is included in the family Bacteroidaceae?

A. Bacteroides B. Fusobacterium

C. Leptotrichia D. All of these

Ans. D.

1444. The bacteria which is predominant flora of the human gut is

A. E.coli B. Clostridium perfringens

C. Bacteroides D. Actinomyces

Ans. B.

1445. The current genus name of a saccharolytic group of Bacteroides is

A. Porphyromonas B. Bacteroides

C. Prevotella D. None of these

Ans. A.

1446. Colonies resembling molar teeth are produced by

A. Nocardia brasiliensis B. N. asteroids

C. Actinomyces israelii D. Actinomadura madurae

Ans. C.

1447. Which of the following bacterial colonies fluoresce brick-red in UV light?

A. B. gingivalis B. B. melaninogenicus

C. Bacteroides fragilis D. B. levii

Ans. B.

1448. Which of the following bacteria is acid-fast ?

A. Actinomyces B. Nocardia

C. Streptomyces D. Corynebacterium

Ans. B.

1449. Lactobacilli constitute the normal flora of

A. Prepubertal vagina B. Adult vagina

C. Post-menopausal vagina D. None of these

Ans. B.

1450. Which of the following bacteria is gram-negative cocci ?

A. Veillonella B. Peptococcus

C. Peptostreptococcus D. Sporosarcina

Ans. A.

1451. The commonest species of Bacteroides in fragilis group, which causes human infection, is

A. B vulgates B. B fragilis

C. B ovatus D. B merdae

Ans. B.

1452. The commonest bacterial cause of cervicofacial actinomycosis is

A. A. Naeslundii B. A. Viscosus

C. A. Israelii D. A. Meyeri

Ans. C.

1453. Which of the following bacteria is moderately saccharolytic?

A. Bacteriodes fragilis B. B. gingivalis

C. B.melaninogenicus D. B. levii

Ans. C.

1454. Which of the following can be identified by milk ring test?

A. Brucellosis B. Salmonellosis

C. Bovine tuberculosis D. All of these

Ans. A.

1455. For brucellosis, 2 ME agglutination test is used to identify

A. IgG B. IgM

C. IgA D. IgE

Ans. A.

1456. Human transmission of Brucellae occurs by

A. Ingestion of contaminated meat B. Direct contact with animal tissues

C. Ingestion of infected milk D. All of these

Ans. D.

1457. Agglutination test for Brucella mainly identifies which class of antibodies ?

A. IgG B. IgM

C. IgA D. IgE

Ans. B.

1458. The most pathogenic Brucella spp for man is

A. B. melitensis B. B. abortus

C. B. suis D. B. canis

Ans. A.

1459. Brucella are

A. Cocci B. Rods

C. Coccobacilli D. Very short rods

Ans. D.

1460. Which of the following medium are used to differentiate the colonies of Vibrio cholerae and V. parahaemolyticus?

A. Alkaline bile salt B. Thiosulphate-citrate-bile-sucrose

C. MacConkey D. All of the above

Ans. B.

1461. Which of the followings can be used to differentiate between classical and El Tor biotypes of Vibrio cholerae?

A. Sensitivity to Mukerjee's group IV phage

B. Agglutination of fowl RBCs

C. Sensitivity to polymyxin B

D. All of these

Ans. D.

1462. Which of the following biotypes of Vibrio cholerae are prevalent in India?

A. EI Tor B. Classical

C. Both A & B D. None of these

Ans. A.

1463. Which of the following bacteria is associated with food poisoning due to consumption of sea fish?

A. Vibrio parahaemolyticus B. V. alginolyticus

C. V. vulnificus D. All of these

Ans. A.

1464. Which of the following conditions can be caused by Plesiomonas ?

A. Septicaemia B. Septicaemia

C. Cellulites D. All of these

Ans. D.

1465. Acute diarrhoeal disease resembling cholera can be caused due to

A. Aeromonas hydrophila B. Vibrio vulnificus

C. V. Alginolyticus D. All of these

Ans. A.

1466. The transport medium for Vibrio cholerae can be

A. Venkatraman-Ramakrishnan medium

B. Selenite F broth

C. Tetrathionate broth

D. Nutrient broth

Ans. A.

1467. Which of the following does not cause wound infection following exposure to sea water or infected shellfish?

A. Vibrio vulnificus

B. V. Alginolyticus

C. V. Cholera

D. Aeromonas

Ans. C.

1468. The test(s) used for the assay of cholera toxin is/are

A. Radioimmunoassay

B. Enzyme-linked immunosorbent assay

C. Morphological changes in Chinese hamster ovary cells

D. All of the above

Ans. D.

1469. The DNA coding for the production of cholera toxin in Vibrio cholerae is on the

A. Phage

B. Plasmid

C. Chromosome

D. Transposon

Ans. C.

1470. The halophilic bacteria is/are

A. V. Alginolyticus

B. V. Vulnificus

C. Vibrio parahaemolyticus

D. All of these

Ans. D.

1471. Which of the following toxin resembles cholera toxin?

A. Stable toxin of E.coli

B. Diphtheria toxin

C. Labile toxin of E.coli

D. Tetanus toxin

Ans. C.

1472. The plasmid-mediated properties is/are

A. Fermentation of lactose

B. Production of enterotoxin

C. Resistance to antibiotics

D. All of these

Ans. D.

1473. In the extracellular medium, DNA-degrading enzymes would likely be to prevent transfer of DNA by

A. Conjugal transfer by a self transmissible plasmid

B. Generalized phage transduction

C. Natural transformation

D. None of these

Ans. C.

1474. What is the term used for a segment of DNA with one or more genes in the centre and the two ends carrying inverted repeat sequences of nucleotides?

A. Plasmid

B. Transpososn

C. Insertion sequence

D. None of these

Ans. B.

1475. The plasmids can be eliminated from a cell by the process known as

A. Curing

B. Breaking

C. Fixing

D. Expulsion

Ans. A.

1476. Recombination of virus genomes occurs

A. By transduction

B. By transcription

C. Simultaneous infection of a host cell by two viruses with homologous chromosomes

D. By transformation

Ans. C.

1477. The type of recombination that commonly occurs between a pair of homologous DNA sequences is

A. Mutagenic recombination

B. Site-specific recombination

C. Replicative recombination

D. General recombination

Ans. D.

1478. Which of the following statement describes plasmids ?

A. Another name for a protoplast

B. A complex membrane structure that covers the chromosome of bacteria

C. Small, circular DNA molecules that can exist independently of chromosomes commonly found in bacteria

D. None of the above

Ans. C.

1479. In lysogeny

A. A bacteriophage transfers bacterial DNA

B. A bacteriophage transfers bacterial DNA

C. DNA-degrading enzymes in the extracellular medium would stop the process

D. A bacteriophage genome is integrated into the bacterial genome

Ans. D.

1480. A microarray differs from a gene fusion in that, it

A. Carries DNA segments from many different genes

B. Is not constructed by cloning

C. Gives direct measurement of mRNA level

D. All of the above

Ans. D.

1481. Who discovered transposons (jumping genes)?

A. Abelson B. Harvey

C. McClintock D. Griffith

Ans. C.

1482. Which type of plasmid can exist with or without being integrated into the host's chromosome?

A. Medisome B. Lysosome

C. Lysogen D. Episome

Ans. D.

1483. The main difference between a self-transmissible and a mobilizable plasmid is that the self-transmissible plasmid

A. Transfers both strands of the plasmid DNA

B. Carries genes encoding the mating apparatus

C. Transfers antibiotic resistance genes

D. Usually has a transposon inserted into it

Ans. B.

1484. Which of the following is the cause for drug resistance in tuberculosis ?

A. Mutation B. Transduction

C. Transformation D. Conjugation

Ans. A.

1485. The transposase gene encodes an enzyme that facilitate

A. Viral replication within a genome

B. General recombination

C. Site-specific integration of transposable elements

D. None of the above

Ans. C.

1486. The term used for plasmids possessing both RTF and r determinants is

A. Non self-transmissible plasmids B. Non conjugative plasmids

C. Conjugative plasmids D. None of these

Ans. C.

1487. Diagnostic DNA probes have been developed for

A. M. tuberculosis B. Hepatitis B virus

C. HIV D. All of the above

Ans. D.

1488. Which of the following statement(s) is/are true in regards to F^+ x F^- mating events?

A. DNA is transferred from F^- to F^+ cells

B. DNA is transferred from F^+ to F^- cells

C. No DNA is transferred because F^- cells are unable to perform conjugation

D. No DNA is transferred because F^+ cells are unable to perform conjugation

Ans. B.

1489. Which of the following type of recombination does not require homologous sequences and is important for the integration of viral genomes into bacterial chromosomes?

A. Mutagenic recombination B. Site specific recombination

C. Replicative recombination D. General recombination

Ans. B.

1490. What information can be generated by interrupted mating experiments?

A. Levels of DNA homology B. Bacterial maps

C. DNA nucleotide sequences D. Proteomics of the bacteria

Ans. B.

1491. Which of the following transport bacterial DNA to other bacteria via bacteriophages?

A. Conjugation B. Transduction

C. Transformation D. Translation

Ans. B.

1492. When composite transposons are formed

A. A small deletion occurs in the transposase gene of an IS element

B. A small deletion occurs in the transposase gene of an IS element and plasmid is integrated

C. An IS element integrates with another IS element with the help of a plasmid

D. Two IS elements integrate into a chromosome with only a small distance separating them

Ans. D.

1493. Which of the following plasmids do not possess information for self transfer to another cell?

A. Cryptic plasmids B. Conjugative plasmids

C. Non-conjugative plasmids D. None of these

Ans. C.

1494. The term used for acquisition of naked DNA from its environment and its incorporation in their genome by a bacterium is

A. Transformation B. Lysogenic conversion

C. Conjugation D. Transduction

Ans. A.

1495. What is term used for a bacterial cell that is able to take up naked DNA?

A. Complementary B. Liable

C. Competent D. Infected

Ans. C.

1496. Penicillin resistance in Staphylococci is acquired due to

A. Conjugation B. Mutation

C. Transformation D. Transduction

Ans. D.

1497. The plasmid which makes the host more pathogenic is

A. F factors B. Metabolic plasmid

C. Virulence plasmid D. None of these

Ans. C.

1498. The expression of gene X (which has promoter Px) is to be monitored. A gene fusion construction for carrying this work will

A. Have Px but not the rest of the X coding region

B. Have the promoter of lacZ or some other reporter gene

C. Allow to monitor the expression of all genes with a promoter similar in sequence to Px

D. Give the same information as from a microarray

Ans. A.

1499. The transducing particles carry only specific portions of the bacterial genome in which of the following transduction?

A. Specialized transduction B. General transduction
C. Abortive transduction D. None of these

Ans. A.

1500. The correct term for the transfer of genetic material between bacteria in direct physical contact is

A. Conjugation B. Transformation
C. Replication D. Transduction

Ans. A.

1501. Plasmid that carries genes encoding enzymes, which degrade substances such as aromatic compounds, pesticides or sugar are

A. F factors B. Metabolic plasmid
C. Virulence plasmid D. None of these

Ans. B.

1502. R factors involved in plant-microbe interactions are

A. Plant proteins
B. Bacterial proteins
C. Essential for transfer of DNA to plant cells
D. Also called opines

Ans. A.

1503. Which of the following is used by microbial geneticists as a tool ?

A. Bacteriophage B. Plasmids
C. Transposable elements D. All of these

Ans. D.

1504. Which of the following type of recombination does not require homologous sequences and is utilized by mobile genetic elements that move about chromosomes?

A. Mutagenic recombination B. Site specific recombination
C. Replicative recombination D. General recombination

Ans. C.

1505. Which of the following term describes the relationship between a virus and host where no new viral particles are produced and the viral genome is replicated along with host chromosome?

A. Lysogeny B. Lysis
C. Transformation D. Conjugation

Ans. A.

1506. Inverted repeat sequences at each end and a gene encoding transposase is contained in which of the following transposable element?

A. Composite transposon
B. Insertion element
C. Virus
D. Plasmid

Ans. B.

1507. F factor plasmids play a major role in

A. Conjugation
B. Replication
C. Transduction
D. Transcription

Ans. A.

1508. Which of the following genetic elements carry the genes required for integration into host chromosomes?

A. Replicon
B. Plasmids
C. Transposons
D. Tandons

Ans. C.

1509. The chromosomal genes, possessing fertility factor is known as

A. R factor
B. F prime factor
C. Hfr
D. F factor

Ans. B.

1510. Which of the following statement can describe horizontal transfer ?

A. The synthesis of protein in RNA
B. The transmission of genetic information from one independent, mature organism to another
C. The transmission of genetic information from parent to offspring
D. The synthesis of RNA from a DNA template

Ans. B.

1511. Genetic variations are

A. Temporary
B. Influenced by the environment
C. Stable
D. Not heritable

Ans. C.

1512. The mutation which will not affect the length of a protein is

A. Nonsense mutation
B. Missense mutation
C. Frameshift mutation
D. All of these

Ans. B.

1513. Changes in which of the following characterizes mutations ?

A. Phenotype
B. Genotype
C. Both A & B
D. None of these

Ans. C.

1514. Which of the following(s) is/are steps in excision repair mechanisms ?

A. Excision
B. Incision
C. Ligation
D. All of these

Ans. D.

1515. The whole-genome shotgun sequencing approach depends primarily on

A. Rapidly sequencing thousands of small randomly cloned fragments
B. Methodical sequencing a few large cloned fragments of DNA
C. Sequencing the bacterial chromosome while it is still intact
D. All of the above

Ans. A.

1516. What was the first eukaryotic chromosome to be sequenced ?

A. Yeast chromosome III
B. Yeast chromosome XI
C. Arabidopsis chromosome IV
D. None of these

Ans. A.

1517. Which of the following mutations arise without exposure to external agents ?

A. Spontaneous mutations
B. Analogous mutations
C. Induced mutations
D. None of these

Ans. A.

1518. Due to which of the following DNA repair mechanisms, one is able to distinguish newly synthesized DNA strands from older one?

A. New strands do not contain cytosine bases
B. New strands are lower in molecular size
C. Old strands are methylated while new strands are not
D. New strands are methylated while old strands are not

Ans. C.

1519. Which of the following bacterial genome was sequenced first ?

A. E.coli
B. S. pneumoniae
C. H. influenzae
D. S. thermophilus

Ans. C.

1520. A nonsense mutation may result into

A. An abnormal elongation of a polypeptide

B. A large deletion within the reading frame of a gene

C. A premature termination of the synthesis of a polypeptide

D. Modification of mRNA

Ans. C.

1521. Which of the following mutation affects only a single nucleotide?

A. Aerial mutation
B. Site mutation

C. Point mutation
D. Regional mutation

Ans. C.

1522. When mutations involve vital functions so that the mutants are nonviable, it is a

A. Nonsense mutation
B. Lethal mutation

C. Transversion
D. None of these

Ans. B.

1523. A mutagen is defined as

A. An enzyme that repairs mutations

B. A chemical or physical agent that induces mutations

C. An inhibitor of gene modification

D. A molecule which stabilizes DNA thus prevents mutations from occurring

Ans. B.

1524. The DNA sequences of rRNA genes can be used to

A. Assess relatedness of eukaryotes but not prokaryotes

B. Obtain a tentative identification of a new microorganism

C. Predict the pulsed field gel pattern of a microorganism

D. Predict whether a bacteria will be gram-positive or gram-negative

Ans. B.

1525. A nonsense mutation introduced into the DNA sequence of a gene may

A. Cause premature termination of the mRNA

B. Shorten the length of the protein encoded by the gene

C. Have no effect on the transcript or protein made

D. Cause a shift in reading frame

Ans. B.

1526. Which of these mechanisms for thymine dimers repair lead to mutations?

A. Excision repair B. Photoreactivation

C. SOS repair D. Never leads to mutation

Ans. C.

1527. Frame shift mutation may occur as a result of

A. Formation of a thymine dimer B. Deamination of cytosine to Uracil

C. Conversion of guanine to xanthine D. None of the above

Ans. D.

1528. Thymine dimers are directly repaired with the help of visible light by process known as

A. Phosphorylation B. Excision repair

C. Photosynthesis D. Photoreactivation

Ans. D.

1529. The promoter on an expression vector used to overproduce proteins in bacteria is

A. A bacterial promoter

B. Expressed both in bacteria and mammalian cells

C. Not a regulated promoter

D. The natural promoter of the gene being cloned

Ans. A.

1530. Differentiation of four different bases in automated sequencing systems is that each base has

A. Different radioactive tag B. Cytosine at start

C. Unique antibody bound to it D. Distinctive fluorescent tag

Ans. D.

1531. Which binding is inhibited by pactamycin ?

A. Aminoacyl-tRNA to the A-site of 30S subunit

B. Initiator-tRNA to 30S/40S initiation complexes

C. Peptidyl t-RNA to the 50S subunit

D. Formation of peptide bond in P site

Ans. B.

1532. Which of the following act as the blueprint or template for the process of protein synthesis that takes place on ribosomes?

A. rRNA B. DNA

C. tRNA D. mRNA

Ans. D.

1533. Negative regulation of protein synthesis is accomplished by

A. Allosteric inhibition

B. The binding of RNA polymerase to the promoter

C. The binding of a repressor to the DNA

D. The binding of a repressor to the RNA polymerase

Ans. C.

1534. Site in the ribosome from which the tRNA donates amino acids to the growing polypeptide chain is

A. P site B. O site

C. T site D. A site

Ans. A.

1535. When was the genetic code completed ?

A. 1958 B. 1952

C. 1966 D. 1968

Ans. C.

1536. Which stop codon has been found to encode selenocysteine ?

A. UAA B. UAG

C. UGA D. AGA

Ans. C.

1537. Which of the following is a nontranslated sequence located between the transcription and the translation start site?

A. Ending frame B. Leader sequence

C. Trailer sequence D. Reading frame

Ans. B.

1538. Which phage always carries a small piece of E.coli genome ?

A. Lambda B. Mu

C. T4 D. T3

Ans. B.

1539. The final step of gene expression is protein synthesis, which is also known as

A. Replication B. Translation

C. Transcription D. None of these

Ans. B.

1540. What is the maximum number of different amino acids in a polypeptide chain coded by the synthetic polyribonucleotides (UCAG) 5?

A. One
B. Two
C. Three
D. Four

Ans. C.

1541. What is the direct cause of cell death by diphtheria toxin ?

A. Formation of an ion channel in the cell membrane
B. Inactivation of a translational elongation factor
C. Induction of apoptosis
D. None of these

Ans. B.

1542. The development of global regulatory systems in prokaryotes

A. Determines the exact location of the cell on the globe
B. Aids in DNA replication
C. Determines the exact location of the replication site
D. Regulates many genes under varying environmental conditions

Ans. D.

1543. The interaction between the mRNA and tRNA determined the position of amino acid in a polypeptide sequence.This is called the

A. Stagerivity
B. Wobble hypothesis
C. Promiscuity
D. Adaptor hypothesis

Ans. D.

1544. What are the Svedberg values for the subunits of the 70S ribosomes of E.coli ?

A. 40S and 30S
B. 50S and 20S
C. 50S and 30S
D. 40S and 20S

Ans. C.

1545. Which of the following three codons translate as serine (Ser) ?

A. AGU
B. CGA
C. CAU
D. AUG

Ans. A.

1546. The role of molecular chaperones is to

A. Facilitate binding of ribosomes to mRNA
B. Degrade newly synthesized polypeptides that contain inaccurate sequences
C. Facilitate binding of RNA polymerase to DNA
D. Aid a newly synthesized polypeptide in folding to its proper shape

Ans. D.

1547. What is the action of tetracycline in prokaryotes?

A. It blocks translocation reaction on ribosomes

B. It blocks peptidyl transferase reaction on ribosomes

C. It blocks the binding of amino-acyl tRNA to the A site of ribosomes

D. Not known with certainty

Ans. C.

1548. A quorum sensing system

A. Detects a signal from the external environment

B. Senses a compound produced by the bacterium itself

C. Consists of a sensor component that phosphorylates a regulatory protein

D. Controls the activity of ribosomes directly

Ans. B.

1549. The Shine-Delgarno sequence is

A. Trailer sequence

B. A stop codon

C. The reading frame of a gene

D. A short sequence that acts as a ribosomal binding site

Ans. D.

1550. Which of the following statement is correct?

A. The size and sequence of introns can be deduced from the cDNA sequence

B. Restriction endonuclease can cleave ss and dsDNA both

C. Restriction fragment length polymorphism (RFLP) is usually formed in coding sequence of a gene

D. Amino acid sequence of a protein can be deduced from corresponding cDNA nucleotide

Ans. D.

1551. What was the first bacterial genome sequenced and made public?

A. Bacillus subtilis

B. Escherichia coli

C. Haemophilus influenzae

D. No bacterial genome has been sequenced yet

Ans. C.

1552. Which of the following modified amino acid is used at the starting of most prokaryotic proteins?

A. N-formylserine
B. N-formylmethionine
C. N-formylleucine
D. N-formylalanine

Ans. B.

1553. During amino acid activation a(n)

A. Amino acid is bound to tRNA
B. Amino acid is bound to mRNA
C. Methyl group is attached to rRNA
D. Methyl group is attached to an amino acid

Ans. A.

1554. The nonsense codon (s) is/are

A. UAG
B. UAA
C. UGA
D. all of these

Ans. D.

1555. Which of the following defines an open reading frame (ORF)?

A. A sequence of genome in bacteriophage
B. The sequence of a complete genome
C. A plasmid vector used in genome sequencing
D. A possible gene predicted by DNA sequencing

Ans. D.

1556. Three stop codons, which aids in termination of translation are also known as

A. Pause codons
B. Nonsense codons
C. Missense codons
D. Antisense codons

Ans. B.

1557. The ribosome binding site

A. Forms a stem-loop structure in the RNA
B. Is located upstream of the promoter sequence
C. Is located immediately upstream of the start codon
D. Is more likely to be associated with an operon than with a gene encoding a single protein

Ans. C.

1558. Which of the following molecule catalyzes the transpeptidation reaction?

A. RNA polymerase
B. Peptidyl transferase
C. DNA ligase
D. DNA polymerase

Ans. B.

1559. Which of the termination codon is called amber?

A. UAA B. UAG

C. UGA D. AUG

Ans. B.

1560. Which of the following infection(s) can be diagnosed by the use of polymerase chain reaction?

A. HIV-1 and HIV-2 B. Hepatitis B virus

C. M. tuberculosis D. All the above

Ans. D.

1561. Polymerase chain reaction basically consists of

A. 2 steps B. 3 steps

C. 4 steps D. 5 steps

Ans. B.

1562. The PCR/sequencing approach to rRNA is most likely to give information about

A. The species to which the bacteria are most closely related

B. Morphology of the bacterium

C. The type of energy metabolism the bacterium has

D. Whether the bacterium is motile

Ans. A.

1563. The efficiency of amplification in PCR in later cycles is reduced due to

A. Reduction in substrate concentration

B. Insufficient enzyme and time to synthesize mass quantity of DNA

C. Build up of PCR product which competes with primers for hybrid formation

D. All of these

Ans. D.

1564. The original enzyme(s) used in PCR reaction is/are known as

A. E. coli DNA polymerase B. E. coli RNA polymerase

C. Taq polymerase D. All of these

Ans. A.

1565. RNA populations can also be used as PCR templates after reverse transcription into

A. cDNA B. tRNA

C. mDNA D. rRNA

Ans. A.

1566. The cloning step in PCR/sequencing analysis of microbial communities is necessary for

A. The amplification process

B. Preventing contamination by outside DNA

C. Separating the different rRNA gene sequences in the mixture

D. None of these

Ans. C.

1567. The template for PCR is

A. RNA

B. ssDNA

C. dsDNA

D. either B or C

Ans. D.

1568. Large parasites such as helminthes may be killed extracellularly by the action of

A. Basophils

B. Monocytes

C. Eosinohils

D. Neutrophils

Ans. C.

1569. Which of the following is correct for CD8 T cells?

A. CD8 T cells only recognize virus-infected cells

B. CD8 T cell receptor recognizes epitopes that are also commonly recognized by B cells

C. In the thymus, CD8 T cells undergo positive selection only, whereas CD4 T cells undergo negative selection only

D. CD8 T cells can kill individual virus-infected cells in a contact dependent fashion

Ans. D.

1570. Passive immunization is done for

A. Tuberculosis

B. Diphtheria

C. Enteric fever

D. All of these

Ans. B.

1571. Which of the following is correct for isoantigens ?

A. They are antigens found in all members of different species

B. They are antigens found in some members of a species

C. They are antigens found in all members of a species

D. They are antigens found in some members of different species

Ans. B.

1572. Numerous antibodies can be prepared, against one antigen, each binds to unique epitopes. How is this antibody diversity generated?

A. By rearrangements of the DNA encoding the variable regions of the heavy and light chains

B. By the combination of different heavy and light chains that form the antigen binding site

C. Antibody proteins can physically change their shape to bind different epitopes

D. Both A and B

Ans. D.

1573. Which of the following expresses CD3 surface antigen?

A. Granulocytes B. T cells

C. Monocytes D. B cells

Ans. B.

1574. Polymorphonuclear leukocytes (or PMNs)

A. Can be attracted to the site of an infection following activbation of complement

A. Are derived from bone marrow stem cells

C. Are a type of phagocyte that can engulf and kill bacteria

D. All of the above

Ans. D.

1575. Major Histocompatibility Complex (MHC) is a collection of genes arrayed on

A. Chromosome 21 in man, chromosome 6 in mice

B. Chromosome 6 in man, chromosome 21 in mice

C. Chromosome 17 in man, chromosome 6 in mice

D. Chromosome 6 in man, chromosome 17 in mice

Ans. D.

1576. CD8 surface antigen is present in

A. T_c cells B. T_s cells

C. Both A and B D. None of these

Ans. C.

1577. Treatment with bacterial endotoxins results blast formation in

A. B cells B. T cells

C. Monocytes D. None of these

Ans. A.

1578. Cytotoxic T-cells can be recognized by which of the following cell surface marker?

A. CD4 B. CD7

C. CD8 D. CD9

Ans. C.

1579. Which is not an antigen-presenting cell (or APC) ?

A. B cells

B. Polymorphonuclear leukocyte (or PMN)

C. Dendritic cells

D. All of the above

Ans. B.

1580. Chemically an antigen may be

A. Lipid B. Protein

C. Polysaccharide D. Any of these

Ans. D.

1581. T cell receptors (or TCR) on CD4+ T cells

A. Recognize peptides not associated with MHC molecules

B. Recognize peptides associated with MHC class I molecules

C. Recognize peptides associated with MHC class II molecules

D. Are secreted out into the environment to bind antigens

Ans. C.

1582. Which of the following proteins would not need localization signal?

A. A nuclear protein

B. A cytosolic protein

C. A protein bound to the endoplasmic reticulum membrane

D. A cell surface protein

Ans. B.

1583. Following are the defences of the colon except

A. sIgA B. Fast flow rate

C. Dense resident microbiota D. Mucus

Ans. B.

1584. Natural killer cells are involved in

A. Tumour rejection

B. Allograft rejection

C. Nonspecific killing of virus transformed target cells

D. All of these

Ans. D.

1585. Which of the following(s) is/are the determinants of antigenicity?

A. Chemical nature
B. Size of the antigen
C. Foreignness
D. All of these

Ans. D.

1586. Which of the following is correct ?

A. All T Cells are CD4+
B. An epitope can have multiple antigens
C. T Cell receptors are generated by random assortment of gene cassettes
D. MHC Class II molecules are generated by random assortment of gene cassettes

Ans. C.

1587. Immunity is not long lasting to

A. Influenza
B. Whooping cough
C. Diphtheria
D. Mumps

Ans. A.

1588. Lysozyme is present in

A. Sweat
B. CSF
C. Urine
D. Saliva

Ans. D.

1589. Macrophages are professional antigen- presenting cells. The protein molecule through which they present antigen in human is

A. Actin
B. Interleukin
C. HLA
D. CD8

Ans. D.

1590. The role of the M cell is to

A. Trap virus in mucus and prevent entry
B. Induce apoptosis in virus-infected small intestinal epithelia cells
C. Pass bacteria or virus to underlying macrophages for processing and presentation of antigen
D. Use their cilia to propel mucus out of the small intestine

Ans. C.

1591. Which of the following statements is false regarding B cells?

A. B cells can undergo class switching and produce a different antibody type

B. Bone marrow stem cells migrate to the thymus and develop into B cells

C. B cells synthesize antibodies and put them on their cell surface

D. B cells that recognize high concentrations of antigens (self) in the absence of other signals undergo apoptosis in the bone marrow

Ans. B.

1592. Why the bacterium Treponema pallidum is difficult to culture?

A. Because it requires a great deal of water to reproduce

B. Because it is unable to use carbohydrates as an energy source

C. Because it lacks the genes needed for TCA cycle and oxidative phosphorylation

D. Because it requires extremely low temperature at which water freezes

Ans. C.

1593. What is the range of minimum set of genes required for life?

A. 50-100 genes B. 250-350 genes

C. 1000-1500 genes D. 155-2000 genes

Ans. B.

1594. The flow of genetic material in microbial cells usually takes place from

A. RNA through DNA to proteins B. Proteins through RNA to DNA

C. DNA through RNA to proteins D. None of these

Ans. C.

1595. Which of the following is used for determining the location of specific genes within the genome?

A. Genomics B. Annotation

C. Cloning D. Proteomics

Ans. B.

1596. Proteomics is

A. The study of algal genomes

B. A branch of quantum physics dealing with proteins

C. The study of formation of lipo-protein in animals

D. The study of the entire collection of proteins expressed by an organism

Ans. D.

1597. Which of the following is concerned with the management and analysis of biological data using computers?

A. Biophysics
B. Bioinformatics
C. Genomics
D. Biomechanics

Ans. B.

1598. Which type of genomics studies the transcripts and proteins expressed by a genome?

A. Comparative genomics
B. Structural genomics
C. Proteogenomics
D. Functional genomics

Ans. D.

1599. Which of the following is the study of the molecular organization of genomes, their information content and the gene products they encode?

A. Genetics
B. Ergonomics
C. Genomics
D. Bioinformatics

Ans. C.

1600. The word, used for the small solid supports onto which are spotted hundreds of thousands of tiny drops of DNA that can be used to screen gene expression, is

A. Southern blot
B. Cloning library
C. DNA microarrays
D. Northern blot

Ans. C.

1601. Which of the following organisms has the smallest genome?

A. H. influenzae
B. M. genitalium
C. M. tuberculosis
D. None of these

Ans. B.

1602. Studies of similarities and differences among the genomes of multiple organisms is carried out in

A. Comparative genomics
B. Proteomics
C. Functional genomics
D. Structural genomics

Ans. A.

1603. Tissue plasminogen activator is

A. A vitamin
B. An enzyme
C. A chemical that stimulates tissue differentiation
D. Amino acid

Ans. B.

1604. Always present known disease is

A. Pandemic B. Prodemic

C. Endemic D. Epidemic

Ans. C.

1605. Long term degenerative diseases are including

A. Coronary Heart Disease (CHD) B. Malnutrition

C. Mental diseases D. Sickle cell anaemia

Ans. A.

1606. Protocyst are known to cause

A. Cholera

B. Acquired Immune Deficiency Syndrome (HIV/AIDS)

C. Malaria

D. Measles

Ans. C.

1607. Vaccination is a major control measure for

A. Infectious diseases B. Genetic diseases

C. Long term degenerative diseases D. Deficiency diseases

Ans. A.

1608. Viruses do not cause

A. Acquired Immune Deficiency Syndrome (HIV/AIDS)

B. Small pox

C. Measles

D. Malaria

Ans. D.

1609. A patient suffering from pneumonia and tuberculosis was found to have very low CD4+ T cells. In all probability the primary causative infectious agent belongs to

A. Klebsiella family B. Mycobacterium family

C. Retrovirus family D. Streptococci family

Ans. C.

1610. Milk is deficient in which vitamins?

A. Vitamin C B. Vitamin A

C. Vitamin B2 D. Vitamin K

Ans. A.

1611. Milk is deficient of which mineral?

A. Phosphorus B. Sodium

C. Iron D. Potassium

Ans. C.

1612. A characteristic feature of marasmus is

A. Severe hypoalbuminemia B. Normal epinephrine level

C. Mild muscle wasting D. Low insulin and high cortisol level

Ans. D.

1613. Obesity generally reflects excess intake of energy and is often associated with the development of

A. Nervousness

B. Non-insulin dependent diabetes mellitus

C. Hepatitis

D. Colon cancer

Ans. B.

1614. Atherosclerosis and coronary heart diseases are associated with the diet

A. High in total fat and saturated fat B. Low in protein

C. High in protein D. High in carbohydrate

Ans. A.

1615. Cerebrovasular disease and hypertension is associated with

A. High calcium intake B. High salt intake

C. Low calcium intake D. Low salt intake

Ans. B.

1616. Clearly defined nucleus, mitochondria in a large central vacuole and chloroplasts, indicate the group of organisms from

A. Bacteria B. Fungi

C. Plants D. Animals

Ans. C.

1617. In which of the following cell types more cellular detail can be observed using an electron microscope compared to a light microscope?

A. Animal B. Bacterial

C. Protist D. All of these

Ans. D.

1618. BRACl, an inherited form of breast cancer, regulates cell division by
   A. Binding to a DNA sequence
   B. Complexing with cyclins
   C. Binding to the cell outer membrane
   D. Binding to the protein RAD 51 which repairs DNA damage

Ans. D.

1619. Metastasis involves
   A. Ability of cells to dissolve cellular matrix
   B. Metalloprotein levels
   C. Decreased levels of proteins that regulate metalloproteins
   D. All of the above

Ans. D.

1620. Why Deinococcus radiodurans is able to survive massive exposure to radiation ?
   A. Because it produces a thick shell which acts as a shield from the radiation
   B. Because it has unique DNA repair mechanisms
   C. Because its cell wall contains radioactive elements
   D. Because it has many copies of genes encoding DNA repair

Ans. D.

1621. Which of the following types of Clostridium perfringens produces alpha toxin most abundantly?
   A. Type A
   B. Type B
   C. Type C
   D. Type D

Ans. A.

1622. Humulin is
   A. Carbohydrate
   B. Protein
   C. Fat
   D. Antibiotic

Ans. B.

1623. Which of the following can be application of fermentation ?
   A. Tanning of leather
   B. Curing of tea
   C. Production of vine
   D. All of these

Ans. D.

1624. Enzyme immobilization is
   A. Conversion of an active enzyme into inactive form
   B. Providing enzyme with protective covering
   C. Changing a soluble enzyme into insoluble state
   D. Changing pH so that enzyme is not able to carry out its function

Ans. B.

1625. Biogas is produced by

A. Aerobic breakdown of biomass

B. Anaerobic break down of biomass

C. With the help of methanogenic bacteria

D. Both B and C

Ans. D.

1626. Virulence of a microorganism can be best described as

A. The ability to penetrate into the host tissue

B. The ability to colonize in the host

C. The ability to produce a pathological symptom

D. The ability to utilize the machinery of the host

E. All the above

Ans. C.

1627. A common type of nosocomial infection is

A. Urinary tract infection B. Meningitis

C. Cellulitis D. Gastroenteritis

Ans. A.

1628. Pathogens

A. Are plant diseases B. Are not animal diseases

C. Cause infectious diseases D. Are known to cause carcinogens

Ans. C.

1629. Which of the following is predominantly proteolytic?

A. C. sporogenes B. C. histolyticum

C. Both A and B D. C. septicum

Ans. C.

1630. Which of the following properties are the characteristics of tetanospasmin?

A. It is a heat labile protein B. It is a neurotoxin

C. It can be toxoided D. All of these

Ans. D.

1631. Types of exotoxin, most commonly associated with botulism in man, is/are?

A. Type A B. Type B

C. Type E D. All of these

Ans. D.

1632. Nagler's reaction is useful for the identification of

A. C. tetani
B. C. perfringens
C. C. botulinum
D. C. Difficile

Ans. B.

1633. The most toxic exotoxin is

A. Tetanus toxin
B. Diphtheria toxin
C. Botulinum toxin
D. Cholera toxin

Ans. C.

1634. Which of the following species of Clostridium is predominantly sacchrolytic?

A. C. septicum
B. C. perfringens
C. C. novyi
D. All of these

Ans. D.

1635. Stormy clot reaction is useful in identification of

A. C. tetani
B. C. botulinum
C. C. perfringens
D. C. difficile

Ans. C.

1636. Food poisoning strains of Clostridium perfringens belong to

A. Type A
B. Type B
C. Type C
D. Type D

Ans. A.

1637. Reddening of meat in cooked meat broth is produced by

A. C. tetani
B. C. histolyticum
C. Clostridium perfringens
D. C. sporogenes

Ans. C.

1638. Clostridium botulinum food poisoning is due to

A. Invasion of bacteria in the intestine
B. Preformed toxin
C. Both A and B
D. None of these

Ans. B.

1639. Drumstick appearance is characteristic of

A. C. tetanomorphum
B. C. tetani
C. C. sphenoides
D. All of these

Ans. D.

1640. Blackening of meat in cooked meat broth is through

A. C.histolyticum
B. Clostridium perfringens
C. C. tetani
D. all of these

Ans. A.

1641. Typical drumstick appearance of bacilli is generally seen in

A. Clostridium perfringens
B. C. botulinum
C. C. tetani
D. C. histolyticum

Ans. C.

1642. Which of the following(s) is/are obligate anaerobes ?

A. C. septicum
B. C.novyi
C. C. tetani
D. All of these

Ans. D.

1643. The nonsymbiotic bacteria which fix nitrogen live in the soil independently are

A. Azotobacter
B. Clostridium
C. Cyanobacteria
D. All of the above

Ans. D.

1644. Nitrogen fixation by the microorganisms can be detected by adopting the approach of

A. Demonstrating growth in a nitrogen free medium
B. Cultivating the microorganisms in the presence of nitrogen labeled with isotropic nitrogen
C. Measuring $^{15}N_2$ by mass spectrometer
D. All of the above

Ans. D.

1645. Which of the following is not the biofertilisers producing bacteria?

A. Nostoc
B. Anabaena
C. Both A and B
D. Clostridium

Ans. D.

1646. Which of the following is capable of oxidizing sulfur to sulfates?

A. Thiobacillus thiooxidans
B. Desulfotomaculum
C. Rhodospirillum
D. Rhodomicrobium

Ans. A.

1647. Most soil protozoa are flagellates or amoebas, having their dominant mode of nitrogen as

A. Ingestion of bacteria
B. Ingestion of mold
C. Ingestion of fungi
D. All of these

Ans. A.

1648. Which of the following microorganism use H_2S as the electron donor to reduce carbon dioxide?

A. Chromaticum
B. Chlorobium
C. Both A and B
D. Rhodomicrobium

Ans. C.

1649. Nitrifying bacteria can not be isolated directly by the usual techniques employed to isolate hetrotrophic bacteria. The reasons may be due to

A. Slow growth
B. Medium growth
C. Fast growth
D. None of these

Ans. A.

1650. Bacteria, as a group, are responsible for

A. Nitrogen oxidation
B. Sulphur oxidation
C. Iron oxidation
D. All of these

Ans. D.

1651. The phenomenon of commensalism refers to a relationship between organisms in which

A. One species of a pair benefits
B. Both the species of a pair benefit
C. One species of a pair is more benefitted
D. None of the above

Ans. A.

1652. The population of algae in soil is ——— that of either bacteria or fungi.

A. Generally smaller than
B. Generally greater than
C. Equal to
D. None of these

Ans. A.

1653. The transformation of nitrates to gaseous nitrogen is accomplished by microorganisms in a series of biochemical reactions. The process is known as

A. Nitrification
B. Denitrification
C. Nitrogen fixation
D. Ammonification

Ans. B.

1654. Nitrogen fixation refers to the direct conversion of atmospheric nitrogen gas into

A. Ammonia B. Glucose

C. ATP D. Nitrate

Ans. A.

1655. The diagnostic enzyme for denitrification is

A. Nitrate reductase B. Nitrate oxidase

C. Nitrooxidoreductase D. None of these

Ans. A.

1656. A heterocyst is

A. A type of spore

B. A terminally differentiated cell that fixes nitrogen

C. The progenitor of cyanobacterial vegetative cells

D. A cell that carries out oxygenic photosynthesis

Ans. B.

1657. The groups of symbiotic bacteria, which have the ability to fix nitrogen

A. Derive their food and minerals from the legume, and in turn they supply the legume with some or all of its nitrogen

B. Grow together for a mutual benefit is called symbiosis and so these bacteria are called symbiotic nitrogen-fixing bacteria

C. These bacteria are from the genus, Rhizobium

D. All of these

Ans. D.

1658. Nitrogen oxidation (nitrification)refers to the

A. Conversion of ammonium ions into nitrates through the activities of certain bacteria

B. Changing of atmospheric nitrogen (N_2) to nitrogen compounds

C. Sulfur is oxidized to the sulfate form through Thiobacillus bacteria

D. None of the above

Ans. A.

1659. An example of a symbiotic nitrogen fixer is

A. Azotobacter B. Beijerinckia

C. Clostridium D. Rhizobium

Ans. D.

1660. Which of the following is correct?

A. Mycorrhizae are fungi that form a mutually beneficial (symbiotic) relationship with plant roots

B. The fungi aid in transmitting nutrients and water to the plant roots

C. The increased nutrient availability from mycorrhizae is thought to be due to the additional absorbing surface provided by the fungi

D. All of the above

Ans. D.

1661. In the process of nitrogen fixation, which of the following microorganism is involved?

A. Non symbiotic microorganisms only

B. Symbiotic microorganisms only

C. Non symbiotic and symbiotic microorganisms only

D. None of the above

Ans. C.

1662. Which of the following statement is not true about composition of biogas?

A. It is composed almost exclusively of methane and carbon dioxide

B. It also contains traces of H_2S, N_2, $H_2$and CO

C. It also contains traces of O_2 and Cl_2

D. Both A and B

Ans. C.

1663. The physical structure of soil is improved by the accumulation of

A. Mold mycelium

B. Minerals

C. Water

D. All of these

Ans. A.

1664. ———————- play a key role in the transformation of rock to soil.

A. Cyanobacteria

B. Pectin decomposing bacteria

C. Nitrifying bacteria

D. Denitrifying bacteria

Ans. A.

1665. The groups of bacteria which have the ability to fix nitrogen from air to soil are

A. Symbiotic

B. Nonsymbiotic

C. Both A and B

D. None of these

Ans. C.

1666. The nitrogenase consists of

A. Dinitrogenase B. Dinitrogenase reductase

C. Both A and B D. None of these

Ans. C.

1667. The crops which are involved in nitrogen fixation are

A. Alfalfa and clover B. Soybean

C. Bean and lupine D. All of these

Ans. D.

1668. Denitrification may be distinguished as

A. Dissimilative B. Assimilative

C. Both A and B D. Blue baby syndrome

Ans. C.

1669. The conversion of molecular nitrogen into ammonia is known as

A. Nitrification B. Denitrification

C. Nitrogen fixation D. Ammonification

Ans. C.

1670. The breakdown of cattle manure in biogas is accomplished by which of the following type of bacteria?

A. Hydrolytic B. Transitional

C. Methanogenic D. All of these

Ans. D.

1671. Which of the following species of different genera of bacteria are not capable of transforming nitrate to nitrogen?

A. Achromobacter B. Agrobacterium

C. Alcaligenes D. None of these

Ans. D.

1672. Some microorganisms have the ability to increase the nitrogen content of soils, are called as

A. Nitrogen fixation B. Denitrification

C. Nitrification D. All of these

Ans. A.

1673. Nitrogen fixation changes the free nitrogen to a

A. Form usable by plants

B. Nitrogen compounds, mostly amines such as NH_2

C. Both A and B

D. Fix the free nitrogen (N_2) by which it should not be usable by plants

Ans. C.

1674. For rapid decomposition by microbes, the substrate should have a C/N ratio of

A. 10-20 B. 20-30

C. 30-40 D. 60-80

Ans. C.

1675. Which are the main source of biofertilisers ?

A. Cyanobacteria B. Bacillus

C. Streptococcus D. None of these

Ans. A.

1676. The organisms responsible for the characteristic musty or earth odour of a freshly ploughed field is/are

A. Nocardia B. Streptomyces

C. Micromonospora D. All of these

Ans. D.

1677. Denitrification is

A. Reduction of nitrate (NO_3^-) to nitrogen gas

B. Reduction of nitrate to organic nitrogen compounds

C. Both A and B

D. Changing of atmospheric nitrogen (N_2) to nitrogen compounds

Ans. C.

1678. Degree of compost maturity can be assessed by

A. Infrared technique B. Germination test

C. Both A and B D. None of the above

Ans. C.

1679. The energy value of biogas is typically

A. 400-700 BTU/ft^3 B. 1,000 BTU/ft^3

C. 1500 BTU/ft^3 D. more than 5000 BTU/ft^3

Ans. A.

1680. The microbial ecosystem of soil includes

A. Biotic components of soil

B. Abiotic components of soil

C. Biotic and abiotic components of soil

D. None of the above

Ans. C.

1681. Denitrification is carried out

A. Usually by facultative anaerobes B. Predominantly by Pseudomonas spp

C. Predominantly by Bacillus spp D. All of the above

Ans. D.

1682. Which of the following soil microorganism is involved in the reduction of sulfates to H_2S?

A. Thiobacillus thiooxidans B. Desulfotomaculum

C. Rhodospirillum D. Rhodomicrobium

Ans. B.

1683. The diagnostic enzyme for nitrogen-fixing organisms is

A. Nitrogenase B. Nitrate reductase

C. Nitrate oxidase D. None of these

Ans. A.

1684. Which of the following fungi on infecting crop roots can improve their uptake of phosphorus and other nutrients?

A. Saccharomyces cerevisiae B. VA Mycorrhiza

C. Candida torulopsis D. Aspergillus niger

Ans. B.

1685. Syntrophism involves

A. Exchange of nutrients between two species

B. Exchange of nutrients among species

C. No exchange of nutrients between two species

D. No exchange of nutrients among species

Ans. A.

1686. Assimilative denitrification is done by

A. Plants B. Fungi

C. Prokaryotes D. All of these

Ans. D.

1687. An excessively high temperature in the fermentation of sauerkraut may inhibit the growth of

A. Leuconostoc B. Pediococcus cerevisiae

C. Both A and B D. None of these

Ans. A.

1688. Which statement is true about flavouring materials spices, garlic etc added to Dill pickles?

A. These markedly stimulate or inhibit the acid forming bacteria

B. They may be source of considerable numbers of undesirable micro-organisms and cause off-fermentations or spoilage of pickles

C. They may improve texture of the pickle

D. None of these

Ans. B.

1689. Gassy spoilage of green olives is usually caused by

A. Enterobacter spp B. Bacillus spp

C. Clostridium spp D. All of these

Ans. D.

1690. Abnormal fermentation of cabbage may result in a cheese like odour caused by

A. Propionic acid B. Butyric acid

C. Caprioc acid and valeric acid D. All of these

Ans. D.

1691. Too long a fermentation of sauerkraut may favour the growth of

A. Lactobacillus lactis B. Lactobacillus brevis

C. Bacillus subtilis D. None of these

Ans. B.

1692. Blackening in pickles occurs due to

A. The formation of hydrogen sulfide by bacteria

B. Growth of penicillium

C. Both a and b

D. None of these

Ans. A.

1693. Soft pickles are made so by pectolytic enzymes mostly from

A. Moulds B. Yeasts

C. Bacteria D. None of these

Ans. A.

1694. The growth of black-pigmented Bacillus nigrificans, a causative agent of black pickle is favoured by

A. Presence of carbohydrate like glucose

B. Low level of available nitrogen

C. Neutral or slightly alkaline brine

D. All of the above

Ans. D.

1695. Slimy or ropy kraut is caused by

A. Encapsulated varieties of lactobacillus plantarum

B. Lactobacillus lactis

C. Encapsulated varieties of lactobacillus brevis

D. None of the above

Ans. A.

1696. The most important bacterium developing acidity in both low and high salt brines is

A. L. lactis B. L. plantarum

C. L. brevis D. B.subtilis

Ans. B.

1697. The elimination of the scum of yeasts in the brine during the fermentation include

A. Agitation of the surface B. Addition of the mustard oil

C. Addition of sorbic acid D. All of these

Ans. D.

1698. Cloudiness of brine of glass-packed olives may be caused by

A. The lactics if fermentation of residual sugar resumes

B. Salt tolerant bacteria

C. Film yeasts or moulds if air is available

D. All of the above

Ans. D.

1699. Which of the following strain(s), that grow in the jellies and candid fruits, are able to grow in sugar concentration upto 67.5%?

A. Aspergillus B. Penicillium

C. Citromyces D. All of these

Ans. D.

1700. The ability of B.coagulans to grow in tomato juice depends upon the

A. Number of spores present B. The availability of oxygen

C. The pH of the juice D. All of these

Ans. D.

1701. Flat sour spoilage of acid foods is caused by

A. B. coagulans B. B. pepo

C. Both A and B D. B. stearothermophillus

Ans. A.

1702. The most important kind of chemical spoilage of canned foods is the hydrogen swell which is favored by

A. Increasing acidities of foods

B. Increasing temperature of storage

C. Imperfection in the tinning and lacquering

D. All of these

Ans. D.

1703. Canned sweetened condensed milk may become thickened by

A. Bacillus species
B. Clostridium species
C. Micrococcus species
D. Saccharomyces species

Ans. C.

1704. The canned acid foods such as pineapple, tomatoes and pears have been found spoiled by C.pasteurianum. Such spoilage is more likely when the pH of the food is

A. >4.5
B. <4.5
C. >5.3
D. <5.3

Ans. A.

1705. Which of the following species can cause bitterness, acidity and curdling in canned milk, cream and evaporated milk?

A. Bacillus
B. Clostridium
C. Both A and B
D. Saccharomyces

Ans. A.

1706. Acid foods with a pH between 4.5 and 3.7 usually are spoiled by

A. B.coagulans
B. Saccharolytic anaerobe
C. Both A and B
D. None of these

Ans. C.

1707. The butyric acid type of fermentation in acid or medium acid foods, with swelling of the container by the carbon dioxide and hydrogen gas is caused by

A. C. butyricum
B. C. pasteurianum
C. Both A and B
D. C. sporogenes

Ans. C.

1708. Which of the following(s) is/are proteolytic or putrefactive decomposing proteins with the production of malodorous compounds such as H_2S, mercaptans, ammonia, indole and skatole?

A. C. sporogenes
B. C. putrifaciens
C. Both A and B
D. C. butyricum

Ans. C.

1709. Canned poultry is more often spoiled by

A. Putrefactive than by Saccharolytic Clostridia

B. Saccharolytic Clostridia than by putrefactive

C. Saccharomyces species

D. Micrococcus species

Ans. A.

1710. Canned meat and fish exhibit spoilage by

A. Bacillus species B. Clostridium species

C. Both A and B D. Saccharomyces

Ans. C.

1711. High acid foods with a pH < 3.7 undergo spoilage by

A. Saccharolytic anaerobe

B. B. coagulans

C. Both A and B

D. Do not undergo spoilage by microorganisms

Ans. D.

1712. The putrefactive anaerobes grow best in the

A. Low acid canned foods B. Medium acid canned foods

C. High acid canned foods D. Any of these

Ans. A.

1713. High acid foods with a pH above 5.3 are especially subjected to

A. Flat sour spoilage B. Putrefaction

C. Both A and B D. TA spoilage

Ans. C.

1714. Which of the following disinfectants act by disrupting microbial membranes?

A. Cationic detergents B. Halogens

C. Heavy metals D. Aldehydes

Ans. A.

1715. Which of the following is best to sterilize heat labile solutions?

A. Dry heat B. Autoclave

C. Membrane filtration D. Pasteurization

Ans. C.

1716. The time required to kill 90% of the microorganisms in a sample at a specific temperature is the

A. Decimal reduction time
B. Thermal death point
C. F value
D. D value

Ans. D.

1717. Which of the following is best used for long term storage of microbial samples when carried out properly?

A. Storage in a freezer at -10°C
B. Storage in a freezer at ultra low temperatures (-70°C)
C. Storage in a refrigerator on an agar slant
D. Storage on a petri plate at room temperature

Ans. B.

1718. Which of the following is not a disinfectant containing a heavy metal ?

A. Silver nitrate
B. Mercurochrome
C. Copper sulphate
D. Chlorine

Ans. D.

1719. Which is the most important surface active disinfectants?

A. Amphoteric compounds
B. Cationic compounds
C. Non-ionic compounds
D. Anionic compounds

Ans. B.

1720. Which disinfectant would be most effective against Staphylococcus found in a blood spill?

A. Phenol
B. Cetylpyridinium chloride
C. Hexachlorophene
D. None of these

Ans. D.

1721. Which of the following substances can sterilize?

A. Alcohol
B. Cetylpyridinium chloride
C. Ethylene oxide
D. Chlorine

Ans. C.

1722. Milk is pasteurized in batch method by keeping it at

A. 63°C for 30 minutes
B. 72°C for 60 seconds
C. 73°C for 30 minutes
D. 72°C for 6 minutes

Ans. A.

1723. Preservation of foods by using salts and sugars works by

A. Raising pH
B. Lowering osmotic pressure
C. Creating a hypertonic environment
D. Creating a hypotonic environment

Ans. C.

1724. Which of the following items could be sterilized by dry heat sterilization?

A. Intravenous solution
B. Plastic IV bags
C. Glass pipettes
D. Rubber gloves

Ans. C.

1725. Which of the following does not kill endospores?

A. Autoclave
B. Incineration
C. Hot air sterilization
D. Pasteurization

Ans. D.

1726. Which disinfectant was the most effective against Salmonella ?

A. Phenol
B. Cetylpyridinium chloride
C. Hexachlorophene
D. Merthiolate

Ans. D.

1727. If a canning procedure is not properly followed, which type of microbe is most likely to grow in the canned food?

A. Obligate aerobe
B. Acidophile
C. Mesophile
D. Obligate anaerobe

Ans. D.

1728. Bactericidal concentration of phenol is

A. 0.25%
B. 0.5%
C. 0.75%
D. 1%

Ans. D.

1729. Which of the following is most effective for sterilizing mattresses and plastic petri plates?

A. Chlorine
B. Ethylene oxide
C. Glutaraldehyde
D. UV radiation

Ans. B.

1730. Which of the following skin disinfectant(s) is/are most frequently used ?

A. Isopropyl alcohol
B. Ethyl alcohol
C. Both A and B
D. None of these

Ans. C.

1731. All of the following are sporicidal except

A. Glutaraldehyde
B. Ethylene oxide
C. Formaldehyde
D. Alcohol

Ans. D.

1732. Which of the following describes the effect of ionizing radiation on microbes?

A. Changes the 3-dimensional structure of proteins to a 2-dimen-sional form
B. Substantially decreases enzymatic activity, slowing microbial reproduction
C. Induces electrons and protons to jump out of the molecules of the microbe
D. None of the above

Ans. C.

1733. The process of making an object free from living organisms including bacterial and fungal spores and viruses is known as

A. Pasteurization
B. Antisepsis
C. Disinfection
D. Sterilization

Ans. D.

1734. Media containing spores and thermolabile constituents are sterilized by

A. Pasteurization
B. UV radiation
C. Dry heat
D. Tyndalization

Ans. B.

1735. A(n)——is used to prevent infection by killing or inhibiting pathogen growth on animal tissues

A. Bacteriostatic agent
B. Sanitizer
C. Disinfectant
D. Antiseptic

Ans. D.

1736. One drawback to the use of ultraviolet light as a sterilizing agent is its

A. Failure to kill bacteria
B. Failure to bacterial spores
C. Failure to kill microbes in a closed environment
D. Failure to kill microbes located in the center of an object

Ans. D.

1737. Ethylene oxide is used to destroy or kill which of the following microbes?

A. Bacteria
B. Spores
C. Fungi
D. All of these

Ans. D.

1738. Which of the following was the first widely used antiseptic and disinfectant?

A. Chlorine B. Phenol

C. Iodine D. Alcohol

Ans. B.

1739. If a 1:600 dilution of a test compound kills a standard population of Staphylococcus aureus in 10 minutes but not 5 minutes while a 1:60 dilution of phenol kills the population in the same time, what is the phenol coefficient of the test compound?

A. 1 B. 5

C. 10 D. 50

Ans. C.

1740. Microbes can be removed from a liquid solution by the process of

A. Filtration B. Freeze drying

C. Osmosis D. Dessication

Ans. A.

1741. Which of the following is bactericidal?

A. Membrane filtration B. Ionizing radiation

C. Freeze drying D. Deep freezing

Ans. B.

1742. Which of the following process can be efficiently carried out by incineration?

A. Sterilization of scalpel blades and needles

B. Sterilization of all glass syringes

C. Sterilization of points of forceps

D. Destruction of contaminated materials

Ans. D.

1743. The organisms retained in the fluids filtered by Seitz filter is

A. Proteus B. Staphylococcus

C. Clostridium D. None of these

Ans. D.

1744. Which of the following material is sterilized by heating at 160°C in a hot air oven for one hour?

A. Swab sticks B. All glass syringes

C. Oils and jellies D. All of these

Ans. B.

1745. For sterilization of which material gamma rays can be used?

A. Catheters
B. Plastic syringes
C. Canulas
D. None of these

Ans. C.

1746. Which of the following is sterilized with the help of glutaraldehyde?

A. Thermometers
B. Bronchoscopes
C. Cystoscopes
D. All of these

Ans. D.

1747. The time in minutes at a specific temperature needed to kill a population of cells is the

A. Decimal reduction time
B. Thermal death point
C. Thermal death temperature
D. F value

Ans. D.

1748. Which of the following is a limitation of the autoclave?

A. It takes too long to sterilize
B. It lacks the ability to inactivate viruses
C. It lacks the ability to kill endospores
D. It will destroy heat labile materials

Ans. D.

1749. Which of the following has most heat resistant spores?

A. Clostridium histolyticum
B. Clostridium perfringens
C. Bacillus stearothermophilus
D. Bacillus cereus

Ans. C.

1750. The lowest temperature that kills all microorganisms in a liquid suspension in 10 minutes is known as the

A. Decimal reduction time
B. Thermal death point
C. Thermal death temperature
D. Thermal death time

Ans. B.

1751. Which of the following tests is designed to simulate the natural conditions under which the disinfectants are used in hospitals?

A. Phenol coefficient test
B. Minimum inhibitory concentration test
C. Capacity test
D. None of these

Ans. C.

1752. Steam exposure of a material at 100°C for 20 minutes for three consecutive days is known as

A. Inspissations
B. Tyndallisation
C. Autoclaving
D. None of these

Ans. B.

1753. Which of the following material is sterilized by use of red heat?

A. Soiled dressings
B. Inoculating wires and loops
C. Glass slides
D. All glass syringes

Ans. B.

1754. Which of the following methods will not sterilize?

A. Aqueous glutaraldehyde for 10 hours
B. Dry heat at 171°C for 1 to 2 hours
C. 121°C at 15 lb/in pressure for 15 to 20 minutes
D. 100°C boiling water for 30 minutes

Ans. D.

1755. Which of the following is/are vapour-phase disinfectant/s?

A. Formaldehyde
B. Ethylene oxide
C. Both A and B
D. None of these

Ans. C.

1756. Sweet and salty foods frequently don't require refrigeration to prevent spoilage because they have

A. Insufficient nutrients
B. Low pH
C. High concentration of solutes
D. Toxic alkaline chemicals

Ans. C.

1757. Iodophores are mixture of

A. Iodine and aldehydes
B. Iodine and surface active agents
C. Iodine and alcohols
D. Iodine and phenols

Ans. B.

1758. Which of the following compounds are commonly used as general antiseptics to treat cuts and scratches?

A. Aldehydes
B. Ethylene oxide
C. Halogens
D. None of these

Ans. C.

1759. Complete destruction of the microorganisms is commonly known as

A. Disinfection B. Sterilization

C. Antisepsis D. None of these

Ans. B.

1760. Synovial fluid contains

A. Heparin B. Hyaluronic acid

C. Chondroitin sulphate D. All of the above

Ans. B.

1761. Which of the following is incorrect?

A. Adenine always pairs thymine

B. In DNA double helix, two strands of the DNA are bound with each other with the bases

C. None of the above

D. Guanine always pairs with the cytosine

Ans. C.

1762. What is the approximate size (in kb) of the E.coli genome?

A. 4500 kilobase B. 3000 kilobase

C. 6500 kilobase D. 5500 kilobase

Ans. A.

1763. Enzymes, responsible for unraveling short segments of DNA is

A. Helicase B. DNA polymerase

C. Primase D. DNA ligase

Ans. A.

1764. The overall conclusion of the Hershey-Chase experiment was that

A. Proteins and DNA were responsible for heredity

B. DNA was responsible for heredity

C. Phage DNA was similar to bacterial DNA

D. The ratio of Adenine to Thymine was always the same

Ans. B.

1765. In DNA double helix, the two DNA chains are held together by

A. Hydrogen bonds between the pair of bases

B. Covalent bonds between the pair of bases

C. None of the above

D. Ionic bond between the pair of bases

Ans. A.

1766. What is the only common methylation in the DNA of eukaryotes?

A. Guanosine in ApGpA trinucleotides

B. Adenosine in GpA dinucleotides

C. None of the above

D. Cytosine in CpG dinucleotides

Ans. D.

1767. Which is the largest among the followings?

A. Nitrogenous base
B. Nucleotide
C. Carbon
D. Phosphate

Ans. B.

1768. PDM is the acronym for:

A. Product data management
B. Project data manipulation
C. Product drawing manipulation
D. Project drawing management

Ans. A.

1769. All infections do not cause fever and all fevers are not due to infections which of the following is an example of non-infections cause of fever?

A. Chicken pox
B. Typhoid
C. Malaria
D. Rheumatic disease

Ans. D.

1770. Mucus helps in protecting against pathogens by

A. Facilitating the growth of normal flora

B. Lowering the pH

C. Sequestering iron

D. Blocking access and attachment of pathogens to mucosal surfaces

Ans. D.

1771. Pink rots in eggs is caused by the strains of

A. Pseudomonas fluorescens
B. Pseudomonas aeruginosa
C. None of the above
D. Species of Micrococcus or Bacillus

Ans. A.

1772. More spoilage of eggs is caused by

A. Molds than bacteria
B. Bacteria than molds
C. None of these
D. Synergistically

Ans. B.

1773. Colorless rots in eggs is caused by

A. Pseudomonas fluorescens
B. Pseudomonas alcaligenes
C. All of these
D. Both A and B

Ans. B.

1774. The spoilage of eggs by fungi goes through stages of mold growth that give the defects their names. Very early mold growth is termed

A. Fungal rotting
B. Pin spot molding
C. Any of these
D. Superficial fungal spoilage

Ans. B.

1775. Vacuum packaged meats are spoiled by

A. Lactobacilli
B. Thermosphacta
C. None of these
D. Both A and B

Ans. C.

1776. In storage atmospheres of high humidity variety of molds may cause

A. Bacterial spoilage
B. Superficial fungal spoilage
C. None of these
D. Both A and B

Ans. B.

1777. Which of the following is recommended for the improvement in flavor during ageing of beef under controlled conditions?

A. Rhizopus
B. Thamnidium
C. M. mucedo
D. T. elegans

Ans. B.

1778. The organisms responsible for the characteristic musty or earth odour of a freshly ploughed field is/are

A. Streptomyces
B. Nocardia
C. All of these
D. Micromonospora

Ans. C.

1779. Which of the following species of different genera of bacteria are not capable of transforming nitrate to nitrogen?

A. Agrobacterium
B. Achromobacter
C. None of these
D. Alcaligenes

Ans. C.

1780. The physical structure of soil is improved by the accumulation of

A. Minerals B. Mold mycelium

C. All of these D. Water

Ans. B.

1781. The conversion of molecular nitrogen into ammonia is known as

A. Denitrification B. Nitrification

C. Ammonification D. Nitrogen fixation

Ans. D.

1782. Nitrogen fixation refers to the direct conversion of atmospheric nitrogen gas into

A. Glucose B. Ammonia

C. Nitrate D. ATP

Ans. B.

1783. Which are the main source of biofertilisers?

A. Bacillus B. Cyanobacteria

C. None of these D. Streptococcus

Ans. B.

1784. A parenteral route of drug administration refers to

A. Nonoral B. Oral

C. Intramuscularly D. Intravenously

Ans. A.

1785. Exponential phase of growth curve of bacteria is of limited duration because of

A. Accumulation of toxic metabolites B. Rise in cell density

C. All of these D. Exhaustion of nutrients

Ans. C.

1786. Which of the following conditions can be caused by Plesiomonas?

A. Gastroenteritis B. Septicaemia

C. All of these D. Cellulites

Ans. C.

1787. Treponema species from human oral cavity can be selected by using

A. Incubation temperature B. pH of the medium

C. All of these D. Cell size and motility

Ans. D.

1788. Intestinal bacteria can grow in the presence of———— whereas nonintestinal bacteria are usually inhibited.

A. Low concentration of various dyes B. Bile salts

C. Low levels of nitrogen D. Sugars

Ans. B.

1789. In the process of freeze drying, a dense cell suspension is placed in small vials and is frozen at

A. -20 to 30°C B. -60 to -78 °C

C. -48 to 58 °C D.-30 to -48 °C

Ans. B.

1790. Which of the following problem makes it impossible to satisfy all of Koch's postulates?

A. Microorganism can not be isolated in pure culture

B. Microorganism causes serious symptoms in humans

C. Genes from the microorganism can not be amplified by PCR

D. Species of microorganism is in question

Ans. A.

1791. For the selection of lactobacilli present in cheddar cheese, the pH of the medium is maintained at

A. 5.35 B. 6.35

C. 5.75 D. 4.35

Ans. A.

1792. All bacteria that inhabit the human body are

A. Chemolithotrophs B. Heterotrophs

C. Phototrophs D. Autotrophs

Ans. B.

1793. Which of the following bacteria dies quickly after drying?

A. M. tuberculosis B. Treponema palladum

C. Pseudomonas aeruginosa D. Staphylococcus aureus

Ans. B.

1794. When a substance is added to a liquid medium which inhibits the growth of unwanted bacteria and favors the growth of wanted bacteria, it is known as

A. Enriched medium B. Differential medium

C. Selective medium D. Enrichment medium

Ans. D.

1795. The growth of Streptomyces on straw or elsewhere near the egg may produce

A. Hay odour
B. Musty or earthy flavours
C. Cabbage water flavour
D. Fishy flavour

Ans. B.

1796. Yellow discolorations in meat are caused by bacteria with yellow pigments, usually species of

A. Flavobacterium
B. Micrococcus
C. Pseudomonas syncyanea
D. Both A and B

Ans. D.

1797. Which of the following is responsible for a musty or earthy flavor ?

A. Flavobacterium
B. Actinomycetes
C. Pseudomonas syncyanea
D. Both A and B

Ans. B.

1798. In the time since E.coli and Salmonella diverged evolutionarily

A. There has been little change in either genome
B. E.coli has acquired many genes via horizontal transfer
C. E.coli has lost approximately 50% of its genome
D. None of these

Ans. C.

1799. Which of the following theory is supported by the genomic sequence of the obligate intracellular parasite Rickettsia prowazekii ?

A. Parasitic bacteria have very large genomes
B. Parasites have a definite genomic sequence similar to viruses
C. Mitochondria have evolved from endosymbiotic bacteria
D. All bacteria evolved from viruses

Ans. C.

1800. The physical nature of genomes is studied under

A. Structural genomics
B. Comparative genomics
C. Proteogenomics
D. Functional genomics

Ans. A.

1801. The species of bacteria, which possesses 250 genes for lipid biosynthesis is

A. M. genitalium
B. M. tuberculosis
C. E.coli
D. H. influenzae

Ans. B.

1802. Why the bacterium Treponema pallidum is difficult to culture?

A. Because it requires a great deal of water to reproduce

B. Because it is unable to use carbohydrates as an energy source

C. Because it lacks the genes needed for TCA cycle and oxidative phosphorylation

D. Because it requires extremely low temperature at which water freezes

Ans. C.

1803. What is the range of minimum set of genes required for life ?

A. 50-100 genes B. 250-350 genes

C. 1000-15000 genes D. 1500-2000 genes

Ans. B.

1804. The flow of genetic material in microbial cells usually takes place from

A. RNA through DNA to proteins B. Proteins through RNA to DNA

C. DNA through RNA to proteins D. None of these

Ans. C.

1805. Which of the following is used for determining the location of specific genes within the genome?

A. Genomics B. Annotation

C. Cloning D. Proteomics

Ans. B.

1806. Proteomics is

A. The study of algal genomes

B. A branch of quantum physics dealing with proteins

C. The study of formation of lipoprotein in animals

D. The study of the entire collection of proteins expressed by an organism

Ans. D.

1807. Which of the following is concerned with the management and analysis of biological data using computers?

A. Biophysics B. Bioinformatics

C. Genomics D. Biomechanics

Ans. B.

1808. Which type of genomics studies the transcripts and proteins expressed by a genome?

A. Comparative genomics B. Structural genomics

C. Proteogenomics D. Functional genomics

Ans. D.

1809. Which of the following is the study of the molecular organization of genomes, their information content and the gene products they encode?

A. Geneties
B. Ergonomics
C. Genomics
D. Bioinformatics

Ans. C.

1810. The word, used for the small solid supports onto which are spotted hundreds of thousands of tiny drops of DNA that can be used to screen gene expression, is

A. Southern blot
B. Cloning library
C. DNA microarrays
D. Northern blot

Ans. C.

1811. Which of the following organisms has the smallest genome?

A. H. influenzae
B. M. genitalium
C. M. tuberculosis
D. None of these

Ans. B.

1812. Studies of similarities and differences among the genomes of multiple organisms is carried out in

A. Comparative genomics
B. Proteomics
C. Functional genomics
D. Structural genomics

Ans. A.

1813. Why Deinococcus radiodurans is able to survive massive exposure to radiation?

A. Because it produces a thick shell which acts as a shield from the radiation
B. Because it has unique DNA repair mechanisms
C. Because its cell wall contains radioactive elements
D. Because it has many copies of gene encoding DNA repair

Ans. D.

1814. The process by which phage reproduction is initiated in lysogenized culture is called

A. Infection
B. Integration
C. Repression
D. Induction

Ans. D.

1815. Area of lysis on a bacterial lawn culture produced by a phage is known as

A. Pock
B. Plaque
C. Pox
D. All of these

Ans. B.

1816. The procapsid is assembled with the aid of———— proteins.

A. Ladder
B. Framing
C. Scaffolding
D. Form

Ans. C.

1817. Which of the following is/are synthesized from late mRNA?

A. Phage structural proteins
B. Proteins that help with phage assembly without becoming part of the virion structure
C. Proteins involved in cell lysis and phage release
D. All of the above

Ans. D.

1818. ————protein keeps the prophage dormant and prevents virus reproduction.

A. Operator
B. Promoter
C. Repressor
D. Enhancer

Ans. C.

1819. "All animals are made of cells" was suggested by

A. Schneider
B. Schwann
C. Hooke
D. Virchow

Ans. B.

1820. Virchow's theory of cell division was surfaced in

A. 1655
B. 1808
C. 1838
D. 1855

Ans. D.

1821. "All plants are made of cells". It was suggested by

A. Schneider
B. Schwann
C. Hooke
D. Virchow

Ans. A.

1822. Cells arise from pre-existing cells by cell division was suggested by

A. Schneider
B. Schwann
C. Hooke
D. Virchow

Ans. D.

1823. Common example of fermented dairy product is

A. Bread and buns
B. Cheese and yogurt
C. Pickles
D. Beer

Ans. B.

1824. Procedure in which oxidation-reduction of glucose ($C_6H_{12}O_6$) is incomplete is called

A. Fertilization
B. Reduction
C. Oxidation
D. Fermentation

Ans. D.

1825. Bacterium which is able to synthesize human growth hormone is known as

A. E. coli bacterium
B. H. coli bacterium
C. X. coli bacterium
D. I. coli bacterium

Ans. A.

1826. Manufacturing of useful services or products by using living organisms is classified as

A. Transgenic engineering
B. Biotechnology
C. Bioengineering
D. Genome engineering

Ans. B.

1827. Bacteria which carries lactic acid fermentation is

A. Lactobacillus
B. Lactobacillus cerevisiae
C. Wilmot cerevisiae
D. Saccharomyces cerevisiae

Ans. A.

1828. Hormone created by genetic engineering which is effective for lung and brain cancer is known as

A. Esomeprazole
B. Atorvastatin
C. Thymosin
D. Thyroxin

Ans. C.

1829. Formic acid is used at industry level for the

A. Production of plastics
B. Leather treatment
C. Production of vinegar
D. Production of cosmetics

Ans. B.

1830. Alcoholic fermentation is carried by yeast known as

A. Wilmot cerevisiae
B. Saccharomyces cerevisiae
C. Lactobacillus
D. Lactobacillus cerevisiae

Ans. B.

1831. Human genome project was published in

A. 1999 B. 2008

C. 2005 D. 2002

Ans. D.

1832. Device which provides environment to microorganisms to interact with substrate is called

A. Producer B. Fermenter

C. Industrializer D. All of above

Ans. B.

1833. Organisms that have modified genetic set-up are classified as

A. Bio enzymes B. Transgenic

C. Genomes D. Microbes

Ans. B.

1834. Attached interest gene and vector DNA (Deoxyribonucleic Acid) are collectively known as

A. Expressed DNA B. Restricted DNA

C. Isolated DNA D. Recombinant DNA

Ans. D.

1835. Anti-viral proteins that are produced by virus infected cells are called

A. Interferon B. Thymosin

C. Beta-endorphin D. Urokinase

Ans. A.

1836. Considering fermentation at industrial level, microorganism Bacillus is used to form

A. Ethanol B. Formic acid

C. Acrylic acid D. Glycerol

Ans. C.

1837. Addition, repair and removal of genetic material is classified as

A. Genetic engineering B. Bioengineering

C. Genome engineering D. Transgenic engineering

Ans. A.

1838. Substrate used by microorganisms to produce single-cell proteins includes

A. Methane gas B. Industrial wastes

C. Agricultural wastes D. All of above

Ans. D.

1839. In carbohydrate ($C_nH_{2m}O_m$) fermentation, glucose molecule ($C_6H_{12}O_6$) is broken into molecules of

A. Pyruvic acid
B. Nitric acid
C. Sulphuric acid
D. Hydrochloric acid

Ans. A.

1840. Types of carbohydrate fermentation includes

A. Lactic acid fermentation
B. Alcoholic fermentation
C. Pyruvic acid
D. Both a and b

Ans. D.

1841. E. coli bacterium was created in

A. 1981
B. 1977
C. 1985
D. 1979

Ans. B.

1842. Pain killer produced with help of genetic engineering for brain is known as

A. Alpha-endorphin
B. Delta-endorphin
C. Gamma-endorphin
D. Beta-endorphin

Ans. D.

1843. By using single-cell protein, amount of protein produced by 50 kgs of yeast is

A. 180 tons
B. 100 tons
C. 300 tons
D. 250 tons

Ans. D.

1844. Protein content which is extracted from mixed or pure cultures of yeasts, bacteria, algae and fungi is called

A. Triple cell protein
B. Single cell protein
C. Double cell protein
D. Tetra cell protein

Ans. B.

1845. Lactic acid ($C_3H_6O_3$) fermentation is used in production of

A. Malted drinks
B. Beer production
C. Brown bread
D. Many types of cheese

Ans. D.

1846. Ethanol is used at industry level for the

A. Production of vinegar
B. Production of cosmetics
C. Production of plastics
D. Leather treatment

Ans. A.

1847. pH (power of Hydrogen) value of black coffee is

A. 7 B. 8

C. 3 D. 5

Ans. D.

1848. When a metal replaces hydrogen atom then compound form is

A. Oxide B. Ether

C. Salt D. Alcohol

Ans. C.

1849. KOH is used in making of

A. Drain cleaner B. Antacid

C. Cement D. Liquid soap

Ans. D.

1850. If concentration of H^+ is greater than 1×10^{-7} then solution is

A. Neutral B. Basic

C. Acidic D. Aqueous

Ans. C.

1851. Acid used for manufacture of fertilizers and explosives is

A. Nitric acid B. Sulphuric acid

C. Phosphoric acid D. Hydrochloric acid

Ans. A.

1852. pH at which methyl red changes color is

A. 7 B. 5.5

C. 3.8 D. 9

Ans. B.

1853. Substances that react with both acids and bases are called

A. Neutral B. Conjugate bases

C. Amphoteric substances D. Conjugate acids

Ans. C.

1854. Acids ionize in water to produce

A. OH^- ions B. H^+ ions

C. SO_4^{-2} ions D. H_2O molecules

Ans. B.

1855. Corrosive effect on skin is caused by

A. Acids B. Bases

C. Water D. Mercury

Ans. A.

1856. pH of water is

A. 8 B. 3

C. 2 D. 7

Ans. D.

1857. In pure water, concentrations of

A. H^+ and OH^- ions are equal B. H^+ ions is more

C. OH^- ions is more D. Cl^- is more

Ans. A.

1858. Phenolphthalein in acidic solution is

A. Colorless B. Pink colored

C. Yellow colored D. Orange colored

Ans. A.

1859. If pH value is greater than 7, then solution is

A. Acidic B. Basic

C. Neutral D. Salty

Ans. B.

1860. When acid reacts with metal carbonate, products are

A. Salt B. Water

C. Carbon dioxide D. All of above

Ans. D.

1861. Amount of hydrochloric acid (HCl) secreted daily by gastric glands is

A. 1 lit B. 3 lit

C. 2 lit D. 4 lit

Ans. C.

1862. Bronsted-Lowery acid in reaction $H_2O + NH_3\ NH^+{}_4 + OH^-$ is

A. H_2O B. NH_3

C. OH^- D. $NH^+{}_4$

Ans. A.

1863. A substance that donates a pair of electrons to form coordinate covalent bond is called

A. Lewis acid B. Lewis base

C. Bronsted-Lowry acid D. Bronsted-Lowry base

Ans. B.

1864. A species which is able to accept a proton is called

A. Acid B. Base

C. Neutral compound D. Cation

Ans. B.

1865. Preservatives are used to preserve

A. Food B. Acids

C. Bases D. Water

Ans. A.

1866. Bases leaves blue litmus

A. Red B. Pint

C. Black D. Unchanged

Ans. D.

1867. Salt among following is

A. HCl B. KCl

C. HNO_3 D. H_3PO_4

Ans. B.

1868. As an electrolyte, water is

A. Strong B. Neutral

C. Weak D. A good insulator

Ans. C.

1869. Process in which acids (H^+) and bases (OH^-) react to form salts and water is called

A. Neutralization B. Hydrogenation

C. Halogenation D. Sublimation

Ans. A.

1870. Amplification of rRNA genes occurs during development of

A. DNA B. RNA

C. Ova D. None of above

Ans. C.

1871. Increase in number of copies of genes is called

A. Gene duplication B. Gene amplification

C. Gene cloning D. Gene location

Ans. B.

1872. Error in DNA replication that can produce duplications of short genetic sequence is called

A. Ectopic recombination B. Replication slippage

C. Retotransposition D. Aneuploidy

Ans. B.

1873. A mechanism through which new genetic material is generated during molecular evolution is called

A. Gene duplication B. Gene amplification

C. Gene cloning D. All of above

Ans. A.

1874. Gene amplification usually occurs in

A. Meiosis B. Mitosis

C. Replication D. Transcription

Ans. A.

1875. Within chromosomes, DNA is held in complexes with

A. Vitamins B. Amino acids

C. Structural proteins D. Minerals

Ans. C.

1876. Structural proteins organize DNA in to a compact structure called

A. Chromosomes B. Chromatin

C. Ribosomes D. Organelles

Ans. B.

1877. Group of proteins that read and interpret genetic "blueprint" in DNA are called

A. Translation factors B. Replication factors

C. Transcriptional factors D. None of above

Ans. C.

1878. A disk shaped complex which contains two complete turns of DNA is called

A. Nucleotide B. Nucleosome

C. Nucleus D. None of above

Ans. B.

1879. Sequence-specific DNA-binding proteins generally interact with major group of

A. B-DNA B. A-DNA

C. Z-DNA D. C-DNA

Ans. A.

1880. A foreign macromolecule that binds selectively to an antibody is called

A. Stem cell B. Antigen

C. Antibody D. Lymph

Ans. B.

1881. Cells which kills cells that display foreign motifs on their surface are

A. Plasma cells B. Red blood cells

C. Antigens D. Cytotoxic T lymphocytes

Ans. D.

1882. Antibodies are secreted by

A. Stem cells B. Tissue cells

C. Plasma cells D. Membranous cells

Ans. C.

1883. Soluble proteins that function as recognition elements that bind foreign molecules and serve as markers signaling foreign invasion are called

A. Antigens B. Antibodies

C. Fighters D. Epitope

Ans. B.

1884. Immune system comprises of

A. Two parallel systems B. Three parallel systems

C. Two anti parallel systems D. Three anti parallel systems

Ans. A.

1885. Human tintin gene has largest number of

A. Sticky ends B. Axons

C. Exons D. mRNA

Ans. C.

1886. Types of RNA polymerases in eukaryotic cells are

A. 2 B. 3

C. 4 D. 5

Ans. B.

1887. After synthesis eukaryotic mRNA undergo extensive modifications including

A. Capping B. Polyadenylation

C. Splicing D. All of above

Ans. D.

1888. Longest primary transcript is produced by

A. Tintin gene B. Dystrophin gene

C. Centromere protein A D. Neuromedin u

Ans. B.

1889. Sequences remaining after splicing are

A. Axons B. Exons

C. Axioms D. Sticky ends

Ans. B.

1890. Fatty acids which are not directly released in to intestinal capillaries are

A. Long chain fatty acids B. Short chain fatty acids

C. Medium chain fatty acids D. All of above

Ans. A.

1891. Triglycerides are coated with cholesterol and protein in to a compound called

A. Chylomicron B. Lacteal

C. Lipoproteins D. Pyruvic acid

Ans. A.

1892. When released from adipocytes, fatty acids exist in blood as

A. Saturated fatty acids B. Unsaturated fatty acids

C. Bound fatty acids D. Free fatty acids

Ans. D.

1893. Within cell, chylomicron is released in to a lymphatic capillary called

A. Duct B. Lacteal

C. Villi D. Bladder

Ans. B.

1894. Amplification of rRNA genes occurs during development of

A. DNA B. RNA

C. Ova D. None of above

Ans. C.

1895. Increase in number of copies of genes is called

A. Gene duplication B. Gene amplification

C. Gene cloning D. Gene location

Ans. B.

1896. Error in DNA replication that can produce duplications of short genetic sequence is called

A. Ectopic recombination B. Replication slippage

C. Retotransposition D. Aneuploidy

Ans. B.

1897. A mechanism through which new genetic material is generated during molecular evolution is called

A. Gene duplication B. Gene amplification

C. Gene cloning D. All of above

Ans. A.

1898. Gene amplification usually occurs in

A. Meiosis B. Mitosis

C. Replication D. Transcription

Ans. A.

1899. Degeneracy of genetic code was identified by

A. Watson B. Crick

C. Lagervist D. Darwin

Ans. C.

1900. Degeneracy results because there are more codons than

A. Decodable amino acids B. Encodable amino acids

C. Encodable DNA D. Encodable RNA

Ans. B.

1901. Glutamic acid is specified by

A. GAA B. GAG

C. both A and B D. UCA

Ans. C.

1902. Pairing between two nucleotides in RNA that does not follow Watson-Crick base pair rules is called

A. Degeneracy B. Base pairing

C. Lagervist pairing D. Wobble pairing

Ans. D.

1903. Hypoxanthine is nucleobase of

A. Cytocine B. Inosine

C. Trypsin D. None of above

Ans. B.

1904. In eukaryotes genetic recombination can lead to a novel set of genetic information that can be passed on from parents to offspring during

A. Mitosis B. Meiosis

C. Genetic expression D. Replication

Ans. B.

1905. Enzymes that catalyse strand transfer step during recombination are called

A. Recombinases B. Transferases

C. Helicase D. Gyraze

Ans. A.

1906. In both meiotic and mitotic cells, recombination between homologous chromosomes is a common mechanism used in

A. DNA replication B. Transcription

C. DNA repair D. Translation

Ans. C.

1907. During meiosis, genetic recombination involves pairing of

A. Non homologous chromosomes B. Super coiled chromosomes

C. Loosely coiled chromosomes D. Homologous chromosomes

Ans. D.

1908. λ phage vector can carry up to

A. 20 kb fragments B. 30 kb fragments

C. 40 kb fragments D. 50 kb fragments

Ans. A.

1909. Genomic library is normally made by

A. α phage vectors B. λ phage vectors

C. β phage vectors D. γ phage vectors

Ans. B.

1910. Long probes are usually made by

A. Gene expression B. Cloning

C. Hybridization D. All of above

Ans. B.

1911. Types of DNA libraries are

A. 4 B. 3

C. 6 D. 2

Ans. D.

1912. DNA library which lack DNA sequences corresponding to genomic sequence are

A. cDNA library B. Genomic DNA library

C. aDNA library D. bDNA library

Ans. A.

1913. In disaccharides, two monosaccharides are linked together by

A. Ionic bond B. Covalent bond

C. Hydrogen bond D. Glycosidic bond

Ans. D.

1914. Lactose is an example of

A. Polysaccharides B. Monosaccharides

C. Oligosaccharides D. All of above

Ans. C.

1915. Gene is molecular unit of

A. Heredity B. DNA

C. RNA D. Genotype

Ans. A.

1916. Genes evolve due to

A. Natural selection B. Artificial selection

C. Random selection D. Gene selection

Ans. A.

1917. Mutations in sequence of genes are known as

A. Locus B. Population

C. Alleles D. Gene sequence

Ans. C.

1918. Region of DNA that encodes a functional RNA or protein product is called

A. Clone B. Gene

C. Phenotype D. Genotype

Ans. B.

1919. Visible genetic traits include

A. Hair color B. Eye color

C. Number of limbs D. All of above

Ans. D.

1920. Condensation of two monosaccharides yields

A. Disaccharides B. Polysaccharides

C. Large amino acid chains D. Large β sheets

Ans. A.

1921. Non-reducing disaccharides include

A. Sucrose B. Trehalose

C. Both A and B D. Maltose

Ans. C.

1922. Number of types of disaccharides are

A. 3 B. 4

C. 2 D. 1

Ans. C.

1923. Difference in disaccharides is due to

A. Number of H atoms B. Arrangement of atoms within

C. Number of C atoms D. Number of O atoms

Ans. B.

1924. Milk sugar is made from

A. Maltose and fructose B. Sucrose and fructose

C. Glucose and fructose D. Glucose and galactose

Ans. D.

1925. A technique that measures degree of genetic similarity between pools of DNA sequences is called

A. Annealing B. Denaturation

C. Hybridization D. None of above

Ans. C.

1926. Enzyme used in formation of cDNA from mRNA is

A. Helicase B. Polymerase

C. Reverse transcriptase D. Gyrase

Ans. C.

1927. cDNA is produced from

A. tRNA B. mRNA
C. Protein chain D. DNA

Ans. B.

1928. Tail which distinguishes mRNA from tRNA and rRNA is

A. Poly C-tail B. Poly B-tail
C. Poly Z-tail D. Poly A-tail

Ans. D.

1929. To express eukaryotic genes in prokaryotes library used is

A. cDNA library B. bDNA library
C. aDNA library D. zDNA library

Ans. A.

1930. Name of antibiotic which is used to lower blood cholesterol made by a fungi is

A. Azomycin B. Clindamycin
C. Tetracycline D. Lovastatin

Ans. D.

1931. Some fungi are poisonous such as death angel(amanita) and Jack-o' lantern mushroom, they are termed as

A. Toadstools B. Poisonous
C. Harmful D. Toxic

Ans. A.

1932. Aflatoxins are most carcinogenic toxins which are produced by

A. Aspergillus B. Spergillus
C. Carcinogillus D. Thombogillus

Ans. A.

1933. An average of 15-50% of world's food is destroyed each year due to attack of

A. Algae B. Hydra
C. Parasites D. Fungi

Ans. D.

1934. Suspension cultures consist of cells and cell aggregates, growing dispersed in

A. Liquid medium B. Solid nutrient medium
C. Solid or liquid medium D. None of these

Ans. A.

1935. Yeast which had been used for genetic research is

A. Neurospore B. Spore

C. Paraspore D. Regrow

Ans. A.

1936. Vector for leishmaniasis is

A. Tick B. Mite

C. Sand fly D. Tsetse fly

Ans. C.

1937. Which of the following is most severely affected in Kala-azar?

A. Liver B. Spleen

C. Adrenal gland D. Bone marrow

Ans. B.

1938. In India, malaria most often spreads by

A. Anopheles crucifaciens B. Anopheles fluvatis

C. Anopheles stephensi D. Anopheles minimus

Ans. A.

1939. Man is intermediate host for

A. Guinea Worm B. Filaria

C. Malaria D. Kala-azar

Ans. C.

1940. Which of the following organisms can infect humans if improperly cooked meat is used?

A. Trichinella spiralis B. Taenia saginata

C. Taenia solium D. Diphyllobothrium latum

E. Both a and c

Ans. E.

1941. The parasite related to Ancylostoma duodenale is

A. Wuchereria bancrofti B. Necatur americanus

C. Loa loa D. Trichinella spiralis

Ans. B.

1942. Which of the following amoeba does not live in large intestine ?

A. Entamoeba coli B. Entamoeba histolytica

C. Endolimax nana D. Entamoeba gingivalis

Ans. D.

1943. NaCl can act as

A. Antagonist at optimal concentrations

B. Synergistically if added in excess of optimum level

C. Both (a) and (b)

D. None of the above

Ans. C.

1944. The different ACC's between food categories reflect the

A. Expected level of contamination of the raw material

B. Potential for microbial growth during storage

C. Potential shelf life

D. All of the above

Ans. D.

1945. The site of energy production in a cell

A. Micro body

B. Chromosome

C. Ribosome

D. Mitochondria

Ans. D.

1946. Thylakoid is present in

A. Mitochondria

B. Chloroplast

C. ER

D. Golgi apparatus

Ans. B.

1947. The photorespiration involves

A. Calvin cycle

B. Hatch-Slack cycle

C. Glycolate cycle

D. Kreb's cycle

Ans. C.

1948. Mesosomes are also known as

A. Mitochondria

B. Chloroplasts

C. Golgi complex

D. Chondroids

Ans. D.

1949. The enzymes responsible for decomposition is

A. Lipolytic

B. Proteolytic

C. Lysozyme

D. Both a and b

Ans. B.

1950. The largest protozoa is –

A. Balantidium coli B. Entamoeba coli

C. Trichomonus vaginalis D. Toxoplasma gondii

Ans. A.

1951. Premunition is particularly seen in –

A. Ascaris B. Giardia

C. Plasmodium D. None of these

Ans. C.

1952. Meningitis is an infection of

A. The peripheral nervous system

B. The spinal cord and brain

C. The covering of the spinal cord and brain

D. The blood brain barrier

Ans. C.

1953. The microscope with high resolution and low magnification is better than a microscope with low resolution and high magnification ?

A. True B. False

Ans. A.

1954. Filariasis is caused when mosquitoes deliver worms that end up blocking ?

A. Digestive system B. Lymphatic system

C. Circulatory system D. Nervous system

Ans. B.

1955. Mucus helps in protecting against pathogens by

A. Lowering the pH

B. Facilitating the growth of normal flora

C. Blocking access and attachment of pathogens to mucosal surfaces

D. Sequestering Iron

Ans. C.

1956. Which is not a major defence mechanism in the stomach?

A. Proteolytic enzymes B. Low pH

C. Dense normal flora D. All of these

Ans. C.

1957. What is common in catheters and ventilators?

A. They bypass important defenses of the body

B. Bacteria responsible for associated infections are usually susceptible to antibiotics

C. They predispose patients to viral rather than bacterial infections

D. They are used primarily in neonatal intensive care units

Ans. A.

1958. An important host defence of human beings is a dense resident microbiota associated with

A. Lungs
B. Bladder
C. Uterus
D. Vagina

Ans. D.

1959. Lactoferrin helps to protect against pathogens by

A. Sequestering iron
B. Blocking sebum production
C. Lowering the pH
D. Facilitating the growth of normal flora

Ans. A.

1960. Evolutionary relationships between groups of organisms are determined using which of the following type of information?

A. Comparisons of nucleotide sequences

B. Comparisons of biochemical pathways

C. Comparisons of structural features

D. All of the above

Ans. D.

1961. Which of the following is not true for eukaryotic cells?

A. Nucleus is bounded by nuclear membrane

B. Chromosomes contain histones

C. Chloroplasts and mitochondria contains 70S ribosomes

D. Gas vacuoles are present

Ans. D.

1962. Which of the following organelles contain DNA, divides and possesses some degree of autonomy?

A. Golgi apparatus
B. Ribosome
C. Chloroplast
D. Peroxisomes

Ans. C.

1963. Who was the inventor of the Petri dish?

A. R.J. Petri, an assistant of R. Koch

B. A famous French cook

C. Italian glass blower from Petri, Italy

D. None of the above

Ans. A.

1964. Which of the following is not an intrinsic factor in food spoilage?

A. pH

B. Moisture content

C. Available nutrients

D. Temperature

E. Physical structure

Ans. D.

1965. Example of aeration device includes

A. A sparger

B. An impeller

C. A cooling jacket

D. Internal coils

Ans. A.

1966. Biogas contains

A. Carbon monoxide

B. Carboxy acids

C. Methane

D. Ethane

Ans. C.

1967. Pellets

A. Are made from dead plants

B. Are made from dead animals

C. Are obtained through fungal action

D. Are obtained through mixing ethanol and bacteria

Ans. B.

1968. During penicillin production, temperature is maintained at

A. Room temperature

B. 26 °C

C. 36 °C

D. 46 °C

Ans. B.

1969. Hormones and enzymes can be developed through

A. Virus

B. Bacteria

C. Fungus

D. Amoeba

Ans. C.

1970. In dough, starch is digested into sugar through

A. Amylase
B. Protease
C. Maltase
D. Lactase

Ans. A.

1971. Fermenters are designed for

A. Aerobic processes
B. Anaerobic processes
C. Both aerobic and anaerobic respiration
D. Antirobic processes

Ans. C.

1972. Traditional breeding methods are

A. Selective breeding
B. Cell fusion
C. Mutation breeding
D. All of above

Ans. D.

1973. Beer may be produced by

A. Germinating barley
B. Fermenting grape
C. Fermentation of rice
D. All of these

Ans. A.

1974. Link between composers and decomposers is called as

A. Nitrogen cycle
B. Water cycle
C. Carbon cycle
D. Fertility restoration process

Ans. C.

1975. Due to lack of protoplasm, these are not considered cells

A. Bacteria
B. Virus
C. Fungi
D. All of these

Ans. B.

1976. Which of the following characteristic differentiate lysosome from other cell organelles ?

A. Lysosome is a microorganelle
B. Lysosome is a single membrane bound organelle
C. Lysosomes present only in plants
D. All of the above

Ans. B.

1977. The main function of carotenoid in photosynthesis is

A. Light absorption

B. Prevention of photooxidation of chlorophyll

C. Acts as light absorbing centre

D. Acts as the source of electrons

Ans. B.

1978. Most essential features required to maintain a plasmid to a host cell is

A. Ability to transfect cells

B. Antibiotic resistance

C. Origin of replication and marker for selection

D. Capacity to insert into the host genome

Ans. C.

1979. In Pisum sativum, the pair of contrasting characters studied by Mendel was actually located on

A. One chromosome B. Two chromosomes

C. Four chromosomes D. Seven chromosomes

Ans. C.

1980. The exact reason for Mendel's law of independent assortment is

A. Linkage B. Crossing over

C. Disjunction D. Nondisjunction

Ans. C.

1981. The number of linkage groups in an organism will be equal to

A. Number of autosomes B. Number of haploid set

C. Number of diploid set D. 2X number of diploid set

Ans. B.

1982. BIAcore is a detection system patented by Pharmacia Biosensor to detect a ligand binding to a target. What is the name of the phenomenon used in this procedure ?

A. Nuclear magnetic resonance B. Electron spin resonance

C. Surface Plasmon resonance D. Scintillation proximate assay

Ans. C.

1983. There are several sources and methods of discovering new compounds. Which of the following is most likely to lead to the discovery of a complex structure quite unlike any other previously discovered ?

A. Combinatorial chemistry
B. Database mining
C. Screening plant extracts
D. Me too drugs

Ans. C.

1984. Which source has been particularly fruitful in finding novel antitumour agents such as bryostatins and dolostatins ?

A. Marine sources
B. Venoms and toxins
C. Combinatorial chemistry
D. Animals

Ans. A.

1985. Which of the following drugs was not isolated from a natural source ?

A. Quinine
B. Morphine
C. Isoniazid
D. Artemisinin

Ans. C.

1986. Yeast are most likely to grow in frozen fruits during

A. Slow thawing
B. Refrigeration
C. Ambient temperature
D. None of these

Ans. A.

1987. Watery soft rot is found mostly in

A. Fruits
B. Vegetables
C. Cereals
D. All of these

Ans. B.

1988. Black mold rot is caused by

A. A.flavus
B. A.niger
C. Trichoderma
D. Trichothecium roseum

Ans. B.

1989. Concentrate of fruits and vegetable juices

A. Favor the growth of A.niger and A.flavus species
B. Favour the growth of yeast and of acid and sugar tolerant Leuconostoc and Lactobacillus species
C. Favor the growth of Saprophytic bacteria
D. None of the above

Ans. B.

1990. The predominant micro-organisms in frozen foods are

A. Bacteria
B. Micro-coccus
C. Yeast and moulds
D. None of these

Ans. C.

1991. Anthracnose is a defect which can be observed as

A. Spotting of leaves
B. Spotting of seedpods
C. Spotting of fruits
D. All of these

Ans. D.

1992. Stem and rots caused by species of molds involve

A. Leaves of fruits
B. Stem ends of fruits
C. Spotting on vegetables
D. Spotting on fruits

Ans. B.

1993. Species of ———— are predominant on thawing vegetables like sweet corn and peas when the temperature of thawing is fairly low.

A. Streptococcus
B. Micrococcus
C. Both a and B
D. None of these

Ans. B.

1994. Under what conditions food poisoning bacteria may grow and produce toxins in vegetables?

A. When thawed vegetables are held at refrigerated temperature for any considerable period
B. When thawed vegetables are held at room temperature for any considerable period
C. When thawed vegetables are held below refrigerated temperature for any considerable period
D. None of the above

Ans. B.

1995. Bacterial soft rot is caused due to

A. Fermentation of pectin
B. Fermentation of sugars
C. Formation of ketones
D. Formation of amino acids

Ans. A.

1996. Saprophytic bacteria cause

A. Sliminess or souring in piled, wet and heating vegetables
B. Brown rot in vegetables
C. Black rot in fruits
D. Bacterial soft rot

Ans. A.

1997. The micro-organism which is present in both fresh and frozen juices is

A. E.coli
B. Entereobacter aerogenes
C. P. chrysogenum
D. None of these

Ans. B.

1998. The technique first described to determine the incipient spoilage in meat was

A. Homogenate extract volume (HEV)
B. Agar Plate Count (APC)
C. Extract Release Volume (ERV)
D. None of the above

Ans. C.

1999. Which of the following is responsible for a musty or earthy flavor?

A. Actinomycetes
B. Flavobacterium
C. Both (a) and (b)
D. Pseudomonas syncyanea

Ans. A.

2000. Molds causing spoilage of eggs include species of

A. Cladosporium
B. Mucor
C. Thamnidium
D. All of these

Ans. D.

2001. Which of the following strain(s), that grow in the jellies and candid fruits, are able to grow in sugar concentration upto 67.5%?

A. Aspergillus
B. Penicillium
C. Citromyces
D. All of these

Ans. D.

2002. The Redfield ratio is an index of concentration of

A. Carbon, hydrogen and oxygen
B. Nitrogen, potassium and iron
C. Carbon, nitrogen and phosphorous
D. Carbon, phosphorous and sulfur

Ans. C.

2003. Removal of solids is generally considered as a

A. Primary treatment
B. Secondary treatment
C. Tertiary treatment
D. None of these

Ans. A.

2004. Which of the following lymphokine(s) is secreted by delayed-type-hypersensitivity cells?

A. Macrophage stimulating factor B. Migration inhibiting factor

C. Macrophage activating factor D. All of the above

Ans. D.

2005. Which of the following is an example of autoimmune disease?

A. Rheumatoid arthritis B. Systemic lupus erythematosus

C. Polyarteritis nodosa D. All of the above

Ans. D.

2006. Immunosuppressive agent(s) is/are

A. Cyclosporine B. Methotrexate

C. Anti-lymphocytic serum D. All of these

Ans. D.

2007. Induction of tolerance mechanism(s) is/are

A. Suppression B. Clonal deletion

C. Clonal anergy D. All of these

Ans. D.

2008. Number of asymmetric carbon atoms in glucose is

A. One B. Two

C. Three D. Four

Ans. D.

2009. β-1,4 glycosidic bond is present in

A. Maltose B. Lactose

C. Sucrose D. None of the above

Ans. B.

2010. Number of steroisomers of glucose is

A. 4 B. 8

C. 16 D. None of the above

Ans. C.

2011. A homopolysaccharide made up of fructose is

A. Glycogen B. Dextrin

C. Cellulose D. Inulin

Ans. D.

2012. Aglycone portion in methyl glucoside is

A. Glucose
B. Methanol
C. Both of the above
D. None of the above

Ans. B.

2013. Identical osazones are formed by

A. Glucose and fructose
B. Glucose and mannose
C. Mannose and fructose
D. All of the above

Ans. D.

2014. Maltose can be formed by hydrolysis of

A. Starch
B. Dextrin
C. Glycogen
D. All of the above

Ans. D.

2015. α-1, 6 glycosidic bond is not present in

A. Glycogen
B. Dextrin
C. Amylose
D. Amylopectin

Ans. C.

2016. Sulphated iduronic acid is present in

A. Hyaluronic acid
B. Chondroitin sulphate
C. Heparin
D. All of the above

Ans. C.

2017. Monosaccharide can be separated by

A. Electrophoresis
B. Chromatography
C. Salting out
D. None of the above

Ans. B.

2018. Fructose is present in hydrolysis of

A. Sucrose
B. Inulin
C. Both of the above
D. Neither of the above

Ans. C.

2019. N-acetylgalactosamine sulphate is present in

A. Hyaluronic acid
B. Heparin
C. Chondroitin sulphate
D. None of the above

Ans. C.

2020. Invertase catalyses the hydrolysis of

A. Maltose B. Lactose

C. Sucrose D. None of the above

Ans. C.

2021. In fructofuranose anomeric carbon atom is

A. Carbon 1 B. Carbon 2

C. Carbon 3 D. Carbon 4

Ans. B.

2022. A carbohydrate found in DNA is

A. Ribose B. Deoxyribose

C. Ribulose D. All of the above

Ans. B.

2023. A monosaccharide not having D- and L- isomers is

A. Ribose B. Deoxyribose

C. Erythrose D. Dihydroxyacetone

Ans. D.

2024. Which of the following preferably infects reticulocytes?

A. P. ovale B. P. vivax

C. P. falciparum D. P. malaria

Ans. B.

2025. In which type of malarial parasite in the exoerythrocytic stage absent?

A. P. ovale B. P. vivax

C. P. falciparum D. P. malariae

Ans. C.

2026. In falciparum malaria, all of the following stages are seen except

A. Ring stage B. Schizont

C. Gametocyte D. None of these

Ans. B.

2027. Sporozite vaccine in malaria has

A. Induces antibodies

B. Prevents only asexual forms with reproduction

C. No effects on clinical illness

D. None of the above

Ans. A.

2028. Growing trophozoites and schizonts are not seen in the peripheral blood in malaria due to

A. P. falciparum
B. P. vivax
C. P. ovale
D. P. malaria

Ans. A.

2029. The radical treatment of malaria is to half

A. Gametocyte
B. Exo-erythrocytic phase
C. Erythrocytic phase
D. All of these

Ans. C.

2030. Kawasaki syndrome is

A. Most prevalent in Japan and Hawaii
B. Patients show rickettsia like bacteria in skin biopsies
C. Strain involved may be propionibacterium
D. All of these

Ans. D.

2031. A study involving analysis of risk for genetic defects in a family is

A. Genetic Engineering
B. Genetic counselling
C. Genetic drift
D. Genetic equilibrium

Ans. D.

2032. Kinetosomes are observed in

A. Algae
B. Fungi
C. Protozoa
D. Viruses

Ans. C.

2033. Black water fever is caused by

A. P. vivax
B. P. falciparum
C. P. ovale
D. None of these

Ans. B.

2034. Amoebic dysentery in humans is caused by

A. Plasmodium
B. Paramecium
C. Yeast
D. Entamoeba histolytica

Ans. D.

2035. Cytochromes are

A. Oxygen acceptors
B. ATP acceptors
C. Electron acceptors
D. Protein acceptors

Ans. C.

2036. The capacity of a given strain of microbial species to produce disease is known as

A. Pathogen
B. Virulence
C. Infection
D. None of these

Ans. B.

2037. Glucans, Mannans and Chitin are found to be present in the cell wall of

A. Plants
B. Eubacteria
C. Fungi
D. Actinomyces

Ans. C.

2038. Communicable means

A. Spread while staying at a hospital
B. Disease that spread by direct contact
C. Disease that is easily spread
D. Inanimate object

Ans. B.

2039. Sterilization is defined as

A. Removal of microbial contamination
B. Complete destruction of all forms of life
C. Completes removal of vegetative cells
D. Removal of most microorganisms

Ans. B.

2040. A substance that has been pasterized could also be considered to be sterilized.

A. True
B. False

Ans. B.

2041. Legionaires disease affect ——— system.

A. Respiratory
B. Urogenital
C. Nervous, fever, eyes
D. Gastrointestinal
E. Skin
F. Muscle

Ans. A.

2042. Which one of the following is true in respect to pyrogens ?

A. Kills cells infected with virus
B. Stimulates fever
C. Oily glue on the skin
D. Kills Gm+ bacteria

Ans. B.

2043. The agent responsible for causing mad cow disease is thought to be a

A. Fungus
B. Protozoan
C. Prion
D. Virus

Ans. C.

2044. All infections do not cause fever and all fevers are not due to infections which of the following is an example of non-infections cause of fever?

A. Typhoid
B. Chicken pox
C. Rheumatic disease
D. Malaria

Ans. C.

2045. Which of the following is not true for prokaryotic organism?

A. Nucleus is not bounded by nuclear membrane
B. Chromosomes does not contain histones
C. 80S ribosomes are distributed in cytoplasm
D. Cell wall contains peptidoglycan as one of the major component

Ans. C.

2046. A newly discovered microscopic structure is hypothesized to be a living organism. Which of the following lines of evidence would support the contention that this organism may be alive?

A. It contains DNA
B. It is made of a single cell
C. It utilizes energy
D. All the above

Ans. C.

2047. Which one is not studied in microbiology?

A. Bacteria
B. Animal behaviour
C. Fungi
D. Algae

Ans. B.

2048. Cell theory includes all of the following except

A. All organisms are composed of one or more cells
B. The cell is the most primitive form of life
C. The cell is the structural unit of life
D. Cells arise by division of preexisting cells

Ans. B.

2049. The five-kingdom system of classification was set up by

A. Louis Pasteur
B. Robert Whittaker
C. Robert Koch
D. Masaki Ogata

Ans. B.

2050. Despite efforts to eliminate spoilage organisms during canning, sometimes canned foods are spoiled. This may be due to

A. Spoilage before canning

B. Underprocessing during canning

C. Leakage of contaminated water through can seams during cooling.

D. All of the above

E. None of the above

Ans. D.

2051. The effectiveness of many chemical preservatives depends primarily on the food

A. Temperature
B. pH
C. Water content
D. Acidity
E. All of the above

Ans. B.

2052. Sodium nitrite is responsible for

A. Protecting against botulism
B. Reducing rate of spoilage
C. Maintenance of red color in meat
D. All of the above
E. None of the above

Ans. D.

2053. Which of the following refers to the addition of microorganisms to the diet in order to provide health benefits beyond basic nutritive value?

A. Antibiotics
B. Adjuvants
C. Probiotics
D. Prebiotics
E. Symbiotics

Ans. C.

2054. The significance of the plasma membrane is that

A. It selectively allows some molecules to pass into the organism

B. It prevents movement of molecules out of the organism

C. It is the site of protein synthesis

D. All of the above

Ans. D.

2055. In bacterial cells, ribosomes are packed into the cytoplasmic matrix and also loosely attached to the plasma membrane. What is the function of ribosomes?

A. Site of energy production
B. Site of protein synthesis
C. Site of genetic reproduction

Ans. B.

2056. Biogas is

A. Methane rich fuel
B. Ecofriendly and pollution free source
C. Propane rich fuel
D. Both A and C

Ans. D.

2057. High value of BOD (Biological Oxygen demand) shows

A. Water is normal
B. Water is highly polluted
C. Water is less polluted
D. None of these

Ans. B.

2058. Rennet is used in

A. Bread making
B. Fermentation
C. Cheese making
D. Antibiotic synthesis

Ans. C.

9

Public Health

1. Which one of the following statement is true regarding pathogenicity of *Mycobacteria species?*

   A. *M. tuberculosis* is more pathogenic than *M. bovis* to humans

   B. *M. Kansasii* can cause a disease indistinguishable from tuberculosis

   C. *M . Africanum* infection is acquired from an environmental source

   D. *M. Marinum* is responsible for tubercular lymphadenopathy

Ans. B. *M. tuberculosis* and *M. bovis* are equally pathogenic to humans. *M Africanum* is part of M. tuberculosis complex together with *M. tuberculosis*, *M. bovis* and *M. microti.* Environmental sources are present in case of non tuberculous mycobacteria and atypical mycobacteria. They are not seen in case of bacteria belonging to *M.tuberculosis* complex.

2. A patient admitted to an ICU is on central venous line for the last one week. He is on ceftazidime and amikacin. After 7 days of antibiotics he develops a spike of fever an his blood culture is positive for gram positive cocci in chains, which are catalase negative. Following this, vancomycin was started but the culture remained positive for the same organism even after 2 weeks of therapy. The most likely organism causing infection is:

   A. *Staphylococcus aureus*

   B. *Viridans streptococci*

   C. *Enterococcus faecalis*

   D. Coagulase negative Staphylococcus

Ans. C.

3. With reference to Bacteroides fragilis the following statements are true except-

   A. *B. fragilis* is the most frequent anaerobe isolated from clinical samples

   B. *B. fragilis* is not uniformly sensitive to metronidazole

   C. The lipopolysaccharide formed by *B. fragilis* is structurally and functionally different from the conventional endotoxin

   D. Shock and disseminated intravascular coagulation are common in Bacteriodes bacteremia

Ans. **D. Bacteroides: Gram negative anaerobic bacilli. Most common anaerobic pathogen isolated from clinical specimens. Virulence factors include capsular polysaccharides and lipopolysaccharide endotoxin Lipopolysaccharide endotoxin is much less toxic compared to other gram negative bacteria.**

Hence infections do not directly produce signs of sepsis, which is common in other gram negative bacteri. Some are resistant to metronidazole.

4. A child had pustular lesion on leg. On gram staining gram positive cocci are seen. To establish the diagnosis of Group A streptococcal erythroderma, the test used is

A. Bile solubility test B. Catalase test

C. Optochin sensitivity D. Bacitracin sensitivity

Ans. **D.**

5. A veterinary doctor had pyrexia of unknown origin. His blood culture in special laboratory media was positive for gram-negative short bacilli which was oxidase positive. Which one of the following is the likely organism grown in culture?

A. *Pasteurella spp* B. *Francisella spp*

C. *Bartonella spp* D. *Brucella spp*

Ans. **D. Brucella is a gram negative bacillus and is oxidase positive. Infection is associated with exposure to infected animals or their products. Individuals at high risk of acquiring infection are farmers, veterinarians and workers in slaughter houses. Patients frequently present with pyrexia of unknown origin.**

6. A young boy had a flea bite while working in a wheat grain godown. After 5 days he developed fever and had axillary lymphadenopathy. A smear was sent to the laboratory to perform a specific staining. Which one of the following staining method would help in the identification of the suspected pathogen:

A. Albert staining B. Ziehl Neelsen staining

C. McFadyen's staining D. Wayson staining

Ans. **D. Flea bite might have been by a rat flea as wheat grain godowns are frequented by rats. Fever and axillary lymphadenopathy are characteristic features of bubonic plague – which is spread by bite of rat flea. Wayson stain is used to demonstrate *Yersinia pestis* which is the causative organism for plague.**

7. An infant had high grade fever and respiratory distress at the time of presentation to the emergency room. The sample collected for blood culture was subsequently positive showing growth of a haemolytic colonies. On Gram staining these were gram positive cocci. In the screening test for identification, the suspected pathogen is likely to be susceptible to the following agent:

A. Bacitracin
B. Novobiocin
C. Optochin
D. Oxacillin

Ans. C.

8. A VDRL reactive mother gave birth to an infant. All of the following would help in determining the risk of transmission to the infant except:
   A. TPHA test on the serum sample of the mother
   B. TPHA test on the serum sample of the infant
   C. VDRL on the paired serum sample of the infant and mother
   D. Time interval between the treatment of the mother and her delivery

Ans. B. Serological testing for syphilis is not reliable in case of neonates. Negative serology does not rule out the possibility of infection.

9. Cholera toxin:
   A. Increases the levels of intracellular cylic GMP
   B. Acts through the opoid receptors
   C. Causes continued activation of adenylate cyclase
   D. Inhibits the enzyme phosphodiesterase

Ans. C.

10. In the gut, anaerobic bacteria outnumber the aerobes by a ratio of
   A. 10:1
   B. 100:1
   C. 1000:1
   D. 10000:1

Ans. C.

11. Vector of the agent of scrub typhus
   A. Larval stage of lice
   B. Larval stage of mites
   C. Adult stage of lice
   D. Adult stage of mites
   E. Fleas

Ans. B.

12. _____ causes post-operative infection after breast augmentation
   A. *M. kansasii*
   B. *M. fortuitum*
   C. *M. chelonae*
   D. *M. asiaticum*
   E. B and C

Ans. B.

13. Susceptible to sulphonamides
   A. *C. trachomatis*
   B. *C. psittaci*
   C. *C. pneumonia*
   D. All of the above

Ans. A.

14. A milder decontaminating solution allowing longer time period for decontamination

A. NALC-NaOH method

B. Benzalkonium Chloride-Trisodium Phosphate Method

C. Modfied Benzalkonium Chloride-Trisodium Phosphate Method

D. All of the above

E. A & B

Ans. B.

15. Which is NOT true?

A. *C. trachomatis* causes trachoma

B. *C. trachomatis* has 18 species specific Ag while *C. psittaci* has 15

C. Chlamydia has tropism for columnar cells

D. Inclusion conjunctivitis is caused by *C. trachomatis*

E. Lymphogranuloma venereum is caused by *C. psittaci*

Ans. E.

16. Which is NOT correctly matched?

A. *M. tuberculosis* - tapered ends

B. MOTT - thicker and more beaded

C. M. avium-intracellulare - short and coccobacillary

D. M. kansasii - barber's pole appearance

E. None of the above

Ans. E.

17. *Treponema pallidum* is cultivated

A. In vitro

B. In footpads of mice

C. Armadillo

D. Testicles of rabbits

E. B and C

Ans. D.

18. Diagnosed by the cold hemagglutination test

A. *C. trachomastis*

B. *C. psittaci*

C. *C. pneumonia*

D. *M. pneumoniae*

E. *R. tsutsugamushi*

Ans. D.

19. Which is NOT true?

A. Mycoplasma lacks a true cell wall

B. Mycoplasma is a pleuropneuominia-like organism

C. Mycoplasma has a fried egg appearance

D. Mycoplasma hyrdolyzes urea

E. Mycoplasma pneumoniae has a mulberry appearance in mod. NYC medium

Ans. D.

20. True to Weil-Felix reaction

A. Diagnoses Weil's disease

B. Uses Proteus vulgaris antigen OX-19, OX-2 and Proteus mirabilis OX-K

C. False (+) in leptospirosis

D. A and B

E. B and C

Ans. E.

21. Which is NOT true to leptospira?

A. Is an obligate aerobe

B. Culture medium = Stewart's medium, Fletcher's medium and EMJH medium

C. Best specimen during the first week of infection is urine

D. Causes Weil's disease

E. None of the above

Ans. C.

22. Which is a mucolytic agent in decontamination and concentration ?

A. N-Acetyl-L-Cystein

B. NaOH

C. Zerphiran Chloride

D. Trisodium Phosphate

E. A and B

Ans. A.

23. Causes lyme disease

A. *B. hermsii*

B. *B. recurrentis*

C. *B. burgdorferi*

D. Borrelia with 7-11 axial fibrils/cell

E. C and D

Ans. E.

24. Which is NOT true for *C. pneumonia* ?

A. Causes walking pneumonia

B. Specimen of choice is sputum

C. Culture in Hep 2 cells and HL cells

D. Inactivated at RT

E. All of the above

Ans. A.

25. Runyon's classification of NTM are based on

A. Colony texture

B. Colonial pigmentation

C. Epidemiology

D. Rate of growth

E. B & D

Ans. E.

26. Which is NOT true

A. Rickettsia and Ehrlichia do not undergo intracellular development cycle

B. Tsutsugamushi disease can be caused by *R. orientalis*

C. Scrub typhus is transmitted by the larva of trombiculid mites

D. Small cell variant and large cell variant of Coxiella are both infectious

E. Coxiella divides by transverse fission

Ans. A.

27. Which one is true ?

A. *T. pallidum* subsp. pertenue causes syphilis

B. Treponema has intracytoplasmic tubules

C. *T. carateum* causes pinta

D. B and C

E. A & B.

Ans. D.

28. Which does NOT develop pigment following exposure to light after being grown in the dark for more than 7 days?

A. *M. asiaticum*

B. *M. kansasii*

C. *M. szulgai*

D. A and B

E. All the above

Ans. C.

29. The habitat of *M. scrofulaceum* is

A. Soil
b. Water
C. Raw milk
d. Dairy products
E. All the above

Ans. E.

30. ————has a fried egg appearance except

A. *Mycoplasma genitalium*
B. *Ureaplasma urealyticum*
C. *Mycoplasma pneuomoniae*
D. *Mycoplasma genitalium*
E. *Mycoplasma hominis*

Ans. C.

31. —— causes Rickettsial pox

A. *R. akari*
B. *R. rickettsii*
C. *R. tsutsugamushi*
D. *E. sennetsu*
E. A & B

Ans A.

32. ——— has cauliflower colonies

A. *M. tuberculosis*
B. *M. bovis*
C. *M. bovis* BCG
D. *M. africanum*
E. All the above

Ans. A.

33. Which does NOT belong to the *Mycobacterium avium* complex?

A. *M. avium*
B. *M. lepraemurium*
C. *M. silvaticum*
D. *M. leprae*
E. *M. intracellulare*

Ans. D.

34. *Calymmatobacterium granulomatis* —

A. Causes granuloma inguinale
B. Forms painless lesions which bleed easily
C. Causes Donovanosis
D. Has a safety pin appearance
E. All the above

Ans. E.

35. Chlamydia are

A. Cell wall deficient
B. Produce endotoxin and exotoxin
C. Obligate intracellular parasites
D. All the above
E. Only A & C

Ans. C.

36. Which is not a desirable specimen for mycobacteria?

A. Gastric aspirate
B. Blood
C. CSF
D. 24 hour urine
E. Semen

Ans. D.

37. Reservoir of *M. kansasii*

A. Humans with cavitary diseases
B. Tap water
C. Children
D. Natural waters
E. None of the above

Ans. B.

38. *M. leprae* is cultivated

A. In vitro
B. In footpads of mice
C. Armadillo
D. In footpads of guineapigs
E. B & C

Ans. E.

39. Which is not true ?

A. For culture, use 2 solid media and 1 liquid media
B. Voided urine does not require decontamination
C. Bottle caps should be loose in the first 2 weeks of incubation
D. NaOH is a toxic decontaminating agent
E. B and D

Ans. B.

40. Excellent medium for MOTT (Mycobacteria other than tuberculosis) especially MAC

A. Lowenstein-Jensen with pyruic acid
B. L-J with iron
C. Bactec 12B medium
D. Mitchison's selective 7H 11
E. Wallenstein

Ans. E.

41. Which moves sluggishly with a drifting motion and flexous movements?

A. Treponema
B. Borrelia
C. Leptospira
D. All of the above
E. None of the above

Ans. A.

42. Uses reagin and cardiolipin

A. VDRL
B. Weil-Felix Reaction
C. Wasserman test
D. RPR
E. None of the above

Ans. C.

43. Which is/are rapid growers ?

A. *M. fortuitum*
B. *M. gordonae*
C. *M. chelonae*
D. B and C
E. A & C

Ans. E.

44. Inhibited by thiophene-2-carboxylic acid hydrazide

A. *M. marinum*
B. *M. bovis*
C. *M. tuberculosis*
D. *M. asiaticum*
E. None of the above

Ans. B.

45. Which is not true ?

A. *M. gordonae* is nonpathogenic
B. Mycobacteria are slow growers
C. Mycobacteria are nonpigmented
D. Mycobacteria contain N-acteylmuramic acid in their cell wall
E. Tuberculin testing is the primary means of identifying individuals with *M. tuberculosis*

Ans. D.

46. Specimen of choice for MAC in AIDS patients

A. Blood
B. CSF
C. Stool
D. Sputum
E. A and D

Ans. A.

47. Media for mycoplasma

A. SP-4 medium
B. Edward Hayflick agar
C. EMJH medium
D. Barbour-Stoenner-Kelly medium
E. A & B

Ans. E.

48. Reiters syndrome is associated with

A. *C. trachomatis*
B. *C. psittaci*
C. *C. pneumonia*
D. *M. pneumoniae*
E. *R. tsutsugamushi*

Ans. A.

49. Levinthal-Cole-Lillie bodies are inclusions in

A. *C. trachomatis*
B. *C. psittaci*
C. *C. pneumonia*
D. All the above
E. None of the above

Ans. B.

50. Specimen of choice for NTM (Non tuberculous mycobacteria)

A. Sputum
B. Gastric aspirate
C. Urine
D. Fecal specimen
E. Bronchial washings

Ans. E.

51. Which is NOT true?

A. Translucent or tranparent colonies of MAC are more virulent than opaque colonies
B. M. leprae cannot be cultivated in vitro
C. Numerous AFB (acid fast bacilli) can be obtained from lesions of Tuberculoid leprosy
D. Wade-Fite technique is used for acid fast staining of paraffinized tissue
E. M. marinum grows at RT

Ans. C.

52. Cell lines used in culture for *C. trachomatis*

A. HL cell line
B. HeLa cells
C. Hep 2 cells
D. McCoy cells
E. B & D

Ans. E.

53. A buff colored, slow growing, rough colony, and a positive niacin test is a preliminary ID for

A. *M. tuberculosis*

B. *M. bovis*

C. *M. kansasii*

D. MAC

E. MOTT (Mycobacteria other than tuberculosis)

Ans. A.

54. Has pear shaped elemental bodies

A. *C. psittaci*

B. *C. trachomatis*

C. *C. pneumoniae*

D. All the above

E. A & B

Ans. C.

55. Heating at 68 degress Celsius for 20min inactivates catalase in

A. *M. bovis*

B. *M. tuberculosis*

C. *M. gastri*

D. *M. haemophlium*

E. All the above

Ans. E.

56. Which does NOT reduce nitrate?

A. *M. tuberculosis*

B. *M. scrofulaceum*

C. *M. szulgai*

D. *M. fortuitum*

E. *M. kansasii*

Ans. B.

57. Not true to the Weil-Felix reaction

A. Uses proteus antigens

B. Significant titer is >1:160

C. There are false (-) reaction in proteus infections

D. It is used as a test for Ricketssia

E. All the above

Ans. C.

58. True to leptospira

A. Have Diaminopimelic acid

B. Do not have hooked ends

C. Microaerophilic

D. Use CHO as their carbon source

E. All of the above

Ans. A.

59. What is caused by *Coxiella burnetti*

A. Scrub typhus
B. Q fever
C. Rocky mountain spotted fever
D. Sennetsu fever
E. A & B

Ans. B.

60. Which are incubated in the dark?

A. Mycobacterium
B. Chlamydia
C. Leptospira
D. All the above
E. A & B

Ans. E.

61. Individuals with lower incomes and levels of education have a shorter life span on average. Which of the following determinants of health best describes this situation?

A. Behavior
B. Geography
C. Genetics
D. Environment
E. Socio-economic

Ans. E.

62. Mold and cockroaches are believed to be related to the development of asthma. Which of the following determinants of health best describes this situation?

A. Behavior
B. Geography
C. Genetics
D. Environment
E. Socio-economic

Ans. D.

63. Cigarette smoking is a major cause of premature births. Which of the following determinants of health best describes this situation?

A. Behavior
B. Geography
C. Genetics
D. Environment
E. Socio-economic

Ans. A.

64. Radon reduction is required for homes that have a high level of radon emissions prior to sale of the home. Which of the following public health strategies best describes this approach?

A. Reducing high risk- focusing on groups at highest risk to reduce their risk leaving others unchanged

B. Improving the average- focusing on the entire population

C. Narrowing the spread - reducing high risk groups by increasing the risk for low risk groups

D. None of the above

Ans. A.

65. Salt is gradually reduced in processed foods and in restaurant menus over the course of a decade. Which of the following public health strategies best describes this approach?

A. Reducing high risk- focusing on groups at highest risk to reduce their risk leaving others unchanged

B. Improving the average- focusing on the entire population

C. Narrowing the spread - reducing high risk groups by increasing the risk for low risk groups

D. None of the above

Ans. B.

66. A site of airborne pollution affecting a nearby community is addressed by building a higher chimney that disperses the pollution over a wider area. Which of the following public health strategies best describes this approach?

A. Reducing high risk- focusing on groups at highest risk to reduce their risk leaving others unchanged

B. Improving the average- focusing on the entire population

C. Narrowing the spread - reducing high risk groups by increasing the risk for low risk groups

D. None of the above

Ans. C.

67. Taxes on soft drinks containing sugar are raised in an effort to discourage consumption. Which of the following types of population health interventions best describes this approach?

A. Healthcare system intervention
B. Traditional public health intervention
C. Social policy intervention
D. None of the above

Ans. C.

68. Vaccinations are provided without cost sharing as part of health insurance. Which of the following types of population health interventions best describes this approach

A. Healthcare system intervention
B. Traditional public health intervention
C. Social policy intervention
D. None of the above

Ans. A.

69. Which of the following is/are currently considered a vulnerable population?

A. Pregnant women and children B. Workers in high risk profession

C. HIV positive individuals D. All of the above

Ans. D.

70. Which of the following are potential definitions of a population?

A. All the individuals living in a country, state or other geographic area

B. Members of an insurance plan

C. Students at a university including those taking distance education courses

D. All of the above

E. None of the above

Ans. D.

71. Which of the following is true of the resistance of bacteria to antibiotics?

A. Resistance is a new phenomenon that has only been recognized in the 21st century.

B. Resistance of TB to drugs is rare.

C. Antibiotic resistant staphylococcus is now widespread outside hospitals

D. New antibiotics are believed to be the best solution to the problem of antibiotic resistance.

Ans. C.

72. Which of the following is/are true of the role that treatment of disease can play in reducing communicability?

A. Treatment of HIV reduces the blood level of the virus and thus reduces its communicability.

B. Epidemiological treatment of disease based upon exposure can be an effective means of controlling the spread of sexually transmitted diseases such as gonorrhoea

C. HIV is most easily transmitted prior to the presence of a positive standard test making treatment of infected individuals a less effective method for controlling spread of the disease.

D. All of the above

Ans. D.

73. Which of the following statements about vaccines (live and/or killed) is true?

A. Vaccines have only been shown to be effective before contact with a disease

B. Vaccines have only been shown to be effective against virus and bacteria

C. Vaccines have only been shown to be effective for those who receive the vaccine

D. Vaccines like medications have benefits and harms

Ans. D.

74. This type of immunization produces immunity that resembles that produced by infection with the pathogen against which the vaccine is directed. This statement best describes which of the following types of immunization

A. Live vaccine

B. Killed vaccine

C. Passive immunity

D. None of the above

Ans. A.

75. This type of immunization utilizes components of the pathogen to generate specific antibodies that provide protection which may be of short duration. This statement best describes which of the following type of immunization?

A. Live vaccine

B. Killed vaccine

C. Passive immunity

D. None of the above

Ans. B.

76. This type of immunization utilizes preformed antibodies to provide temporary protection similar to the protection provided by a mother to her newborn child. This statement best describes which of the following type of immunization?

A. Live vaccine

B. Killed vaccine

C. Passive immunity

D. None of the above

Ans. C.

77. Which of the following is the most accurate statement about the eradication of disease

A. Smallpox and polio are the only diseases that are can potentially be eradicated.

B. Eradication is likely to be the primary method of disease prevention in the future

C. The optimum conditions for eradication of a disease include the absence of animal reservoirs, the absence of long-term carrier states, and the development of potent long term protection through natural infection or vaccination.

D. Eradication is made easier if the disease can be transmitted before the appearance of symptoms

Ans. C.

78. Which of the following is a true statement about influenza?

A. The rapid mutation of influenza requires annual changes in seasonal influenza vaccine

B. Live influenza vaccines are now available for nasal administration.

C. Influenza's short incubation period and ability to be readily transmitted through the air before the appearance of symptoms gives it the potential for epidemic spread.

D. All of the above

Ans. D.

79. Which of the following is the most accurate statement about rabies vaccine?

A. Rabies vaccine must be administered before exposure to be effective

B. Rabies vaccine is now grown in human tissue and has a safety record comparable to most other vaccines

C. Rabies can potentially be eradicated through the use of vaccines

D. None of the above is true.

Ans. B.

80. Which of the following is NOT true of HIV and drugs?

A. Post exposure treatment with drugs has been shown to be effective for needle stick exposure

B. Drugs have been shown to be effective in reducing the viral load of HIV

C. Drugs have been shown to extend the life span of those with HIV

D. Drugs have been shown to cure HIV

Ans. D.

81. Most spoilage bacteria grow at

A. Acidic pH b. Alkaline pH

C. Neutral pH d. Any of the pH

Ans. C.

82. The microbiological examination of coliform bacteria in foods preferably use

A. MacConkey broth B. Violet red bile agar

C. Eosin Methylene blue agar D. All of these

Ans. D.

83. Which of the following acid will have higher bacteriostatic effect at a given pH?

A. Acetic acid B. Tartaric acid

C. Citric acid D. Maleic acid

Ans. A.

84. Which of the following is not true for the thermal resistance of the bacterial cells?

A. Cocci are usually more resistant than rods

B. Higher the optimal and maximal temperatures for growth, higher the resistance

C. Bacteria that clump considerably or form capsules are difficult to kill

D. Cells low in lipid content are harder to kill than other cells

Ans. D.

85. Water activity can act as

A. An intrinsic factor determining the likelihood of microbial proliferation

B. A processing factor

C. An extrinsic factor

D. All of the above

Ans. D.

86. The different ACC's between food categories reflect the

A. Expected level of contamination of the raw material

B. Potential for microbial growth during storage

C. Potential shelf life

D. All of the above

Ans. D.

87. Examination of the presence / absence of organisms refers to

A. Incubation of a food suspension in an enrichment medium followed by inoculation on to a suitable selective medium

B. Incubation of a food suspension in an enrichment medium followed by inoculation on to a non-selective medium

C. Incubation of a food suspension in an enrichment medium

D. None of the above

Ans. A.

88. Plate count of bacteria in foods generally use the plating medium consisting of

A. Peptone, yeast extract, glucose, sodium chloride, agar and distilled water

B. Yeast extract, glucose, sodium chloride, agar and distilled water

C. Peptone, glucose, sodium chloride, agar and distilled water

D. Peptone, yeast extract, glucose, sodium chloride and distilled water

Ans. A.

89. What are the intrinsic factors for the microbial growth?

A. pH
B. Moisture
C. Oxidation-Reduction Potential
D. All of these

Ans. D.

90. Yeast and mould count determination requires-

A. Nutrient agar
b. Acidified potato glucose agar
C. Mac Conkey agar
D. Violet Red Bile agar

Ans. B.

91. The time temperature combination for HTST paterurization of 71.1°C for 15 sec is selected on the basis of

A. *Coxiella burnetii*
B. *E. coli*
C. *B. subtilis*
D. *C. botulinum*

Ans. A.

92. Aerobic Colony Count (ACC), is also known as

A. Total viable count (TVC)
B. Aerobic plate count (APC)
C. Standard plate count (SPC)
D. All of these

Ans. D.

93. Which of the following is true about ISO 2002 method for Salmonella detection?

A. Selenite cystine (SC) broth is replaced by Muller Kauffmann tetrathionate novobiocin broth (MKTTn)
B. Rappaport Vassiliadis (RV) broth has been replaced by Rappaport Vassiliadis Soya (RVS) broth
C. XLD is the first isolation medium rather than BGA
D. All of these

Ans. D.

94. Suspected colonies of *Staphylococcus aureus* when grown on Baird-Parker medium shall show

A. Coagulase activity
b. Protease activity
C. Catalase activity
D. None of these

Ans. A.

95. A psychrophilic halophile would be a microbe that prefers

A. Cold temperatures and increased amounts of salt
B. Warm temperatures and increased amounts of pressure
C. Cold temperatures and the absence of oxygen
D. Warm temperatures and increased amounts of acid

Ans. A.

96. NaCl can act as

A. Antagonist at optimal concentrations

B. Synergistically if added in excess of optimum level

C. Both (a) and (b)

D. None of the above

Ans. C.

97. The cells which act as parasite in the body.

A. Schwann cells
B. Hepatocytes
C. Kupffer's cells
D. Cancer cells

Ans. D.

98. TAB vaccine is useful against

A. Polio
B. Diphtheria
C . Typhoid
D. Pertussis

Ans. C.

99. Which one of the following is tested the most for the detection of carrier of typhoid ?

A. Urine
B. blood
C. Faeces
D. Sputum

Ans. C.

100. The pathogen of typhoid is transmitted through

A. Urine
B. Water
C. Blood
D. CSF

Ans. B.

101. A sexually transmitted bacterial disease is

A. AIDS
B. Syphilis
C. Herpes
D. Hepatitis

Ans. B.

102. Sarcoma is cancer of

A. Bone

B. Adipose tissue

C. Connective tissue and muscular tissue

D. All the above

Ans. D.

103. Most of the tumours are

A. Malignant
B. Benign
C. Related to carcinoma
D. Sample boils

Ans. B.

104. Inactive cancer gene is called

A. Transposon
B. Proto-oncogene
C. Tumour promoter gene
D. Tumour suppressor gene

Ans. B.

105. ELISA is helpful for the detection of

A. Malaria
B. AIDS
C. Leprosy
D. Cancer

Ans. B.

106. The symptoms of typhoid called intestinal haemorrhage occurs in ——— weeks of infection.

A. 1st
B. 2nd
C. 3rd
D. 4th

Ans. C.

107. AIDS day

A. May 1
B. December 20
C. June 1
D. December 1

Ans. D.

10

Virology

1. Which of the following hepatitis viruses is not RNA virus?

A. Hepatitis A virus B. Hepatitis B virus

C. Hepatitis E virus D. Hepatitis G virus

Ans. B.

2. Which of the following nucleic acid is present in hepatitis B virus?

A. dsDNA B. ssRNA

C. ssDNA D. dsRNA

Ans. A.

3. Hepatitis G virus belongs to the family ——.

A. Caliciviridae B. Flaviviridae

C. Hepadnaviridae D. Coronaviridae

Ans. B.

4. Transmission of hepatitis G virus is ——.

A. Parenterally B. Sexually

C. Both A and B D. None of these

Ans. C.

5. Which of the following disinfectant is effective against viruses?

A. Hydrogen peroxide B. Hypochloride

C. Formaldehyde D. All the above

Ans. D.

6. Viruses largely lack metabolic machinery of their own to generate energy or to synthesize

A. Protein B. Carbohydrate

C. Alcohol D. All the above

Ans. A.

7. Viruses require __________ for growth.

A. Bacteria
B. Plants
C. Animals
D. Living cells

Ans. D.

8. Reverse transcriptase is a useful enzyme to have when

A. An RNA virus converts its RNA to DNA
B. There are no host cells present
C. Nutrients are scarce
D. Spikes are forming in the new virion

Ans. A.

9. Which of the following is the agent associated with the development of neurodegenerative disease in livestock and humans?

A. Prions
B. Viriods
C. Virions
D. Virinos

Ans. A.

10. The __________ of the influenza-enveloped virus appear to be involved in attachment to the host cell receptor site.

A. Fimbriae
B. Flagellae
C. Haemagglutinin
D. Neuraminidase

Ans. C.

11. Intracellular structures formed during many viral infections, called __________, which can directly disrupt cell structure.

A. Prokaryotes
B. Chromosomal disruptions
C. Inclusion bodies
D. Cytocidal bodies

Ans. C.

12. Animal viruses with capsids displaying helical symmetry include

A. Measles and mumps
B. Influenza
C. Rabies
D. All of these

Ans. D.

13. Icosahedral viruses are generally

A. Polioviruses
B. Adenoviruses
C. Both A &B
D. None of these

Ans. C

14. Negative strand ssRNA viruses need to have a preformed replicase when they invade a mammalian cell because they

    A. Use it to terminate transcripts when they copy host cell mRNA

    B. Have to make a positive strand copy that can be translated

    C. Use it to modify host enzymes that are recruited for viral replication

    D. None of the above

Ans. B.

15. Which of the following reflects the correct order of events that take place during the multiplication of a virus?

    A. Attachment, penetration, maturation, biosynthesis, release

    B. Penetration, attachment, biosynthesis, maturation, release

    C. Attachment, penetration, biosynthesis, maturation, release

    D. Attachment, release, biosynthesis, maturation, penetration

Ans. C.

16. Influenza virus undergoes antigenic shift resulting in major antigenic changes by which of the following mechanisms?

    A. Somatic recombination of heavy and light chains

    B. Expression of several different capsule types

    C. Changing the receptor binding canyon that docks with the host receptor

    D. Reassortment of RNA segments from different influenza viruses

Ans. D.

17. The nucleocapsid is covered by an outer membrane like structure called

    A. Envelope B. Covering

    C. Membronocapsid D. All of these

Ans. A.

18. Which type of interferon is produced by virus-infected cells?

    A. α B. β

    C. Both A & B D. None of these

Ans. C.

19. Viral matrix proteins are

    A. Exposed on the surface of the virus

    B. Found mainly on naked viruses

    C. Anchor the envelope of enveloped viruses

    D. Part of the nucleoprotein core of viruses

Ans. C.

20. Mumps vaccine is prepared from the cultures of

A. Chick fibroblasts B. African green monkey cells

C. Healthy calves D. Sheep

Ans. A.

21. The microbes which are most likely to be completely dependent on a plant or animal host are

A. Viruses B. Bacteria

C. Fungi D. Algae

Ans. A.

22. The two major components of viruses are

A. Fat and protein B. Nucleic acid and protein

C. Carbohydrate and nucleic acid D. Fat and carbohydrate

Ans. B.

23. The transcription of the viral nucleic acid into mRNA is not necessary in case of

A. RNA viruses B. ds DNA viruses

C. ss DNA viruses D. All of these

Ans. A.

24. West Nile virus can cause a disease in human beings that may be transmitted from an infected bird to a person by a mosquito. This is an example of

A. Endogenous infection B. Fomite borne disease

C. Arthropod borne D. Nosocomial infection

Ans. C.

25. What does the positive strand in double stranded RNA viruses stands for?

A. rRNA B. tRNA

C. mRNA D. None of these

Ans. C.

26. Which of the following characteristics would not be used to classify viruses?

A. Type of cell wall structure B. Type of nucleic acid

C. Presence of an envelope D. Symmetry

Ans. A.

27. Intranuclear inclusion bodies are found in cells infected with

A. Parvovirus B. Adenovirus

C. Herpesvirus D. All of these

Ans. D.

28. The reovirus and influenza virus contain

A. 10 different segments of dsRNA and 8 different segments of ssRNA respectively

B. 8 different segments of dsRNA and 10 different segments of ssRNA respectively

C. 5 different segments of dsRNA and 7 different segments of ssRNA respectively

D. 7 different segments of dsRNA and 5different segments of ssRNA respectively

Ans. A.

29. Intracytoplasmic inclusion bodies are found in cells infected with

A. Rabies virus
B. Vaccinia virus
C. Fowlpox virus
D. All of these

Ans. D.

30. What is the function of positive strand in double stranded RNA viruses?

A. Synthesis of protein
B. Production of ribosomes
C. Both (a) and (b)
D. None

Ans. A.

31. Which of the following virus is transmitted by the respiratory route?

A. Rhinovirus
B. Coronavirus
C. Measles virus
D. All of these

Ans. D.

32. The predominant lipid substance found in the viral envelope is

A. Phospholipids
B. Glycolipids
C. Neural fat
D. All of these

Ans. A.

33. Which of the following viruses has not been associated with human cancer?

A. Hepatitis C virus
B. Hepatitis B virus
C. Varicella-Zoster virus
D. HSV 2

Ans. C.

34. The viral nucleocapsid is the combination of

A. Genome & capsid
B. Capsid & spike
C. Envelope & capsid
D. Capsomere & genome

Ans. A.

35. Edward Jenner began inoculating humans with material from __________ lesions.

A. Smallpox
B. Avianpox
C. Cow pox
D. Chickenpox

Ans. C.

36. The viruses in an attenuated vaccine

A. The viruses in an attenuated vaccine
B. Continue to replicate
C. Are usually larger than bacteria
D. Is altered with chemicals

Ans. B.

37. Enveloped viruses have a __________ shape

A. Icosahedral
B. Helical
C. Roughly spherical
D. Complex

Ans. C.

38. The envelope of which of the following viruses is derived from the host cell nucleus?

A. Paramyxoviruses
B. Retroviruses
C. Orthomyxoviruses
D. Herpesviruses

Ans. D.

39. Which of the following viruses belong to family Flaviviridae?

A. Rubella virus
B. Yellow fever virus
C. Hepatitis C virus
D. All the above

Ans. D.

40. Which of the following viruses show/s transformation of infected cells ?

A. HBV
B. HTLV
C. EBV
D. All of these

Ans. D.

41. Which of the following statements is not true of viruses?

A. Viruses have been successfully grown in pure cultures in test tubes
B. All viruses are obligatory intracellular parasites
C. All viruses have either DNA or RNA as their genetic material
D. Viruses probably arose from small fragments of cellular chromosomes

Ans. A.

42. Which of the following viruses belong/s to family Caliciviridae?

A. Hepatitis B virus
B. Hepatitis D virus
C. Hepatitis E virus
D. All of these

Ans. C.

43. In the simplest capsid, there is a capsomere at each of the 12 vertices; this capsomere, which is surrounded by five other capsomeres, is termed a

A. Penton
B. Polyhedral
C. Icosahedral
D. Helical

Ans. A.

44. The size of viruses is usually measured in

A. mm
B. nm
C. micrometer
D. cm

Ans. B.

45. Enzyme neuraminidase is carried by which of the following viruses?

A. HIV
B. EBV
C. Influenza virus
D. Adenovirus

Ans. C.

46. Which of the following virus is susceptible to chloroform?

A. Herpes virus
B. Influenza virus
C. Measles
D. All of these

Ans. D.

47. Group E phages have

A. ssDNA
B. ssDNA
C. ssRNA
D. dsRNA

Ans. C.

48. The bacterial viruses having head made up of large capsomeres, but no tail is morphologically classified as

A. A
B. B
C. C
D. D.

Ans. D.

49. Which of the following is not true of virions?

A. Reproduce independently
B. Contains DNA
C. Contains RNA
D. Are extracellular

Ans. A.

50. Bacteriophages have been used widely in genetic research, since they are the smallest and simplest biological entities capable of

A. Self replication B. Duplication

C. Self duplication D. Multiplication

Ans. A.

51. Lesions on chorioallantoic membrane are produced by

A. HBV B. Vaccinia virus

C. HSV D. All of these

Ans. D.

52. Which one is not useful in the treatment of viruses except

A. Acyclovir B. IFN

C. Penicillin D. Antibodies

Ans. C.

53. The infected cells continue to reproduce themselves as well as the virus, and the mature virions are extruded from the cell surface continuously over a long period of time. This type of release mechanism is called a

A. Productive infection B. Inductive infection

C. Resultant infection D. All of these

Ans. A.

54. What kind of embryo is often used for viral assays?

A. Mouse B. Rat

C. Cat D. Chicken

Ans. D.

55. The envelope of an enveloped virus is derived from

A. The mitochondrion of the cell

B. The cell membrane

C. The endoplasmic reticulum of the cell

D. None of these

Ans. B.

56. The most popular indirect method of counting virus particles is by

A. Hemagglutination assay B. Plaque-assay

C. Counting plaque forming units D. Colony counting

Ans. A.

57. Which of the following viruses belong to family Hepadnaviridae ?

A. Hepatitis A virus
B. Hepatitis B virus
C. Hepatitis D virus
D. All of these

Ans. B.

58. Inclusion bodies of measles virus are

A. Intracytoplasmic
B. Intranuclear
C. Both A & B
D. None of these

Ans. C.

59. The most efficient way to enclose a space is within a/an

A. Sphere
B. Cube
C. Icosahedron
D. Helix

Ans. C.

60. The function of a viral capsid is

A. Protection against the viral genome from physical and enzymatic destruction
B. Providing binding sites that enable the virus to attach to specific receptor sites on the host cell
C. Serving as a vehicle of transmission from one host to another
D. All of these

Ans. D.

61. Which of the following oncogenic viruses was first detected?

A. RSV
B. HTLV
C. EBV
D. HSV-2

Ans. A.

62. The yield of phage per bacterium is called the

A. Eclipse size
B. Latent size
C. Burst size
D. None of these

Ans. C.

63. Which of the following viruses are relatively thermostable ?

A. HIV
B. Rubella
C. HAV
D. Influenza virus

Ans. C.

64. The time from infection until lysis is called as

A. Eclipse period
B. Latent period
C. Burst size
D. Rise period

Ans. B.

65. Virus reproduces in living cells by

A. Replication B. Duplication

C. Multiplication D. All of these

Ans. A.

66. Which of the following virus is enveloped?

A. Adenovirus B. Herpes virus

C. Poliovirus D. None of these

Ans. B.

67. Which of the following viruses can rescue adenovirus in simian cells?

A. Rabies B. Vaccinia

C. SV40 D. Cytomegalovirus

Ans. C.

68. The phage components begin to assemble into mature phages only after the synthesis of

A. Protein B. Nucleic acid

C. Both A & B D. Amino acid

Ans. C.

69. Which of the following bacteriophage is said to have banal symmetry?

A. T2 B. T4

C. T6 D. All of these

Ans. D.

70. Which of the following statements is correct?

A. Up to 10% of human tumours have a viral risk factor

B. Up to 40% of human tumours have a viral risk factor

C. Up to 30% of human tumours have a viral risk factor

D. Up to 20% of human tumours have a viral risk factor

Ans. D.

71. Which of the following viral infections is associated with the development of hydrophobia?

A. Rabies B. Influenza

C. Polio D. Hepatitis

Ans. A.

72. Which of the following viruses is star-shaped in outline and transmitted by the faecal-oral route?

A. Astrovirus B. Calicivirus

C. Hepatitis E D. Hepatitis D.

Ans. A.

73. What is the shape of rabies virus?

A. Spherical B. Polygonal

C. Bullet shaped D. Tubular

Ans. C.

74. The species of animals which is most susceptible to rabies infection is

A. Dog B. Cat

C. Fowl D. Cow

Ans. B.

75. The mode of transmission of hepatitis E is through

A. Infected syringes and needles B. Faecally contaminated drinking water

C. Sexually D. None of these

Ans. B.

76. Which of the following viral agents can cause diarrhoea?

A. Rotavirus B. Norwalk virus

C. Astrovirus D. All of these

Ans. D.

77. The virus(es) which has club-shaped peplomers and infects the respiratory tract is/are

A. Coronavirus B. Astrovirus

C. Norwalk agent D. All of these

Ans. A.

78. Which of the following clinical specimens can be used for the demonstration of rabies antigen by direct immunofluorescence antemortem?

A. Saliva smear B. Corneal smear

C. Conjunctival smear D. All of these

Ans. D.

79. Which of the following is a drug that interferes with the process of DNA production in the virus that causes genital herpes?

A. Erythromycin B. Vancomycin

C. Amantidine D. Acyclovir

Ans. D.

80. More promising chemotherapeutic agents for treating viral diseases is

A. Leukocytic interferon
B. Fibroblast interferon
C. Interferon
D. Nystatin

Ans. C.

81. Which of the following infection(s) can be diagnosed by the use of polymerase chain reaction?

A. HIV-1 and HIV-2 viruses
B. Hepatitis B virus
C. *Mycobacterium tuberculosis*
D. All of these

Ans. D.

82. Polymerase chain reaction basically consists of

A. 2 steps
B. 3 steps
C. 4 steps
D. 5 steps

Ans. B.

83. The disease(s) caused by genus *Orthopoxvirus* is/are

A. Vaccinia
B. Smallpox
C. Cowpox
D. All of these

Ans. D.

84. The virus(es) which can cause aseptic meningitis is/are

A. Polioviruses
B. Coxsackieviruses
C. Echo viruses
D. All of these

Ans. D.

85. Which of the following genera can cause disease in humans?

A. Orthopoxvirus
B. Parapoxvirus
C. Molluscipoxvirus
D. All of these

Ans. D.

86. Which of the coxsackieviruses can cause herpangina?

A. Group A
B. Group B
C. Both (a) and (b)
D. None of these

Ans. A.

87. Which of the following genera is included in the family Picornaviridae?

A. Enterovirus
B. Rhinovirus
C. Hepatovirus
D. All of these

Ans. D.

88. Transmission of *Molluscum contagiosum* virus is through

A. Direct contact B. Sexual contact

C. Both (a) and (b) D. None of these

Ans. C.

89. Which of the following viruses are acid-labile?

A. Rhinoviruses B. Echoviruses

C. Polioviruses D. Coxsackieviruses

Ans. A.

90. The symmetry of nucleocapsid of poxvirus is

A. Complex B. Icosahedral

C. Helical D. All of these

Ans. A.

91. The cell lines which can support the growth of polioviruses is/are

A. Human amnion B. Monkey kidney

C. HeLa D. All of these

Ans. D.

92. Which one of the following immunization should be administered immediately after birth?

A. DPT vaccine B. HIB vaccine

C. Oral polio vaccine D. HBV vaccine E. HIV vaccine

Ans. C.

93. All the following picornaviruses are resistant to the acidity of the stomach except

A. Coxsackie virus A B. Coxsackie virus B

C. ECHO virus D. Poliovirus

E. Rhinovirus

Ans. E.

94. Which of the following is not a RNA virus ?

A. HAV B. HBV

C. HCV D. HGV

Ans. B.

95. What is the minimum infective dose of FMD to infect a cattle by tongue epithelium and respiratory routes?

Ans. 1 I.U. by tongue epithelium route and 10-100 I.U. by aerosol route.

96. What is the minimum infective dose of FMD to infect a pig ?

Ans. 1-10 I.U. when inoculated into bulb of the heel and > 1000 I.U by intranasal route.

97. What is the minimum infective dose of FMD to infect a sheep ?

Ans. 10,000 I.U. by intranasal and intratracheal route.

98. What is the duration of carrier state in buffalo, cattle sheep and goat ?

Ans. 24 years or life time in buffaloes, 3 years in cattle, 9 months in sheep and 6 months in goats.

99. What are the different inactivants used to inactivate the FMDV ?

Ans. Previously HCHO was used.Subsequently, acetylethylenimine (AEI) and more recently binary ethylenimine (BEI) is used.

100. What are the different adjuvants used to prepare the FMDV vaccine?

Ans. Al(OH)3, saponin or oil adjuvant (Montanide). Al(OH)3 based FMD vaccine is effective only in ruminants whereas oil adjuvanted vaccine is effective against ruminants and pigs. Al(OH)3 based vaccine gives 6 months protection whereas oil adjuvanted vaccine gives 1 year protection.

101. How much antigenic mass in the vaccine is required to obtain optimum protection in respective to different FMD virus serotypes ?

Ans. Per dose 166 ng in case O, 5.4 ng in case of C and 4.5 ng in case of A is required.

102. The mouse blood brain barrier remains firmly closed in the case of infection with a virulent rabies virus strains (True/False).

Ans. True.

103. The mouse blood brain barrier opens when infection with an attenuated rabies virus strains occur (True/False)..

Ans. True.

104. In Europe ———————— is the principal rabies vector and reservoir.

Ans. Red fox.

105. In North America ————, ———— and ———————— are principal reservoirs of rabies.

Ans. Raccoons, skunks, coyotes and various fox species.

106. What is the full form of GARC ?

Ans. Global Alliance for Rabies control formed in 2007.

107. What is the full form of PRP ?

Ans. Partners for rabies prevention formed in 2008.

108. Phylogenetic evidence indicates that lyssaviruses infected terrestrial mammals before they infected bats (True/False).

Ans. False. Reverse is true. Bats were infected first then terrestrial mammals.

109. In China ———— million people get vaccinated after rabies exposure or take post exposure antirabies vaccine.

Ans. 15 million.

110. Which Asian countries are free from canine rabies ?

Ans. In Asia, canine rabies has been eliminated in Malaysia in 1954, Japan in 1956 and Taiwan in 1961.

111. Which South American countries have not reported canine or human rabies or reported free from rabies recently ?

Ans. Coloumbia, Costa Rica, Chile, Ecuador, Panama, Paraguay and Uruguay.

112. What are the rabies related viruses ?

Ans. Lagosbat virus, Mokola virus, Duvenhage virus, EBLV-1, EBLV-2 and ABLV-1.

113. Name some recently discovered rabies related viruses ?

Ans. Aravan virus, Khujand virus, Irkut virus, West Caucasian bat virus, Shimoni bat lyssavirus, Bokeloh bat lyssavirus, Ikoma lyssa virus.

114. What are different viruses under the group I, II and III coronavirus ?

Ans. Group I Coronavirus : Canine coronavirus, feline coronavirus type I and type II, Transmissible gastroenteritis virus, porcine respiratory coronavirus, porcine epidemic diarrhoea virus.

Group II coronavirus : SARS, canine respiratory coronavirus

Group III coronavirus : Infectious bronchitis virus.

115. What are the causative agents of the canine infectious respiratory disease ?

Ans. Canine respiratory coronavirus along with B.bronchoseptica, CAV-1, CAV-2, canine parainfluenza virus, canine herpes virus, reovirus and influenza virus.

116. What are the different members under the genus Pestivirus and family Flaviviridae?

Ans. Bovine viral diarrhoea virus, classical swine fever virus and border disease virus.

117. What are the two biotypes of BVDV ?

Ans. Cytopathic (CP) and non-cytopathic (NCP). Both are responsible for severe disease outbreaks.

118. What are the agents responsible for bovine respiratory disease complex ?

Ans. *P. multocida*, *M. haemolytica*, PI-3, BRSV and BVDV.

119. What is the effect of BVDV during early pregnancy ?

Ans. During one and half month of gestation, there is early embryonic death.

120. What is the effect of BVDV during late pregnancy ?

Ans. It can cross blood brain barrier and causes cerebellar hypoplasia.

121. How the persistently infected (PI) and mucosal disease infected animals are produced ?

Ans. In utero exposure to NCP strain of BVDV before the development of foetal immunocompetence (generally by 125 days of gestation) can result in a PI calf. Superinfection of PI animals with homologous CP strains of BVDV may result in MD infected animals.

122. What is the prevalence of Mucosal disease (MD) of BVD and how it is characterized ?

Ans. The prevalence of MD is very low but mortality is very high. It is characterized by upper gastrointestinal tract ulceration and haemorrhagic lesions in the abomasums and elsewhere.

123. BVD PI animals are primary reservoir of BVDV and serves as the major source of infection to other cattle through direct contact with infected material (True/False).

Ans. True.

124. BVD PI infected animals do not mount an antibody response to the infecting strain of virus (True/False).

Ans. True.

125. BVDV-1 based vaccines are cross protective against BVDV-2 (True/False).

Ans. True.

126. Both BVDV-1 and BVDV-2 based vaccines are available (True/False).

Ans. True.

127. CSF disease is more severe with high mortality than BVD (True/False).

Ans. True.

128. Persistent infection (PI) is also a feature of CSF like bovine vial diarrhoea and border disease(True/False).

Ans. True. It occurs when infection occurs during 50-70 days of gestation.

129. Antibodies to ruminant pestiviruses (BVDV and BDV) do not cross react with those of CSFV(True/False).

Ans. False.

130. BVDV mainly affect sheep but goats are also affected occasionally(True/False).

Ans. True.

131. Persistent infection in sheep occurred in BDV infection like BVDV infection in bovine (True/False).

Ans. True. When infection occurs between 21-72 days of gestation period.

132. Persistently infected lamb due to BDV infection is called ———— due to typical neurological and fleece abnormalities.

Ans. Hairy shaker.

133. Vaccines are available against BDV (border disease virus) infection (True/False).

Ans. True.

134. ————(Species of animal) is more susceptible to FMD.

Ans. Cattle.

135. ——— (Species of animal) is considered as amplifier host of FMDV.

Ans. Pigs.

136. ——————(disease) is most infectious human or animal disease agent known.

Ans. FMDV.

137. How many different genotypes of CPV have been reported ?

Ans. 8 (CPV-2, 2a, 2b, 2c, New CPV-2a, New CPV-2b and Asp (300) CPV-2a, Asp (300) 2b.

138. What is the rate of nucleotide substitution in CPV genome ?

Ans. 10^{-4} substitution/site /year.

139. CPV-2c mainly affect adult dogs with severe clinical symptoms and higher mortality (True/False).

Ans. True.

140. Cross bred dogs are less susceptible to CPV-2 infection than pure breeds (True/False).

Ans. True. Pure breeds like Rottweilers, Doberman Pinchers, English Springer, Spaniels and German Shepherd are more susceptible. Exception Toy Poodles and Cocker Spaniels which are pure breed but less susceptible.

141. Myocarditis in pups is an important feature of CPV-2 infections (True/False).

Ans. True.

142. Canine parvovirus have spike (22A°) at ——(axis), canyon (15A°) at ——— (axis) and dimple (15A°) at —— (axis)

Ans. 3', 5' and 2'.

143. Which amino acid changes in VP2 protein of CPV-2 cause the CPV-2 to replicate in cats?

Ans. 87 (Met to Leu), 300 (Ala to Gly), 305 (Asp to Tyr).

144. What is Zika ?

Ans. Zika is a virus. First identified in 1947 in rhesus monkeys in Uganda, it was found in humans in 1952 in Uganda and Tanzania. Outbreaks of Zika virus infection have been reported in Africa, Asia, and the Pacific islands, and most recently in the Americas.

145. What does Zika mean ?

Ans. Zika means "*overgrown*" in the Uganda language.

146. Does the Zika virus cause microcephaly ?

Ans. It is unclear.

147. The causative agent of 'Zika' fever is

A. Mosquito B. DNA virus

C. RNA virus D. Bacteria

Ans. C.

148. Zika disease is named after

A. Zika virus that causes the disease

B. Zika forest in Uganda

C. Zika mosquito, the vector of the disease

D. Zika, the scientist who first reported the disease

Ans. B.

149. Zika virus first identified in

A. Rhesus monkey B. Chimpanzee

C. Gibbon D. Humans

Ans. A.

150. Zika virus belongs to the family

A. Adenoviridae B. Flaviviridae

C. Filoviridae D. Geminiviridae

Ans. B.

151. The vector of Zika virus is

A. A.aegypti B. A.albopictus

C. Both A and B D. Other species of mosquitoes

Ans. C.

152. The diagnosis of Zika fever include

A. Blood or body fluid for the presence of viral DNA

B. Blood or body fluid for the presence of viral RNA

C. Blood or body fluid for the presence of Zika viral protein

D. All of the above

Ans. B.

153. Zika disease is treated using

A. Vaccines

B. Antibiotics

C. Interferons

D. No specific treatment currently available

Ans. D.

154. Which of the following is false regarding Zika disease

A. Zika disease is life threatening

B. Recently Zika is reported in more than 13 countries

C. Zika disease is often a mild disease

D. Recent Zika outbreak was first reported in Brazil

Ans. A.

155. Two major diseases that seem to have relationship with Zika disease is

A. Guillain-Barre Syndrome and Microencephaly in babies

B. Guillain-Barre Syndrome and Turner syndrome in babies

C. Microencephaly and Turner syndrome in babies

D. Turner and Downs syndrome in babies

Ans. A.

156. The best preventive strategy of Zika virus is

A. Use anti-viral drugs B. Protect against mosquito bite

C. Use of interferons and vaccines D. All of the above

Ans. B.

157. Can someone without symptoms spread Ebola?

Ans. No.

158. Is Ebola an airborne disease?

Ans. No.

159. Can people survive from Ebola?

Ans. Yes.

160. Can mosquitoes spread Ebola?

Ans. No.

161. What is the level of risk associated with Ebola virus contaminating rivers and drinking water sources ?

A. High B. Medium

C. Low

Ans. C.

162. I was in close contact with an Ebola infected person. How long should I check my health for?

A. 7 days B. 14 days

C. 21 days

Ans. C.

163. Can I get vaccinated for Ebola?

Ans. No.

164. Can people who have died from Ebola infect others?

Ans. Yes.

165. Name the genus and family of Ebola virus.

Ans. Ebolavirus ; Filoviridae.

166. How many different virus species are there under Ebolavirus ?

Ans. 5. The five known virus species are named for the region where each was originally identified: *Bundibugyo ebolavirus*, *Reston ebolavirus*, *Sudan ebolavirus*, *Taï Forest ebolavirus* (originally *Côte d'Ivoire ebolavirus*), and *Zaire ebolavirus*. Each species of the genus *Ebolavirus* has one member virus, and four of these cause Ebola virus disease (EVD) in humans, a type of hemorrhagic fever having a very high case fatality rate; the fifth, Reston virus, has caused EVD in other primates. *Zaire ebolavirus* is the type species (reference or example species) for *Ebolavirus*, and has the highest mortality rate of the ebolaviruses, and is also responsible for the largest number of outbreaks of the five known members of the genus, including the 1976 Zaire outbreak and the outbreak with the most deaths (2014).

167. Where was first outbreak of Ebola virus reported ?

Ans. Ebola viruses were first described after outbreaks of EVD in southern Sudan in June 1976 and in Zaire in August 1976. The

name *Ebolavirus* is derived from the Ebola River in Zaire (now the Democratic Republic of the Congo), the location of the 1976 outbreak, and the taxonomic suffix *-virus* (denoting a viral genus). This genus was introduced in 1998 as the "Ebola-like viruses". In 2002 the name was changed to *Ebola virus* and in 2010, the genus was emended. Ebola viruses are closely related to Marburg viruses.

168. Are fruit bats susceptible to Ebolavirus infection ?

Ans. The evidence of Ebola infection in three species of fruit bat has been reported. The bats show no symptoms of the disease, indicating that they may be the main natural reservoirs of the Ebolavirus. It is possible that there are other reservoirs and vectors. The researchers found that bats of three species—*Hypsignathus monstrosus*, *Epomops franqueti*, and *Myonycteris torquata*—had either genetic material from the Ebola virus, known as RNA sequences, or evidence of an immune response to the disease. The bats showed no symptoms themselves.

169. Hepatitis B virus is under the genus ———— and family ————.

Ans. Orthohepadnavirus and Hepadnaviridae.

170. Other viruses under Orthohepadnavirus are ————, ———— &— ————.

Ans. Ground squirrel hepatitis virus, Woodchuck hepatitis virus, and the Woolly monkey hepatitis B virus.

171. Which primates are infected with hepatitis B like viruses ?

Ans. Viruses similar to hepatitis B have been found in all apes (orangutan, gibbons, gorillas and chimpanzees), in Old World monkeys, and in a New World woolly monkeys.

172. How many serotypes are there under hepatitis B virus ?

Ans. The virus is divided into four major serotypes (adr, adw, ayr, ayw) based on antigenic epitopes present on its envelope proteins.

173. How many genotypes and subtypes are there under hepatitis B virus ?

Ans. The viral strains have also been divided into ten genotypes (A–J) and forty subgenotypes according to overall nucleotide sequence variation of the genome.

174. The hepatitis C virus is under the genus ———— and family ————.

Ans. Hepacivirus and Flaviviridae. It is a small, enveloped, single stranded positive sense RNA virus.

175. How many different genotypes of hepatitis C are there ?

Ans. 7 (1-7). In the United States, about 70% of cases are caused by genotype 1, 20% by genotype 2 and about 1% by each of the other genotypes. Genotype 1 is also the most common in South America and Europe.

176. How the hepatitis C virus is transmitted ?

Ans. It is transmitted through blood contact, I/V drug use, unsafe medical procedure.

177. AIDS patients show substantial decrease in their disease progression if they are infected with hepatitis G virus (True/False).

Ans. True.

178. Every cell in our body contains viral DNA. Human endogenous retroviruses make up about —— % of our DNA.

Ans. 5-8%.

179. Virus has been derived from Latin word which means ———.

Ans. Poison.

180. Inclusion bodies in the form of clumps of ribosomes is virus found in——— virus.

Ans. Arenavirus.

181. Inclusion bodies in the form of clumps of chromatin is found in———— virus.

Ans. Herpesvirus.

182. What is virome ?

Ans. The collection of all viruses in a specific environment such as sewage, the human body or the intestinal tract.

183. Koala retrovirus is a γ retrovirus related to gibbon ape leukemia and feline leukemia viruses (True/False).

Ans. True.

184. There are a million of virus particles/ml of sea water and total of 10^{30} virions (True/False).

Ans. True.

185. ————————— discovered the first human virus, yellow fever virus in 1901.

Ans. Walter Reed.

186. ——————— virus contains ———— genes. Its genome is twice as big as that of any other known virus and bigger than that of many bacteria.

Ans. Mimivirus ; 900 genes.

187. ———— virus was found inside an amoeba in a Paris cooling tower.

Ans. Mamavirus.

188. Mamavirus has its dependent satellite virus known as —————.

Ans. Sputnik.

189. Virus particle with different structures in different host.

Ans. Dengue. In mosquito cell it grows at 28^{0}C and mammalian cells at 37^{0}C.

190. —————————— in 1970 provided the first evidence for the existence of an RNA dependent DNA polymerase activity in retrovirus particles.

Ans. Temin and Baltimore.

191. Most of the plant RNA viruses contain

A. dsRNA

B. + ssRNA

C. –ssRNA

D. None of the above

Ans. B.

192. Reverse transcriptases (RTs) are the enzyme that synthesize DNA from both DNA and RNA (True/False).

Ans. True.

193. Reverse transcriptases (RTs) is an error prone process as RT lacks proof reading activity (True/False).

Ans. True.

194. Retroviral particles are considered to be pseudodiploid (True/False).

Ans. True.

195. Retroviral genomes like those of other RNA viruses accumulate mutations at much higher rates than do cellular genomes (True/False).

Ans. True.

196. RTs not only are error prone but also lack an endonuclease capable of excising mispaired nucleotides (True/False).

Ans. True.

197. The error rate of RT is 1 per 10^4 to 10^6 nucleotide polymerized (True/False).

Ans. True.

198. The error rate is 1 per 10^4 to 10^6 nucleotide polymerized in case of cellular DNA replication (True/False).

Ans. True.

199. What are retroid viruses?

Ans. Hepadnavirus, Retrovirus and some plant virus such as Caulimoviruses synthesize DNA via RNA intermediate and called retroid viruses.

200. Which Indian Ocean Island countries are free from FMD without vaccination ?

Ans. Madagascar, Mauritius and Seychelles.

201. How many topotypes are there under SAT-1, SAT-2 & SAT-3 serotypes of FMDV?

Ans. 8, 14 and 6.

202. How many wildlife species are susceptible to FMD ?

Ans. 70.

203. How many countries in the world are still affected with FMD virus infections in the animals ?

Ans. More than 100 countries.

204. How 'O', 'A' in respect to FMD virus have been derived ?

Ans. FMDV 'O' for the department of 'Oise' in France, A for Allemagre (the French word for Germany).

205. Where the FMDV serotype 'Asia-1" was first detected and isolated ?

Ans. Asia-1 was detected in a water buffalo at 'Okara', Punjab, Pakistan in 1954.

206. How many times ELISA is sensitive to CFT to provide FMD diagnosis ?

Ans. 125 times.

207. ——— and ——— cell lines are used for isolation of FMDV.

Ans. BHK-21 and IBRS-2.

208. Which FMDV serotype is most diverse serotype ?

Ans. FMDV serotype 'O'.

209. Which FMDV serotype is lease diverse serotype ?

Ans. Asia-1.

210. The RGD receptor binding motif of Asia-1 viruses is more variable than O and A of FMDV (True/False).

Ans. True.

211. Where and when was the last outbreak of serotype C of FMDV ?

Ans. Ethiopia in 2005.

212. Where and when the FMDV SAT-1 outbreak was reported outside South Africa?

Ans. Middle East in 1962-1965 and 1969-1970 and in Greece in 1962.

213. Where and when the FMDV SAT-2 outbreak was reported outside South Africa?

Ans. Yemen in 1990, Kuwait and Saudi Arabia in 2000 and Palestine in 2012 and Bahrain.

214. Where and when the Asia-1 outbreak was reported outside South east Asia ?

Ans. Greece in 1984.

215. FMD was once present in Australia and now it is free from FMD. When was last outbreak reported ?

Ans. 1872.

216. The pandemic serotype O virus designated as (PanAsia strain) belong to the ——— topotype which has spread rapidly and vigorously.

Ans. ME-SA topotype.

217. The Pan Asia serotype O of FMD virus was first detected in India in ———.

Ans. 1982.

218. How many regional pools of FMD virus have been reported throughout the world?

Ans. 7 regional pools.

219. Which two countries have shared viruses belonging to two different pools ?

Ans. Egypt and Libya.

220. Anti-NSP antibodies of FMDV can persist for a long period and do not necessarily indicate recent FMD virus infection (True/False).

Ans. True.

221. What percentage of polio virus infections exhibit paralysis ?

Ans. 0.1 to 1%.

222. The following antiviral agents is active against the following virus (True/False).

A. Lamivudine and HIV : B. Lamivudine and HBV:

C. Amantidine and influenza B virus D. Ribavirin and RSV :

E. Acyclovir and HSV :

Ans. A. True B. True

C. False D. True

E. True.

223. Herpes simplex encephalitis (True/False).

A. Commonly affect temporal lobe :

B. Is usually diagnosed by culture of the CSF:

C. May be diagnosed by PCR of the CSF :

D. Should be treated with IV Ganciclovir :

E. May be diagnosed by detecting specific antibody in the CSF :

Ans. A : True B. False

C. True D. False

E. True.

224. Varicella zoster virus (True/False).

A. Causes a maculopapular rash :

B. Responds to AZT therapy :

C. Remains latent in sensory ganglion following primary infection :

D. Patients with shingles are not infectious :

E. VZV causes vesicular rash.

Ans. A False B. False

C. True D. False

E. True.

225. HPV-16 and HPV-18 are associated with genital cancers (True/False).

Ans. True.

226. The following viruses are transmitted from animals to humans (True/False).

A. Rabies B. Poliovirus:

C. CMV D. Hantavirus

E. Lassa fever virus

Ans. A. True B. False

C. False D. True

E. True.

227. Viruses routinely establish latent infections in human sensory ganglia (True/False).

A. EB virus B. HSV-1

C. HSV-2 D. VZ virus

Ans. A. False B. True

C. True D. True

228. DEAFF test is carried out to detect ———— disease.

Ans. CMV.

229. The following viruses cause gastroenteritis (True/False).

A. Enterovirus B. Adenovirus

C. Norwalk virus D. Astrovirus

E. Rotavirus

Ans. A. False B. True

C. True D. True

E. True.

230. Following viruses are transmitted from animals to humans (True/False).

A. Influenza A
B. HTLV-1
C. Hantavirus
D. Poliovirus
E. Rabies

Ans. A. True
B. False
C. True
D. False
E. True.

231. A chronic carrier state may occur in the following (True/False).

A. Hepatitis A
B. Hepatitis B
C. Hepatitis C
D. Hepatitis delta
E. Hepatitis E

Ans. A. False
B. True
C. True
D. True
E. False

232. The following viruses are transmitted by blood (True/False).

A. Rubella
B. HIV
C. Measles
D. Hepatitis BV
E. Hepatitis CV

Ans. A. False
B. True
C. False
D. True
E. True.

233. Hepatitis C virus (True/False).

A. May be transmitted by blood
B. Associated with hepatocellular carcinoma
C. May respond to IFN therapy
D. Has one genotype only
E. May cause chronic infection

Ans. A. True
B. True
C. True
D. False
E. False.

234. Hepatitis B virus infection (True/False).

A. May result in chronic infection

B. May result in cirrhosis of liver

C. May result in hepatocellular carcinoma

D. Is highly infectious when positive for HBeAg

E. May respond to IFN therapy

Ans. A. True B. True

C. True D. True

E. True.

235. Hepatitis A infection (True/False).

A. May result in chronic infection

B. May be prevented by Ig

C. May be prevented by vaccination

D. Is highly infectious during jaundice phase

Ans. A. False B. True

C. True D. False

236. HIV may respond to (True/False).

A. Nucleoside analogues B. Protease inhibitors

C. Neuraminidase inhibitors D. RT inhibitors

E. Acyclovir

Ans. A. True B. True

C. False D. True

E. True.

237. Respiratory syncytial virus (True/False).

A. Cause disease mainly in adults B. May cause bronchiolitis

C. May be prevented by vaccination D. May be treated by amantidine

E. May cause latent infections

Ans. A. False B. True

C. False D. False

E. False

238. Write true or false about the following sentences (True/False).

A. Influenza A may undergo antigenic shift

B. Influenza B may undergo antigenic shift

C. Influenza A may undergo antigenic drift

D. Influenza B may undergo antigenic drift

E. Influenza B may respond to amantidine

Ans. A. True B. False

C. True D. True

E. False

239. Write true or false about the following thought to cause gastroenteritis (True/False).

A. Enterovirus B. Calicivirus

C. Norwalk like virus D. Astrovirus

E. Paramyxovirus

Ans. A. False B. True

C. True D. True

E. False

240. Viral DNA is resistant to DNase of the host cell because it contains

A. 5'-HMC B. 5'-HMA

C. 5'-CHM D. 5'MHC

Ans. A.

241. 'Reye's syndrome' is caused by

A. St. pneumoniae B. *St. pyogenes*

C. Influenza D. None of these

Ans. C.

242. German measles is also known as

A. Rubella / 2-day measles B. Rubella / 3day measles

C. Rubella / 4-day measles D. Rubella / 1-day measles

Ans. B.

243. The commonest cause of rubella in new born

A. Congenital rubella

B. Post natal rubella

C. Expanded rubella syndrome (ERS)

D. Both a and c

Ans. D.

244. Measles is characterized by

A. Negri bodies
B. Babes-Ernest granules
C. Koplik's spots
D. Fever

Ans. C.

245. In India, Japanese B encephalitis was first isolated from the mosquitoes of the

A. Culex tritaeriorhynchus
B. Culex annulirostris
C. Culex vishnui
D. None of these

Ans. C.

246. Dengue virus is transmitted from man to man by the

A. Sand fly
B. Ticks
C. *Aedes aegypti*
D. *Culex sp.*

Ans. C.

247. Epidemic pleurodynia and myocarditis of new born infants are both caused by

A. Coxsackie B virus
B. Reovirus
C. Polyomavirus
D. Cytomegalovirus

Ans. A.

248. Following virus is known to establish latent infections:

A. Adenovirus
B. Varicella-zoster virus
C. Cytomegalovirus
D. Hepes simplex virus
E. All of these

Ans. E.

249. Viruses which have teratogenic property are

A. Herpes simplex virus
B. Cytomegalovirus
C. Rubella virus
D. All of these

Ans. D.

250. First genetically engineered and biotechnologically produced vaccine was against

A. AIDS
B. Small pox
C. Herpes simplex
D. Hepatitis B

Ans. D.

251. A patient attends the surgery with bilateral swelling of the parotid salivary glands. Which condition is he suffering from?

A. Diphtheria
B. Measles
C. Mumps
D. Poliomyelitis
E. Rubella

Ans. C.

252. Virus will contain

A. Cell membrane B. Cell wall

C. DNA D. DNA or RNA

Ans. D.

253. Koplic spots observed in the mucous membrane is characteristic feature of the disease

A. Rubella B. Measles

C. Mumps D. Influenza

Ans. B.

254. What are virulent phages, temperate phages and prophage ?

Ans. ***Phages* that replicate only via the *lytic* cycle are known as *virulent phages* while *phages* that replicate using both *lytic* and *lysogenic* cycles are known as *temperate phages*. In the *lysogenic* cycle, the *phage* DNA first integrates into the bacterial chromosome to produce the *prophage*.**

255. Virion means

A. Infectious virus particles B. Non-infectious particles

C. Incomplete particles D. Defective virus particles

Ans. A.

256. Bacteriophage capable of only lytic growth is called

A. Temperate B. Avirulent

C. Virulent D. None of these

Ans. C.

257. HIV is belonging to

A. Retroviridae B. Rhabdoviridae

C. Togaviridae D. Paramyxoviridae

Ans. A.

258. Special feature of Retro viruses

A. Reverse transcriptase B. Two copies genomic RNA

C. Both a & b D. Boils

Ans. C.

259. Which of the following organisms is most commonly associated with AIDS patients?

A. Klebsiella B. Str. pneumonia

C. Mycoplasma D. *Mycobacterium tuberculosis*

Ans. D.

260. Sero conservation in HIV infection takes place in

A. 3 weeks B. 6 weeks

C. 9 weeks D. 12 weeks

Ans. C.

261. Following is the marker of HIV infection in blood:

A. Reverse transcriptase B. DNA polymerase

C. RNA polymerase D. None of these

Ans. A.

262. Which of the following is the most specific in diagnosis of AIDS?

A. IHA B. Western blot

C. ELISA D. Immunoelectrophoresis

Ans. B.

263. The interval period between HIV infection and appearance of antibodies in serum is called

A. Intrinsic period B. Incubation period

C. Window period D. None of these

Ans. C.

264. Screening test for AIDS is

A. Western blot test B. ELISA test

C. Both a and b D. VDRL test

Ans. B.

265. Confirmatory test for AIDS is

A. Western blot test B. ELISA test

C. Karpas test D. Fujerbio test

Ans. A.

266. The most common infection in AIDS is

A. LGV B. CMV

C. Pneumocystis carinii D. Syphilis

Ans. C.

267. During AIDS, HIV infects

A. CD3 lymphocytes B. CD4 lymphocytes

C. CD2 lymphocytes D. B lymphocytes

Ans. B.

268. All of the following are DNA viruses except

A. Parvovirus B. Paramyxovirus

C. Herpes virus D. Pox virus

Ans. B.

269. The dengue fever virus is

A. Flavivirus B. Echovirus

C. Enterovirus D. Orthomyxovirus

Ans. A.

270. Dengue fever is caused by

A. Bacteria B. Virus

C. Fungi D. Rickettsia

Ans. B.

271. Example for DNA viruses:

A. Adenovirus

B. Bacteriophage T1, T2, T3, T4, T5, T6

C. Papovavirus

D. Herpes virus and cauliflower mosaic virus

E. All of the above

Ans. E.

272. The nucleic acid of polio viruses is

A. DNA B. + sense RNA

C. tRNA D. mRNA

Ans. B.

273. Rabies virus is

A. Naked RNA virus B. Naked DNA virus

C. Enveloped RNA virus D. Enveloped DNA virus

Ans. C.

274. Example for DNA virus:

A. Polio virus B. Adenovirus

C. Echo virus D. Coronavirus

Ans. B.

275. Negri bodies produced by rabies virus show characteristic _____ inner granules

A. Basophilic B. Eosinophilic

C. Neutrophilic D. Acidophilic

Ans. B.

276. AIDS disease is çaused by a virus which belongs to

A. Retro virus group
B. Rhabdovirus group
C. Hepatitis virus group
D. Adenovirus group

Ans. A.

277. Kuru disease in Humans is caused by

A. Bacteria
B. Viroides
C. Prions
D. Mycoplasma

Ans. C.

278. What is the peculiarity of pandoravirus ?

A. Largest virus
B. Largest viral genome
C. Smallest virus
D. Smallest viral genome

Ans. B.

279. Which type of interferon is produced by T lymphocytes?

A. α
B. β
C. γ
D. γ and β

Ans. C.

280. Mice latently infected with some murine herpesvirus are resistant to infections with *L. monocytogens* and *Y. pestis (*True/false).

Ans. True.

281. RNA viruses have genome that consists of RNA. What must a positive strand RNA virus do before it can replicate ?

A. Nothing, it is ready to start translating protein
B. It must make a positive strand RNA to be translated
C. It must use reverse transcriptase to convert RNA to DNA
D. It must become a prophage before replicating

Ans. A.

282. The hepatic cell carcinoma is associated with acute form of HBV infection.

A. True
B. False

Ans. B.

283. Which of the following hepatitis viruses is not RNA virus?

A. Hepatitis A virus
B. Hepatitis B virus
C. Hepatitis E virus
D. Hepatitis G virus

Ans. B.

284. Which of the following nucleic acid is present in hepatitis B virus?

A. dsDNA B. ssRNA

C. SSDNA D. dsRNA

Ans. A.

285. The agent representing an isolate of hepatitis G virus is

A. GBA-A B. GBV-B

C. GBV-C D. None of these

Ans. C.

286. Hepatitis G virus belongs to the family

A. Caliciviridae B. Flaviviridae

C. Hepadnaviridae D. Coronaviridae

Ans. B.

287. Transmission of hepatitis G virus is

A. Parenterally B. Sexually

C. Both A and B D. None of these

Ans. C.

288. The most serious infection is

A. Superinfection of an HBsAg carrier by HDV

B. Infection with HBV alone

C. Coinfection of HBVand HDV

D. None of the above

Ans. A.

289. Which of the following specimens contain/s hepatitis B virus in an infected person?

A. Blood B. Semen

C. Saliva D. All of these

Ans. D.

290. Vertical transmission may be seen in

A. Hepatitis B virus B. Hepatitis C virus

C. Hepatitis D virus D. All of these

Ans. D.

291. Which of the following viral infections can result in chronic carrier state?

A. HBV B. HCV

C. HDV D. All of these

Ans. D.

292. Most reliable test for detection of hepatitis E infection is

A. ELISA test for IgM anti-HEV

B. Western blot assay for IgM anti-HEV

C. Polymerase chain reaction for detection of HEV RNA

D. ELISA test for IgG anti-HEV

Ans. C.

293. The defective satellite virus is

A. Hepatitis B

B. Hepatitis C

C. Hepatitis D

D. Hepatitis A

Ans. C.

294. All of the following viruses are enveloped except

A. Hepatitis A virus

B. Hepatitis B virus

C. Hepatitis C virus

D. Hepatitis D virus

Ans. A.

295. The diagnosis of hepatitis A virus infection is based on

A. Aminotransferase levels

B. Detection of faecal HAV by immunoelectron microscopy

C. Both (a) and (b)

D. Detection of IgM anti-HAV by ELISA

Ans. D.

296. Which of the following is not correct for hepatitis A virus?

A. It can be grown in cell cultures of primate and human cells

B. It is one of the most stable viruses infecting humans

C. It may cause hepatocellular carcinoma

D. None of the above

Ans. C.

297. Which of the following characteristic of the Rotavirus was important for the construction of the Rotashield vaccine?

A. The possession of a segmented RNA genome

B. A limited number of capsule types

C. The ability of monkey Rotavirus strains to cause serious illness (diarrhea) in human beings

D. The ability of the Rotavirus to be transmitted faster

Ans. A.

298. The nature of the poliovirus gives for oral vaccination (Sabin vaccine) as part of the eradication programme is

A. Heat killed virus

B. Live attenuated strains of all three immunological types

C. Small dosage of wild-type live viruses

D. Formalin-inactivated viruses

Ans. B.

299. The influenza vaccine is administered each year because

A. Mutations in the viral hemagglutinin may allow the virus to evade the immune response elicited by previous vaccines

B. It is a polysaccharide vaccine that does not confer long-term protection

C. The vaccine is sufficiently toxic to make it necessary to administer only a small amount at any one time

D. None of the above

Ans. A.

300. Which of the following disease is caused by DNA viruses?

A. Poliomyelitis B. Yellow fever

C. Measles D. Small pox

Ans. D.

301. The disease(s) caused by genus *Orthopoxvirus* is/are

A. Vaccinia B. Small pox

C. Cowpox D. All of these

Ans. D.

302. The virus(es) which can cause aseptic meningitis is/are

A. Polioviruses B. Coxsackieviruses

C. Echo viruses D. All of these

Ans. D.

303. Which of the following genera can cause disease in humans?

A. Orthopoxvirus B. Parapoxvius

C. Molluscipoxvirus D. All the above

Ans. D.

304. Which of the coxsackieviruses can cause herpangina?

A. Group A B. Group B

C. Both A & B D. None of the above

Ans. A.

305. Which of the following genera is included in the family Picornaviridae?

A. Enterovirus B. Rhinovirus

C. Hepatovirus D. All of these

Ans. D.

306. Transmission of *Molluscum contagiosum* virus is through

A. Direct contact B. Sexual contact

C. Both A & B D. None of these

Ans. C.

307. Which of the following viruses are acid labile ?

A. Rhinoviruses B. Echoviruses

C. Polioviruses D. Coxsackieviruses

Ans. A.

308. The symmetry of nucleocapsid of poxvirus is

A. Complex B. Icosahedral

C. Helical D. All of these

Ans. A.

309. The cell lines which can support the growth of polioviruses is/are

A. Human amnion B. Monkey kidney

C. HeLa D. All of these

Ans. D.

310. Fatalities following influenza infection are usually due to the

A. Dehydration B. Bacterial superinfection

C. Damage to the heart muscle D. Formation of granulomas in the lung

Ans. B.

311. What type of mosquitoes are responsible for the spread of dengue?

A. Female Aedes mosquitoes B. Male Anopheles mosquitoes

C. Male Aedes mosquitoes D. Female Culex mosquito

Ans. A.

312. Which of the following viruses are responsible for causing dengue?

A. DEN-1 B. DEN-2

C. DEN-3 D. DEN-4

E. All of the above

Ans. E.

313. Dengue usually attack people who have

A. Low levels of proteins in their body

B. High levels of proteins in their body

C. Low levels of immunity

D. Low levels of calcium in their body

Ans. C.

314. Which of the following statements about dengue is incorrect?

A. Infection by one dengue virus provides lifelong immunity against all dengue viruses

B. Dengue fever results in intense joint pains

C. Dengue fever can occur many times

Ans. C.

315. Symptoms of dengue appear the next day after the bite of an infected mosquito

A. True B. False

Ans. B.

316. Which of the following is a symptom of Dengue Hemorrhagic Fever?

A. Small red or purple blisters under the skin

B. Fever with rash

C. Bleeding in the nose or gums

D. All of the above

Ans. D.

317. Dengue Fever is also known as

A. Black Fever B. Yellow Fever

C. Red Fever D. Breakbone Fever or Dandy Fever

Ans. D.

318. How many days are required for the incubation of dengue virus in a mosquito?

A. Eight to ten days B. Five to ten days

C. Ten to twenty days D. Eight to twelve days

Ans. A.

319. For how many days does the dengue virus circulate in the blood of infected human beings?

A. Ten to twelve days B. Two to seven days

C. Ten to fifteen days D. Ten to twenty days

Ans. B.

320. Bleeding in dengue occurs due to

A. A decrease in red blood cells
B. A decrease in white blood cells
C. A decrease in platelet levels
D. Eating spicy foods

Ans. C.

321. The antibiotics are useful in treating dengue infection.

A. True
B. False

Ans. B.

322. The dengue can be spread by direct contact with an infected patient.

A. True
B. False

Ans. B.

323. Vaccines are available to prevent dengue.

A. True
B. False

Ans. B.

324. What time does the mosquitoes that spread dengue usually bite?

A. During the night
B. During the day
C. Early in the morning

Ans. B.

325. West Nile virus belongs to a group of viruses known as flaviviruses. How are these viruses spread?

A. Through contaminated water
B. By mosquitoes
C. By sneezing or coughing
D. Through raw or undercooked meat

Ans. B.

326. People aren't the usual host of the mosquitoes that carry the West Nile virus. What is?

A. Raccoons
B. White tail deer
C. Skunks
D. Crow and jays

Ans. D.

327. Which group of people is at higher risk of becoming seriously ill with West Nile virus?

A. Infants
B. Teenagers
C. People over 60
D. A & C.

Ans. D.

328. Which of these may be a symptom of West Nile virus infection in a healthy person?

A. Fever B. Headache

C. Nausea D. Skin rash E. All of the above

Ans. E.

329. Which of these is a serious complication of West Nile virus infection?

A. Encephalitis B. Meningitis

C. Arthritis D. A & B.

Ans. D.

330. Which of these is a treatment for West Nile virus infection?

A. Antibiotics B. Antihistamines

C. Vitamins D. None of the above

Ans. D.

331. Which of these are ways to prevent getting infected with West Nile virus?

A. Wear long sleeves and long pants when outdoors

B. Stay indoors at dawn and dusk

C. Use an insect repellent that contains DEET

D. All of the above

Ans. D.

332. Which one of the following arbovirus diseases has not been reported in India ?

A. Japanese encephalitis B. Yellow fever

C. Chikungunya fever D. Kyasanur forest disease

Ans. B.

333. Which one of the following viral infections is transmitted by tick ?

A. Japanese encephalitis B. Yellow fever

C. Dengue D. Kyasanur forest disease

Ans. D.

334. Which one of the following vaccine is contraindicated in pregnancy ?

A. Hepatitis B B. Cholera

C. Rabies D. Yellow fever

Ans. D.

335. The incubation period for yellow fever is —

A. 3-6 days B. 1-2 days

C. 3-4 weeks D. 8-10 weeks

Ans. A.

336. Which of the following viral infections is associated with the development of hydrophobia?

A. Rabies B. B.Influenza

C. Polio D. Hepatitis

Ans. A.

337. Which of the following viruses is star-shaped in outline and transmitted by the faecal-oral route?

A. Astrovirus B. Calicivirus

C. Hepatitis E virus D. Hepatitis D virus

Ans. A.

338. The species of animals which is most susceptible to rabies infection is

A. Dog B. Cat

C. Fowl D. Cow

Ans. B.

339. Which of the following clinical specimens can be used for the demonstration of rabies antigen by direct immunofluorescence antemortem?

A. Saliva smears B. Corneal smears

C. Conjunctival smears D. All of these

Ans. D.

340. The mode of transmission of hepatitis E is through

A. Infected syringes and needles B. Faecally contaminated drinking water

C. Sexual intercourse D. None of these

Ans. B.

341. Which of the following viral agents can cause diarrhea?

A. Rotaviruses B. Norwalk virus

C. Astrovirus D. All of these

Ans. D.

342. The virus(es) which has club-shaped peplomers and infects the respiratory tract is/are

A. Coronavirus B. Astrovirus

C. Norwalk virus D. All of these

Ans. A.

343. What is the most common cause of aseptic meningitis of viral etiology?

A. Enteroviruses
B. Herpesviruses
C. Arboviruses
D. Retroviruses
E. Orthomyxoviruses

Ans. A.

344. Which one of the following immunizations should be administered immediately after birth?

A. Diphtheria-pertusis-tetanus (DPT) vaccine
B. Haemophilus influenzae type b vaccine
C. Hepatitis B vaccine
D. HIV Vaccine
E. Oral Polio virus

Ans. C.

345. Which one of the following infection routes is most often involved in the neonatal transmission of hepatitis B virus (HBV)?

A. Blood transfusion
B. Fetal contact with infected blood during childbirth
C. Ingestion of the virus via maternal breast milk
D. Transmission of the virus from hospital personnel during childbirth
E. Transplacental transmission of the virus

Ans. E.

346. The finding of large, multinucleated, clumps of cells in the bronchial secretions of a 2 year old girl with acute bronchopneumonia suggests that this infection is caused by

A. Bordetella pertusis
B. Epstein-Barr virus
C. Mycoplasma hominis
D. Rhinovirus
E. Respiratory syncytial virus (RSV)

Ans. E.

347. All of the following picornaviruses are resistant to the acidity of the stomach except:

A. Coxsackievirus A
B. Coxsackievirus B
C. Echo virus
D. Poliovirus
E. Rhinovirus

Ans. E.

348. In a chronic carrier of hepatitis B virus (HBV), which positive test is most indicative of high infectivity? Hepatitis B Antigens

A. Hepatitis B Surface Antigen (HbsAg)

B. Hepatitis B Core Antigen (HbcAg)

C. Hepatitis B e Antigen (HbeAg)

D. Anti-HBsAg

E. Anti-HBeAg

Ans. C.

349. West Nile, western equine Encephalitis, EEE are all zoonotic encephalitis. Man get this disease from mosquitoes that have bitten infected

A. Horses B. Birds

C. Humans D. Mice and other rodents

Ans. B.

350. The Reservoir host is WEE and EEE is:

A. The horse B. Man

C. Birds D. Mice and other rodents

E. Mosquito

Ans. C.

351. The Reservoir host is WEE and EEE is:

A. The horse B. Man

C. Birds D. Mice and other rodents

E Mosquito

Ans. C.

352. The tissue and body systems affected by panleukopenia virus (distemper) in the cat is similar to which virus

A. Canine distemper B. Canine parvo

C. Canine hepatitis D. Canine parainfluenza

E. Canine corona

Ans. B.

353. Which of the following is least characteristic of panleukopenia

A. Dehydration B. Icterus

C. Neurologic signs including ataxia D. Abortion

E. Very low WBC

Ans. B.

354. Considering the tissues affected, clinical signs and etiology which of the following treatments would be least indicated for a panleukopenia cat

A. Antitussives B. Antiemetics

C. ABs D. Blood transfusions

E. Iv fluids

Ans. A.

355. Which disease is transmitted by cat biting one another.

A. Panleukopenia B. FIP

C. FLV D. FIV

E. FIA

Ans. D.

356. A cat displaying ascites progressively should be considered for:

A. Panleukopenia B. FIP

C. FIV D. FLV

E. FIA

Ans. B.

357. What is the main route of entry for Chlamydial infection in cats

A. Oral B. Aerosol

C. In-utero D. Via milk

E. Contact with mucus membranes of the eyes

Ans. E.

358. Which one of the following is a herpes virus known to infect the upper respiratory tract of cats

A. Calici virus B. Chlamydia

C. Panleukopenia D. Rhinopnumonitis

E. Rhinotracheitis

Ans. E.

359. The etiology for FIP is:

A. Parvovirus B. Corona virus

C. Protozoan D. Bacteria

E. Mycoplasma

Ans. B.

360. Which disease is transferred from flea bites

A. Panleukopenia
B. FIP
C. FLV
D. FIV
E. FIA

Ans. E.

361. Which disease has highly fatal clinical manifestations resulting from the reaction of the cats immune system

A. Panleukopenia
B. FIP
C. FLV
D. FIV
E. FIA

Ans. B.

362. The bubonic plague in felines refer to.

A. Pneumonia
B. Lymphadenopathy
C. Infection from mice
D. Septicemic infection
E. Highly fatal form

Ans. B.

363. Which of the cat respiratory disease pathology is also associated with human conjunctivitis

A. Calicivirus
B. Rhinotracheitis virus
C. *Chlamydia psittaci*
D. All three

Ans. C.

364. How do horses get West Nile Virus:

A. Aerosol only
B. Aerosol and oral only
C. Bite from mosquito only
D. Bite from large fly
E. None of the above

Ans. C.

365. Canine Parvovirus infection carries an approx 15-35% mortality even with treatment (True or false)

Ans. True.

366. A litter of 1 1/2 week old puppies presents with pronounced lethargy and diarrhoea and a very marked mucopurulent oculonasal exudate and dyspnoea.Two of the litter had already stopped eating and had died, this clinical picture is most characteristic of which of the following:

A. Leptospirosis
B. Hepatitis
C. Parvovirus
D. Herpes virus
E. Distemper

Ans. E.

367. The body fluid considered most contagious in a leptospirosis case is:

A. Urine B. Blood

C. Faeces D. Discharge from coughing

E. All of the above

Ans. A.

368. What is another name for swamp fever ?

Ans. Equine infectious anaemia.

369. Who is the one awarded with Nobel Prize for contribution towards elucidation of 3D structure of DNA along with Watson and Crick?

A. Rosalind Franklin B. Maurice Wilkins

C. Linus Pauling D. Temin

Ans. B.

370. Andrew Z Fire and Craig C Mello got Nobel Prize in medicine for the discovery of

A. Split genes B. Transposons

C. Ribozymes D. RNA interference mechanism

Ans. D.

371. Stanley Prusiner, Nobel winner of 1997 discovered bizarre infectious protein particle called as

A. Prions B. Viroids

C. Virusoids D. Proteomes

Ans. A.

372. The key enzyme that helped Kary Mullis in the invention of PCR was

A. Ligase B. Taq Polymersae

C. Restriction endonuclease D. Vent polymerase

Ans. B.

373. "All enzymes are proteins" this was the concept before the discovery of ribozymes or catalytic RNAs by

A. Roberts and Sharp B. Cech and Altman

C. Alwin and Towbin D. Sanger

Ans. B.

374. Bacterial conjugation was discovered by

A. Beadle and Tatum B. Meselson and Stahl

C. Lederberg and Tatum D. Griffith

Ans. C.

375. The first confirmation regarding the status of DNA as genetic material was given by the work of Avery, Macleod and McCarty on

A. E.coli
B. Diplococcus pneumoniae
C. Klebsiella
D. T2 phage

Ans. B.

376. DNA finger printing using β KM-DNA probe was developed by

A. Alec Jeffrey
B. Kary Mullis
C. Watson
D. Lalji Singh

Ans. D.

377. 'Central dogma of Biology' was put forward by

A. Watson
B. Crick
C. Temin
D. Khorana

Ans. B.

378. The discovery of restriction enzyme actually paved way towards the development of modern biotechnology or rDNA technology. The discoverers are

A. Kary Mullis and Mc Clintock
B. Arber, Nathans and Smith
C. Milstein and Saiki
D. Sanger, Maxam and Gilbert

Ans. B.

379. Shape of bacteriophage is

A. Brick shape
B. Bullet shape
C. Helical shape
D. Tadpole shape

Ans. D.

380. Which of the following is not true for viruses?

A. No growth on inanimate culture media
B. Not sensitive to antibiotics
C. No energy producing enzymes
D. Insensitive to interferon

Ans. D.

381. Main causative organism of chicken pox is

A. Fox virus
B. Mumps virus
C. Measles virus
D. None of these

Ans. D.

382. Double stranded RNA is seen in

A. Reovirus B. Rhabdovirus

C. Parvovirus D. Retrovirus

Ans. A.

383. IFN has an innate ability to fight viral infections and is always circulating in the body ?

A. True B. False

Ans. B.

384. Hepatitis viruses attack the liver and cause following symptoms except

A. Jaundice B. Dark urine

C. Light colored faeces D. Macropapular rash

Ans. D.

385. Polio is primarily a disease that affects ?

A. G.I. tract B. CNS

C. Musle and skeleton D. The respiratory system

Ans. B.

386. A condition called West Nile fever may develop in one who ?

A. Has consumed raw beef

B. Has been bitten by an infected mosquitoes

C. Walks on warm most soil without shoes

D. Uses manure in the farm fields

Ans. B.

387. Haemoorhagic viruses often kill by what mechanism ?

A. Systemic shock B. Dehydration

C. Bleeding to death D. Pneumonia

Ans. C.

388. The vaccine for herpes simplex virus II is

A. Expensive B. Given in multiple doses

C. Can result i a positive skin test D. Nonexistent

Ans. D.

389. Coxsackie virus B3, a subgroup of enteroviruses, commonly causes

A. Acute hemorrhagic conjunctivitis B. Muscular dystrophy

C. Myocarditis D. Gastroenteritis

Ans. C.

390. Which part of the body is affected in mumps ?

A. My humps
B. The ears
C. Reproductive organs
D. Parotid glands

Ans. D.

391. The major groups of arthropod borne viruses include

A. Togaviruses, Flaviviruses and Bunyaviruses
B. Togaviruses, Rhabdoviruses and Reoviruses
C. Reoviruses, Enteroviruses and Rhabdoviruses
D. Retroviruses, Enteroviruses and Togaviruses

Ans. A.

392. The major pathological features in Yellow fever include

A. Midzonal hepatic necrosis and Councilman bodies
B. Midzonal hepatic necrosis and Negri bodies
C. Glomerular and renal papillary necrosis
D. Midzonal hepatic necrosis and diffuse encephalitis

Ans. A.

393. The pathogenesis of dengue haemorrhagic shock syndrome is distinguished from that of uncomplicated dengue by

A. Excitotoxic injury of neurones
B. Development of dengue virus meningitis
C. Immune enhancement of infection
D. Neurotropic spread of virus

Ans. C.

394. Rabies virus reaches the CNS by

A. Hematogenous distribution
B. Neurotropic spread
C. Entry into brain within macrophages
D. Both A and B.

Ans. B.

395. Creutzfeldt-Jacob disease is caused by

A. JC virus
B. Pumuula virus
C. Prions
D. SV40 virus

Ans. C.

396. Rabies virus produces infection of

A. Astrocytes
B. Oligodendrocytes
C. Neurones
D. Macrophages

Ans. C.

397. The most common cause of viral meningitis in USA is

A. Enterovirus
B. Rhabdovirus
C. Adenovirus
D. LCM virus

Ans. A.

398. Common symptoms of hepatitis include

A. Fever, nausea and diarrhoea
B. Malaise, anorexia and jaundice
C. Nausea, vomiting, abdominal pain
D. Clear urine, dark coloured stool and anorexia

Ans. B.

399. Hepatitis A can be transmitted by

A. Changing diapers on an infected baby
B. Having sex with someone who is infected
C. Eating cooked meat
D. Needle injury contaminated with infected person's blood

Ans. A.

400. A 29 years old patient comes in with symptoms of hepatitis. The following serological results are obtained : Hepatitis A IgM antibody negative, Hepatitis A IgG antibody positive, Hepatitis B surface antigen positive, Hepatitis B surface antibody negative. The patient has acute

A. Hepatitis A
B. Hepatitis B
C. Hepatitis C
D. Hepatitis A and B

Ans. B.

401. A major characteristic of hepatitis C is

A. It is transmitted by eating raw oysters
B. It is highly likely to cause chronic ongoing infection
C. Most patients have severe symptoms when first infected
D. It is a DNA virus

Ans. B.

402. HIV is the same as

A. HTLV III
B. HTLV II
C. HTLV I
D. None of the above

Ans. A.

403. The likelihood of HIV being transmitted from a pregnant woman to her infant in the absence of antiretroviral therapy is about

A. 1 to 5%
B. 5-10%
C. 20-25%
D. 50-75%

Ans. C.

404. Serologic conversion to a positive test for HIV infection occurs

A. In2-3 days
B. In 3-4 weeks
C. In 3-6 months
D. May take up to 10 years

Ans. B.

405. One of the key differences between amantidine/rimantidine and the newer neuraminidase inhibitor influenza virus drugs is

A. Drug allergy
B. Antimetabolic effect on host cells due to lack of specificity for viral enzymes
C. Rate of development of drug resistance
D. Drug-drug interactions associated with competition for cytochrome P450 enzymes

Ans. C.

406. Which of the following best characterizes antiviral chemotherapy in comparison to bacterial chemotherapy ?

A. Few drug targets, toxicity problematic
B. Sensitivity tests of limited value
C. Toxicity a minor problem, multiple enzymatic targets
D. many more drug options are available to treat viral infections

Ans. A.

407. HIV reverse transcriptase, a critical target in modern antiretroviral chemotherapy, performs which critical function for the virus

A. Cleaves polyprotein precursor leading to functional assembly of viral core
B. Cleaves sialic acid residue form glycoprotein permitting attachment and entry into cell
C. Transcribes RNA into DNA
D. Activates 2'-5' oligoadenylate synthetase

Ans. C.

408. Foscarnet interacts with which of the following viral enzymes

A. Pyrophosphate binding site of the polymerase

B. Protease

C. Nucleoside reductase

D. Reverse transcriptase

Ans. A.

409. Enteroviruses are most closely related to which of the following viruses

A. Herpes virus

B. Hepatitis C

C. Hepatitis A

D. Rotavirus

E. Rubella

Ans. C.

410. The following statements are clearly true about enteroviruses except

A. There are many serotypes

B. They can cause a variety of diseases which imitate bacterial infection

C. They are an important cause of meningitis

D. They are an important cause of diarrhoea

Ans. D.

411. All of the following are syndromes associated with enteroviruses except

A. Conjunctivitis

B. Coronary artery disease

C. Myocarditis

D. Pericarditis

E. Pleuritis

Ans. B.

412. Antiviral drugs currently in the market including acyclovir and pencyclovir are active against enteroviruses

A. True

B. False

Ans. B.

413. All of the following statements regarding viruses are true except

A. They contain both DNA and RNA

B. The nucleic acid may be single or double stranded

C. They are obligate intracellular parasite

D. They reproduce using host cell machinery

Ans. A.

414. A cytolytic virus would be expected to cause cytopathic effect in cell culture

A. True B. False

Ans. A.

415. The haemagglutinin of infleunza virus plays a role in which of the following phases of viral replication

A. Uncoating B. Virion assembly

C. Release by budding D. Adsorption

E. Production of mRNA

Ans. D.

416. Which of the followiing statemets is true regarding naked viruses ?

A. They release from infected cells by budding

B. They are almost exclusively RNA viruses

C. Their release from the infected cells after cell lysis

D. All alphaviruses are naked

Ans. C.

417. Foot and mouth disease (FMD) of animals is caused by

A. RNA virus B. DNA virus

C. Bacteria D. Protozoa

Ans. A.

418. Viruses can only be destroyed by

A. Antibodies in our blood B. White blood cells in host's body

C. Red blood cells in host's body D. Both A and B

Ans. D.

419. In order to combat virus-produced diseases,

A. Antibiotics shall be administered

B. Depressant drugs shall be administered

C. Amphetamines shall be administered

D. Body's own immunity system shall combat

Ans. D.

420. Tadpole shaped viruses are largely

A. Tobacco mosaic virus B. Bacteriophages

C. Influenza virus D. May cause death

Ans. B.

421. Example of rod-shaped viruses include

A. Influenza virus
B. Bacteriophages
C. Tobacco mosaic virus
D. Norwalk virus

Ans. C.

422. Viruses are not considered cells because

A. They can not divide
B. They do not have a nucleus
C. They do not have a protoplasm
D. They are non-living things

Ans. C.

423. Outside host cells, viruses do not

A. Replicate
B. Feed
C. Respire
D. All of these

Ans. D.

424. Viruses only replicate and divide

A. When they are on bread
B. When they are in an environment they can find a host cells
C. When once they are inside host cell
D. In night

Ans. C.

425. Koplic's spots will develop in

A. HIV
B. Measles
C. Mumps
D. Rubella

Ans. B.

426. The extra cellular infectious virus particle is called

A. Capsid
B. Nucleocapsid
C. Virion
D. None of these

Ans. C.

427. MMR protects against which 3 diseases ?

A. Measles, malaria and rabies
B. Monkey pox, malaria and rabies
C. Measles, mumps and rubella
D. None of the above

Ans. C.

428. Pathogen for Measles is known as

A. Variola Virus
B. Vibrio Cholerae
C. Plasmodium
D. Morbillivirus

Ans. D.

429. Variola virus has been known to cause

A. Malaria B. Measles

C. Smallpox D. Chickenpox

Ans. C.

430. The genetic material of retroviruses such as HIV is

A. DNA B. RNA

C. Protein D. All of these

Ans. B.

431. Retroviruses replicate via __________ intermediate

A. RNA B. DNA

C. mRNA D. rDNA

Ans. B.

432. The viruses that can achieve neoplastic transformation are called

A. DNA tumor viruses B. RNA tumor viruses

C. retroviruses HIV D. None of these

Ans. A.

433. Which of the following is correct?

A. HIV is a retrovirus that kills human helper T cells

B. Causes acquired immune deficiency syndrome (AIDS)

C. Cripples the immunity systems

D. All of the above

Ans. D.

434. Animal viruses with capsids displaying helical symmetry include

A. Measles and mumps B. Influenza

C. rabies D. All the above

Ans. D.

435. Icosahedral viruses are generally

A. Poliovirus B. Adenoviruses

C. Both A and B D. None of these

Ans. C.

436. Negative strand ssRNA viruses need to have a preformed replicase when they invade a mammalian cell because they

A. Use it to terminate transcripts when they copy host cell mRNA

B. Have to make a positive strand copy that can be translated

C. Use it to modify host enzymes that are recruited for viral replication

D. None of these

Ans. B.

437. Which of the following reflects the correct order of events that take place during the multiplication of a virus?

A. Attachment, penetration, maturation, biosynthesis, release

B. Penetration, attachment, biosynthesis, maturation, release

C. Attachment, penetration, biosynthesis, maturation, release

D. Attachment, release, biosynthesis, maturation, penetration

Ans. C.

438. What can be coated to the plastic dish if an ELISA is performed to directly detect polio virus?

A. Patient serum

B. Anti-polio antibody

C. Polio capsid protein

D. Colored substrate

Ans. B.

439. Influenza virus undergoes antigenic shift resulting in major antigenic changes by which of the following mechanisms?

A. Somatic recombination of heavy and light chains

B. Expression of several different capsule types

C. Changing the receptor binding canyon that docks with the host receptor

D. Reassortment of RNA segments from different influenza viruses

Ans. D.

440. The nucleocapsid is covered by an outer membrane like structure called

A. Envelope

B. Covering

C. Membranocapsid

D. All of these

Ans. A.

441. Which type of interferon is produced by virus-infected cells ?

A. α

B. β

C. Both A and B

D. None of these

Ans. C.

442. Fluorescence microscopy can be used for the diagnosis of
   A. Subacute sclerosing panencephalitis
   B. Herpes simplex encephalitis
   C. Rabies
   D. All of these

Ans. D.

443. Viral matrix proteins are
   A. Exposed on the surface of the virus
   B. Present in naked virus
   C. Anchor the envelope of enveloped viruses
   D. Part of the nucleoprotein core of viruses

Ans. C.

444. Mumps vaccine is prepared from the cultures of
   A. Chicken fibroblasts
   B. African Green monkey cells
   C. Healthy calves
   D. Sheep

Ans. A.

445. The microbes which are most likely to be completely dependent on a plant or animal host are
   A. Viruses
   B. Bacteria
   C. Fungi
   D. Algae

Ans. A.

446. The two major components of viruses are
   A. Fat and protein
   B. Nucleic acid and protein
   C. Carbohydrate and nucleic acid
   D. Fat and carbohydrate

Ans. B.

447. The transcription of the viral nucleic acid into mRNA is not necessary in case of
   A. + sense ssRNA viruses
   B. dsDNA viruses
   C. ssDNA viruses
   D. All of these

Ans. A.

448. West Nile virus can cause a disease in human beings that may be transmitted from an infected bird to a person by a mosquito. This is an example of
   A. Endogenous infection
   B. Fomite borne disease
   C. Arthropod borne disease
   D. Nosocomial infection

Ans. C.

449. What does the positive strand in double stranded RNA viruses stands for ?
A. rRNA
B. tRNA
C. mRNA
D. None of these

Ans. C.

450. Which of the following characteristics would not be used to classify viruses ?
A. Type of cell wall structure
B. Type of nucleic acid
C. Presence of an envelope
D. Symmetry

Ans. A.

451. Interanuclear inclusion bodies are found in cells infected with
A. Parvoviruses
B. Herpesviruses
C. Adenoviruses
D. All of these

Ans. D.

452. The reovirus and influenza virus contain
A. 10 different segments of dsRNA and 8 different segments of ssRNA respectively
B. 8 different segments of dsRNA and 10 different segments of ssRNA respectively
C. 5 different segments of dsRNA and 7 different segments of ssRNA respectively
D. 7 different segments of dsRNA and 5different segments of ssRNA respectively

Ans. A.

453. Intracytoplasmic inclusion bodies are found in cells infected with
A. Rabies virus
B. Vaccinia virus
C. Fowl pox virus
D. All of these

Ans. D.

454. What is the function of positive strand in double stranded RNA viruses?
A. Synthesis of protein
B. Production of ribosomes
C. Both A and B
D. None of these

Ans. A.

455. Which of the following virus is transmitted by the respiratory route?
A. Rhinovirus
B. Coronavirus
C. Measles virus
D. All of these

Ans. D.

456. The predominant lipid substance found in the viral envelope is
A. Phospholipids
B. Glycolipids
C. Neutral fats
D. All of these

Ans. A.

457. Supercoiling refers to the extra turns in the structure of dsDNA due to the action of

A. DNA gyrase
B. DNA pyrase
C. RNA gyrase
D. RNA pyrase

Ans. A.

458. The tissue structure deteriorates as the virus multiplies. This deterioration is called

A. Aneuploidy
B. Protopathic effect
C. Cytopathic effect
D. None of these

Ans. C.

459. The penetration of animal viruses into attached cells occur by mechanisms consisting of engulfment of whole virions by the cells in a phagocytic process called

A. Vitropexis
B. Viropexis
C. Ectodesmata
D. Vivopexis

Ans. B.

460. Viropexis takes place in the phagocytic vacuoles and is due to the action of enzymes

A. DNA gyrase
B. Lysosomal protease
C. Lysosomal lipase
D. All of these

Ans. B.

461. Negri bodies are found in cells infected with

A. Paramyxoviruses
B. Vaccinia virus
C. Fowl pox virus
D. Rabies virus

Ans. D.

462. The uncontrolled proliferation of cells is termed as

A. Hyperplasia
B. Anaplasia
C. Metastasis
D. All of these

Ans. A.

463. Which of the following virus is transmitted by genital route?

A. Papillomaviruses
B. Herpes simplex virus type 2
C. Hepatitis B virus
D. All of these

Ans. D.

464. The RNA sarcoma viruses, the most strongly transforming viruses may transform which of the following cells in a culture?

A. Fibroblasts
B. Myoblasts
C. Iris epithelial
D. All of these

Ans. D.

465. Plant viruses penetrate host cells through transient pores called

A. Ectodesmata B. Endodesmata

C. Cytodesmata D. Protodesmata

Ans. A.

466. HIV can infect

A. Microglial cells B. M cells

C. CD4+ T lymphocytes D. All of these

Ans. D.

467. Parasitic infection/s frequently observed in HIV disease is / are

A. Cryptosporidiosis B. Toxoplasmosis

C. Isosporiasis D. All of these

Ans. D.

468. What is the average incubation period for development of AIDS?

A. One year B. Five years

C. Ten years D. Twenty years

Ans. C.

469. The commonest bacterial infection in HIV disease is/are

A. Mycobacterial infection B. Salmonella infection

C. Bartonella infection D. All of these

Ans. A.

470. Viral infections frequently observed in HIV disease is /are

A. Herpes simplex B. Varicella-Zoster

C. Cytomegalovirus D. All of these

Ans. D.

471. The commonest opportunistic infection in AIDS patient in India is

A. Cryptosporidiosis B. Toxoplasmosis

C. Tuberculosis D. Cryptococcosis

Ans. C.

472. HIV belongs to the family retroviridae and sub-family

A. Oncovirinae B. Lentivirinae

C. Spumavirinae D. None of these

Ans. B.

473. HIV or Human Immunodeficiency Virus is considered unique because each virus contains:

A. More than 100 copies of the viral genome

B. A genome made up of both DNA and RNA components

C. A viral enzyme known as reverse transcriptase

D. Sticky proteins that allow it to bind tightly to host cells

Ans. C.

474. Which of the following is transmembrane pedicle antigen of HIV-I?

A. gp41 B. gp140

C. gp120 D. gp 36

Ans. A.

475. The confirmatory test(s) for HIV infection is/are

A. Virus isolation B. Detection of p24 antigen

C. Detection of viral nucleic acid D. All of the above

Ans. D.

476. A viral load test detects the

A. Provirus of HIV in infected cells

B. Total amount of virus in the infected host

C. Number of viruses being released by each infected cell

D. Amount of bacteriophage being produced by *E. coli* cells

Ans. A.

477. Fungal infection/s frequently observed in HIV disease is /are:

A. Candidiasis B. Cryptococcosis

C. Aspergillosis D. All of these

Ans. D.

478. The screening test/s for diagnosis of HIV infection is/are

A. ELISA B. Latex agglutination

C. Dot blot assay D. All of these

Ans. D.

479. The problem(s) associated with development of a vaccine against HIV is/are

A. Antibody alone may be insufficient

B. Rapid mutation of HIV

C. Virus can spread from cell to cell by fusion to produce syncytia

D. All of these

Ans. D.

480. The commonest mode of transmission of HIV is

A. Parental B. Perinatal

C. Sexual D. Oral

Ans. C.

481. The cells most often infected by HIV are

A. Null cells B. CD8+ T lymphocytes

C. CD4+ T lymphocytes D. None of these

Ans. C.

482. Which of the following is the spike antigen of HIV-I?

A. gp120 B. gp140

C. gp36 D. gp41

Ans. A.

483. Which of the following articles can be sterilized in an autoclave?

A. Gloves B. Culture media

C. Dressing material D. All of these

Ans. D.

484. Which of the following hepatitis viruses is not RNA virus?

A. Hepatitis B virus B. Hepatitis A virus

C. Hepatitis G virus D. Hepatitis E virus

Ans. A.

485. Most reliable test for detection of hepatitis E infection is

A. Western blot assay for IgM anti-HEV

B. ELISA test for IgM anti-HEV

C. ELISA test for IgG anti-HEV

D. PCR for detection of HEV RNA

Ans. D.

486. The agent representing an isolate of hepatitis G virus is

A. GBV-B B. GBA-A

C. None of the above D. GBV-C

Ans. D.

487. Which of the following viral infections can result in chronic carrier state?

A. HCV B. HBV

C. All of these D. HDV

Ans. C.

488. Transmission of hepatitis G virus is

A. Sexually B. Parenterally

C. None of these D. Both A and B

Ans. D.

489. Hepatitis G virus belongs to the family

A. Flaviviridae B. Caliciviridae

C. Coronaviridae D. Hepadnaviridae

Ans. A.

490. The most serious infection is

A. Infection with hbv alone

B. Superinfection of an HBsAG carrier by HDV

C. None of the above

D. Coinfection of HBV and HDV

Ans. B.

491. Which of the following specimens contain/s hepatitis B virus in an infected person?

A. Semen B. Blood

C. All of these D. Saliva

Ans. C.

492. Recombinant vaccine for Hepatitis B virus has been synthesized against which of the following antigen?

A. Viral surface antigen (HBsAg) B. Viral antigen (HBcAg)

C. All of these D. E antigen (HBeAg)

Ans. A.

493. In India first genetically engineered vaccine against HBV was developed by

A. Shantha Biotechnics Pvt Ltd B. Ranbaxy Pvt Ltd

C. Glaxo Pvt Ltd D. Dabur Pvt Ltd

Ans. B.

494. Recombinant vaccine for HBV was produced by cloning viral genes in

A. Cosmids B. Plasmids

C. Phagemids D. Autonomously replicating plasmid of yeast

Ans. D.

495. More promising chemotherapeutic agents for treating viral diseases is

A. Fibroblast interferon
B. Leukocytic interferon
C. Nystatin
D. Interferon

Ans. D.

496. Which capsid symmetry is exhibited by most of the phages?

A. Helical
B. Icosahedral
C. Complex
D. None of these

Ans. B.

497. Which of the following is the necessary step for cultivating the microorganisms?

A. Preparing a culture medium for the growth of microorganisms
B. Sterilizing in order to eliminate all living microorganisms in vessel
C. Inoculating the microorganisms in the prepared medium
D. All of the above

Ans. D.

498. Contractile sheath of the tail is present in which of the following phages?

A. T3
B. T2
C. P22
D. All of these

Ans. B.

499. One of the first enzymes synthesized by many bacteriophage is ————, an RNA-dependent RNA polymerase

A. RNA transcriptase
B. RNA polymerase
C. RNA ligase
D. RNA replicase

Ans. D.

500. In viruses with envelopes

A. The envelope and the embedded proteins are encoded by the viral nucleic acid
B. The envelope is derived from the host but it contains embedded proteins coded by the viral nucleic acid
C. The envelope is coded by the viral nucleic acids, but the proteins come from the host's membrane proteins
D. The envelope and its imbedded proteins are derived from the host's membranes

Ans. B.